T0306136

A Pharmacology Primer

Fourth Edition

A Pharmacology Primer
Techniques for More Effective and Strategic Drug Discovery

Fourth Edition

Terry P. Kenakin, PhD
Professor
Department of Pharmacology
University of North Carolina School of Medicine, USA

AMSTERDAM • BOSTON • HEIDELBERG • LONDON • NEW YORK • OXFORD • PARIS
SAN DIEGO • SAN FRANCISCO • SINGAPORE • SYDNEY • TOKYO
Academic Press is an imprint of Elsevier

Academic Press is an imprint of Elsevier
525 B Street, Suite 1800, San Diego, CA 92101-4495, USA
32 Jamestown Road, London NW1 7BY, UK
225 Wyman Street, Waltham, MA 02451, USA

Copyright © 2014, 2009, 2006, 2004 Elsevier Inc. All rights reserved

No part of this publication may be reproduced, stored in a retrieval system, or transmitted in any form
or by any means electronic, mechanical, photocopying, recording or otherwise without the prior
written permission of the publisher.

Permissions may be sought directly from Elsevier's Science & Technology Rights Department in Oxford, UK:
phone (+44) (0) 1865 843830; fax (+44) (0) 1865 853333; email: permissions@elsevier.com. Alternatively,
visit the Science and Technology Books website at www.elsevierdirect.com/rights for further information.

Notice
No responsibility is assumed by the publisher for any injury and/or damage to persons, or property
as a matter of products liability, negligence or otherwise, or from any use or operation of any methods,
products, instructions or ideas contained in the material herein. Because of rapid advances in the medical
sciences, in particular, independent verification of diagnoses and drug dosages should be made.

British Library Cataloguing-in-Publication Data
A catalogue record for this book is available from the British Library

Library of Congress Cataloging-in-Publication Data
A catalog record for this book is available from the Library of Congress

ISBN: 978-0-12-407663-1

For information on all Academic Press publications
visit our website at elsevierdirect.com

Typeset by MPS Limited, Chennai, India
www.adi-mps.com

Printed and bound in China

14 15 16 17   10 9 8 7 6 5 4 3 2 1

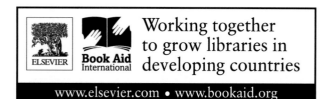

Working together
to grow libraries in
developing countries

www.elsevier.com • www.bookaid.org

As always . . . for Debbie

Contents

Preface   xiii
Preface to the Third Edition   xv
Preface to the Second Edition   xvii
Preface to the First Edition   xix

1. What Is Pharmacology?

1.1 About This Book   1
1.2 What Is Pharmacology?   1
1.3 The Receptor Concept   3
1.4 Pharmacological Test Systems   5
1.5 The Nature of Drug Receptors   7
1.6 Pharmacological Intervention and the
     Therapeutic Landscape   8
1.7 System-Independent Drug Parameters:
     Affinity and Efficacy   9
1.8 What is Affinity?   11
1.9 The Langmuir Adsorption Isotherm   13
1.10 What is Efficacy?   15
1.11 Dose-Response Curves   16
     1.11.1 Potency and Maximal Response   17
     1.11.2 p-Scales and the Representation
             of Potency   18
1.12 Chapter Summary and Conclusions   19
1.13 Derivations: Conformational Selection
     as a Mechanism of Efficacy   20
     References   20

2. How Different Tissues Process Drug Response

2.1 Drug Response as Seen Through the
     "Cellular Veil"   21
2.2 The Biochemical Nature of Stimulus-
     Response Cascades   23
2.3 The Mathematical Approximation
     of Stimulus-Response Mechanisms   25
2.4 System Effects on Agonist Response:
     Full and Partial Agonists   27
2.5 Differential Cellular Response to
     Receptor Stimulus   30
     2.5.1 Choice of Response Pathway   31

     2.5.2 Augmentation or Modulation
            of Stimulus Pathway   31
     2.5.3 Differences in Receptor Density   32
     2.5.4 Target-Mediated Trafficking
            of Stimulus   33
2.6 Receptor Desensitization and
     Tachyphylaxis   35
2.7 The Measurement of Drug Activity   37
2.8 Advantages and Disadvantages
     of Different Assay Formats   37
2.9 Drug Concentration as an Independent
     Variable   38
     2.9.1 Dissimulation in Drug
            Concentration   38
     2.9.2 Free Concentration of Drug   40
2.10 Chapter Summary and Conclusions   40
2.11 Derivations   41
     2.11.1 Series Hyperbolae Can Be
             Modeled by a Single Hyperbolic
             Function   41
     2.11.2 Successive Rectangular Hyperbolic
             Equations Necessarily Lead to
             Amplification   41
     2.11.3 Saturation of Any Step in a Stimulus
             Cascade by Two Agonists Leads to
             Identical Maximal Final Responses
             for the Two Agonists   41
     2.11.4 Procedure to Measure Free Drug
             Concentration in the Receptor
             Compartment   42
     References   42

3. Drug-Receptor Theory

3.1 About This Chapter   45
3.2 Drug-Receptor Theory   46
3.3 The Use of Mathematical Models in
     Pharmacology   47
3.4 Some Specific Uses of Models in
     Pharmacology   47
3.5 Classical Model of Receptor Function   49
3.6 The Operational Model of Receptor
     Function   50
3.7 Two-State Theory   51
3.8 The Ternary Complex Model   52
3.9 The Extended Ternary Complex Model   52

3.10 Constitutive Receptor Activity and
Inverse Agonism   53
3.11 The Cubic Ternary Complex Model   55
3.12 Multistate Receptor Models and
Probabilistic Theory   56
3.13 Chapter Summary and Conclusions   57
3.14 Derivations   57
   3.14.1 Radioligand Binding to Receptor
Dimers Demonstrating Cooperative
Behavior   58
   3.14.2 Effect of Variation in an HIV-1
Binding Model   58
   3.14.3 Derivation of the Operational
Model   59
   3.14.4 Operational Model Forcing
Function for Variable Slope   60
   3.14.5 Derivation of Two-State Theory   60
   3.14.6 Derivation of the Extended Ternary
Complex Model   61
   3.14.7 Dependence of Constitutive
Activity on Receptor Density   61
   3.14.8 Derivation of the Cubic Ternary
Complex Model   61
   References   62

4. Pharmacological Assay Formats:
Binding

4.1 The Structure of This Chapter   63
4.2 Binding Theory and Experiment   63
   4.2.1 Saturation Binding   65
   4.2.2 Displacement Binding   67
   4.2.3 Kinetic Binding Studies   71
4.3 Complex Binding Phenomena: Agonist
Affinity from Binding Curves   72
4.4 Experimental Prerequisites for Correct
Application of Binding Techniques   75
   4.4.1 The Effect of Protein Concentration
on Binding Curves   75
   4.4.2 The Importance of Equilibration
Time for Equilibrium between
Two Ligands   77
4.5 Chapter Summary and Conclusions   78
4.6 Derivations   79
   4.6.1 Displacement Binding: Competitive
Interaction   79
   4.6.2 Displacement Binding: Noncompetitive Interaction   79
   4.6.3 Displacement of a Radioligand
by an Allosteric Antagonist   80
   4.6.4 Relationship between IC_{50} and K_I
for Competitive Antagonists   80
   4.6.5 Maximal Inhibition of Binding
by an Allosteric Antagonist   81
   4.6.6 Relationship between IC_{50} and K_I
for Allosteric Antagonists   81

   4.6.7 Two-Stage Binding Reactions   81
   4.6.8 Effect of G-protein Coupling on
Observed Agonist Affinity   82
   4.6.9 Effect of Excess Receptor
in Binding Experiments: Saturation
Binding Curve   82
   4.6.10 Effect of Excess Receptor in Binding
Experiments: Displacement
Experiments   82
   References   82

5. Agonists: The Measurement of Affinity
and Efficacy in Functional Assays

5.1 Functional Pharmacological Experiments   85
5.2 The Choice of Functional Assays   86
5.3 Recombinant Functional Systems   90
5.4 Functional Experiments: Dissimulation
in Time   93
5.5 Experiments in Real Time Versus
Stop-Time   95
5.6 Quantifying Agonism: The Black-Leff
Operational Model of Agonism   96
   5.6.1 Affinity-Dependent versus
Efficacy-Dependent Agonist Potency   98
   5.6.2 Secondary and Tertiary Testing
of Agonists   101
5.7 Biased Signaling   102
   5.7.1 Receptor Selectivity   107
5.8 Null Analyses of Agonism   107
   5.8.1 Partial Agonists   107
   5.8.2 Full Agonists   110
5.9 Chapter Summary and Conclusions   114
5.10 Derivations   114
   5.10.1 Relationship Between the EC_{50}
and Affinity of Agonists   114
   5.10.2 Method of Barlow, Scott, and
Stephenson for Affinity of Partial
Agonists   115
   5.10.3 Maximal Response of a Partial
Agonist Is Dependent on Efficacy   115
   5.10.4 System Independence of Full
Agonist Potency Ratios   115
   5.10.5 Measurement of Agonist Affinity:
Method of Furchgott   115
   References   116

6. Orthosteric Drug Antagonism

6.1 Introduction   119
6.2 Kinetics Of Drug-Receptor Interaction   120
6.3 Surmountable Competitive Antagonism   122
   6.3.1 Schild Analysis   122
   6.3.2 Patterns of Dose-Response Curves
That Preclude Schild Analysis   126

6.3.3   Best Practice for the Use of Schild
        Analysis   127
6.3.4   Analyses for Inverse Agonists in
        Constitutively Active Receptor
        Systems   128
6.3.5   Analyses for Partial Agonists   131
6.3.6   The Method of Lew and Angus:
        Nonlinear Regressional Analysis   133
6.4   Noncompetitive Antagonism   134
6.5   Agonist-Antagonist Hemi-Equilibria   138
6.6   Resultant Analysis   139
6.7   Antagonist Receptor Coverage: Kinetics
      of Dissociation   141
      6.7.1   Estimating Antagonist Dissociation
              with Hemi-Equilibria   142
6.8   Blockade of Indirectly Acting
      Agonists   144
6.9   Irreversible Antagonism   144
6.10 Chemical Antagonism   146
6.11 Chapter Summary and Conclusions   149
6.12 Derivations   149
      6.12.1   Derivation of the Gaddum
               Equation for Competitive
               Antagonism   149
      6.12.2   Derivation of the Gaddum
               Equation for Noncompetitive
               Antagonism   150
      6.12.3   Derivation of the Schild
               Equation   150
      6.12.4   Functional Effects of an Inverse
               Agonist with the Operational
               Model   150
      6.12.5 pA_2 Measurement for Inverse
               Agonists   151
      6.12.6   Functional Effects of a Partial
               Agonist with the Operational
               Model   151
      6.12.7 pA_2 Measurements for Partial
               Agonists   151
      6.12.8   Method of Stephenson for
               Partial Agonist Affinity
               Measurement   152
      6.12.9   Derivation of the Method of
               Gaddum for Noncompetitive
               Antagonism   152
      6.12.10 Relationship of pA_2 and pK_B for
               Insurmountable Orthosteric
               Antagonism   152
      6.12.11 Resultant Analysis   153
      6.12.12 Blockade of Indirectly Acting
               Agonists   153
      6.12.13 Chemical Antagonism:
               Abstraction of Agonist
               Concentration   153
      6.12.14 Chemical Antagonism:
               Abstraction of Antagonist
               Concentration   154
References   154

7. Allosteric Modulation

7.1   Introduction   155
7.2   The Nature of Receptor Allosterism   155
7.3   Unique Effects of Allosteric Modulators   158
7.4   Functional Study of Allosteric Modulators   162
      7.4.1   Phenotypic Allosteric Modulation
              Profiles   166
      7.4.2   Allosteric Agonism   166
      7.4.3   Affinity of Allosteric Modulators   167
      7.4.4   Negative Allosteric Modulators
              (NAMs)   168
      7.4.5   Positive Allosteric Modulators
              (PAMs)   172
      7.4.6   Optimal Assays for Allosteric
              Function   174
7.5   Methods for Detecting Allosterism   175
7.6   Chapter Summary and Conclusions   177
7.7   Derivations   178
      7.7.1   Allosteric Model of Receptor
              Activity   178
      7.7.2   Effects of Allosteric Ligands on
              Response: Changing Efficacy   178
      7.7.3   Schild Analysis for Allosteric
              Antagonists   179
      References   179

8. The Optimal Design of Pharmacological Experiments

8.1   Introduction   181
8.2   The Optimal Design of Pharmacological
      Experiments   181
      8.2.1   Drug Efficacy   182
      8.2.2   Affinity   188
      8.2.3   Orthosteric vs. Allosteric
              Mechanisms   195
      8.2.4   Target Coverage *In Vivo*   196
8.3   Null Experiments and Fitting Data
      to Models   197
8.4   Interpretation of Experimental Data   199
8.5   Predicting Therapeutic Activity
      in All Systems   202
      8.5.1   Predicting Agonism   203
      8.5.2   Predicting Binding   204
      8.5.3   Kinetics of Target Coverage   206
      8.5.4   Drug Combinations *In Vivo*   206
8.6   Summary and Conclusions   208
8.7   Derivations   209
      8.7.1 IC_{50} Correction Factors:
              Competitive Antagonists   209
      8.7.2   Relationship of pA_2 and pK_B for
              Insurmountable Orthosteric
              Antagonism   209
      8.7.3   Relationship of pA_2 and pK_B for
              Insurmountable Allosteric
              Antagonism   210
      References   210

9. Pharmacokinetics

9.1	Introduction	213
9.2	Biopharmaceutics	213
9.3	The Chemistry of "Druglike" Character	214
9.4	Pharmacokinetics	218
	9.4.1 Drug Absorption	219
	9.4.2 Route of Drug Administration	225
	9.4.3 General Pharmacokinetics	227
	9.4.4 Metabolism	229
	9.4.5 Clearance	232
	9.4.6 Volume of Distribution and Half Life	234
	9.4.7 Renal Clearance	240
	9.4.8 Bioavailability	242
9.5	Nonlinear Pharmacokinetics	243
9.6	Multiple Dosing	244
9.7	Practical Pharmacokinetics	247
	9.7.1 Allometric Scaling	247
9.8	Placement of Pharmacokinetic Assays in Discovery and Development	249
9.9	Summary and Conclusions	252
	References	253

10. Safety Pharmacology

10.1	Safety Pharmacology	255
10.2	Hepatotoxicity	261
	10.2.1 Drug-Drug Interactions	261
	10.2.2 Direct Hepatotoxicity	270
10.3	Cytotoxicity	271
10.4	Mutagenicity	272
10.5	hERG Activity and *Torsades De Pointes*	273
10.6	Autonomic Receptor Profiling	273
10.7	General Pharmacology	274
10.8	Clinical Testing	274
10.9	Summary and Conclusions	278
	References	279

11. The Drug Discovery Process

11.1	Some Challenges for Modern Drug Discovery	281
11.2	Target-Based Drug Discovery	282
	11.2.1 Target Validation and the Use of Chemical Tools	283
	11.2.2 Recombinant Systems	285
	11.2.3 Defining Biological Targets	286
11.3	Systems-Based Drug Discovery	291
	11.3.1 Assays in Context	294
11.4	*In vivo* Systems, Biomarkers, and Clinical Feedback	296
11.5	Types of Therapeutically Active Ligands: Polypharmacology	297
11.6	Pharmacology in Drug Discovery	300
11.7	Chemical Sources for Potential Drugs	302
11.8	Pharmacodynamics and High-Throughput Screening	307
11.9	Drug Development	314
11.10	Clinical Testing	316
11.11	Summary and Conclusions	318
	References	318

12. Statistics and Experimental Design

12.1	Structure of This Chapter	321
12.2	Introduction	321
12.3	Descriptive Statistics: Comparing Sample Data	321
	12.3.1 Gaussian Distribution	322
	12.3.2 Populations and Samples	322
	12.3.3 Confidence Intervals	324
	12.3.4 Paired Data Sets	325
	12.3.5 One-Way Analysis of Variance	326
	12.3.6 Two-Way Analysis of Variance	327
	12.3.7 Regression and Correlation	327
	12.3.8 Detection of Single Versus Multiple Populations	329
12.4	How Consistent are Experimental Data with Models?	330
	12.4.1 Comparison of Data to Models: Choice of Model	330
	12.4.2 Curve Fitting: Good Practice	332
	12.4.3 Outliers and Weighting Data Points	334
	12.4.4 Overextrapolation of Data	336
	12.4.5 Hypothesis Testing: Examples with Dose-Response Curves	337
	12.4.6 One Curve or Two? Detection of Differences in Curves	340
	12.4.7 Asymmetrical Dose-Response Curves	341
	12.4.8 Comparison of Data to Linear Models	342
	12.4.9 Is a Given Regression Linear?	342
	12.4.10 One or More Regression Lines? Analysis of Covariance	343
12.5	Comparison of Samples to "Standard Values"	346
	12.5.1 Comparison of Means by Two Methods or in Two Systems	346
	12.5.2 Comparing Assays/Methods with a Range of Ligands	347
12.6	Experimental Design and Quality Control	347
	12.6.1 Detection of Difference in Samples	347
	12.6.2 Power Analysis	348
12.7	Chapter Summary and Conclusions	350
	References	350

13. Selected Pharmacological Methods

13.1 Binding Experiments 351
13.1.1 Saturation Binding 351
13.1.2 Displacement Binding 351
13.2 Functional Assays 353
13.2.1 Determination of Equiactive Concentrations on Dose-Response Curves 353
13.2.2 Method of Barlow, Scott, and Stephenson for Measurement of the Affinity of a Partial Agonist 355
13.2.3 Method of Furchgott for the Measurement of the Affinity of a Full Agonist 356
13.2.4 Schild Analysis for the Measurement of Competitive Antagonist Affinity 357
13.2.5 Method of Stephenson for Measurement of Partial Agonist Affinity 359
13.2.6 Method of Gaddum for Measurement of Noncompetitive Antagonist Affinity 361
13.2.7 Method for Estimating Affinity of Insurmountable Antagonist (Dextral Displacement Observed) 362
13.2.8 Resultant Analysis for Measurement of Affinity of Competitive Antagonists with Multiple Properties 363
13.2.9 Measurement of the Affinity and Maximal Allosteric Constant for Allosteric Modulators Producing Surmountable Effects 364
13.2.10 Method for Estimating Affinity of Insurmountable Antagonist (No Dextral Displacement Observed): Detection of Allosteric Effect 368
13.2.11 Measurement of pK_B for Competitive Antagonists from a pIC_{50} 369

14. Exercises in Pharmacodynamics and Pharmacokinetics

14.1 Introduction 373
14.2 Agonism 373
14.2.1 Agonism: Structure-Activity Relationships 373
14.2.2 Prediction of Agonist Effect 374
14.2.3 "Super Agonists" 375
14.2.4 Atypical Agonists 376
14.2.5 Ordering of Affinity and Efficacy in Agonist Series 376
14.2.6 Kinetics of Agonism 376
14.2.7 Affinity-Dominant versus Efficacy-Dominant Agonists 377
14.2.8 Agonist Affinities and Potencies Do Not Correlate 379
14.2.9 Lack of Agonist Effect 380
14.2.10 Assay-Specific Agonism 382
14.3 Antagonism 383
14.3.1 Antagonist Potency and Kinetics: Part A 383
14.3.2 Antagonist Potency in pIC_{50} Format (Kinetics Part B) 385
14.3.3 Mechanism of Antagonist Action (Kinetics Part C) 386
14.3.4 Mechanism of Antagonist Action: Curve Patterns 386
14.3.5 Mechanism of Action: Incomplete Antagonism 387
14.3.6 pIC_{50} Mode: Antagonism Below Basal 389
14.3.7 Secondary Effects of Antagonists 390
14.3.8 Antagonist Potency Variably Dependent on Agonist Concentration 390
14.4 *In vitro—In vivo* Transitions and General Discovery 391
14.4.1 "Silent Antagonism" 391
14.4.2 Loss of Activity 392
14.4.3 Marking Relevant Agonism 393
14.4.4 *In vitro—In vivo* Correspondence of Activity 394
14.4.5 Divergent Agonist-Dependent Antagonism 395
14.5 SAR Exercises 396
14.5.1 Surrogate Screens 396
14.6 Pharmacokinetics 397
14.6.1 Clearance 397
14.6.2 Drug-Drug Interactions 399
14.6.3 Distribution I 399
14.6.4 Distribution II 399
14.6.5 Half Life I 399
14.6.6 Half Life II 400
14.6.7 Half Life III 400
14.6.8 Renal Clearance I 400
14.6.9 Renal Clearance II 400
14.6.10 Renal Clearance III 401

14.6.11 Absorption   401
14.6.12 Predictive Pharmacokinetics I   401
14.6.13 Predictive Pharmacokinetics II   401
14.6.14 Predictive Pharmacokinetics III   401
14.6.15 Log D and Pharmacokinetics   401
14.7 Conclusions   402
    References   402

Appendices   403
A.1 Statistical Tables of Use for Assessing
Significant Difference   403
A.2 Mathematical Fitting Functions   411

Glossary of Pharmacological Terms   415
Index   421

The usual reason for a new edition to a book of this type is that the information in previous editions is dated to the point where new advances in the field are hampered by absence of the new knowledge, or, worse, the dated knowledge is now known to be erroneous and incorrect future work is predicted. To a certain extent, both of those scenarios are now operable in the pharmacology of drug discovery thereby suggesting that another edition of this book may be relevant. Pharmacology attempts to understand the mechanisms of action of therapeutic molecules on systems of complexity not yet fully understood; at best, pharmacologists constantly are in a mode of approximation. Because of this, new technology becomes the means to learn more about cellular activity and with advancing technology comes a constantly changing view of drug mechanisms. Specifically two ideas, namely receptor signaling bias and receptor allosteric function, have led to a revision in the strategy of new drug

discovery and have revitalized research into receptors as therapeutic targets. In addition, the idea that biased ligands for pleiotropically coupled receptors can cause cell-type dependence of agonist potency ratios effectively negates the use of this basic pharmacologic tool for these molecules. This edition hopefully discusses techniques to capitalize on this new knowledge and address the single most prevalent cause of failure of new drug entities in clinical trials, namely, failure in efficacy. The fact that a discovery and development program can 'do everything right' and still fail to produce a useful therapy suggests that a re-evaluation of what we mean by 'efficacy' is warranted. The application of concepts regarding protein allostery and biased signaling may allow better definition of efficacy and thus a better targeting of new therapies.

Terry P. Kenakin Ph.D.
Chapel Hill, NC 2013

Preface to the Third Edition

It has been an interesting experience as an author and pharmacologist to see the changes that the discipline has experienced through the drug discovery process. While the definition of the human genome has undoubtedly marked pharmacology forever (and advanced it immeasurably), the more we learn, the more we are humbled by nature's complexity. With the genome, knowing the road map is still a long way from completing the journey and recent experience seems to reinforce the idea that pharmacology must be used to understand integrated systems, not just the pieces they are made of.

This edition incorporates a new trend in drug discovery; namely the consideration of pharmacokinetics and ADME properties of drugs (absorption, distribution, metabolism, excretion) early in the process. As prospective new drugs are tested in more complex systems (with concomitantly more complex dependent variable values), the trend in screening is to test fewer compounds of higher ("druglike") quality. Finally, this edition also hopefully fills a previous void whereby the ideas and concepts discussed can be applied to actual problems in pharmacological drug discovery in the form of questions with accompanying answers. The expanded version now spans pharmacology from consideration of the independent variable (drug concentration in the form of pharmacokinetics) to the dependent variable (system-independent measurement of drug activity). As with previous editions, the emphasis of this book is still on the chemist—biologist interface with special reference to the use of pharmacology by non-pharmacologists.

Terry P. Kenakin, Ph.D.
Research Triangle Park, NC, 2008

Preface to the Second Edition

With publication of the human genome has come an experiment in reductionism for drug discovery. With the evaluation of the number and quality of new drug treatments from this approach has come a re-evaluation of target-based versus systems-based strategies. Pharmacology, historically rooted in systems-based approaches and designed to give systems-independent measures of drug activity, is suitably poised to be a major, if not the major, tool in this new environment of drug discovery.

Compared to the first edition, this book now expands discussion of tools and ideas revolving around allosteric drug action. This is an increasingly therapeutically relevant subject in pharmacology as new drug screening utilizes cell function for discovery of new drug entities. In addition, discussion of system-based approaches, drug development (pharmacokinetics, therapeutics), sources of chemicals for new drugs, and elements of translational medicine have been added. As with the first edition, the emphasis of this volume is the gaining of understanding of pharmacology by the nonpharmacologist to the mutual enrichment of both.

Terry P. Kenakin, Ph.D.
Research Triangle Park, NC, 2006

Preface to the First Edition

If scientific disciplines can be said to go in and out of vogue, pharmacology is exemplary in this regard. The flourishing of receptor theory in the 1950s, the growth of biochemical binding technology in the 1970s, and the present resurgence of interest in defining cellular phenotypic sensitivity to drugs have been interspersed with troughs such as that brought on by the promise of the human genome and a belief that this genetic road map may make classical pharmacology redundant. The fallacy in this belief has been found in experimental data showing the importance of phenotype over genotype which underscores a common finding with roadmaps; They are not as good as a guide who knows the way. Pharmacology is now more relevant to the drug discovery process than ever as the genome furnishes a wealth of new targets to unravel. Biological science often advances at a rate defined by the technology of its tools; that is, scientists cannot see new things in old systems without new eyes. A veritable explosion in technology coupled with the great gift of molecular biology have definitely given pharmacologists new eyes to see.

This book initially began as a series of lectures at GlaxoSmithKline Research and Development on receptor pharmacology aimed at increasing the communication between pharmacologists and chemists. As these lectures developed it became evident that the concepts were useful to biologists not specifically trained in pharmacology. In return, the exchange between the chemists and biologists furnished new starting points from which to view the pharmacological concepts. It is hoped that this book will somewhat fill what could be a gap in present biological sciences, namely the study of dose-response relationships and how cells react to molecules.

Terry P. Kenakin, Ph.D.
Research Triangle Park, 2003

Chapter 1

What Is Pharmacology?

I would in particular draw the attention to physiologists to this type of physiological analysis of organic systems which can be done with the aid of toxic agents...

— Claude Bernard (1813−1878)

1.1 About This Book
1.2 What is Pharmacology?
1.3 The Receptor Concept
1.4 Pharmacological Test Systems
1.5 The Nature of Drug Receptors
1.6 Pharmacological Intervention and the Therapeutic Landscape
1.7 System-Independent Drug Parameters: Affinity and Efficacy
1.8 What is Affinity?
1.9 The Langmuir Adsorption Isotherm
1.10 What is Efficacy?
1.11 Dose-Response Curves
1.12 Chapter Summary and Conclusions
1.13 Derivations: Conformational Selection as a Mechanism of Efficacy
References

1.1 ABOUT THIS BOOK

Essentially this is a book about the methods and tools used in pharmacology to quantify drug activity. Receptor pharmacology is based on the comparison of experimental data and simple mathematical models, with a resulting inference of drug behavior to the molecular properties of drugs. From this standpoint, a certain level of understanding of the mathematics involved in the models is useful but not imperative. This book is structured such that each chapter begins with the basic concepts and then moves on to the techniques used to estimate drug parameters, and, finally, for those so inclined, the mathematical derivations of the models used. Understanding the derivation is not a prerequisite for understanding the application of the methods or the resulting conclusion; these are included for completeness and are for readers who wish to pursue exploration of the models. In general, facility with mathematical equations is definitely not required for pharmacology; the derivations can be ignored without any detriment to the use of this book.

Second, the symbols used in the models and derivations, on occasion, duplicate each other (i.e., α is an extremely popular symbol). However, the use of these multiple symbols has been retained, since this preserves the context of where these models were first described and utilized. Also, changing these to make them unique would cause confusion if these methods were to be used beyond the framework of this book. Therefore, care should be taken to consider the actual nomenclature of each chapter.

Third, an effort has been made to minimize the need to cross-reference different parts of the book (i.e., when a particular model is described, the basics are reiterated somewhat to minimize the need to read the relevant but different part of the book in which the model is initially described). While this leads to a small amount of repeated description, it is felt that this will allow for a more uninterrupted flow of reading and use of the book.

1.2 WHAT IS PHARMACOLOGY?

Pharmacology (an amalgam of the Greek *pharmakos*, medicine or drug, and *logos*, study) is a broad discipline describing the use of chemicals to treat and cure disease. The Latin term *pharmacologia* was used in the late 1600s, but the term *pharmacum* was used as early as the fourth century to denote the term *drug* or *medicine*. There are subdisciplines within pharmacology representing specialty areas. *Pharmacokinetics* deals with the disposition of drugs in the human body. To be useful, drugs must be absorbed and transported to their site of therapeutic action. Drugs will be ineffective in therapy if they do not reach the

T. P. Kenakin: A Pharmacology Primer, Fourth edition. DOI: http://dx.doi.org/10.1016/B978-0-12-407663-1.00001-6
© 2014 Elsevier Inc. All rights reserved.

organs(s) to exert their activity; this will be discussed specifically in Chapter 9 of this book. *Pharmaceutics* is the study of the chemical formulation of drugs to optimize absorption and distribution within the body. *Pharmacognosy* is the study of plant natural products and their use in the treatment of disease. A very important discipline in the drug discovery process is *medicinal chemistry*, the study of the production of molecules for therapeutic use. This couples synthetic organic chemistry with an understanding of how biological information can be quantified and used to guide the synthetic chemistry to enhance therapeutic activity. *Pharmacodynamics* is the study of the interaction of the drug molecule with the biological target (referred to generically as the "receptor," *vide infra*). This discipline lays the foundation of pharmacology since all therapeutic application of drugs has a common root in pharmacodynamics (i.e., as a prerequisite to exerting an effect, all drug molecules must bind to and interact with receptors).

The history of pharmacology is tied to the history of drug discovery — see Chapter 8. As put by the great Canadian physician Sir William Osler (1849–1919; the "father of modern medicine"), '...the desire to take medicine is perhaps the greatest feature which distinguishes man from animals...' Pharmacology as a separate science is approximately 120 to 140 years old. The relationship between chemical structure and biological activity began to be studied systematically in the 1860s [1]. It began when physiologists, using chemicals to probe physiological systems, became more interested in the chemical probes than the systems they were probing. By the early 1800s, physiologists were performing physiological studies with chemicals that became pharmacological studies more aimed at the definition of the biological activity of chemicals. The first formalized chair of pharmacology, indicating a formal university department, was founded in Estonia by Rudolf Bucheim in 1847. In North America, the first chair was founded by John Jacob Abel at Johns Hopkins University in 1890. A differentiation of physiology and pharmacology was given by the pharmacologist Sir William Paton [2]:

If physiology is concerned with the function, anatomy with the structure, and biochemistry with the chemistry of the living body, then pharmacology is concerned with the changes in function, structure, and chemical properties of the body brought about by chemical substances

— W. D. M. Paton (1986)

Many works about pharmacology essentially deal in therapeutics associated with different organ systems in the body. Thus, in many pharmacology texts, chapters are entitled drugs in the cardiovascular system, the effect of drugs on the gastrointestinal system, the central nervous system (CNS), and so on. However, the underlying principles for all of these is the same; namely, the pharmacodynamic interaction between the drug and the biological recognition system for that drug. Therefore, a prerequisite to all of pharmacology is an understanding of the basic concepts of dose-response and how living cells process pharmacological information. This generally is given the term *pharmacodynamics* or *receptor pharmacology*, where *receptor* is a term referring to any biological recognition unit for drugs (membrane receptors, enzymes, DNA, and so on). With such knowledge in hand, readers will be able to apply these principles to any branch of therapeutics effectively. This book treats dose-response data generically and demonstrates methods by which drug activity can be quantified across all biological systems irrespective of the nature of the biological target.

A great strength of pharmacology as a discipline is that it contains the tools and methods to convert "descriptive data," i.e., data that serves to characterize the activity of a given drug in a particular system, to "predictive data." This latter information can be used to predict that drug's activity in all organ systems, including the therapeutic one. This defines the drug discovery process which is the testing of new potential drug molecules in surrogate systems (where a potentially toxic chemical can do no lasting harm) before progression to the next step, namely testing in human therapeutic systems. The models and tools contained in pharmacology to convert drug behaviors in particular organs to molecular properties (see Chapter 2) are the main subject of this book and the step-by-step design of pharmacologic experiments to do this are described in detail in Chapter 8 (after the meaning of the particular parameters and terms is described in previous chapters).

The human *genome* is now widely available for drug discovery research. Far from being a simple blueprint of how drugs should be targeted, it has shown biologists that receptor *genotypes* (i.e., properties of proteins resulting from genetic transcription to their amino acid sequence) are secondary to receptor *phenotypes* (how the protein interacts with the myriad of cellular components and how cells tailor the makeup and functions of these proteins to their individual needs). Since the arrival of the human genome, receptor pharmacology as a science is more relevant than ever in drug discovery. Current drug therapy is based on less than 500 molecular targets, yet estimates utilizing the number of genes involved in multifactorial diseases suggest that the number of potential drug targets ranges from 2000 to 5000 [3]. Thus, current therapy is using only 5 to 10% of the potential trove of targets available in the human genome.

A meaningful dialogue between chemists and pharmacologists is the single most important element of the drug discovery process. The necessary link between medicinal chemistry and pharmacology has been elucidated by Paton [2]:

For pharmacology there results a particularly close relationship with chemistry, and the work may lead quite naturally, with no special stress on practicality, to therapeutic application, or (in the case of adverse reactions) to toxicology.

— W. D. M. Paton (1986)

Chemists and biologists reside in different worlds from the standpoint of the type of data they deal with. Chemistry is an exact science with physical scales that are not subject to system variance. Thus, the scales of measurement are transferable. Biology deals with the vagaries of complex systems that are not completely understood. Within this scenario, scales of measurement are much less constant and much more subject to system conditions. Given this, a gap can exist between chemists and biologists in terms of understanding and also in terms of the best method to progress forward. In the worst circumstance, it is a gap of credibility emanating from a failure of the biologist to make the chemist understand the limits of the data. Usually, however, credibility is not the issue, and the gap exists due to a lack of common experience. This book was written in an attempt to limit or, hopefully, eliminate this gap.

1.3 THE RECEPTOR CONCEPT

One of the most important concepts emerging from early pharmacological studies is the concept of the *receptor*.

Pharmacologists knew that minute amounts of certain chemicals had profound effects on physiological systems. They also knew that very small changes in the chemical composition of these substances could lead to huge differences in activity. This led to the notion that something on or in the cell must specifically read the chemical information contained in these substances and translate it into a physiological effect. This something was conceptually referred to as the "receptor" for that substance. Pioneers such as Paul Ehrlich (1854−1915, Figure 1.1A) proposed the existence of "chemoreceptors" (actually he proposed a collection of amboreceptors, triceptors, and polyceptors) on cells for dyes. He also postulated that the chemoreceptors on parasites, cancer cells, and microorganisms were different from healthy host and thus could be exploited therapeutically. The physiologist turned pharmacologist John Newport Langley (1852−1926, Figure 1.1B), during his studies with the drugs jaborandi (which contains the alkaloid pilocarpine) and atropine, introduced the concept that receptors were switches that received and generated signals and that these switches could be activated or blocked by specific molecules. The originator of quantitative receptor theory, the Edinburgh pharmacologist Alfred Joseph Clark (1885−1941, Figure 1.1C), was the first to suggest that the data, compiled from his studies of the interactions of acetylcholine and atropine, resulted from the unimolecular interaction of the drug and a substance on the cell surface. He articulated these ideas in the classic work *The Mode of Action of Drugs on Cells* [4], later

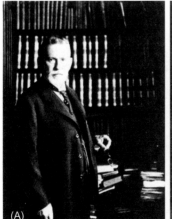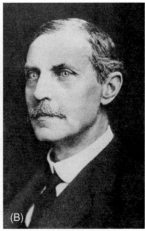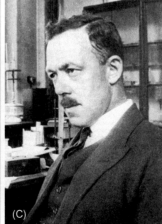

FIGURE 1.1 Pioneers of pharmacology. (A) Paul Ehrlich (1854−1915). Born in Silesia, Ehrlich graduated from Leipzig University to go on to a distinguished career as head of institutes in Berlin and Frankfurt. His studies with dyes and bacteria formed the basis of early ideas regarding recognition of biological substances by chemicals. (B) John Newport Langley (1852−1926). Though he began reading mathematics and history in Cambridge in 1871, Langley soon took to physiology. He succeeded the great physiologist M. Foster to the chair of physiology in Cambridge in 1903 and branched out into pharmacological studies of the autonomic nervous system. These pursuits led to germinal theories of receptors. (C) Alfred J. Clark (1885−1941). Beginning as a demonstrator in pharmacology in King's College (London), Clark went on to become professor of pharmacology at University College London. From there he took the chair of pharmacology in Edinburgh. Known as the originator of modern receptor theory, Clark applied chemical laws to biological phenomena. His books on receptor theory formed the basis of modern pharmacology.

revised as the *Handbook of Experimental Pharmacology* [5]. As put by Clark:

It appears to the writer that the most important fact shown by a study of drug antagonisms is that it is impossible to explain the remarkable effects observed except by assuming that drugs unite with receptors of a highly specific pattern ... No other explanation will, however, explain a tithe of the facts observed.

— A. J. Clark (1937)

Clark's next step formed the basis of receptor theory by applying chemical laws to systems of "infinitely greater complexity" [4]. It is interesting to note the scientific atmosphere in which Clark published these ideas. The dominant ideas between 1895 and 1930 were based on theories such as the law of phasic variation essentially stating that "certain phenomena occur frequently." Homeopathic theories like the Arndt−Schulz law and Weber−Fechner law were based on loose ideas around surface tension of the cell membrane, but there was little physicochemical basis for these ideas [6]. In this vein,

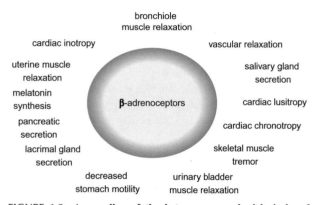

FIGURE 1.2 A sampling of the heterogeneous physiological and pharmacological response to the hormone epinephrine. The concept of receptors links these diverse effects to a single control point, namely the β-adrenoceptor.

prominent pharmacologists of the day, such as Walter Straub (1874−1944), suggested that a general theory of chemical binding between drugs and cells utilizing receptors was "... going too far ... and ... not admissible" [6]. The impact of Clark's thinking against these concepts cannot be overemphasized to modern pharmacology.

It is possible to underestimate the enormous significance of the receptor concept in pharmacology until it is realized how relatively chaotic the study of drug effect was before it was introduced. Specifically, consider the myriad of physiological and pharmacological effects of the hormone epinephrine in the body. As shown in Figure 1.2, a host of responses are obtained; from the CNS, cardiovascular system, smooth muscle, and other organs. It is impossible to see a thread which relates these very different responses until it is realized that all of these are mediated by the activation of a single protein receptor, namely, in this case, the β-adrenoceptor. When this is understood, then a much better idea can be gained as to how to manipulate these heterogeneous responses for therapeutic benefit; the receptor concept introduced order into physiology and pharmacology.

Drug receptors can exist in many forms, including cell surface proteins, enzymes, ion channels, membrane transporters, DNA, and cytosolic proteins (see Figure 1.3). There are examples of important drugs for all of these. This book deals with general concepts which can be applied to a range of receptor types, but most of the principles are illustrated with the most tractable receptor class known in the human genome; namely *seven transmembrane (7TM) receptors*. These receptors are named for their characteristic structure, which consists of a single protein chain that traverses the cell membrane seven times to produce extracellular and intracellular loops. These receptors activate G-proteins to elicit response, thus they are also commonly referred to as *G-protein-coupled receptors (GPCRs)*; this should now be considered a limiting moniker as these proteins signal to a wide

FIGURE 1.3 Schematic diagram of potential drug targets. Molecules can affect the function of numerous cellular components both in the cytosol and on the membrane surface. There are many families of receptors that traverse the cellular membrane and allow chemicals to communicate with the interior of the cell.

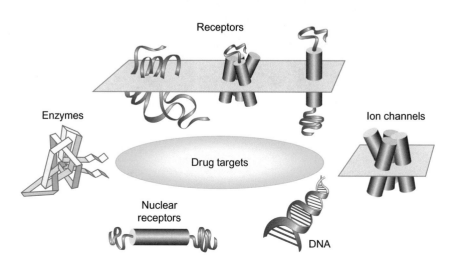

variety of signaling molecules in the cell and are not confined to G-protein effects. There are between 800 and 1000 [7] of these in the genome (the genome sequence predicts 650 GPCR genes, of which approximately 190 [on the order of 1% of the genome of superior organisms] are categorized as known 7TMRs [8] activated by some 70 ligands). In the United States, in 2000, nearly half of all prescription drugs were targeted toward 7TM receptors [3]. These receptors, comprising between 1 and 5% of the total cell protein, control a myriad of physiological activities. They are tractable for drug discovery because they are on the cell surface, and therefore drugs do not need to penetrate the cell to produce effect. In the study of biological targets such as 7TMRs and other receptors, a "system" must be employed that accepts chemical input and returns biological output. It is worth discussing such receptor systems in general terms before their specific uses are considered.

1.4 PHARMACOLOGICAL TEST SYSTEMS

Molecular biology has transformed pharmacology and the drug discovery process. As little as 20 years ago, screening for new drug entities was carried out in surrogate animal tissues. This necessitated a rather large extrapolation to span the differences in genotype and phenotype. The belief that the gap could be bridged came from the notion that the chemicals recognized by these receptors in both humans and animals were the same (*vide infra*). Receptors are unique proteins with characteristic amino acid sequences. While *polymorphisms* (spontaneous alterations in amino acid sequence, *vide infra*) of receptors exist in the same species, in general the amino acid sequence of a natural ligand-binding domain for a given receptor type largely may be conserved. There are obvious pitfalls of using surrogate species receptors for predicting human drug activity, and it never can be known for certain whether agreement for estimates of activity for a given set of drugs ensures accurate prediction for all drugs. The agreement is very much drug and receptor dependent. For example, the human and mouse α_2-adrenoceptors are 89% homologous, and thus considered very similar from the standpoint of amino acid sequence. Furthermore, the affinities of the α_2-adrenoceptor antagonists atipamezole and yohimbine are nearly indistinguishable (atipamezole human α_2-C10K_i = 2.9 ± 0.4 nM, mouse α_2-4H K_i = 1.6 ± 0.2 nM; yohimbine human α_2-C10K_i = 3.4 ± 0.1 nM, mouse α_2-4H K_i = 3.8 ± 0.8 nM). However, there is a 20.9-fold difference for the antagonist prazosin (human α_2-C10K_i = 2034 ± 350 nM, mouse α_2-4H K_i = 97.3 ± 0.7 nM) [9]. Such data highlight a general theme in pharmacological research; namely, that a hypothesis, such as one proposing that two receptors which are identical with respect to their sensitivity to drugs are the

same, cannot be proven, only disproven. While a considerable number of drugs could be tested on the two receptors (thus supporting the hypothesis that their sensitivity to all drugs is the same), this hypothesis is immediately disproven by the first drug that shows differential potency on the two receptors. The fact that a series of drugs tested show identical potencies may mean only that the wrong sample of drugs has been chosen to unveil the difference. Thus, no general statements can be made that any one surrogate system is completely predictive of activity on the target human receptor. This will always be a drug-specific phenomenon.

The link between animal and human receptors is the fact that both proteins recognize the endogenous transmitter (e.g., acetylcholine, norepinephrine), and therefore the hope is that this link will carry over into other drugs that recognize the animal receptor. This imperfect system formed the basis of drug discovery until human *cDNA* for human receptors could be used to make cells express human receptors. These engineered (recombinant) systems are now used as surrogate human receptor systems, and the leap of faith from animal receptor sequences to human receptor sequences is not required (i.e., the problem of differences in genotype has been overcome). However, cellular signaling is an extremely complex process and cells tailor their receipt of chemical signals in numerous ways. Therefore, the way a given receptor gene behaves in a particular cell can differ in response to the surroundings in which that receptor finds itself. These differences in phenotype (i.e., properties of a receptor produced by interaction with its environment) can result in differences in both the quantity and quality of a signal produced by a concentration of a given drug in different cells. Therefore, there is still a certain, although somewhat lesser, leap of faith taken in predicting therapeutic effects in human tissues under pathological control from surrogate recombinant or even surrogate natural human receptor systems. For this reason, it is a primary requisite of pharmacology to derive system-independent estimates of drug activity that can be used to predict therapeutic effect in other systems.

A schematic diagram of the various systems used in drug discovery, in order of how appropriate they are to therapeutic drug treatment, is shown in Figure 1.4. As discussed previously, early functional experiments in animal tissue have now largely given way to testing in recombinant cell systems engineered with human receptor material. This huge technological step greatly improved the predictability of drug activity in humans, but it should be noted that there still are many factors that intervene between the genetically engineered drug testing system and the pathology of human disease.

A frequently used strategy in drug discovery is to express human receptors (through *transfection* with human cDNA) in convenient surrogate host cells (referred

FIGURE 1.4 A history of the drug discovery process. Originally, the only biological material available for drug research was animal tissue. With the advent of molecular biological techniques to clone and express human receptors in cells, recombinant systems supplanted animal isolated tissue work. It should be noted that these recombinant systems still fall short of yielding drug response in the target human tissue under the influence of pathological processes.

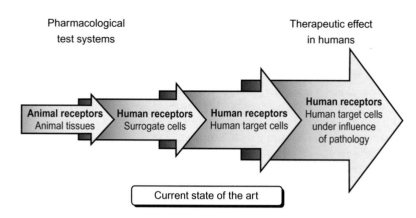

to as "target-based" drug discovery; see Chapter 10 for further discussion). These host cells are chosen mainly for their technical properties (i.e., robustness, growth rate, stability) and not with any knowledge of verisimilitude to the therapeutically targeted human cell type. There are various factors relevant to the choice of surrogate host cell, such as a very low background activity (i.e., a cell cannot be used that already contains a related animal receptor for fear of cross-reactivity to molecules targeted for the human receptor). Human receptors are often expressed in animal surrogate cells. The main idea here is that the cell is a receptacle for the receptor, allowing it to produce physiological responses, and that activity can be monitored in pharmacological experiments. In this sense, human receptors expressed in animal cells are still a theoretical step distanced from the human receptor in a human cell type. However, even if a human surrogate is used (and there are such cells available) there is no definitive evidence that a surrogate human cell is any more predictive of a natural receptor activity than an animal cell when compared to the complex receptor behavior in its natural host cell type expressed under pathological conditions. Receptor phenotype dominates in the end organ, and the exact differences between the genotypic behavior of the receptor (resulting from the genetic makeup of the receptor) and the phenotypic behavior of the receptor (due to the interaction of the genetic product with the rest of the cell) may be cell specific. Therefore, there is still a possible gap between the surrogate systems used in the drug discovery process and the therapeutic application. Moreover, most drug discovery systems utilize receptors as switching mechanisms and quantify whether drugs turn on or turn off the switch. The pathological processes that we strive to modify may be more subtle. As put by pharmacologist Sir James Black [10]:

... angiogenesis, apoptosis, inflammation, commitment of marrow stem cells, and immune responses. The cellular reactions subsumed in these processes are switch like in their behavior ... biochemically we are learning that in all these processes many chemical regulators seem to be involved. From the literature on

synergistic interactions, a control model can be built in which no single agent is effective. If a number of chemical messengers each bring information from a different source and each deliver only a subthreshold stimulus but together mutually potentiate each other, then the desired information-rich switching can be achieved with minimum risk of miscuing.

— J. W. Black (1986)

Such complex end points are difficult to predict from any one of the component processes leading to yet another leap of faith in the drug discovery process. For these reasons, an emerging strategy for drug discovery is the use of natural cellular systems. This approach is discussed in some detail in Chapter 10.

Even when an active drug molecule is found and activity is verified in the therapeutic arena, there are factors that can lead to gaps in its therapeutic profile. When drugs are exposed to huge populations, genetic variations in this population can lead to discovery of *alleles* that code for mutations of the target (isogenes) and these can lead to variation in drug response. Such polymorphisms can lead to resistant populations (i.e., resistance of some asthmatics to the β-adrenoceptor bronchodilators [11]). In the absence of genetic knowledge, these therapeutic failures for a drug could not easily be averted since they in essence occurred because of the presence of new biological targets not originally considered in the drug discovery process. However, as new epidemiological information becomes available these polymorphisms can now be incorporated into the drug discovery process.

There are two theoretical and practical scales that can be used to make system-independent measures of drug activity on biological systems. The first is a measure of the attraction of a drug for a biological target; namely, its *affinity* for a receptor. Drugs must interact with receptors to produce an effect, and the affinity is a chemical term used to quantify the strength of that interaction. The second is much less straightforward and is used to quantify the degree of effect imparted to the biological system after the drug binds to the receptor. This is termed *efficacy*. This property was named by R. P. Stephenson [12] within classical receptor theory as a proportionality factor

Levels of protein (receptor) structure

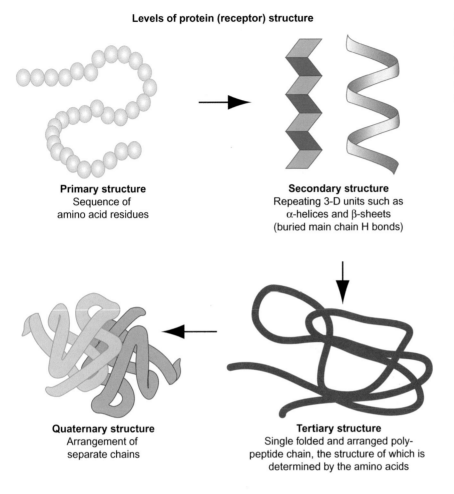

Primary structure
Sequence of
amino acid residues

Secondary structure
Repeating 3-D units such as
α-helices and β-sheets
(buried main chain H bonds)

Quaternary structure
Arrangement of
separate chains

Tertiary structure
Single folded and arranged polypeptide chain, the structure of which is
determined by the amino acids

FIGURE 1.5 **Increasing levels of protein structure.** A protein has a given amino acid sequence to make peptide chains. These adopt a 3-D structure according to the free energy of the system. Receptor function can change with changes in tertiary or quaternary structure.

for the tissue response produced by a drug. There is no absolute scale for efficacy but rather it is dealt with in relative terms (i.e., the ratio of the efficacy of two different drugs on a particular biological system can be estimated and, under ideal circumstances, will transcend the system and be applicable to other systems as well). It is the foremost task of pharmacology to use the translations of drug effect obtained from cells to provide system-independent estimates of affinity and efficacy. Before specific discussion of affinity and efficacy, it is worth considering the molecular nature of biological targets.

1.5 THE NATURE OF DRUG RECEPTORS

While some biological targets such as DNA are not protein in nature, most receptors are. It is useful to consider the properties of receptor proteins to provide a context for the interaction of small molecule drugs with them. An important property of receptors is that they have a 3-D structure. Proteins are usually composed of one or more peptide chains; the composition of these chains makes up the primary and secondary structure of the protein. Proteins also are described in terms of a tertiary structure, which defines their shape in 3-D space, and a quarternary structure, which defines the molecular interactions between the various components of the protein chains (Figure 1.5). It is this 3-D structure which allows the protein to function as a recognition site and effector for drugs and other components of the cell; in essence, the ability of the protein to function as a messenger, shuttling information from the outside world to the cytosol of the cell. For 7TMRs the 3-D nature of the receptor forms binding domains for other proteins such as G-proteins (these are activated by the receptor and then go on to activate enzymes and ion channels within the cell; see Chapter 2) and endogenous chemicals such as neurotransmitters, hormones, and autacoids that carry physiological messages. This important class of drug target is named for a characteristic structure consisting of seven transmembrane domains looping into the extracellular and intracellular space — see Figure 1.6. These molecules are the main transfer points of information from the outside to the inside of the cell, and such transfers occur through changes in the conformation of the receptor protein (*vide infra*). For other receptors, such as ion channels and single transmembrane enzyme receptors, the conformational change *per se* leads to a response; either through an opening of a channel to allow the flow of ionic current or the initiation of enzymatic activity. Therapeutic advantage can be taken by designing small molecules to utilize these binding domains or other 3-D binding domains on the receptor protein in order to modify physiological and pathological processes.

1.6 PHARMACOLOGICAL INTERVENTION AND THE THERAPEUTIC LANDSCAPE

It is useful to consider the therapeutic landscape with respect to the aims of pharmacology. As stated by Sir William Ossler (1849−1919) "... the prime distinction between man and other creatures is man's yearning to

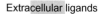

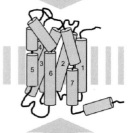

FIGURE 1.6 Depiction of the structure of seven transmembrane domain receptors, one of the most if not the most important therapeutic targets available in the human genome. Chemicals access the receptor through the extracellular space by binding to the extracellular domains of the protein. This causes a conformational change in the protein that alters the interaction of signaling proteins in the cell cytosol. This latter process results in the initiation of cellular signaling.

take medicine." The notion that drugs can be used to cure disease is as old as history. One of the first written records of actual "prescriptions" can be found in the Ebers Papyrus (circa 1550 B.C.): "... for night blindness in the eyes ... liver of ox, roasted and crushed out ... really excellent!" − see Figure 1.7. Now it is known that liver is an excellent source of vitamin A, a prime treatment for night blindness, but that chemical detail was not known to the ancient Egyptians. Disease can be considered under two broad categories: those caused by invaders such as pathogens and those caused by intrinsic breakdown of normal physiological function. The first generally is approached through the invader (i.e., the pathogen is destroyed, neutralized, or removed from the body). The one exception of where the host is treated when an invader is present is the treatment of HIV-1 infection leading to AIDS. In this case, while there are treatments to neutralize the pathogen, such as antiretrovirals to block viral replication, a major new approach is the blockade of the interaction of the virus with the protein that mediates viral entry into healthy cells, the chemokine receptor CCR5. In this case, CCR5 antagonists are used to prevent HIV fusion and subsequent infection. The second approach to disease requires an understanding of the pathological process and repair of the damage to return to normal function.

The therapeutic landscape onto which drug discovery and pharmacology in general combat disease can generally be described in terms of the major organ systems of the body and how they may go awry. A healthy cardiovascular system consists of a heart able to pump deoxygenated blood through the lungs and to pump oxygenated blood throughout a circulatory system that does not unduly resist blood flow. Since the heart requires a high

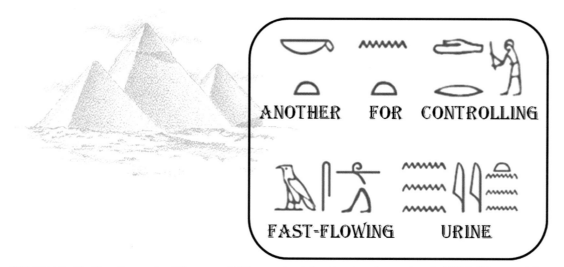

FIGURE 1.7   The Ebers Papyrus is a 110-page scroll (20 meters long) thought to have been written in 1550 B.C. but containing information dating from 3400 B.C. It is a record of Egyptian medicine and contains numerous 'prescriptions' some of which, though empirical, are valid therapeutic approaches to diseases.

degree of oxygen itself to function, myocardial ischemia can be devastating to its function. Similarly, an inability to maintain rhythm (arrhythmia) or loss in strength with concomitant inability to empty (congestive heart failure) can be fatal. The latter disease is exacerbated by elevated arterial resistance (hypertension). A wide range of drugs are used to treat the cardiovascular system, including coronary vasodilators (nitrates), diuretics, renin-angiotensin inhibitors, vasodilators, cardiac glycosides, calcium antagonists, beta and alpha blockers, antiarrhythmics, and drugs for dyslipidemia. The lungs must extract oxygen from the air, deliver it to the blood, and release carbon dioxide from the blood into exhaled air. Asthma, chronic obstructive pulmonary disease (COPD), and emphysema are serious disorders of the lungs and airways. Bronchodilators (beta agonists), anti-inflammatory drugs, inhaled glucocorticoids, anticholinergics, and theophylline analogues are used for treatment of these diseases. The central nervous system controls all conscious thought and many unconscious body functions. Numerous diseases of the brain can occur, including depression, anxiety, epilepsy, mania, degeneration, obsessive disorders, and schizophrenia. Brain functions such as those controlling sedation and pain also may require treatment. A wide range of drugs are used for CNS disorders, including serotonin partial agonists and uptake inhibitors, dopamine agonists, benzodiazepines, barbiturates, opioids, tricyclics, neuroleptics, and hydantoins. The gastrointestinal (GI) tract receives and processes food to extract nutrients and removes waste from the body. Diseases such as stomach ulcers, colitis, diarrhea, nausea, and irritable bowel syndrome can affect this system. Histamine antagonists, proton pump blockers, opioid agonists, antacids, and serotonin uptake blockers are used to treat diseases of the GI tract.

The inflammatory system is designed to recognize self from non-self, and to destroy non-self to protect the body. In diseases of the inflammatory system, the self-recognition can break down, leading to conditions in which the body destroys healthy tissue in a misguided attempt at protection. This can lead to rheumatoid arthritis, allergies, pain, COPD, asthma, fever, gout, graft rejection, and problems with chemotherapy. Nonsteroidal anti-inflammatory drugs (NSAIDs), aspirin and salicylates, leukotriene antagonists, and histamine receptor antagonists are used to treat inflammatory disorders. The endocrine system produces and secretes hormones crucial to the body for growth and function. Diseases of this class of organs can lead to growth and pituitary defects; diabetes; abnormality in thyroid, pituitary, adrenal cortex, and androgen function; osteoporosis; and alterations in estrogen-progesterone balance. The general approach to treatment is through replacement or augmentation of secretion. Drugs used are replacement hormones, insulin, sulfonylureas, adrenocortical steroids, and oxytocin. In addition to the major organ

and physiological systems, diseases involving neurotransmission and neuromuscular function, ophthalmology, hemopoiesis and hematology, dermatology, immunosuppression, and drug addiction and abuse are amenable to pharmacological intervention.

Cancer is a serious malfunction of normal cell growth. In the years from 1950 through 1970, the major approach to treating this disease was to target DNA and DNA precursors according to the hypothesis that rapidly dividing cells (cancer cells) are more susceptible to DNA toxicity than normal cells. Since that time, a wide range of new therapies based on manipulation of the immune system, induction of differentiation, inhibition of angiogenesis, and increased killer T-lymphocytes to decrease cell proliferation has greatly augmented the armamentarium against neoplastic disease. Previously lethal malignancies such as testicular cancer, some lymphomas, and leukemia are now curable.

Three general treatments of disease are surgery, genetic engineering (still an emerging discipline), and pharmacological intervention. While early medicine was subject to the theories of Hippocrates (460−357 B.C.), who saw health and disease as a balance of four humors (i.e., black and yellow bile, phlegm, and blood), by the sixteenth century pharmacological concepts were being formulated. These could be stated concisely as the following [13]:

- Every disease has a cause for which there is a specific remedy.
- Each remedy has a unique essence that can be obtained from nature by extraction ("doctrine of signatures").
- The administration of the remedy is subject to a dose-response relationship.

The basis for believing that pharmacological intervention can be a major approach to the treatment of disease is the fact that the body generally functions in response to chemicals. Table 1.1 shows partial lists of hormones and neurotransmitters in the body. Many more endogenous chemicals are involved in normal physiological function. The fact that so many physiological processes are controlled by chemicals provides the opportunity for chemical intervention. Thus, physiological signals mediated by chemicals can be initiated, negated, augmented, or modulated. The nature of this modification can take the form of changes in the type, strength, duration, or location of signal.

1.7 SYSTEM-INDEPENDENT DRUG PARAMETERS: AFFINITY AND EFFICACY

The process of drug discovery relies on the testing of molecules in systems to yield estimates of biological activity in an iterative process of changing the structure

TABLE 1.1 Some Endogenous Chemicals Controlling Normal Physiological Function

Neurotransmitters		
Acetylcholine	2-Arachidonylglycerol	Anandamide
ATP	Corticotropin-releasing hormone	Dopamine
Epinephrine	Aspartate	Gamma-aminobutyric acid
Galanin	Glutamate	Glycine
Histamine	Norepinephrine	Serotonin
Hormones		
Thyroid-stimulating hormone	Follicle-stimulating hormone	Luteinizing hormone
Prolactin	Adrenocorticotropin	Antidiuretic hormone
Thyrotropin-releasing hormone	Oxytocin	Gonadotropin-releasing hormone
Growth-hormone-releasing hormone	Corticotropin-releasing hormone	Somatostatin
Melatonin	Thyroxin	Calcitonin
Parathyroid hormone	Glucocorticoid(s)	Mineralocorticoid(s)
Estrogen(s)	Progesterone	Chorionic gonadotropin
Androgens	Insulin	Glucagon
Amylin	Erythropoietin	Calcitriol
Calciferol	Atrial-natriuretic peptide	Gastrin
Secretin	Cholecystokinin	Neuropeptide Y
Insulin-like growth factor	Angiotensinogen	Ghrelin
	Leptin	

of the molecule until optimal activity is achieved. It will be seen in this book that there are numerous systems available to do this, and that each system may interpret the activity of molecules in different ways. Some of these interpretations can appear to be in conflict with each other, leading to apparent capricious patterns. For this reason, the way forward in the drug development process is to use only system-independent information. Ideally, scales of biological activity should be used that transcend the actual biological system in which the drug is tested. This is essential to avoid confusion and also because it is quite rare to have access to the exact human system under the control of the appropriate pathology available for *in vitro* testing. Therefore, the drug discovery process necessarily relies on the testing of molecules in surrogate systems and the extrapolation of the observed activity to all systems. The only means to do this is to obtain system-independent measures of drug activity; namely, affinity and efficacy.

If a molecule in solution associates closely with a receptor protein, it has affinity for that protein. The area where it is bound is the binding *domain* or *locus*. If the same molecule interferes with the binding of a physiologically active molecule such as a hormone or a neurotransmitter (i.e., if the binding of the molecule precludes activity of the physiologically active hormone or neurotransmitter), the molecule is referred to as an *antagonist*. Therefore, a pharmacologically active molecule that blocks physiological effect is an antagonist. Similarly, if a molecule binds to a receptor and produces its own effect it is termed an *agonist*. It also is assumed to have the property of efficacy. Efficacy is detected by observation of pharmacological response. Therefore, agonists have both affinity and efficacy.

Classically, agonist response is described in two stages, the first being the initial signal imparted to the immediate biological target; namely, the receptor. This first stage is composed of the formation, either through interaction with an agonist or spontaneously, of an active state receptor conformation. This initial signal is termed the *stimulus* (Figure 1.8). This stimulus is perceived by the cell and processed in various ways through successions of biochemical reactions to the end point; namely, the response. The sum total of the subsequent reactions is referred to as the stimulus-response mechanism or cascade (see Figure 1.8).

Efficacy is a molecule-related property (i.e., different molecules have different capabilities to induce a physiological response). The actual term for the molecular aspect of response-inducing capacity of a molecule is *intrinsic efficacy* (see Chapter 3 for how this term evolved). Thus, every molecule has a unique value for its intrinsic efficacy (in cases of antagonists this could be zero). The different abilities of molecules to induce response are illustrated in Figure 1.9. This figure shows dose-response curves for four 5-HT (serotonin) agonists in rat jugular vein. It can be seen that if response is plotted as a function of the percent receptor occupancy, different receptor occupancies for the different agonists lead to different levels of response. For example, while 0.6 g force can be generated by 5-HT by occupying 30% of the receptors, the agonist 5-cyanotryptamine requires twice the receptor occupancy to generate the same response (i.e., the capability of 5-cyanotryptamine to induce response

is half that of 5-HT [14]). These agonists are then said to possess different magnitudes of intrinsic efficacy.

It is important to consider affinity and efficacy as separately manipulatable properties. Thus, there are chemical features of agonists that pertain especially to affinity and other features that pertain to efficacy. Figure 1.10 shows a series of key chemical compounds made en route to the histamine H_2 receptor antagonist cimetidine (used for healing gastric ulcers). The starting point for this discovery program was the knowledge that histamine, a naturally occurring autacoid, activates histamine H_2 receptors in the stomach to cause acid secretion. This constant acid secretion is what prevents the healing of lesions and ulcers. The task was then to design a molecule that would antagonize the histamine receptors mediating acid secretion and prevent histamine H_2 receptor activation to allow the ulcers to heal. This task was approached with the knowledge that molecules, theoretically, could be made that retained or even enhanced affinity but decreased the efficacy of histamine (i.e., these were separate properties). As can be seen in Figure 1.10, molecules were consecutively synthesized with reduced values of efficacy and enhanced affinity until the target histamine H_2 antagonist cimetidine was made. This was a clear demonstration of the power of medicinal chemistry to separately manipulate affinity and efficacy for which, in part, the Nobel Prize in Medicine was awarded in 1988.

1.8 WHAT IS AFFINITY?

The affinity of a drug for a receptor defines the strength of interaction between the two species. The forces controlling the affinity of a drug for the receptor are thermodynamic (enthalpy as changes in heat and entropy as

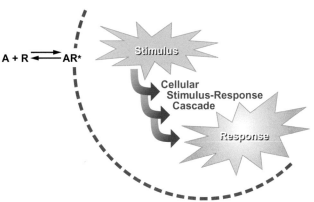

FIGURE 1.8 **Schematic diagram of response production by an agonist.** An initial stimulus is produced at the receptor as a result of agonist–receptor interaction. This stimulus is processed by the stimulus-response apparatus of the cell into observable cellular response.

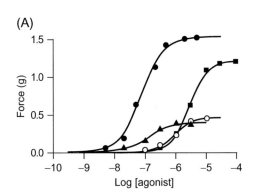
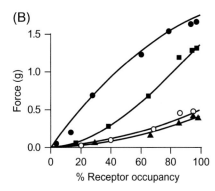

FIGURE 1.9 **Differences between agonists producing contraction of rat jugular vein through activation of 5-HT receptors.** (A) Dose-response curves to 5-HT receptor agonists, 5-HT (filled circles), 5-cyanotryptamine (filled squares), N,N-dimethyltryptamine (open circles), and N-benzyl-5-methoxytryptamine (filled triangles). Abscissae: logarithms of molar concentrations of agonist. (B) Occupancy response curves for curves shown in panel A. Abscissae: percent receptor occupancy by the agonist as calculated by mass action and the equilibrium dissociation constant of the agonist–receptor complex. Ordinates: force of contraction in g. Data drawn from [14].

FIGURE 1.10 Key compounds synthesized to eliminate the efficacy (burgundy red) and enhance the affinity (green) of histamine for histamine H_2 receptors to make cimetidine, one of the first histamine H_2 antagonists of use in the treatment of peptic ulcers. Quotation from James Black [10].

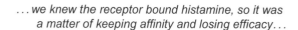

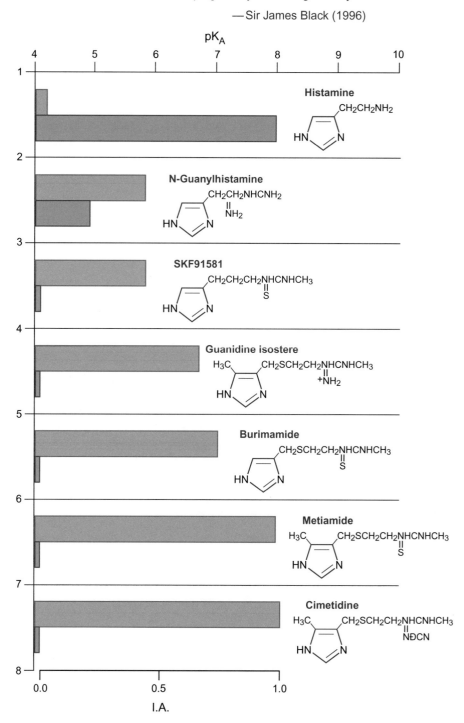

changes in the state of disorder). The chemical forces between the components of the drug and the receptor vary in importance in relation to the distance of the drug from the receptor's binding surface. Thus, the strength of electrostatic forces (attraction due to positive and negative charges and/or complex interactions between polar groups) varies as a function of the reciprocal of the distance between the drug and the receptor. Hydrogen bonding (the sharing of a hydrogen atom between an acidic and basic group) varies in strength as a function of the fourth power of the reciprocal of the distance. Also involved are van der Waals' forces (weak attraction

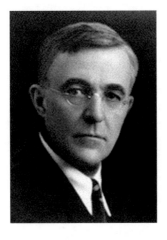

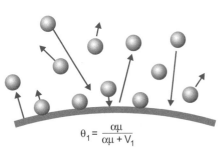

$$\theta_1 = \frac{\alpha\mu}{\alpha\mu + V_1}$$

FIGURE 1.11 **The Langmuir adsorption isotherm representing the binding of a molecule to a surface.** Photo shows Irving Langmuir (1881–1957), a chemist interested in the adsorption of molecules to metal filaments for the production of light. Langmuir devised the simple equation still in use today for quantifying the binding of molecules to surfaces. The equilibrium is described by condensation and evaporation to yield the fraction of surface bound (θ_1) by a concentration μ.

between polar and nonpolar molecules) and hydrophobic bonds (interaction of nonpolar surfaces to avoid interaction with water). The combination of all of these forces causes the drug to reside in a certain position within the protein binding pocket. This is a position of minimal free energy. It is important to note that drugs do not statically reside in one uniform position. As thermal energy varies in the system, drugs approach and dissociate from the protein surface. This is an important concept in pharmacology as it sets the stage for competition between two drugs for a single binding domain on the receptor protein. The probability that a given molecule will be at the point of minimal free energy within the protein binding pocket thus depends on the concentration of the drug available to fuel the binding process and also the strength of the interactions for the complementary regions in the binding pocket (affinity). Affinity can be thought of as a force of attraction and can be quantified with a very simple tool, first used to study the adsorption of molecules onto a surface; namely, the Langmuir adsorption isotherm.

1.9 THE LANGMUIR ADSORPTION ISOTHERM

Defined by the chemist Irving Langmuir (1881–1957, Figure 1.11), the model for affinity is referred to as the *Langmuir adsorption isotherm*. Langmuir, a chemist at General Electric was interested in the adsorption of molecules onto metal surfaces for the improvement of lighting filaments. He reasoned that molecules had a characteristic rate of diffusion toward a surface (referred to as *condensation* and denoted α in his nomenclature) and also a characteristic rate of dissociation (referred to as *evaporation* and denoted as V_1; see Figure 1.11). He assumed that the amount of surface that already has a molecule bound is not available to bind another molecule. The surface area bound by molecule is denoted θ_1, expressed as a fraction of the total area. The amount of

free area open for the binding of molecule, expressed as a fraction of the total area, is denoted as $1 - \theta_1$. The rate of adsorption toward the surface therefore is controlled by the concentration of drug in the medium (denoted μ in Langmuir's nomenclature) multiplied by the rate of condensation on the surface and the amount of free area available for binding:

$$\text{Rate of diffusion toward surface} = \alpha\mu(1 - \theta_1). \quad (1.1)$$

The rate of evaporation is given by the intrinsic rate of dissociation of bound molecules from the surface multiplied by the amount already bound:

$$\text{Rate of evaporation} = V_1\theta_1. \quad (1.2)$$

Once equilibrium has been reached, the rate of adsorption equals the rate of evaporation. Equating (1.1) and (1.2) and rearranging yields:

$$\theta_1 = \frac{\alpha\mu}{\alpha\mu + V_1}. \quad (1.3)$$

This is the Langmuir adsorption isotherm in its original form. In pharmacological nomenclature, it is rewritten according to the convention:

$$\rho = \frac{[AR]}{[R_t]} = \frac{[A]}{[A] + K_A}, \quad (1.4)$$

where [AR] is the amount of complex formed between the ligand and the receptor and [R_t] is the total number of receptor sites. The ratio ρ refers to the fraction of maximal binding by a molar concentration of drug [A] with an equilibrium dissociation constant of K_A. This latter term is the ratio of the rate of offset (in Langmuir's terms V_1 and referred to as k_2 in receptor pharmacology) divided by the rate of onset (in Langmuir's terms α denoted k_1 in receptor pharmacology).

It is amazing to note that complex processes such as drugs binding to protein, activation of cells, and observation of syncytial cellular response should apparently so closely follow a model based on these simple concepts.

This was not lost on A. J. Clark in his treatise on drug-receptor theory *The Mode of Action of Drugs on Cells* [4]:

It is an interesting and significant fact that the author in 1926 found that the quantitative relations between the concentration of acetylcholine and its action on muscle cells, an action the nature of which is wholly unknown, could be most accurately expressed by the formulae devised by Langmuir to express the adsorption of gases on metal filaments.

— A. J. Clark (1937)

The term K_A is a concentration and it quantifies affinity. Specifically, it is the concentration that binds to 50% of the total receptor population (see Equation 1.4 when $[A] = K_A$). Therefore, the smaller is the K_A, the higher is the affinity. Affinity is the reciprocal of K_A. For example, if $K_A = 10^{-8}$ M, then 10^{-8} M binds to 50% of the receptors. If $K_A = 10^{-4}$ M, a 10,000-fold higher concentration of the drug is needed to bind to 50% of the receptors (i.e., it is of lower affinity).

It is instructive to discuss affinity in terms of the adsorption isotherm in the context of measuring the amount of receptor bound for given concentrations of drug. Assume that values of fractional receptor occupancy can be visualized for various drug concentrations. The kinetics of such binding are shown in Figure 1.12. It can

be seen that initially the binding is rapid, in accordance with the fact that there are many unbound sites for the drug to choose. As the sites become occupied, there is a temporal reduction in binding until a maximal value for that concentration is attained. Figure 1.12 also shows that the binding of higher concentrations of drug is correspondingly increased. In keeping with the fact that this is first-order binding kinetics (where the rate is dependent on a rate constant multiplied by the concentration of reactant), the time to equilibrium is shorter for higher concentrations than for lower concentrations. The various values for receptor occupancy at different concentrations constitute a concentration binding curve (shown in Figure 1.13A). There are two areas in this curve of particular interest to pharmacologists. The first is the maximal asymptote for binding. This defines the maximal number of receptive binding sites in the preparation. The binding isotherm Equation 1.4 defines the ordinate axis as the fraction of the maximal binding. Thus, by definition the maximal value is unity. However, in experimental studies real values of capacity are used since the maximum is not known. When the complete curve is defined, the maximal value of binding can be used to define fractional binding at various concentrations and thus define the concentration at which half-maximal binding (binding to 50% of the receptor population) occurs. This is the equilibrium dissociation constant of the drug-receptor complex (K_A), the important measure of drug affinity. This comes from the other important region of the curve; namely, the midpoint. It can be seen from Figure 1.13A that graphical estimation of both the maximal asymptote and the midpoint is difficult to perform with the graph in the form shown. A much easier format to present binding, or any concentration-response data, is a semilogarithmic form of the isotherm. This allows better estimation of the maximal asymptote and places the midpoint in a linear portion of the graph where intrapolation can be done (see Figure 1.13B). Dose-response curves for binding are not often visualized, as they require a means to detect bound (over unbound) drug. However, for drugs that produce a pharmacological response (i.e., agonists) a signal proportional to bound drug can be observed. The true definition

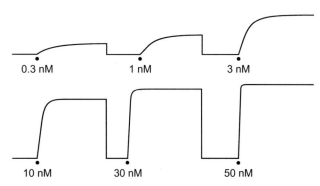

FIGURE 1.12 Time course for increasing concentrations of a ligand with a K_A of 2 nM. Initially the binding is rapid but slows as the sites become occupied. The maximal binding increases with increasing concentrations as does the rate of binding.

FIGURE 1.13 Dose-response relationship for ligand binding according to the Langmuir adsorption isotherm. (A) Fraction of maximal binding as a function of concentration of agonist. (B) Semilogarithmic form of curve shown in panel A.

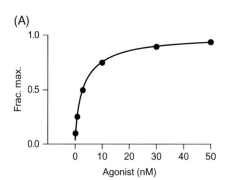

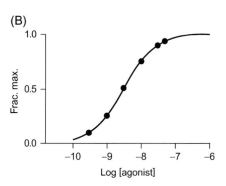

of a dose-response curve is the observed *in vivo* effect of a drug given as a dose to a whole animal or human. However, it has entered into the common pharmacological jargon as a general depiction of drug and effect. Thus, a dose-response curve for binding is actually a binding concentration curve, and an *in vitro* effect of an agonist in a receptor system is a *concentration-response curve*.

1.10 WHAT IS EFFICACY?

The property that gives a molecule the ability to change a receptor, such that it produces a cellular response, is termed *efficacy*. Early concepts of receptors likened them to locks and keys. As stated by Paul Ehrlich:

"Substances can only be anchored at any particular part of the organism if they fit into the molecule of the recipient complex like a piece of mosaic finds its place in a pattern."

This historically useful but inaccurate view of receptor function has in some ways hindered development models of efficacy. Specifically, the lock-and-key model implies a static system with no moving parts. However, one feature of proteins is their malleability. While they have structure, they do not have a single structure but rather many potential shapes referred to as *conformations*. A protein stays in a particular conformation because it is energetically favorable to do so (i.e., there is minimal free energy for that conformation). If thermal energy enters the system, the protein may adopt another shape in response. Stated by Lindstrom-Lang and Schellman [15]:

... a protein cannot be said to have "a" secondary structure but exists mainly as a group of structures not too different from one another in free energy ... In fact, the molecule must be conceived as trying every possible structure...
— Lindstrom and Schellman (1959)

Not only are a number of conformations for a given protein possible, but the protein samples these various conformations constantly. It is a dynamic and not a static entity. Receptor proteins can spontaneously change conformation in response to variations in the energy of the system. An important concept here is that small molecules, by interacting with the receptor protein, can bias the conformations that are sampled. It is in this way that drugs can produce active effects on receptor proteins (i.e., demonstrate efficacy). A thermodynamic mechanism by which this can occur is through what is known as *conformational selection* [16]. A simple illustration can be made by reducing the possible conformations of a given receptor protein to just two. These will be referred to as the "active" (denoted $[R_a]$) and "inactive" (denoted $[R_i]$) conformation.

Thermodynamically it would be expected that a ligand may not have identical affinity for both receptor conformations. This was an assumption in early formulations of conformational selection. For example,

differential affinity for protein conformations was proposed for oxygen binding to hemoglobin [17] and for choline derivatives and nicotinic receptors [18]. Furthermore, assume that these conformations exist in an equilibrium defined by an allosteric constant L (defined as $[R_a]/[R_i]$) and that a ligand [A] has affinity for both conformations defined by equilibrium association constants K_a and αK_a, respectively, for the inactive and active states:

$$R_i \xleftrightarrow{\text{ L }} R_a$$
$$\uparrow K_a \qquad \uparrow \alpha K_a \qquad (1.5)$$
$$A \qquad\qquad A$$

It can be shown that the ratio of the active species R_a in the presence of a saturating concentration (ρ_∞) of the ligand versus in the absence of the ligand (ρ_0) is given by the following (see Section 1.13):

$$\frac{\rho_\infty}{\rho_0} = \frac{\alpha(1+L)}{(1+\alpha L)}. \qquad (1.6)$$

It can be seen that if the factor α is unity (i.e., the affinity of the ligand for R_a and R_i is equal [$K_a = \alpha K_a$]), then there will be no change in the amount of R_a when the ligand is present. However, if α is not unity (i.e., if the affinity of the ligand differs for the two species), then the ratio necessarily will change when the ligand is present. Therefore, its differential affinity for the two protein species will alter their relative amounts. If the affinity of the ligand is higher for R_a, then the ratio will be >1 and the ligand will enrich the R_a species. If the affinity for the ligand for R_a is less than for R_i, then the ligand (by its presence in the system) will reduce the amount of R_a. For example, if the affinity of the ligand is 30-fold greater for the R_a state, then in a system where 16.7% of the receptors are spontaneously in the R_a state, the saturation of the receptors with this agonist will increase the amount of R_a by a factor of 5.14 (16.7 to 85%).

This concept is demonstrated schematically in Figure 1.14. It can be seen that the initial bias in a system of proteins containing two conformations (square and spherical) lies far toward the square conformation. When a ligand (filled circles) enters the system and selectively binds to the circular conformations, this binding process removes the circles driving the backward reaction from circles back to squares. In the absence of this backward pressure, more square conformations flow into the circular state to fill the gap. Overall, there is an enrichment of the circular conformations when unbound and ligand-bound circular conformations are totaled.

This also can be described in terms of the Gibbs free energy of the receptor-ligand system. Receptor conformations are adopted as a result of attainment of minimal free energy. Therefore, if the free energy of the collection of

FIGURE 1.14 Conformational selection as a thermodynamic process to bias mixtures of protein conformations. (A) The two forms of the protein are depicted as circular and square shapes. The system initially is predominantly square. Gaussian curves to the right show the relative frequency of occurrence of the two conformations. (B) As a ligand (blue dots) enters the system and prefers the circular conformations, these are selectively removed from the equilibrium between the two protein states. The distributions show the enrichment of the circular conformation at the expense of the square one. (C) A new equilibrium is attained in the presence of the ligand favoring the circular conformation because of the selective pressure of affinity between the ligand and this conformation. The distribution reflects the presence of the ligand and the enrichment of the circular conformation.

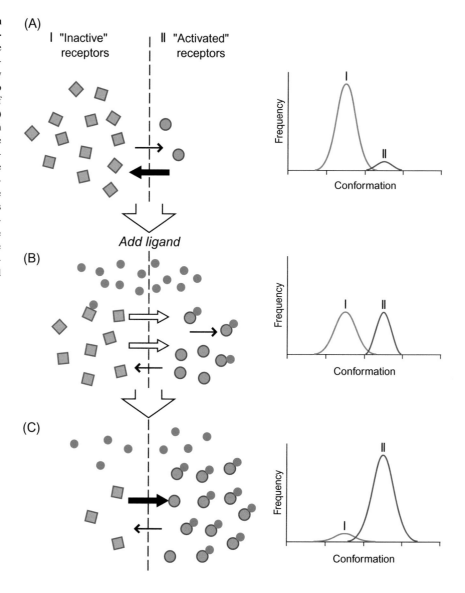

receptors changes, so too will the conformational makeup of the system. The free energy of a system composed of two conformations a_i and a_o is given by the following [19]:

$$\sum \Delta G_i = \sum \Delta G_i^0 - RT \times \sum \ln(1 + K_{a,i}[A])/\ln(1 + K_{a,0}[A]), \quad (1.7)$$

where $K_{a,i}$ and $K_{a,0}$ are the respective affinities of the ligand for states i and O. It can be seen that unless $K_{a,i} = K_{a,0}$ the logarithmic term will not equal zero and the free energy of the system will change $\left(\sum \Delta G_i \neq \sum \Delta G_i^0\right)$. Thus, if a ligand has differential affinity for either state, then the free energy of the system will change in the presence of the ligand. Under these circumstances, a different conformational bias will be formed by the differential affinity of the ligand. From these models comes the concept that binding is not a passive process whereby a ligand simply adheres to a protein without changing it. The act of binding can itself bias the behavior of the protein. This is the thermodynamic basis of efficacy.

1.11 DOSE-RESPONSE CURVES

The concept of "dose-response" in pharmacology has been known and discussed for some time. A prescription written in 1562 for hyoscyamus and opium for sleep clearly states, "If you want him to sleep less, give him less" [13]. It was recognized by one of the earliest physicians, Paracelsus (1493−1541), that it is only the dose that makes something beneficial or harmful: "All things are poison, and nothing is without poison. The Dosis alone makes a thing not poison."

Dose-response curves depict the response to an agonist in a cellular or subcellular system as a function of the agonist concentration. Specifically, they plot response as a function of the logarithm of the concentration. They can be defined completely by three parameters; namely, location along the concentration axis, slope, and maximal asymptote (Figure 1.15). At first glance, the shapes of dose-response curves appear to closely mimic the line predicted by the Langmuir adsorption isotherm, and it is tempting to assume that dose-response curves reflect the first-order binding and activation of receptors on the cell surface. However, in most cases this resemblance is happenstance, and dose-response curves reflect a far more complex amalgam of binding, activation, and recruitment of cellular elements of response. In the end, these may yield a sigmoidal curve but in reality they are far removed from the initial binding of drug and receptor. For example, in a cell culture with a collection of cells with varying thresholds for depolarization, the single-cell response to an agonist may be complete depolarization (in an all-or-none fashion). Taken as a complete collection, the depolarization profile of the culture where the cells all have differing thresholds for depolarization would have a Gaussian distribution of depolarization thresholds – some cells being more sensitive than others (Figure 1.16A). The relationship of depolarization of the complete culture to the concentration of a depolarizing agonist is the area under the Gaussian curve. This yields a sigmoidal dose-response curve (Figure 1.16B), which resembles the Langmuirian binding curve for drug-receptor binding. The slope of the latter curve reflects the molecularity of the drug-receptor interaction (i.e., one ligand binding to one receptor yields a slope of unity for the curve). In the case of the sequential depolarization of a collection of cells, it can be seen that a narrower range of depolarization thresholds yields a steeper dose-response curve, indicating that the actual numerical value of the slope for a dose-response curve cannot be equated to the molecularity of the binding between agonist and receptor. In general, shapes of dose-response curves are completely controlled by cellular factors and cannot be used to discern drug-receptor mechanisms. These must be determined indirectly by null methods.

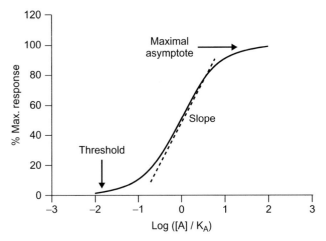

FIGURE 1.15 **Dose-response curves.** Any dose-response curve can be defined by the threshold (where response begins along the concentration axis), the slope (the rise in response with changes in concentration), and the maximal asymptote (the maximal response).

1.11.1 Potency and Maximal Response

There are certain features of agonist dose-response curves that are generally true for all agonists. The first is that the magnitude of the maximal asymptote is totally dependent on the efficacy of the agonist and the efficiency of the

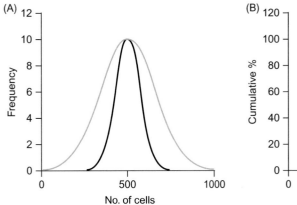
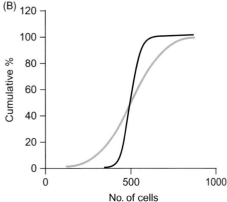

FIGURE 1.16 **Factors affecting the slope of dose-response curves.** (A) Gaussian distributions of the thresholds for depolarization of cells to an agonist in a cell culture. Solid line shows a narrow range of threshold, and the lighter line a wider range. (B) Area under the curve of the Gaussian distributions shown in panel A. These would represent the relative depolarization of the entire cell culture as a function of the concentration of agonist. The more narrow range of threshold values corresponds to the dose-response curve of steeper slope.

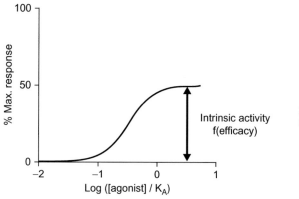

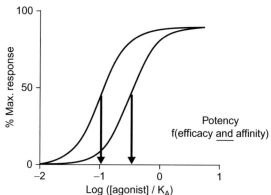

FIGURE 1.17 **Major attributes of agonist dose-response curves.** Maximal responses solely reflect efficacy, while the potency (location along the concentration axis) reflects a complex function of both efficacy and affinity.

biological system to convert receptor stimulus into tissue response (Figure 1.17A). This can be an extremely useful observation in the drug discovery process when attempting to affect the efficacy of a molecule. Changes in chemical structure that affect only the affinity of the agonist will have no effect on the maximal asymptote of the dose-response curve for that agonist. Therefore, if chemists wish to optimize or minimize efficacy in a molecule they can track the maximal response to do so. Second, the location, along the concentration axis of dose-response curves, quantifies the *potency* of the agonist (Figure 1.17B). The potency is the molar concentration required to produce a given response. Potencies vary with the type of cellular system used to make the measurement and the level of response at which the measurement is made. A common measurement used to quantify potency is the EC_{50}; namely, the molar concentration of an agonist required to produce 50% of the maximal response to the agonist. Thus, an EC_{50} value of $1\,\mu M$ indicates that 50% of the maximal response to the agonist is produced by a concentration of $1\,\mu M$ of the agonist (Figure 1.18). If the agonist produces a maximal response of 80% of the system maximal response, then 40% of the system maximal response will be produced by $1\,\mu M$ of this agonist (Figure 1.18). Similarly, an EC_{25} will be produced by a lower concentration of this same agonist; in this case, the EC_{25} is $0.5\,\mu M$.

1.11.2 p-Scales and the Representation of Potency

Agonist potency is an extremely important parameter in drug-receptor pharmacology. Invariably it is determined from log-dose-response curves. It should be noted that since these curves are generated from semilogarithmic plots, the location parameter of these curves are *log normally distributed*. This means that the *logarithms* of the sensitivities (EC_{50}) and *not* the EC_{50} values themselves are normally distributed (Figure 1.19A). Since all

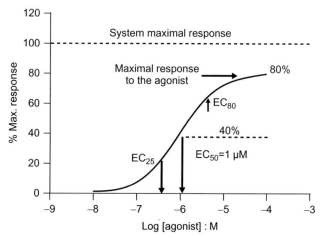

FIGURE 1.18 **Dose-response curves.** Dose-response curve to an agonist that produces 80% of the system maximal response. The EC_{50} (concentration producing 40% response) is $1\,\mu M$, the EC_{25} (20%) is $0.5\,\mu M$, and the EC_{80} (64%) is $5\,\mu M$.

statistical parametric tests must be done on data that come from normal distributions, all statistics (including comparisons of potency and estimates of errors of potency) must come from logarithmically expressed potency data. When log normally distributed EC_{50} data (Figure 1.19B) are converted to EC50 data, the resulting distribution is seriously skewed (Figure 1.19C). It can be seen that error limits on the mean of such a distribution are not equal (i.e., one standard error of the mean unit [see Chapter 12] either side of the mean gives different values on the skewed distribution [Figure 1.19C]). This is not true of the symmetrical normal distribution (Figure 1.19B).

One representation of numbers such as potency estimates is with the p-scale. The p-scale is the negative logarithm of number. For example, the pH is the negative logarithm of a hydrogen ion concentration (10^5 molar $=$ pH $= 5$). It is essential to express dose-response parameters as p-values ($-$ log of the value, as in the pEC_{50})

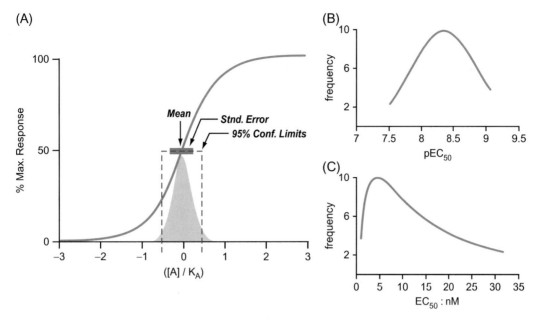

FIGURE 1.19 Log normal distributions of sensitivity of a pharmacological preparation to an agonist. (A) Dose-response curve showing the distribution of the EC_{50} values along the log concentration axis. This distribution is normal only on a log scale. (B) Log normal distribution of pEC_{50} values ($-\log EC_{50}$ values). (C) Skewed distribution of EC_{50} values converted from the pEC_{50} values shown in panel B.

TABLE 1.2 Expressing Mean Agonist Potencies with Error

pEC_{50}[1]	EC_{50} (nM)[2]
8.5	3.16
8.7	2
8.3	5.01
8.2	6.31
8.6	2.51
Mean = 8.46	Mean = 3.8
SE = 0.21	SE = 1.81

[1] Replicate values of $-1/Nlog\ EC_{50}$'s.
[2] Replicate EC_{50} values in nM.

since these are log normal. However, it sometimes is useful on an intuitive level to express potency as a concentration (i.e., the antilog value). One way this can be done and still preserve the error estimate is to make the calculation as p-values and then convert to concentration as the last step. For example, Table 1.2 shows five pEC_{50} values, giving a mean pEC_{50} of 8.46 and a standard error of 0.21. It can be seen that the calculation of the mean as a converted concentration (EC_{50} value) leads to an apparently reasonable mean value of 3.8 nM, with a standard error of 1.81 nM. However, the 95% confidence limits (range of values that will include the true value) of the concentration value is meaningless, in that one of them

(the lower limit) is a negative number. The true value of the EC_{50} lies within the 95% confidence limits given by the mean + 2.57 × the standard error, which leads to the values 8.4 nM and −0.85 nM. However, when pEC_{50} values are used for the calculations this does not occur. Specifically, the mean of 8.46 yields a mean EC_{50} of 3.47 nM. The 95% confidence limits on the pEC_{50} are 7.8 to 9.0. Conversion of these limits to EC_{50} values yields 95% confidence limits of 1 nM to 11.8 nM. Thus, the true potency lies between the values of 1 and 11.8 nM 95% of the time.

1.12 CHAPTER SUMMARY AND CONCLUSIONS

- Some ideas on the origins and relevance of pharmacology and the concept of biological "receptors" are discussed.
- Currently there are drugs for only a fraction of the druggable targets present in the human genome.
- While recombinant systems have greatly improved the drug discovery process, pathological phenotypes still are a step away from these drug testing systems.
- Because of the fact that drugs are tested in experimental, not therapeutic, systems, system-independent measures of drug activity (namely, affinity and efficacy) must be measured in drug discovery.
- Affinity is the strength of binding of a drug to a receptor. It is quantified by an equilibrium dissociation constant.
- Affinity can be depicted and quantified with the Langmuir adsorption isotherm.

- Efficacy is measured in relative terms (having no absolute scale) and quantifies the ability of a molecule to produce a change in the receptor (most often leading to a physiological response).
- Dose-response curves quantify drug activity. The maximal asymptote is totally dependent on efficacy, while potency is due to an amalgam of affinity and efficacy.
- Measures of potency are log normally distributed. Only p-scale values (i.e., pEC_{50}) should be used for statistical tests.

1.13 DERIVATIONS: CONFORMATIONAL SELECTION AS A MECHANISM OF EFFICACY

Consider a system containing two receptor conformations R_i and R_a that coexist in the system according to an allosteric constant denoted L:

$$R_i \underset{}{\overset{L}{\longleftrightarrow}} R_a$$
$$\uparrow K_a \qquad \uparrow \alpha K_a$$
$$A \qquad\qquad A$$

Assume that ligand A binds to R_i with an equilibrium association constant K_a, and R_a by an equilibrium association constant αK_a. The factor α denotes the differential affinity of the agonist for R_a (i.e., $\alpha = 10$ denotes a 10-fold greater affinity of the ligand for the R_a state). The effect of α on the ability of the ligand to alter the equilibrium between R_i and R_a can be calculated by examining the amount of R_a species (both as R_a and AR_a) present in the system in the absence of ligand and in the presence of ligand. The equilibrium expression for $[R_a] + [AR_a]/[R_{tot}]$, where $[R_{tot}]$ is the total receptor concentration given by the conservation equation $[R_{tot}] = [R_i] + [AR_i] + [R_a] + [AR_a]$), is:

$$\rho = \frac{L(1 + \alpha[A]/K_A)}{[A]/K_A(1 + \alpha L) + 1 + L}, \qquad (1.8)$$

where L is the allosteric constant, [A] is the concentration of ligand, K_A is the equilibrium dissociation constant of the agonist-receptor complex ($K_A = 1/K_a$), and α is the differential affinity of the ligand for the R_a state. It can be seen that in the absence of agonist ([A] = 0), $\rho_0 = L/(1 + L)$, and in the presence of a maximal concentration of ligand (saturating the receptors; [A] → ∞), $\rho_\infty = (\alpha(1 + L))/(1 + \alpha L)$. The effect of the ligand on changing the proportion of the R_a state is given by the ratio ρ/ρ_0. This ratio is given by

$$\frac{\rho_\infty}{\rho_0} = \frac{\alpha(1 + L)}{(1 + \alpha L)}. \qquad (1.9)$$

Equation 1.9 indicates that if the ligand has an equal affinity for both the R_i and R_a states ($\alpha = 1$) then ρ_∞/ρ_0 will equal unity and no change in the proportion of R_a will result from maximal ligand binding. However, if $\alpha > 1$, then the presence of the conformationally selective ligand will cause the ratio ρ_∞/ρ_0 to be >1 and the R_a state will be enriched by presence of the ligand.

REFERENCES

[1] Maehle A-H, Prull C-R, Halliwell RF. The emergence of the drug-receptor theory. Nature Rev Drug Disc 2002;1:1637–42.
[2] Paton WDM. On becoming a pharmacologist. Ann Rev Pharmacol and Toxicol 1986;26:1–22.
[3] Drews J. Drug discovery: a historical perspective. Science 2000;287:1960–4.
[4] Clark AJ. The mode of action of drugs on cells. London: Edward Arnold; 1933.
[5] Clark AJ. General pharmacology. In: Heffter A, editor. Handbuch der Experimentellen Pharmakologie, 4. Berlin: Springer; 1937. p. 165–76. Ergansungsweerk band.
[6] Holmstedt B, Liljestrand G. Readings in pharmacology. New York: Raven Press; 1981.
[7] Marchese A, George SR, Kolakowski LF, Lynch KR, O'Dowd BF. Novel GPCRs and their endogenous ligands: expanding the boundaries of physiology and pharmacology. Trends Pharmacol Sci 1999;20:370–5.
[8] Venter JC, Adams MD, Myers EW, Li PW, Mural RJ, Sutton GG, et al. The sequence of the human genome. Science 2001;291:1304–51.
[9] Link R, Daunt D, Barsh G, Chruscinski A, Kobilka B. Cloning of two mouse genes encoding α_2-adrenergic receptor subtypes and identification of a single amino acid in the mouse α_2-C10 homolog responsible for an interspecies variation in antagonist binding. Mol Pharmacol 1992;42:16–7.
[10] Black JW. A personal view of pharmacology. Ann Rev Pharmacol Toxicol 1996;36:1–33.
[11] Buscher R, Hermann V, Insel PA. Human adrenoceptor polymorphisms: evolving recognition of clinical importance. Trends Pharmacol Sci 1999;20:94–9.
[12] Stephenson RP. A modification of receptor theory. Br J Pharmacol 1956;11:379–93.
[13] Norton S. Origins of pharmacology. Mol Interventions 2005;5:144–9.
[14] Leff P, Martin GR, Morse JM. Differences in agonist dissociation constant estimates for 5-HT at 5-HT2-receptors: a problem of acute desensitization?. Br J Pharmacol 1986;89:493–9.
[15] Linderstrom-Lang A, Schellman P. Protein conformation. Enzymes 1959;1:443–71.
[16] Burgen ASV. Conformational changes and drug action. Fed Proc 1966;40:2723–8.
[17] Wyman JJ, Allen DW. The problem of the haem interaction in haemoglobin and the basis for the Bohr effect. J Polymer Sci 1951;7:499–518.
[18] Del Castillo J, Katz B. Interaction at end-plate receptors between different choline derivatives. Proc Roy Soc Lond B 1957;146:369–81.
[19] Freire E. Can allosteric regulation be predicted from structure? Proc Natl Acad Sci USA 2000;97:11680–2.

Chapter 2

How Different Tissues Process Drug Response

[Nature] can refuse to speak but she cannot give a wrong answer.

— Dr. Charles Brenton Hugins (1966)

We have to remember that what we observe is not nature in itself, but nature exposed to our method of questioning...

— Werner Heisenberg (1901–1976)

2.1 Drug Response as Seen Through the "Cellular Veil"
2.2 The Biochemical Nature of Stimulus-Response Cascades
2.3 The Mathematical Approximation of Stimulus-Response Mechanisms
2.4 System Effects On Agonist Response: Full and Partial Agonists
2.5 Differential Cellular Response to Receptor Stimulus
2.6 Receptor Desensitization and Tachyphylaxis
2.7 The Measurement of Drug Activity
2.8 Advantages and Disadvantages of Different Assay Formats
2.9 Drug Concentration as an Independent Variable
2.10 Chapter Summary and Conclusions
2.11 Derivations
References

2.1 DRUG RESPONSE AS SEEN THROUGH THE "CELLULAR VEIL"

If a drug possesses the molecular property of efficacy, then it produces a change in the receptor that may be detected by the cell. However, this can occur only if the stimulus is of sufficient strength and the cell has the amplification machinery necessary to convert the stimulus into an observable response. In this sense, the cellular host system completely controls what the experimenter observes regarding the events taking place at the drug receptor. Drug activity is thus revealed through a "cellular veil" that can, in many cases, obscure or substantially modify drug-receptor activity (Figure 2.1). Minute signals, initiated either at the cell surface or within the cytoplasm of the cell, are interpreted, transformed, amplified, and otherwise altered by the cell to tailor that signal to its own particular needs. In receptor systems where a drug does produce a response, the relationship between the binding reaction (drug + receptor protein) and the observed response can be studied indirectly through observation of the cellular response as a function of drug concentration (dose-response curve). A general phenomenon observed experimentally is that the cellular response most often is not linearly related to receptor occupancy (i.e., it does not require 100% occupation of all of the receptors to produce the maximal cellular response). Figure 2.2A shows a functional dose-response curve for human calcitonin in human embryonic kidney (HEK) cells transfected with cDNA for human calcitonin receptor type 2. The response being measured here is hydrogen ion release by the cells, a sensitive measure of cellular metabolism. Also shown (dotted line) is a curve for calcitonin binding to the receptors (as measured with radioligand binding). A striking feature of these curves is that the curve for function is shifted considerably to the left of

T. P. Kenakin: A Pharmacology Primer, Fourth edition. DOI: http://dx.doi.org/10.1016/B978-0-12-407663-1.00002-8
© 2014 Elsevier Inc. All rights reserved.

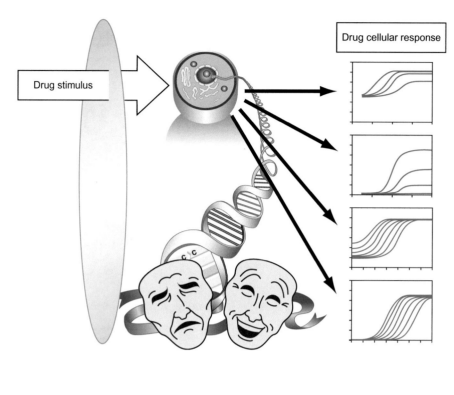

FIGURE 2.1 The cellular veil. Drugs act on biological receptors in cells to change cellular activity. The initial receptor stimulus usually alters a complicated system of interconnected metabolic biochemical reactions, and the outcome of the drug effect is modified by the extent of these interconnections, the basal state of the cell, and the threshold sensitivity of the various processes involved. This can lead to a variety of apparently different effects for the same drug in different cells. Receptor pharmacology strives to identify the basic mechanism initiating these complex events.

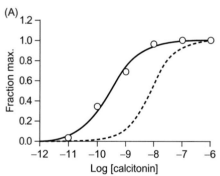

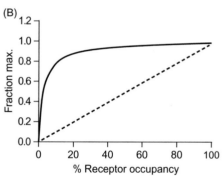

FIGURE 2.2 Binding and dose-response curves for human calcitonin on human calcitonin receptors type 2. (A) Dose-response curves for microphysiometry responses to human calcitonin in HEK cells (open circles) and binding in membranes from HEK cells (displacement of [^{125}I]-human calcitonin). Data from [1]. (B) Regression of microphysiometry responses to human calcitonin (ordinates) upon human calcitonin fractional receptor occupancy (abscissae). Dotted line shows a direct correlation between receptor occupancy and cellular response.

the binding curve. Calculation of the receptor occupancy required for 50% maximal tissue response indicates that less than 50% occupancy, namely, more on the order of 3 to 4%, is needed. In fact, a regression of tissue response upon the receptor occupancy is hyperbolic in nature (Figure 2.2B), showing a skewed relationship between receptor occupancy and cellular response. This skewed relationship indicates that the stimulation of the receptor initiated by binding is amplified by the cell in the process of response production.

The ability of a given agonist to produce a maximal system response can be quantified as a *receptor reserve*.

The reserve refers to the percentage of receptors not required for production of maximal response (sometimes referred to as *spare receptors*). For example, a receptor reserve of 80% for an agonist means that the system maximal response is produced by activation of 20% of the receptor population by that agonist. Receptor reserves can be quite striking. Figure 2.3 shows guinea pig ileal smooth muscle contractions to the agonist histamine before and after irreversible inactivation of a large fraction of the receptors with the protein alkylating agent phenoxybenzamine. The fact that the depressed maximum dose-response curve is observed so far to the right of the

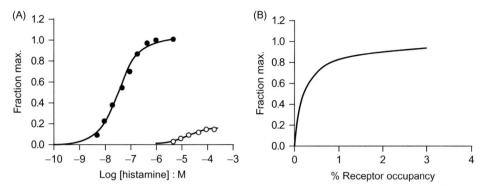

FIGURE 2.3 **Guinea pig ileal responses to histamine.** (A) Contraction of guinea pig ileal longitudinal smooth muscle (ordinates as a percentage of maximum) to histamine (abscissae, logarithmic scale). Responses obtained before (filled circles) and after treatment with the irreversible histamine receptor antagonist phenoxybenzamine (50 μM for 3 minutes; open circles). (B) Occupancy-response curve for data shown in (A). Ordinates are percentage of maximal response. Abscissae are calculated receptor occupancy values from an estimated affinity of 20 μM for histamine. Note that maximal response is essentially observed after only 2% receptor occupancy by the agonist (i.e., a 98% receptor reserve for this agonist in this system). Data redrawn from [2].

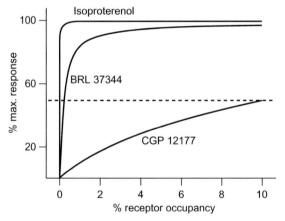

FIGURE 2.4 **Occupancy-response curves for β-adrenoceptor agonists in transfected CHO cells.** Occupancy (abscissae) calculated from binding affinity measured by displacement of [^{125}I]-iodocyanopindolol. Response measured as increases in cyclic AMP. Drawn from [3].

control dose-response curve indicates a receptor reserve of 98% (i.e., only 2% of the receptors must be activated by histamine to produce the tissue's maximal response [Figure 2.3B]). In teleological terms, this may be useful, since it allows neurotransmitters to produce rapid activation of organs with minimal receptor occupancy leading to optimal and rapid control of function.

Receptor reserve is a property of the tissue (i.e., the strength of amplification of receptor stimulus inherent to the cells) *and* it is a property of the agonist (i.e., how much stimulus is imparted to the system by a given agonist receptor occupancy). This latter factor is quantified as the efficacy of the agonist. A high-efficacy agonist need occupy a smaller fraction of the receptor population than a lower-efficacy agonist to produce a comparable stimulus. Therefore, it is incorrect to ascribe a given tissue or

cellular response system with a characteristic receptor reserve. The actual value of the receptor reserve will be unique to each agonist in that system. For example, Figure 2.4 shows the different amplification hyperbolae of Chinese hamster ovary (CHO) cells transfected with β-adrenoceptors in producing cyclic AMP responses to three different β-adrenoceptor agonists. It can be seen that isoproterenol requires many times less receptors to produce 50% response than do both the agonists BRL 37344 and CGP 12177. This underscores the idea that the magnitude of receptor reserves is very much dependent on the efficacy of the agonist (i.e., one agonist's spare receptor is another agonist's essential one).

2.2 THE BIOCHEMICAL NATURE OF STIMULUS-RESPONSE CASCADES

Cellular amplification of receptor signals occurs through a succession of saturable biochemical reactions. Different receptors are coupled to different stimulus-response mechanisms in the cell. Each has its own function and operates on its own timescale. For example, receptor tyrosine kinases (activated by growth factors) phosphorylate target proteins on tyrosine residues to activate protein phosphorylation cascades such as MAP kinase pathways. This process, on a timescale on the order of seconds to days, leads to protein synthesis from gene transcription with resulting cell differentiation and/or cell proliferation. Nuclear receptors, activated by steroids, operate on a timescale of minutes to days and mediate gene transcription and protein synthesis. This leads to homeostatic, metabolic, and immunosuppression effects. Ligand gated ion channels, activated by neurotransmitters, operate on the order of milliseconds to increase the permeability of

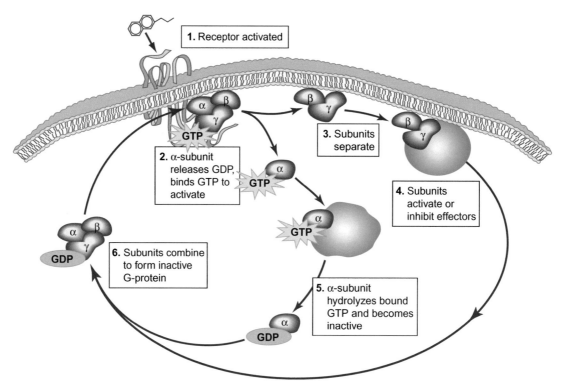

FIGURE 2.5 Activation of trimeric G-proteins by activated receptors. An agonist produces a receptor active state that goes on to interact with the G-protein. A conformational change in the G-protein causes bound GDP to exchange with GTP. This triggers dissociation of the G-protein complex into α- and βγ-subunits. These go on to interact with effectors such as adenylate cyclase and calcium channels. The intrinsic GTPase activity of the α-subunit hydrolyzes bound GTP back to GDP, and the inactived α-subunit reassociates with the βγ-subunits to repeat the cycle.

plasma membranes to ions. This leads to increases in cytosolic Ca^{2+}, depolarization, or hyperpolarization of cells. This in turn results in muscle contraction, release of neurotransmitters, or inhibition of these processes.

G-protein-coupled receptors (GPCRs) react with a wide variety of molecules, from small ones such as acetylcholine, to some as large as the protein SDF-1α. Operating on a timescale of minutes to hours, these receptors mediate a plethora of cellular processes. A common reaction in the activation cascade for GPCRs is the binding of the activated receptor to a trimeric complex of proteins called *G-proteins* (Figure 2.5). These proteins — composed of three subunits named α, β, and γ — act as molecular switches for a number of other effectors in the cell. The binding of activated receptors to the G-protein initiates the dissociation of GDP from the α-subunit of the G-protein complex, the binding of GTP, and the dissociation of the complex into α- and βγ-subunits. The separated subunits of the G-protein can activate effectors in the cell such as adenylate cyclase and ion channels. Amplification can occur at these early stages if one receptor activates more than one G-protein. The α-subunit also is a GTPase, which hydrolyzes the bound GTP to produce its own deactivation. This terminates the action of the α-subunit on the effector. It can be seen that the length of

time for which the α-subunit is active can control the amount of stimulus given to the effector, and that this also can be a means of amplification (i.e., one α-subunit could activate many effectors). The α- and βγ-subunits then reassociate to complete the regulatory cycle (Figure 2.5). Such receptor-mediated reactions generate cellular molecules called *second messengers*. These molecules go on to activate or inhibit other components of the cellular machinery to change cellular metabolism and state of activation. For example, the second messenger (cyclic AMP) is generated by the enzyme adenylate cyclase from ATP. This second messenger furnishes fuel, through protein kinases, for the phosphorylation of serine and threonine residues on a number of proteins such as other protein kinases, receptors, metabolic enzymes, ion channels, and transcription factors (see Figure 2.6). Activation of other G-proteins leads to the activation of phospholipase C. These enzymes catalyze the hydrolysis of phosphatidylinositol 4.5-bisphosphate (PIP2) to 1,2 diacylglycerol (DAG) and inositol 1,4,5-triphosphate (IP3) (see Figure 2.7). This latter second messenger interacts with receptors on intracellular calcium stores, resulting in the release of calcium into the cytosol. This calcium binds to calcium sensor proteins such as calmodulin or troponin C, which then go on to regulate the

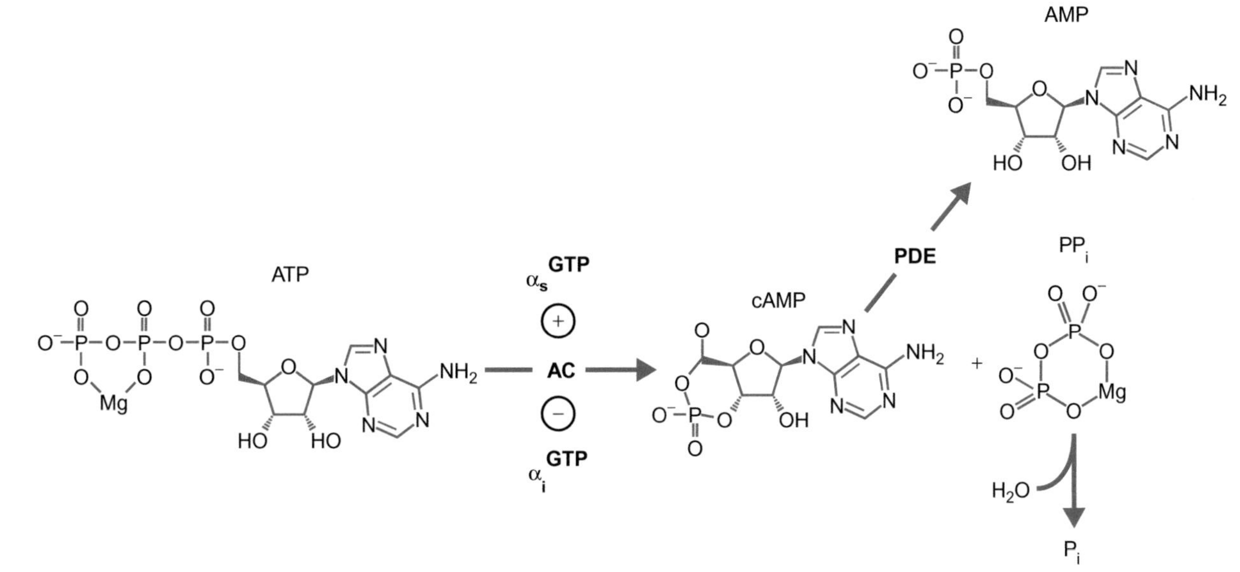

FIGURE 2.6 **Production of cyclic AMP from ATP by the enzyme adenylate cyclase.** Cyclic AMP is a ubiquitous second messenger in cells activating numerous cellular pathways. The adenylate cyclase is activated by the α-subunit of G_s-protein and inhibited by the α-subunit of G_i-protein. Cyclic AMP is degraded by phosphodiesterases in the cell.

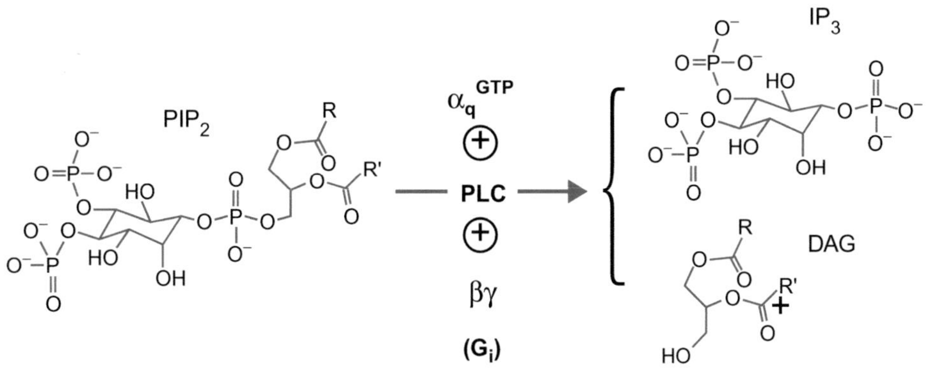

FIGURE 2.7 Production of second messengers inositol 1,4,5-triphosphate (IP$_3$) and diacylglycerol (DAG) through activation of the enzyme phospholipase C. This enzyme is activated by the α-subunit of G_q-protein and also by $\beta\gamma$-subunits of G_i-protein. IP$_3$ stimulates the release of Ca^2 from intracellular stores, while DAG is a potent activator of protein kinase C.

activity of proteins such as protein kinases, phosphatases, phosphodiesterase, nitric oxide synthase, ion channels, and adenylate cyclase. The second messenger DAG diffuses in the plane of the membrane to activate protein kinase C isoforms, which phosphorylate protein kinases, transcription factors, ion channels, and receptors. DAG also functions as a source of arachidonic acid, which goes on to be the source of eicosanoid mediators such as prostanoids and leukotrienes. In general, all these processes can lead to a case where a relatively small amount of receptor stimulation can result in a large biochemical signal. An example of a complete stimulus-response cascade for the β-adrenoceptor production of blood glucose is shown in Figure 2.8.

There are numerous second messenger systems such as those utilizing cyclic AMP and cyclic GMP, calcium and calmodulin, phosphoinositides, and diacylglycerol with accompanying modulatory mechanisms. Each receptor is coupled to these in a variety of ways in different cell types.

Therefore, it can be seen that it is impractical to attempt to quantitatively define each stimulus-response mechanism for each receptor system. Fortunately, this is not an important prerequisite in the pharmacological process of classifying agonists, since these complex mechanisms can be approximated by simple mathematical functions.

2.3 THE MATHEMATICAL APPROXIMATION OF STIMULUS-RESPONSE MECHANISMS

Each of the processes shown in Figure 2.8 can be described by a Michaelis–Menten type of biochemical reaction, a standard generalized mathematical equation describing the interaction of a substrate with an enzyme. Michaelis and Menten realized in 1913 that the kinetics of enzyme reactions differed from those of conventional chemical reactions. They visualized the reaction of

FIGURE 2.8 **Stimulus-response cascade for the production of blood glucose by activation of β-adrenoceptors.** Redrawn from [4].

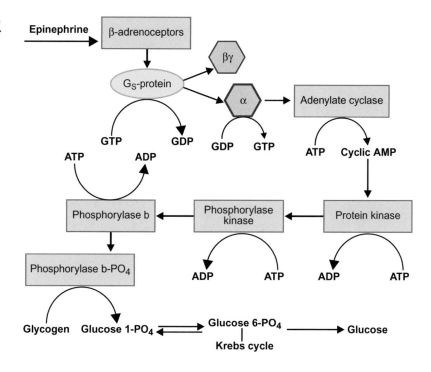

substrate and an enzyme yielding enzyme plus product as a form of this equation: reaction velocity = (maximal velocity of the reaction × substrate concentration)/(concentration of substrate + a fitting constant K_m). The constant K_m (referred to as the Michaelis–Menten constant) characterizes the tightness of the binding of the reaction between substrate and enzyme, essentially a quantification of the coupling efficiency of the reaction. K_m is the concentration at which the reaction is half the maximal value or, in terms of kinetics, the concentration at which the reaction runs at half its maximal rate. This model forms the basis of enzymatic biochemical reactions and can be used as a mathematical approximation of such functions.

As with the Langmuir adsorption isotherm, which in shape closely resembles Michaelis–Menten-type biochemical kinetics, the two notable features of such reactions are the location parameter of the curve along the concentration axis (the value of K_m or the magnitude of the coupling efficiency factor) and the maximal rate of the reaction (V_{max}). In generic terms, Michaelis–Menten reactions can be written in the form:

$$\text{Velocity} = \frac{[\text{substract}] \cdot V_{max}}{[\text{substract}] + K_m} = \frac{[\text{input}] \cdot \text{MAX}}{[\text{input}] + \beta} \quad (2.1)$$

where β is a generic coupling efficiency factor. It can be seen that the velocity of the reaction is inversely proportional to the magnitude of β (i.e., the lower the value of β the more efficiently is the reaction coupled). If it is assumed that the stimulus-response cascade of any given cell is a series succession of such reactions, there are two general features of the resultant that can be predicted mathematically. The first is that the resultant of the total

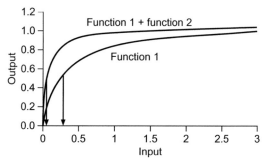

FIGURE 2.9 **Amplification of stimulus through successive rectangular hyperbolae.** The output from the first function ($\beta = 0.3$) becomes the input of a second function with the same coupling efficiency ($\beta = 0.3$), to yield a more efficiently coupled overall function ($\beta = 0.069$). Arrows indicate the potency for input to yield 50% maximal output for the first function and the series functions.

series of reactions will itself be of the form of the same hyperbolic shape (see Section 2.11.1). The second is that the location parameter along the input axis (magnitude of the coupling efficiency parameter) will reflect a general amplification of any single reaction within the cascade (i.e., the magnitude of the coupling parameter for the complete series will be lower than the coupling parameter of any single reaction; see Figure 2.9). The magnitude of β_{total} for the series sum of two reactions (characterized by β_1 and β_2) is given by (see Section 2.11.2):

$$\beta_{total} = \frac{\beta_1 \beta_2}{1 + \beta_2}. \quad (2.2)$$

It can be seen from Equation 2.2 that for positive nonzero values of β_2, $\beta_{total} < \beta_1$. Therefore, the location

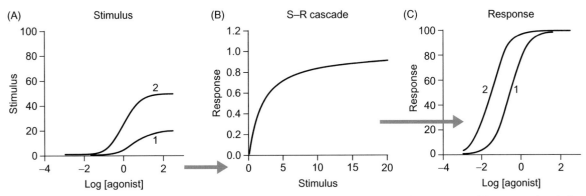

FIGURE 2.10 **The monotonic nature of stimulus-response mechanisms.** (A) Receptor stimulus generated by two agonists designated 1 and 2 as a function of agonist concentration. (B) Rectangular hyperbola characterizing the transformation of receptor stimulus (abscissae) into cellular response (ordinates) for the tissue. (C) The resulting relationship between tissue response to the agonists as a function of agonist concentration. The general rank order of activity (2 > 1) is preserved in the response as a reflection of the monotonic nature of the stimulus-response hyperbola.

parameter of the rectangular hyperbola of the composite set of reactions in series is shifted to the left (increased potency) of that for the first reaction in the sequence (i.e., there is amplification inherent in the series of reactions).

The fact that the total stimulus-response chain can be approximated by a single rectangular hyperbola furnishes the basis of using an end organ response to quantify an agonist effect in a non-system-dependent manner. An important feature of such a relationship is that it is monotonic (i.e., there is only one value of y for each value of x). Therefore, the relationship between the strength of signal imparted to the receptor between two agonists is accurately reflected by the end organ response (Figure 2.10). This is the primary reason that pharmacologists can circumvent the effects of the cellular veil and discern system-independent receptor events from translated cellular events.

2.4 SYSTEM EFFECTS ON AGONIST RESPONSE: FULL AND PARTIAL AGONISTS

For any given receptor type, different cellular hosts should have characteristic efficiencies of coupling, and these should characterize all agonists for that same receptor irrespective of the magnitude of the efficacy of the agonists. Different cellular backgrounds have different capabilities for amplification of receptor stimuli. This is illustrated by the strikingly different magnitudes of the receptor reserves for calcitonin and histamine receptors shown in Figures 2.2 and 2.3. Figure 2.11 shows the response produced by human calcitonin activation of the human calcitonin receptor type 2 when it is expressed in three different cell formats (human embryonic kidney cells [HEK 293 cells], Chinese hamster ovary cells [CHO cells], and *Xenopus laevis* melanophores). From this figure it can be seen that, while only 3% receptor activation by this agonist is required for 50% response in

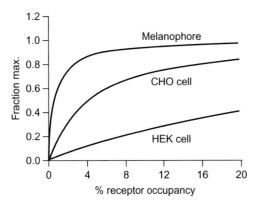

FIGURE 2.11 **Receptor occupancy curves for activation of human calcitonin type 2 receptors by the agonist human calcitonin.** Ordinates: response as a fraction of the maximal response to human calcitonin. Abscissae: fractional receptor occupancy by human calcitonin. Curves shown for receptors transfected into three cell types: human embryonic kidney cells (HEK), Chinese hamster ovary cells (CHO), and *Xenopus laevis* melanophores. It can be seen that the different cell types lead to differing amplification factors for the conversion from agonist receptor occupancy to tissue response.

melanophores, this same occupancy in CHO cells produces only 10% response and even less in HEK cells.

One operational view of differing efficiencies of receptor coupling is to consider the efficacy of a given agonist as a certain mass characteristic of the agonist. If this mass were to be placed on one end of a balance, it would depress that end by an amount dependent on the weight. The amount that the end is depressed would be the stimulus (see Figure 2.12). Consider the other end of the scale as reflecting the placement of the weight on the scale (i.e., the displacement of the other end is the response of the cell). The point along the arm at which this displacement is viewed reflects the relative amplification of the original stimulus (i.e., the closer to the fulcrum, the less the amplification). Therefore, different

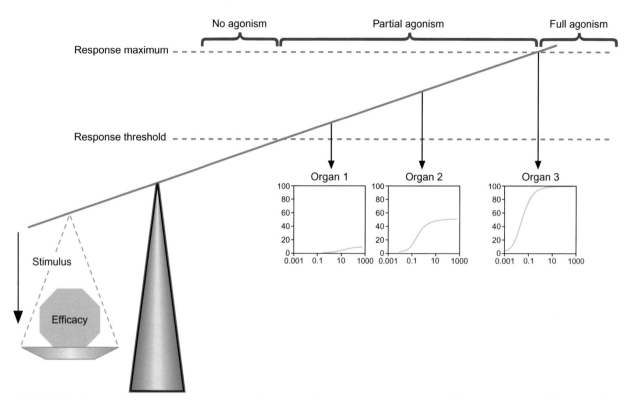

FIGURE 2.12 Depiction of agonist efficacy as a weight placed on a balance to produce displacement of the arm (stimulus) and the observation of the displacement of the other end of the arm as tissue response. The vantage point determines the amplitude of the displacement. Where no displacement is observed, no agonism is seen. Where the displacement is between the limits of travel of the arm (threshold and maximum), partial agonism is seen. Where displacement goes beyond the maximal limit of travel of the arm, uniform full agonism is observed.

vantage points along the displaced end of the balance arm reflect different tissues with different amplification factors (different magnitudes of coupling parameters). The response features of cells have limits (i.e., a threshold for detecting the response and a maximal response characteristic of the tissue). Depending on the efficiency of stimulus-response coupling apparatus of the cell, a given agonist could produce no response, a partially maximal response, or the system maximal response (see Figure 2.12). The observed response to a given drug gives a label to the drug in that system. Thus, a drug that binds to the receptor but produces no response is an *antagonist*, a drug that produces a submaximal response is a *partial agonist*, and a drug that produces the tissue maximal response is termed a *full agonist* (see Figure 2.13). It should be noted that while these labels often are given to a drug and used across different systems as identifying labels for the drug, they are in fact dependent on the system. Therefore, the magnitude of the response can completely change with changes in the coupling efficiency of the system. For example, the low-efficacy β-adrenoceptor agonist prenalterol can be an antagonist in guinea pig extensor digitorum longus muscle, a partial agonist in guinea pig left atria, and nearly a full agonist in right atria from thyroxine-treated guinea pigs (Figure 2.14).

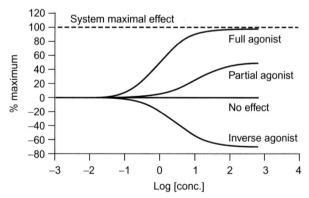

FIGURE 2.13 **The expression of different types of drug activities in cells.** A drug that produces the full maximal response of the biological system is termed a *full agonist*. A drug that produces a submaximal response is a *partial agonist*. Drugs also may produce no overt response or may actively reduce basal response. This latter class of drug is known as an *inverse agonist*. These ligands have negative efficacy. This is discussed specifically in Chapter 3.

As noted previously, the efficacy of the agonist determines the magnitude of the initial stimulus given to the receptor, and therefore the starting point for the input into the stimulus-response cascade. As agonists are tested in systems of varying coupling efficiency, it will be seen

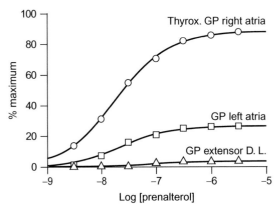

FIGURE 2.14 Dose-response curves to the β-adrenoceptor low-efficacy agonist prenalterol in three different tissues from guinea pigs. Responses all mediated by β₁-adrenoceptors. Depending on the tissue, this drug can function as nearly a full agonist, a partial agonist, or a full antagonist. Redrawn from [5].

that the point at which system saturation of the stimulus-response cascade is reached differs for different agonists. Figure 2.15 shows two agonists, one of higher efficacy than the other. It can be seen that both are partial agonists in tissue A but that agonist 2 saturates the maximal response producing capabilities of tissue B and is a full agonist. The same is not true for agonist 1. In a yet more efficiently coupled system (tissue C), both agonists are full agonists. This illustrates the obvious error in assuming that all agonists that produce the system maximal response have equal efficacy. All full agonists in a given system may not have equal efficacy.

The more efficiently coupled is a given system, the more likely that agonists will produce the system maximum response (i.e., be full agonists). It can also be shown that if an agonist saturates any biochemical reaction within the stimulus-response cascade, it will produce full

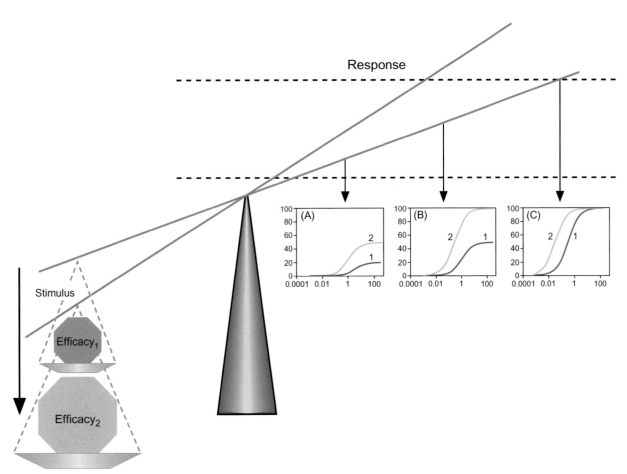

FIGURE 2.15 Depiction of agonist efficacy as a weight placed on a balance to produce displacement of the arm (stimulus) and the observation of the displacement of the other end of the arm as tissue response for two agonists, one of higher efficacy (Efficacy₂) than the other (Efficacy₁). The vantage point determines the amplitude of the displacement. In system A, both agonists are partial agonists. In system B, agonist 2 is a full agonist and agonist 1 a partial agonist. In system C, both are full agonists. It can be seen that the tissue determines the extent of agonism observed for both agonists and that system C does not differentiate the two agonists on the basis of efficacy.

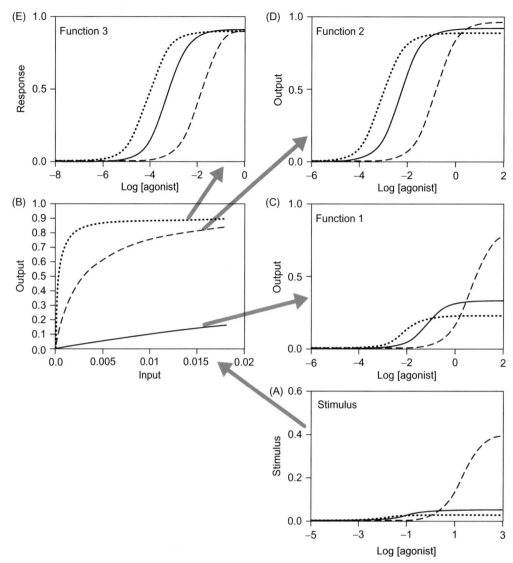

FIGURE 2.16 **Effects of successive rectangular hyperbolae on receptor stimulus.** (A) Stimulus to three agonists. (B) Three rectangular hyperbolic stimulus-response functions in series. Function 1 ($\beta = 0.1$) feeds function 2 ($\beta = 0.03$), which in turn feeds function 3 ($\beta = 0.1$). (C) Output from function 1. (D) Output from function 2 (functions 1 and 2 in series). (E) Final response: output from function 3 (all three functions in series). Note how all three are full agonists when observed as final response.

agonism (see Section 2.11.3). This also means that there will be an increasing tendency for an agonist to produce the full system maximal response the further down the stimulus-response cascade the response is measured. Figure 2.16 shows three agonists, all producing different amounts of initial receptor stimulus. These stimuli are then passed through three successive rectangular hyperbolae simulating the stimulus-response cascade. As can be seen from the figure, by the last step all the agonists are full agonists. Viewing the response at this point gives no indication of differences in efficacy.

2.5 DIFFERENTIAL CELLULAR RESPONSE TO RECEPTOR STIMULUS

As noted in the previous discussion, different tissues have varying efficiencies of stimulus-response coupling. However, within a given tissue there may be the capability of choosing or altering the responsiveness of the system to agonists. This can be a useful technique in the study of agonists. Specifically, the ability to observe full agonists as partial agonists enables the experimenter to compare relative efficacies (see previous material). Also, if stimulus-response capability can be reduced, weak partial agonists can be studied as antagonists to gain measures of affinity. There are three general approaches to add texture to agonism: (1) choice of response pathway, (2) augmentation or modulation of pathway stimulus, and (3) manipulation of receptor density. This latter technique is operable only in recombinant systems where receptors are actively expressed in surrogate systems.

2.5.1 Choice of Response Pathway

The production of second messengers in cells by receptor stimulation leads to a wide range of biochemical reactions. As noted in the previous discussion, these can be approximately described by Michaelis—Menten type reaction curves, and each will have unique values of maximal rates of reaction and sensitivities to substrate. There are occasions where experimenters have access to different end points of these cascades, and with them different amplification factors for agonist response. One such case is the stimulation of cardiac β-adrenoceptors. In general, this leads to a general excitation of cardiac response composed of an increase in heart rate (for right atria), an increased force of contraction (inotropy), and an increase in the rate of muscle relaxation (lusitropy). These latter two cardiac functions can be accessed simultaneously through measurement of isometric cardiac contraction, and each has its own sensitivity to β-adrenoceptor excitation (lusitropic responses being more efficiently coupled to elevation of cyclic AMP than inotropic responses). Figure 2.17 shows the relative sensitivity of cardiac lusitropy and intropy to elevations in cyclic AMP in guinea pig left atria. It can be seen that the coupling of lusitropic response is fourfold more efficiently coupled to cyclic

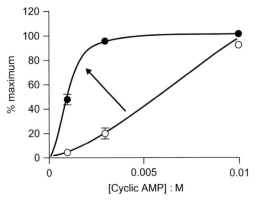

FIGURE 2.17 **Differential efficiency of receptor coupling for cardiac function.** Guinea pig left atrial force of contraction (inotropy, open circles) and rate of relaxation (lusitropy, filled circles) as a function (ordinates) of elevated intracellular cyclic AMP concentration (abscissae). Redrawn from [6].

AMP elevation than is inotropic response. Such differential efficiency of coupling can be used to dissect agonist response. For example, the inotropic and lusitropic responses of the β-adrenoceptor agonists isoproterenol and prenalterol can be divided into different degrees of full and partial agonism (Figure 2.18). It can be seen from Figure 2.18A that there are concentrations of isoproterenol that increase the rate of myocardial relaxation (i.e., 0.3 nM) without changing inotropic state. As the concentration of isoproterenol increases, the inotropic response appears (Figure 2.18B and C). Thus, the dose-response curve for myocardial relaxation for this full agonist is shifted to the left of the dose-response curve for inotropy in this preparation (Figure 2.18D). For a partial agonist such as prenalterol, there is nearly a complete dissociation between cardiac lusitropy and inotropy (Figure 2.18E). Theoretically, an agonist of low efficacy can be used as an antagonist of isoproterenol response in the more poorly coupled system (inotropy) and then compared with respect to efficacy (observation of visible response) in the more highly coupled system.

2.5.2 Augmentation or Modulation of Stimulus Pathway

The biochemical pathways making up the cellular stimulus-response cascade are complex systems with feedback and modulation mechanisms. Many of these are mechanisms to protect against overstimulation. For example, cells contain phosphodiesterase enzymes to degrade cyclic AMP to provide a fine control of stimulus strength and duration. Inhibition of phosphodiesterase therefore can remove this control and increase cellular levels of cyclic AMP. Figure 2.19A shows the effect of phosphodiesterase inhibition on the inotropic response of guinea pig papillary muscle. It can be seen from this figure that whereas 4.5% receptor stimulation by isoproterenol is required for 50% inotropic response in the natural system (where phosphodiesterase modulated intracellular cyclic AMP response), this is reduced to only 0.2% required receptor stimulation after inhibition of phosphodiesterase degradation of intracellular cyclic AMP. This technique can be used to modulate responses as well. Smooth muscle contraction requires extracellular calcium ion (calcium entry mediates contraction). Therefore, reduction of the calcium concentration in the extracellular space causes a modulation of the contractile responses (see example for the muscarinic contractile agonist carbachol, Figure 2.19B). In general, the sensitivity of functional systems can be manipulated by antagonism of modulating mechanisms and control of cofactors needed for cellular response.

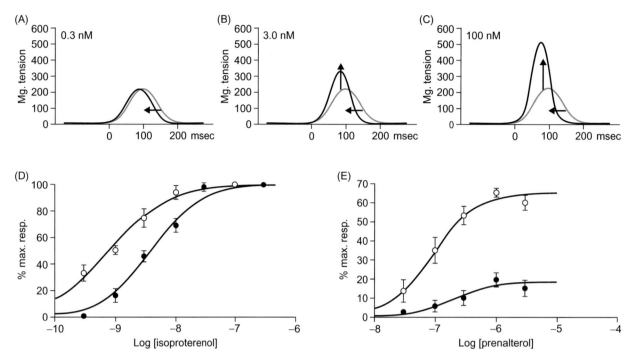

FIGURE 2.18   **Inotropic and lusitropic responses of guinea pig left atria to β-adrenoceptor stimulation.**   Panels A to C: isometric tension waveforms of cardiac contraction (ordinates are mg tension; abscissae are msec). (A) Effect of 0.3 nM isoproterenol on the waveform. The wave is shortened due to an increase in the rate of diastolic relaxation, whereas no inotropic response (change in peak tension) is observed at this concentration. (B) A further shortening of waveform duration (lusitropic response) is observed with 3 nM isoproterenol. This is concomitant with positive inotropic response (increase maximal tension). (C) This trend continues with 100 nM isoproterenol. (D) Dose-response curves for inotropy (filled circles) and lusitropy (open circles) in guinea pig atria for isoproterenol. (E) Dose-response curves for inotropy (filled circles) and lusitropy (open circles) in guinea pig atria for the β-adrenoceptor partial agonist prenalterol. Data redrawn from [6].

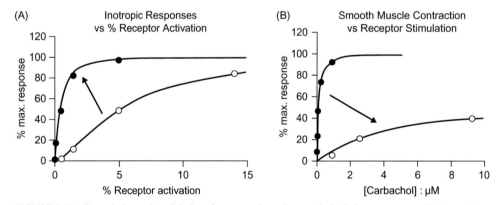

FIGURE 2.19   **Potentiation and modulation of response through control of cellular processes.**   (A) Potentiation of inotropic response to isoproterenol in guinea pig papillary muscle by the phosphodiesterase inhibitor isobutyl-methylxanthine (IBMX). Ordinates: percent of maximal response to isoproterenol. Abscissa: percent receptor occupancy by isoproterenol (log scale). Responses shown in absence (open circles) and presence (filled circles) of IBMX. Data redrawn from [7]. (B) Effect of reduction in calcium ion concentration on carbachol contraction of guinea pig ileum. Responses in the presence of 2.5 mM (filled circles) and 1.5 mM (open circles) calcium ion in physiological media bathing the tissue. Data redrawn from [8].

2.5.3 Differences in Receptor Density

The number of functioning receptors controls the magnitude of the initial stimulus given to the cell by an agonist. Number of receptors on the cell surface is one means by which the cell can control its stimulatory environment.

Thus, it is not surprising that receptor density varies with different cell types. Potentially, this can be used to control the responses to agonists since low receptor densities will produce less response than higher densities. Experimental control of this factor can be achieved in recombinant

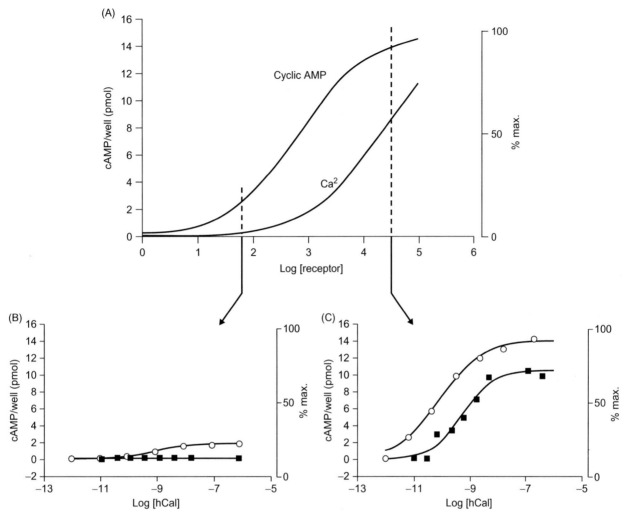

FIGURE 2.20 **Effect of receptor expression level on responses of human calcitonin receptor type 2 to human calcitonin.** (A) Cyclic AMP and calcium responses for human calcitonin activation of the receptor. Abscissae: logarithm of receptor density in fmole/mg protein. Ordinates: pmole cyclic AMP (left-hand axis) or calcium entry as a percentage of maximum response to human calcitonin. Two receptor expression levels are shown: At 65 fmole/mg, there is sufficient receptor to produce only a cyclic AMP response. At 30,000 fmole/mg receptor, more cyclic AMP is produced, but there is also sufficient receptor to couple to G_q-protein and produce a calcium response. (B and C) Dose-response curves to human calcitonin for the two responses in cell lines expressing the two different levels of receptor. Effects on cyclic AMP levels (open circles; left-hand ordinal axes) and calcium entry (filled squares; right-hand ordinal axes) for HEK cells expressing calcitonin receptors at 65 fmole/mg (panel B) and 30,000 fmole/mg (panel C). Data redrawn from [9].

systems. The methods of doing this are discussed more fully in Chapter 5. Figure 2.20 shows the cyclic AMP and calcium responses to human calcitonin activating calcitonin receptors in human embryonic kidney cells. Responses from two different recombinant cell lines of differing receptor density are shown. It can be seen that not only does the quantity of response change with increasing receptor number response (note ordinate scales for cyclic AMP production in Figure 2.20B and C), but also the *quality* of the response changes. Specifically, calcitonin is a pleiotropic receptor with respect to the G-proteins with which it interacts (this receptor can couple to G_s-, G_i-, and G_q-proteins). In cells containing a low number of receptors, there is an insufficient density to activate G_q-proteins, and thus no G_q response (calcium signaling) is observed

(see Figure 2.20B). However, in cells with a higher receptor density, both a cyclic AMP and a calcium response (indicative of concomitant G_s- and G_q-protein activation) is observed (Figure 2.20C). In this way, the receptor density controls the overall composition of the cellular response to the agonist.

2.5.4 Target-Mediated Trafficking of Stimulus

The foregoing discussion is based on the assumption that the activation of the receptor by an agonist leads to uniform stimulation of all cellular pathways connected to that

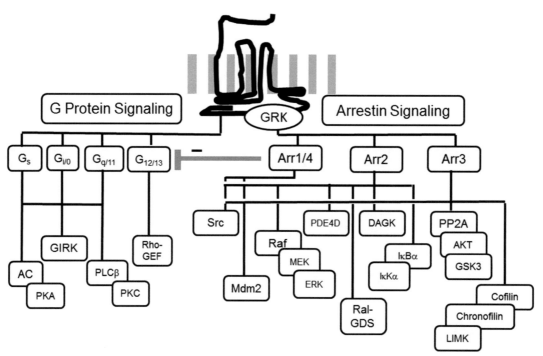

FIGURE 2.21 Seven transmembrane receptor signaling through two major networks. Receptors can interact with G-proteins (G$_s$) to activate adenylate cyclase (AC, and protein kinase A, PKA), G$_q$ to activate phospholipase Cβ (PLCβ) and protein kinase C (PKC), through G$_α$ and G$_{βγ}$ G-protein subunits to interact with gated inwardly rectifying K$^+$ channels (GIRK) and small GTP-ases (Rho-guanine nucleotide exchange factor, Rho-GEF). Receptors also can be phosphorylated by GRKs to subsequently bind arrestins; this process uncouples G-protein signaling but also can form scaffolds for the assembly of signalosomes and internalization of receptors. Arrestin mediated signaling involves the Src family of tyrosine kinases (Src), E3 ubiquitin ligases (Mdm2), ERK1/2 mitogen-activated protein kinase cascades (Raf-MEK-ERK1/2), cyclic AMP phosphodiesterases (PDE4D), Ral-GDP dissociation stimulator (Ral-GDS), diacylglycerol kinases (DAGK), regulators of nuclear factor-κB signaling (IκBα-IκKα), glycogen synthase kinase 3 regulatory complex PP2A-Akt-GSK3 and the actin filament-severing complex cofilin-chronofilin-LIMK. Redrawn from [12].

target. Over the past 15 years, incontrovertible evidence has emerged that for some agonists this is not the case, and that, in fact, some agonists can bias or preferentially activate some pathways linked to the receptor over others [10]. This is in contrast to the previous view of efficacy in pharmacology, which assumed a linear property for agonism, that is, activation of the receptor brought with it all the physiological functions mediated by that receptor. A concomitant view for seven transmembrane receptors was that these primarily couple to G-proteins to elicit response; it is now known that non-G-protein-linked cellular pathways are also a very important means for these receptors to alter cellular metabolism and function [11–14]. A very important major signaling pathway for seven transmembrane receptors is comprised of the binding of a group of intracellular proteins called arrestins. These proteins were thought to only mediate the desensitization and internalization of receptors until it was discovered that they also can function as scaffolds to bind diverse, catalytically-active, intracellular proteins to form "signalosomes" [11], which produce a wide range of cellular signals. Thus, the

recruitment of various protein and lipid kinases, phosphatases, phosphodiesterases and ubiquitin ligase into signalosomes leads to the regulation of members of the Src family of nonreceptor tyrosine kinases, mitogen-activated protein kinases, protein kinase B (AKT), glycogen synthase kinase 3, protein phosphatase 2 A, nuclear factor-κB and other proteins — see Figure 2.21. The activation of these non-G-protein pathways causes a low-level but prolonged response in the cell (referred to as *extracellular receptor-mediated kinase (ERK) activation, external receptor kinase signal*) as opposed to the rapid but transient G-protein-mediated response (see Figure 2.22). It requires different assays to detect this β-arrestin-mediated response; thus, in the absence of such an assay, a molecule may be an undetected β-arrestin agonist. For example, one of the most extensively studied drugs in the world, the β-blocker propranolol (discovered in 1964), was not classified as a β-arrestin ERK agonist until nearly 40 years after its initial discovery [15]; this new activity was detected when ERK assays became available. This underscores the importance of defining agonism in the context

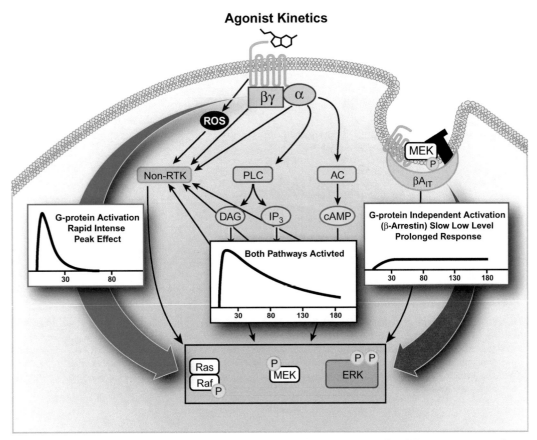

FIGURE 2.22 Schematic diagram of two major cellular signaling pathways mediated by seven transmembrane receptors. A rapid response is generated through the activation of G-proteins (see Figure 2.5), while a more persistent response is mediated by a receptor/β-arrestin complex of kinases intracellularly. Natural endogenous agonists usually activate both of these, while synthetic agonists may be made, in some cases, to selectively activate one pathway or the other.

of the assay. Thus, propranolol is an inverse agonist for cyclic AMP and a positive agonist for ERK activation. In fact, new vantage points to view agonist activity can lead to reclassification of ligands. For example, Figure 2.23 shows a collection of β-blockers reclassified in terms of their activity on β-adrenoceptors as activators of G-proteins and ERK via β-arrestin binding [16,17]. This polyfunctional view of receptors extends beyond cellular signaling, as it is now known that modification of receptor behavior does not require activation of conventional signaling pathways. For example, the internalization (absorption of the receptor into the cytoplasm either to be recycled to the cell surface or degraded) had been thought to be a direct function of activation, yet antagonists that do not activate the receptor are now known to cause active internalization of receptors [18]. The detection of these dichotomous activities is the direct result of having new assays to observe cellular function, in this case, the internalization of receptors. Figure 2.24 shows a number of receptor behaviors that now can be separately monitored with different assays.

2.6 RECEPTOR DESENSITIZATION AND TACHYPHYLAXIS

There is a temporal effect that must be considered in functional experiments; namely, the *desensitization* of the system through sustained or repeated stimulation. Receptor response is regulated by processes of phosphorylation and internalization, which can prevent overstimulation of physiological function in cells. This desensitization can be specific for a receptor, in which case it is referred to as *homologous desensitization*, or it can be related to modulation of a pathway common to more than one receptor and thus is *heterologous desensitization*. In this latter case, repeated stimulation of one receptor may cause the reduction in responsiveness of a number of receptors. The effects of desensitization on agonist dose-response curves are not uniform. Thus, for powerful, highly efficacious agonists, desensitization can cause a dextral displacement of the dose response with no diminution of maximal response (see Figure 2.25A). In contrast, desensitization can cause a depression of the

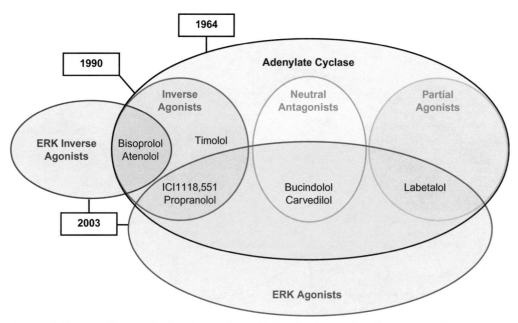

FIGURE 2.23 Venn diagram showing classifications of β-blocking drugs. A uniform property of these drugs is blockade of the β-adrenoceptor. However, within this class of drugs, subclasses exist relating to G-protein function, which can weakly stimulate adenylate cyclase (partial agonists), have a negative effect on elevated basal response (inverse agonists), or have no positive or negative stimulatory effect (neutral antagonists). Another subclass exists relating to extracellular receptor-mediated kinase activity (ERK activity) where some of these are positive and others inverse agonists. Redrawn from [17].

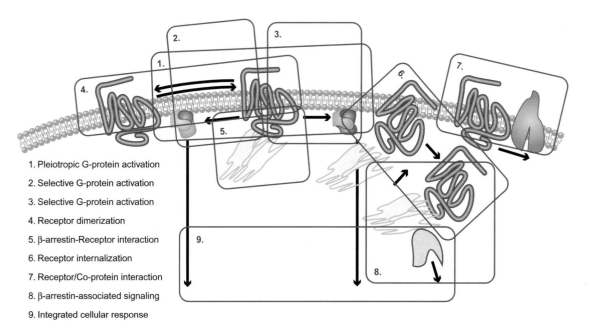

1. Pleiotropic G-protein activation

2. Selective G-protein activation

3. Selective G-protein activation

4. Receptor dimerization

5. β-arrestin-Receptor interaction

6. Receptor internalization

7. Receptor/Co-protein interaction

8. β-arrestin-associated signaling

9. Integrated cellular response

FIGURE 2.24 Schematic showing some of the properties of seven transmembrane receptors. While many of these behaviors are interdependent upon each other, others are not, and receptors can be made to demonstrate partial panels of these behaviors selectively through binding of different ligands. Separate assays can be used to detect these various behaviors.

maximal response to weak partial agonists (see Figure 2.25B). The overall effects of desensitization on dose-response curves relate to the effective receptor reserve for the agonist in a particular system. If the desensitization process eliminates receptor responsiveness where it is essentially irreversible in terms of the time-scale of response (i.e., response occurs in seconds whereas reversal from desensitization may require hours), then the desensitization process will mimic the removal of active receptors from the tissue. Therefore, for an

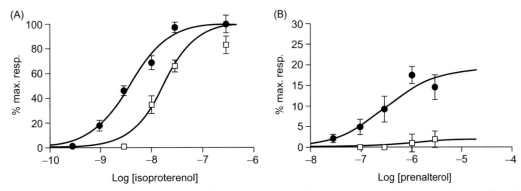

FIGURE 2.25 **Effects of desensitization on inotropic responses of guinea pig atria to isoproterenol (panel A) and prenalterol (panel B).** Ordinates: response as a percent of the maximal response to isoproterenol. Abscissae: logarithms of molar concentrations of agonist (log scale). Responses shown after peak response attained (within 5 minutes, filled circles) and after 90 minutes of incubation with the agonist (open squares). Data redrawn from [6].

agonist with a high receptor reserve (i.e., only a small portion of the receptors are required for production of maximal tissue response), desensitization will not depress the maximal response until a proportion greater than the reserve is affected. In contrast, for an agonist with no receptor reserve, desensitization will produce an immediate decrease in the maximal response. These factors can be relevant to the choice of agonists for therapeutic application. This is discussed more fully in Chapter 5.

2.7 THE MEASUREMENT OF DRUG ACTIVITY

In general there are two major formats for pharmacological experiments: cellular function and biochemical binding. Historically, function has been by far the more prevalent form of experiment. Since the turn of the century, isolated tissues have been used to detect and quantify drug activity. Pioneers such as Rudolph Magnus (1873–1927) devised methods of preserving the physiological function of isolated tissues (i.e., isolated intestine) to allow the observation of drug-induced response. Such preparations formed the backbone of all *in vitro* pharmacological experimental observation and furnished the data to develop drug-receptor theory. Isolated tissues were the workhorses of pharmacology, and various laboratories had their favorite. As put by W. D. M. Paton [19]:

The guinea pig longitudinal muscle is a great gift to the pharmacologist. It has low spontaneous activity; nicely graded responses (not too many tight junctions); is highly sensitive to a very wide range of stimulants; is tough, if properly handled, and capable of hours of reproducible behavior.

— W. D. M. Paton (1986)

All drug discovery relied upon such functional assays until the introduction of binding techniques. Aside from

the obvious shortcoming of using animal tissue to predict human responsiveness to drugs, isolated tissue formats did not allow for high-throughput screening of compounds (i.e., the experiments were labor intensive). Therefore, the numbers of compounds that could be tested for potential activity were limited by the assay format. In the mid-1970s, a new technology (in the form of biochemical binding) was introduced, and this quickly became a major approach to the study of drugs. Both binding and function are valuable and have unique application, and it is worth considering the strengths and shortcomings of both approaches in the context of the study of drug-receptor interaction.

2.8 ADVANTAGES AND DISADVANTAGES OF DIFFERENT ASSAY FORMATS

High-throughput volume was the major reason for the dominance of binding in the 1970s and 1980s. However, technology has now progressed to the point where the numbers of compounds tested in functional assays can equal or even exceed the volume that can be tested in binding studies. Therefore, this is an obsolete reason for choosing binding over function, and the relative scientific merits of both assay formats can now be used to make the choice of assay for drug discovery. There are advantages and disadvantages to both formats. In general, binding assays allow the isolation of receptor systems by use of membrane preparations and selective radioligand (or other traceable ligand; see material following) probes. The interference with the binding of such a probe can be used as direct evidence of an interaction of the molecules with the receptor. In contrast, functional studies in cellular formats can be much more complex, in that the interactions may not be confined to the receptor but rather extend further into the complexities of cellular functions. Since these may be cell-type dependent, some of this information may not be transferable across systems and therefore will not be useful for prediction of therapeutic effects. However, selectivity can be achieved in functional assays through the use of selective agonists. Thus, even in the presence of mixtures of functional receptors, a judicious choice of agonist can be used to select the receptor of interest and reduce nonspecific signals.

In binding, the molecules detected are only those that interfere with the specific probe chosen to monitor receptor activity. There is a potential shortcoming of binding assays in that often the pharmacological probes used to monitor receptor binding are not the same probes that are relevant to receptor function in the cell. For example, there are molecules that may interfere with the physiologically relevant receptor probe (the G-proteins that interact with the receptor and control cellular response to activation of that receptor) but not with the probe used for monitoring receptor binding. This is true for a number of interactions generally classified as *allosteric* (*vide infra*; see Chapters 4 and 7 for details) interactions. Specifically, allosteric ligands do not necessarily interact with the same binding site as the endogenous ligand (or the radioligand probe in binding), and therefore binding studies may not detect them.

Receptor levels in a given preparation may be insufficient to return a significant binding signal (i.e., functional responses are highly amplified and may reveal receptor presence in a more sensitive manner than binding). For example, CHO cells show a powerful 5-HT$_{1B}$ receptor-mediated agonist response to 5-HT that is blocked in nanomolar concentrations by the antagonist ($\pm$)-cyanopindolol [20]. However, no significant binding of the radioligand [^{125}I]-iodocyanopindolol is observed. Therefore, in this case the functional assay is a much more sensitive indicator of 5-HT responses. The physiological relevant probe (one that affects the cellular metabolism) can be monitored by observing cellular function. Therefore, it can be argued that functional studies offer a broader scope for the study of receptors than do binding studies. Another major advantage of function over binding is the ability of the former, and not the latter, to directly observe ligand efficacy. Binding registers only the presence of the ligand bound to the receptor but does not return the amount of stimulation that the bound agonist imparts to the system.

In general, there are advantages and disadvantages to both assay formats, and both are widely employed in pharmacological research. The specific strengths and weaknesses inherent in both approaches are discussed in more detail in Chapters 4 and 5. As a preface to the consideration of these two major formats, a potential issue with both of them should be considered; namely, dissimulations between the concentrations of drugs added to the experimentally accessible receptor compartment and the actual concentration producing the effect.

2.9 DRUG CONCENTRATION AS AN INDEPENDENT VARIABLE

In pharmacological experiments, the independent variable is drug concentration and the dependent (observed) variable is tissue response. Therefore, all measures of drug activity, potency, and efficacy are totally dependent on accurate knowledge of the concentration of drug at the receptor producing the observed effect. With no knowledge to the contrary, it is assumed that the concentration added to the receptor system by the experimenter is equal to the concentration acting at the receptor (i.e., there is no difference in the magnitude of the independent variable). However, there are potential factors in pharmacological experiments that can negate this assumption and thus lead to serious error in the measurement of drug activity. One is error in the concentration of the drug that is able to reach the receptor.

2.9.1 Dissimulation in Drug Concentration

The receptor compartment is defined as the aqueous volume containing the receptor and cellular system. It is assumed that free diffusion leads to ready access to this compartment (i.e., that the concentration within this compartment is the free concentration of drug at the receptor). However, there are factors that can cause differences between the experimentally accessible liquid compartment and the actual receptor compartment. One obvious potential problem is limited solubility of the drug being added to the medium. The assumption is made tacitly that the dissolved drug in the stock solution, when added to the medium bathing the pharmacological preparation, will stay in solution. There are cases where this may not be a valid assumption.

Many drug-like molecules have aromatic substituents and thus have limited aqueous solubility. A routine practice is to dissolve stock drugs in a solvent known to dissolve many types of molecular structures. One such solvent is dimethylsulfoxide (DMSO). This solvent is extremely useful, because physiological preparations such as cells in culture or isolated tissues can tolerate relatively high concentrations of DMSO (i.e., 0.5 to 2%) with no change in function. When substances dissolved in one solvent are diluted into another solvent where the substance has different (lower) solubility, local concentration gradients may exceed the solubility of the substance in the mixture. When this occurs, the substance may begin to come out of solution in these areas of limited solubility (i.e., microcrystals may form). This may in turn lead to a phenomenon known as *nucleation*, whereby the microcrystals form the seeds required for crystallization of the substance from the solution. The result of this process can be the complete crystallization

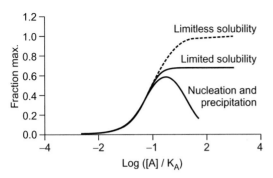

FIGURE 2.26 **Theoretical effects of agonist insolubility on dose-response curves.** Sigmoidal curve partially in dotted lines shows the theoretically ideal curve obtained when the agonist remains in solution throughout the course of the experiment determining the dose-response relationship. If a limit to the solubility is reached, then the responses will not increase beyond the point at which maximal solubility of the agonist is attained (labeled limited solubility). If the precipitation of the agonist in solution causes nucleation that subsequently causes precipitation of the amount already dissolved in solution, then a diminution of the previous response may be observed.

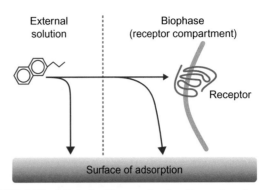

FIGURE 2.27 **Schematic diagram showing the routes of possible removal of drug from the receptor compartment.** Upon diffusion into the compartment, the drug may be removed by passive adsorption en route. This will cause a constant decrease in the steady-state concentration of the drug at the site of the receptor until the adsorption process is saturated.

of the substance from the entire mixture. For this reason, the dilution into the solution of questionable solubility (usually the aqueous physiological salt solution) should be done at the lowest concentration possible to ensure against nucleation and potential loss of solubility of the drug in the pharmacological medium. All dilutions of the stock drug solution should be carried out in the solution of maximal solubility, usually pure DMSO, and the solution for pharmacological testing must be taken directly from these stocks. Even under these circumstances, the drug may precipitate out of the medium when added to the aqueous medium. Figure 2.26 shows the effects of limited solubility on a dose-response curve to an agonist. Solubility limits are absolute. Thus, once the limit is reached, no further addition of stock solution will result in an increased soluble drug concentration. Therefore, the response at that solubility limit defines the maximal response for that preparation. If the solubility is below that required for the true maximal response to be observed (dotted line, Figure 2.25), then an erroneously truncated response to the drug will be observed. A further effect on the dose-response curve can be observed if the drug, upon entering the aqueous physiological solution, precipitates because of local supersaturated concentration gradients. This could lead to nucleation and subsequent crystallization of the drug which had previously dissolved in the medium. This would reduce the concentration below the previously dissolved concentration and lead to a decrease in the maximal response (bell-shaped dose-response curve, Figure 2.26).

Another potential problem causing differences in the concentration of drug added to the solution (and that reaching the receptors) is the sequestration of drug in

TABLE 2.1 Effect of Pretreatment of Surface on Adsorption of [3H]-endorphin

Treatment	fmole Adsorbed	% Reduction over Lysine Treatment
Lysine	615	0
Arginine	511	16.9
Bovine serum albumin	383	38
Choline chloride	19.3	97
Polylysine	1.7	99.5
Myelin basic protein	1.5	99.9

Data from [21].

regions other than the receptor compartment (Figure 2.27). Some of these effects can be due to active uptake or enzymatic degradation processes inherent in the biological preparation. These are primarily encountered in isolated whole tissues and are not a factor in *in vitro* assays composed of cellular monolayers. However, another factor that is common to nearly all *in vitro* systems is the potential adsorption of drug molecules onto the surface of the vessel containing the biological system (i.e., well of a cell culture plate). The impact of these mechanisms depends on the drug and the nature of the surface, being more pronounced for some chemical structures and also more pronounced for some surfaces (i.e., nonsilanized glass). Table 2.1 shows the striking differences in adsorption of [3H]-endorphin with pretreatment of the surface with various agents. It can be seen that a difference of over 99.9% can be observed when the surface is treated with a substance that prevents adsorption such as myelin basic protein.

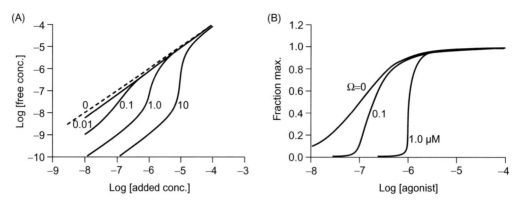

FIGURE 2.28 **Effects of a saturable adsorption process on concentrations of agonist (panel A) and dose-response curves to agonists (panel B).** (A) Concentrations of drug added to system (abscissae, log scale) versus free concentration in solution (ordinates, log scale). Numbers next to curves indicate the capacity of the adsorption process in μM. The equilibrium dissociation constant of the agonist adsorption site is 10 nM. Dotted line indicates no difference between added concentrations and free concentration in solution. (B) Effect of a saturable adsorption process on agonist dose-response curves. Numbers next to curves refer to the maximal capability of the adsorption process. The equilibrium dissociation constant of the agonist adsorption site is 0.1 μM. Curve farthest to the left is the curve with no adsorption taking place.

2.9.2 Free Concentration of Drug

If the adsorption process is not saturable within the concentration range of the experiment, it becomes a sink claiming a portion of the drug added to the medium, the magnitude of which is dependent on the maximal capacity of the sink ($[\Omega]$) and the affinity of the ligand for the site of adsorption ($1/K_{ad}$, where K_{ad} is the equilibrium dissociation constant of the ligand-adsorption site complex). The receptor then interacts with the remaining free concentration of drug in the compartment. The free concentration of drug, in the presence of an adsorption process, is given as follows (see Section 2.11.4):

$$[A_{free}] = [A_T] - \frac{1}{2}\left\{[A_T] + K_{ad} + \Omega \right.$$
$$\left. - \sqrt{([A_T^*] + K_{ad} + \Omega)^2 - 4[A_T]\Omega}\right\} \quad (2.3)$$

The free concentration of a drug $[A_{free}]$ in a system containing an adsorption process with maximal capacity ranging from 0.01 to 10 μM and for which the ligand has an affinity ($1/K_d$) is shown in Figure 2.28A. It can be seen that there is a constant ratio depletion of free ligand in the medium at low concentrations until the site of adsorption begins to be saturated. When this occurs, there is a curvilinear portion of the line reflecting the increase in the free concentration of ligand in the receptor compartment due to cancellation of adsorption-mediated depletion (adsorption sites are fully bound and can no longer deplete the ligand). It is useful to observe the effects such processes can have on dose-response curves of drugs. Figure 2.28B shows the effect of an adsorption process on the observed effects of an agonist in a system

where an adsorption process becomes saturated at the higher concentrations of agonist. It can be seen that there is a change in shape of the dose-response curve (increase in Hill coefficient with increasing concentration). This is characteristic of the presence of an agonist removal process that is saturated at some point within the concentration range of agonist used in the experiment.

In general, it should be recognized that the most carefully designed experimental procedure can be completely derailed by processes causing differences in what is thought to be the concentration of drug at the receptor and the actual concentration producing the effect. Insofar as experiments can be done to indicate that these effects are not operative in a given experiment, they should be.

2.10 CHAPTER SUMMARY AND CONCLUSIONS

- It is emphasized that drug activity is observed through a translation process controlled by cells. The aim of pharmacology is to derive system-independent constants characterizing drug activity from the indirect product of cellular response.
- Different drugs have different inherent capacities to induce response (intrinsic efficacy). Thus, equal cellular responses can be achieved by different fractional receptor occupancies of these drugs.
- Some cellular stimulus-response pathways and second messengers are briefly described. The overall efficiency of receptor coupling to these processes is defined as the stimulus-response capability of the cell.

- While individual stimulus-response pathways are extremely complicated, they all can be mathematically described by hyperbolic functions.
- The ability to reduce stimulus-response mechanisms to single monotonic functions allows relative cellular response to yield receptor-specific drug parameters.
- When the maximal stimulus-response capability of a given system is saturated by agonist stimulus, the agonist will be a full agonist (produce a full system response). Not all full agonists are of equal efficacy; they only all saturate the system.
- In some cases, the stimulus-response characteristics of a system can be manipulated to provide a means to compare maximal responses of agonists (efficacy).
- Receptor desensitization can have differing overall effects on high- and low-efficacy agonists.
- All drug parameters are predicated on an accurate knowledge of the concentration of drug acting at the receptor. Errors in this independent variable negate all measures of dependent variables in the system.
- Adsorption and precipitation are two commonly encountered sources of error in drug concentration.

2.11 DERIVATIONS

- Series hyperbolae can be modeled by a single hyperbolic function (2.11.1).
- Successive rectangular hyperbolic equations necessarily lead to amplification (2.11.2).
- Saturation of any step in a stimulus cascade by two agonists leads to identical maximal final responses for the two agonists (2.11.3).
- Procedure to measure drug concentration in the receptor compartment (2.11.4).

2.11.1 Series Hyperbolae Can Be Modeled by a Single Hyperbolic Function

Rectangular hyperbolae are of the general form:

$$y = \frac{Ax}{x + B}. \tag{2.4}$$

Assume a function:

$$y_1 = \frac{x}{x + \beta_2} \tag{2.5}$$

where the output y_1 becomes the input for a second function of the form:

$$y_2 = \frac{y_1}{y_1 + \beta_2}. \tag{2.6}$$

It can be shown that a series of such functions can be generalized to the form:

$$y_n = \frac{x}{x(1 + \beta_n(1 + \beta_{n-1}(1 + \beta_{n-2}(1 + \beta_{n-3})..)..)...)...) + (\beta_n..\beta_1)} \tag{2.7}$$

which can be rewritten in the form of Equation 2.4, where $A = (1 + \beta_n(1 + \beta_{n-1}(1 + \beta_{n-2}(1 + \beta_{n-3})..)...)..)^{-1}$ and $B = (\beta_n.....\beta_1)/(1 + \beta_n(1 + \beta_{n-1}(1 + \beta_{n-2})..)...)..)$. Thus, it can be seen that the product of a succession of rectangular hyperbolae is itself a hyperbola.

2.11.2 Successive Rectangular Hyperbolic Equations Necessarily Lead to Amplification

Assume a rectangular hyperbola of the form:

$$\rho_1 = \frac{[A]}{[A] + K_A}, \tag{2.8}$$

where $[A]$ is the molar concentration of drug and K_A is the location parameter of the dose-response curve along the concentration axis (the potency). Assume also a second rectangular hyperbola where the input function is defined by Equation 2.8:

$$\rho_2 = \frac{[A]/([A] + K_A)}{([A]/([A] + K_A)) + \beta}. \tag{2.9}$$

The term β is the coupling efficiency constant for the second function. The location parameter (potency) of the second function (denoted K_{obs}) is given by

$$K_{obs} = \frac{K_A \beta}{1 + \beta}. \tag{2.10}$$

It can be seen that for non-zero and positive values of β, $K_{obs} < K_A$ (i.e., the potency of the overall process will be greater than the potency for the initial process).

2.11.3 Saturation of Any Step in a Stimulus Cascade by Two Agonists Leads to Identical Maximal Final Responses for the Two Agonists

For a given agonist $[A]$, the product of any one reaction in the stimulus-response cascade is given by:

$$Output_1 = \frac{[A] \cdot M_1}{[A] + \beta_1} \tag{2.11}$$

where M_1 is the maximal output of the reaction and β_1 is the coupling constant for the reaction. When this product becomes the substrate for the next reaction, the output becomes:

$$Output_2 = \frac{[A] \cdot M_1 M_2}{[A](M_1 + \beta_2) + \beta_1 \beta_2}. \tag{2.12}$$

The maximal output from this second reaction (i.e., as $[A] \to \infty$) is

$$\text{Max}_2 = \frac{M_1 M_2}{M_1 \beta_2}. \tag{2.13}$$

By analogy, the maximal output from the second reaction for another agonist $[A']$ is:

$$\text{Max}_2' = \frac{M_1' M_2}{M_1' + \beta_2}. \tag{2.14}$$

The relative maximal responses for the two agonists are therefore:

$$\text{Relative Maxima} = \frac{\text{Max}_2}{\text{Max}_2'} = \frac{1 + \beta_2/M_1'}{1 + \beta_2/M_1}. \tag{2.15}$$

It can be seen from this equation that if $M_1 = M_1'$ (i.e., if the maximal response to two agonists in any previous reaction in the cascade is equal), the relative maxima of the two agonists in subsequent reactions will be equal $(\text{Max}_2/\text{Max}_2' = 1)$.

2.11.4 Procedure to Measure Free Drug Concentration in the Receptor Compartment

Assume that the total drug concentration $[A_1]$ is the sum of the free concentration $[A_{\text{free}}]$ and the concentration bound to a site of adsorption $[AD]$ (therefore, $[A_{\text{free}}] = [A_T] - [AD]$). The mass action equation for adsorption is:

$$[AD] = \frac{([A_T] - [AD])\Omega}{[A_T] - [AD] + K_{\text{ad}}} \tag{2.16}$$

where the maximal number of adsorption sites is Ω and the equilibrium dissociation constant of the drug site of adsorption is K_{ad}. Equation 2.16 results in the quadratic equation:

$$[AD]^2 - [AD](\Omega + [A_T] + K_{\text{ad}}) + [A_T]\Omega = 0, \tag{2.17}$$

one solution for which is:

$$\frac{1}{2}\left\{ [A_T] + K_{\text{ad}} + \Omega - \sqrt{([A_T^*] + K_{\text{ad}} + \Omega)^2 - 4[A_T]\Omega} \right\}. \tag{2.18}$$

Since $[A_{\text{free}}] = [A_T] - [AD]$, then:

$$[A_{\text{free}}] = [A_T] - \frac{1}{2}\left\{ [A_T] + K_{\text{ad}} + \Omega \right.$$
$$\left. - \sqrt{([A_T^*] + K_{\text{ad}} + \Omega)^2 - 4[A_T]\Omega} \right\} \tag{2.19}$$

REFERENCES

[1] Chen W-J, Armour S, Way J, Chen GC, Watson C, Irving PE, et al. Expression cloning and receptor pharmacology of human calcitonin receptors from MCF-7 cells and their relationship to amylin receptors. Mol Pharmacol 1997;52:1164−75.

[2] Kenakin TP, Cook DA. Blockade of histamine-induced contractions of intestinal smooth muscle by irreversibly acting agents. Can J Physiol Pharmacol 1976;54:386−92.

[3] Wilson S, Chambers JK, Park JE, Ladurner A, Cronk DW, Chapman CG, et al. Agonist potency at the cloned human beta-3 adrenoceptor depends on receptor expression level and nature of assay. J Pharmacol Exp Ther 1996;279:214−21.

[4] Goldberg ND. Cyclic nucleotides and cell function. In: Weissman G, Claiborne R, editors. Cell membranes, biochemistry, cell biology, and pathology. New York: H. P. Publishing; 1975. p. 185−202.

[5] Kenakin TP, Beek D. Is prenalterol (H 133/80) really a selective beta-1 adrenoceptor agonist? Tissue selectivity resulting from differences in stimulus-response relationships. J Pharmacol Exp Ther 1980;213:406−13.

[6] Kenakin TP, Ambrose JR, Irving PE. The relative efficiency of beta-adrenoceptor coupling to myocardial inotropy and diastolic relaxation: organ-selective treatment of diastolic dysfunction. J Pharmacol Exp Ther 1991;257:1189−97.

[7] Kenakin TP, Beek D. The measurement of the relative efficacy of agonists by selective potentiation of tissue responses: studies with isoprenaline and prenalterol in cardiac tissue. J Auton Pharmacol 1984;4:153−9.

[8] Burgen ASV, Spero L. The action of acetylcholine and other drugs on the efflux of potassium and rubidium from smooth muscle of the guinea-pig intestine. Br J Pharmacol 1968;34:99−115.

[9] Kenakin TP. Differences between natural and recombinant G-protein coupled receptor systems with varying receptor G-protein stoichiometry. Trends Pharmacol Sci 1997;18:456−64.

[10] Kenakin TP. Collateral efficacy as pharmacological problem applied to new drug discovery. Expert Opin Drug Disc 2006;1:635−52.

[11] Luttrell LM, Ferguson SSG, Daaka Y, Miller WE, Maudsley S, Della Rocca GJ, et al. β-arrestin-dependent formation of β2 adrenergic-Src protein kinase complexes. Science 1999;283:655−61.

[12] Gesty-Palmer D, Luttrell LM. Refining efficacy: exploiting functional selectivity for drug discovery. Adv Pharmacol 2011;62:79−107.

[13] Lefkowitz RJ, Shenoy SK. Transduction of receptor signals by β-arrestins. Science 2005;308:512−7.

[14] Luttrell LM. Composition and function of G-protein-coupled receptor signalsomes controlling mitogen-activated protein kinase activity. J Mol Neurosci 2005;26:253−63.

[15] Azzi M, Charest PG, Angers S, Rousseau G, Kohout T. β-arrestin-mediated activation of MAPK by inverse agonists reveals distinct active conformations for G-protein-coupled receptors. Proc Natl Acad Sci USA 2003;100:11406−11.

[16] Galandrin S, Bouvier M. Distinct signaling profiles of β1 and β2 adrenergic receptor ligands toward adenylyl cyclase and mitogen-activated protein kinase reveals the pluridimensionality of efficacy. Mol Pharmacol 2006;70:1575−84.

[17] Kenakin TP. Pharmacological onomastics: what's in a name? Br J Pharmacol 2008;153:432−8.

[18] Gray JA, Roth BL. Paradoxical trafficking and regulation of 5-HT$_{2A}$ receptors by agonists and antagonists. *Brain Res*. Bulletin 2001;56:441−51.

[19] Paton WDM. On becoming a pharmacologist. Ann Rev Pharmacol and Toxicol 1986;26:1−22.

[20] Giles H, Lansdell SJ, Bolofo M-L, Wilson HL, Martin GR. Characterization of a 5-HT$_{1B}$ receptor on CHO cells: functional responses in the absence of radioligand binding. Br J Pharmacol 1996;117:1119−26.

[21] Ferrar P, Li CH. β-endorphin: Radioreceptor binding assay. Int J Pept Protein Res 1980;16:66−9.

Drug-Receptor Theory

3.1 About This Chapter
3.2 Drug-Receptor Theory
3.3 The Use of Mathematical Models in Pharmacology
3.4 Some Specific Uses of Models in Pharmacology
3.5 Classical Model of Receptor Function

3.6 The Operational Model of Receptor Function
3.7 Two-State Theory
3.8 The Ternary Complex Model
3.9 The Extended Ternary Complex Model
3.10 Constitutive Receptor Activity and Inverse Agonism

3.11 The Cubic Ternary Complex Model
3.12 Multistate Receptor Models and Probabilistic Theory
3.13 Chapter Summary and Conclusions
3.14 Derivations
References

What is it that breathes fire into the equations and makes a universe for them to describe?

— Stephen W. Hawking (1991)

An equation is something for eternity...

— Albert Einstein (1879−1955)

Casual observation made in the course of a purely theoretical research has had the most important results in practical medicine ... Saul was not the last who, going forth to see his father's asses, found a kingdom.

— Arthur Robertson Cushny (1866−1926)

3.1 ABOUT THIS CHAPTER

This chapter discusses the various mathematical models that have been put forward to link the experimental observations (relating to drug-receptor interactions) and the events taking place on a molecular level between the drug and protein recognition sites. A major link between the data and the biological understanding of drug-receptor activity is the model. In general, experimental data is a sampling of a population of observations emanating from a system. The specific drug concentrations tested control the sample size, and the resulting dependent variables reflect what is happening at the biological target. A model defines the complete relationship for the whole population (i.e., for an infinite number of concentrations). The choice of model, and how it fits into the biology of what is thought to be occurring, is critical to the assessment of the experiment. For example, Figure 3.1A shows a set of dose-response data which have been fitted to two mathematical functions. It can be seen that both equations appear to adequately fit the data. The first curve is defined by:

$$y = 78(1 - e^{-(0.76([A]^{0.75}))}) - 2. \tag{3.1}$$

This is simply a collection of constants in an exponential function format. The constants cannot be related to the interactions at a molecular level. In contrast, the refit of the data to the Langmuir adsorption isotherm:

$$y = \frac{80 \cdot [A]}{[A] + EC_{50}} \tag{3.2}$$

allows some measure of interpretation (i.e., the location parameter along the concentration axis may reflect affinity and efficacy while the maximal asymptote may reflect efficacy; Figure 3.1B). In this case, the model built on chemical concepts allows interpretation of the data in molecular terms. The fitting of experimental data to equations derived from models of receptor function are at least consistent with the testing and refinement of these models with the resulting further insight into biological behavior.

T. P. Kenakin: A Pharmacology Primer, Fourth edition. DOI: http://dx.doi.org/10.1016/B978-0-12-407663-1.00003-X
© 2014 Elsevier Inc. All rights reserved.

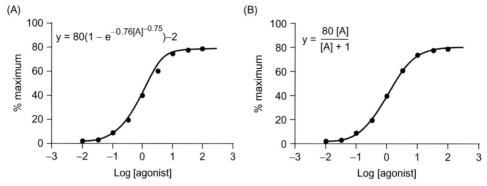

FIGURE 3.1 Data set fit to two functions of the same general shape. (A) Function fit to the exponential Equation 3.1. (B) Function fit to rectangular hyperbola of the form 80*[A]/([A] + 1).

An early proponent of using such models and laws to describe the very complex behavior of physiological systems was A. J. Clark, known as the originator of receptor pharmacology. As put by Clark in his monograph *The Mode of Action of Drugs on Cells* [1]:

The general aim of this author in this monograph has been to determine the extent to which the effects produced by drugs on cells can be interpreted as processes following known laws of physical chemistry.

— A. J. Clark (1937)

A classic example of where definitive experimental data necessitated refinement and extension of a model of drug-receptor interaction involved the discovery of constitutive receptor activity in GPCR systems. The state of the art model before this finding was the ternary complex model for GPCRs, a model that cannot accommodate ligand-independent (constitutive) receptor activity. With the experimental observation of constitutive activity for GPCRs by Costa and Herz [2], a modification was needed. Subsequently, Samama and colleagues [3] presented the extended ternary complex model to fill the void. This chapter discusses relevant mathematical models and generally offers a linkage between empirical measures of activity and molecular mechanisms.

3.2 DRUG-RECEPTOR THEORY

The various equations used to describe the quantitative activity of drugs and the interaction of those drugs with receptors is generally given the name *drug-receptor theory*. The models used within this theory originated from those used to describe enzyme kinetics. A. J. Clark is credited with applying quantitative models to drug action. His classic books *The Mode of Action of Drugs on Cells* [1] and *Handbook of Experimental Pharmacology* [4] served as the standard texts for quantitative receptor pharmacology for many years.

A consideration of the more striking examples of specific drug antagonisms shows that these in many cases follow recognizable laws, both in the case of enzymes and cells.

— A. J. Clark (1937)

With increasing experimental sophistication has come new knowledge of receptor function, and insights into the ways in which drugs can affect that function. In this chapter, drug-receptor theory is described in terms of what is referred to as "classical theory"; namely, the use and extension of concepts described by Clark and other researchers such as Stephenson [5], Ariens [6,7], MacKay [8], and Furchgott [9,10]. In this sense, classical theory is an amalgam of ideas linked chronologically. These theories were originated to describe the functional effects of drugs on isolated tissues and thus naturally involved functional physiological outputs. Another model used to describe functional drug activity, derived by Black and Leff [11], is termed the *operational model*. Unlike classical theory, this model makes no assumptions about the intrinsic ability of drugs to produce a response. The operational model is a very important new tool in receptor pharmacology, and is used throughout this book to illustrate receptor methods and concepts. Another model used primarily to describe the function of ion channels is termed *two-state theory*. This model contributed ideas essential to modern receptor theory, specifically in the description of drug efficacy in terms of the selective affinity for protein conformation. Finally, the idea that proteins translocate within cell membranes [12] and the observation that seven transmembrane receptors couple to separate G-proteins in the membrane led to the ternary complex model. This scheme was first described by DeLean and colleagues [13] and later modified to the extended ternary complex model by Samama and coworkers [3]. These are described separately as a background to discussion of drug-receptor activity and as context for the description of the quantitative tools and methods used in receptor pharmacology to quantify drug effect.

3.3 THE USE OF MATHEMATICAL MODELS IN PHARMACOLOGY

Mathematical models are the link between what is observed experimentally and what is thought to occur at the molecular level. In physical sciences, such as chemistry, there is a direct correspondence between the experimental observation and the molecular world (i.e., a nuclear magnetic resonance spectrum directly reflects the interaction of hydrogen atoms in a molecule). In pharmacology the observations are much more indirect, leaving a much wider gap between the physical chemistry involved in drug-receptor interaction and what the cell does in response to those interactions (through the "cellular veil"; see Figure 2.1). Hence, models become uniquely important.

There are different kinds of mathematical models, and they can be classified in two ways: by their complexity and by the number of estimable parameters they use. The simplest models are cartoons with very few parameters. These – such as the black box that was the receptor at the turn of the century – usually are simple input-output functions with no mechanistic description (i.e., the drug interacts with the receptor and a response ensues). Another type, termed the *Parsimonious model*, is also simple but has a greater number of estimable parameters. These do not completely characterize the experimental situation but do offer insights into mechanism. Models can be more complex as well. For example, complex models with a large number of estimable parameters can be used to simulate behavior under a variety of conditions (simulation models). Similarly, complex models for which the number of independently verifiable parameters is low (termed *heuristic models*) can still be used to describe complex behaviors not apparent by simple inspection of the system.

In general, a model will express a relationship between an independent variable (input by the operator) and one or more dependent variables (output, produced by the model). A ubiquitous form of equation for such input-output functions is curves of the rectangular hyperbolic form. It is worth illustrating some general points about models with such an example. Assume that a model takes on the general form:

$$\text{Output} = \frac{[\text{Input}] \cdot A}{B \cdot [\text{Input}] + C}. \tag{3.3}$$

The form of that function is shown in Figure 3.2. There are two specific parameters that can be immediately observed from this function. The first is that the maximal asymptote of the function is given solely by the magnitude of A/B. The second is that the location parameter of the function (where it lies along the input axis) is given by C/B. It can be seen that when [Input] equals C/B the output necessarily will be 0.5. Therefore, whatever the function, the midpoint of the curve will lie on a point at [Input] = C/B. These ideas are useful since they describe two essential behaviors of any drug-receptor model; namely, the maximal response (A/B) and the potency (concentration of input required for effect; C/B). Many of the complex equations used to describe drug-receptor interaction can be reduced to these general forms, and the maxima and midpoint values can be used to furnish general expressions for the dependence of efficacy and potency on the parameters of the mechanistic model used to furnish the equations.

3.4 SOME SPECIFIC USES OF MODELS IN PHARMACOLOGY

Models can be very useful in designing experiments, predicting drug effect, and describing complex systems. Ideally, models should be composed of species that can be independently quantified. Also, the characteristics of the processes that produce changes in the amounts of these species should be independently verifiable. The difference between a heuristic model and a simulation model is that the latter has independently verifiable constants for at least some of the processes. An ideal model also has internal checks that allow the researcher to determine whether the calculation is or is not following the predicted patterns set out by the model. A classic example of an internal check for a model is the linearity and slope of a Schild regression for simple competitive antagonism (see Chapter 6). In this case, the calculations must predict a linear regression of linear slope or the model of simple competitive antagonism is not operable. The internal check determines the applicability of the model.

Models can also predict apparently aberrant behaviors in systems that may appear to be artifactual (and therefore appear to denote experimental problems) but are in fact perfectly correct behaviors according to a given complex system. Simulation with modeling allows the researcher

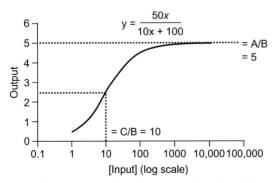

FIGURE 3.2 General curve for an input-output function of the rectangular hyperbolic form (y = 50x/(10x + 100)). The maximal asymptote is given by A/B and the location parameter (along the *x* axis) is given by C/B (see text).

to determine whether the data are erroneous or indicative of a correct system activity. For example, consider a system in which the receptors can form dimers, and where the affinity of a radioligand (radioactive molecule with affinity for the receptor allowing measurement of ligand-receptor complex binding to be measured) differs between the single receptor and the dimer. It is not intuitively obvious how the system will behave when a nonradioactive ligand that also binds to the receptor is added. In a standard single receptor system, preincubation with a radioligand followed by addition of a nonradioactive ligand will produce displacement of the radioligand. This will cause a decrease in the bound radioactive signal. The result usually is a sigmoidal dose-response curve for displacement of the radioligand by the nonradioactive ligand (see Figure 3.3). This is discussed in some detail in Chapter 4. The point here is that addition of the same nonradioactive ligand to a system of prebound radioligand would be expected to produce a decrease in signal. However, in the case of dimerization, if the combination of two receptors forms a "new" receptor of higher affinity for the radioligand, addition of a nonradioligand may actually increase the amount of radioligand bound before decreases are observed [14]. This is an apparent paradox (addition of a nonradioactive species actually increasing the binding of a radioactive species to a receptor). The equation for the amount of radioactive ligand [A*] bound (signal denoted ω) in the presence of a range of concentrations of nonradioactive ligand [A] is (Section 3.14.1).

$$\omega = \frac{\begin{aligned}([A^*]/K_d + \alpha[A^*][A]/K_d^2 + 2\alpha([A^*]/K_d)^2) \\ (1 + [A^*]/K_d + \alpha([A^*]/K_d)^2)\end{aligned}}{\begin{aligned}(1 + [A]/K_d + [A^*]/K_d + \alpha[A^*][A]/K_d^2 + \alpha([A^*]/K_d)^2 \\ + \alpha([A]/K_d)^2)([A^*]/K_d + 2\alpha([A^*]/K_d)^2)\end{aligned}}$$

(3.4)

As shown in Figure 3.3, addition of the nonradioactive ligand to the system can increase the amount of bound radioactivity in a system where the affinity of the ligand is higher for the dimer than it is for the single receptor. The prediction of this effect by the model changes the interpretation of a counterintuitive finding to one that conforms to the experimental system. Without the benefit of the modeling, observation of increased binding of radioligand with the addition of a nonradioactive ligand might have been interpreted erroneously.

Models also can assist in experimental design and the determination of the limits of experimental systems. For example, it is known that three proteins mediate the interaction of HIV with cells; namely, the chemokine receptor CCR5, the cellular protein CD4, and the viral coat protein gp120. An extremely useful experimental system to study this interaction is one in which radioactive CD4, prebound to soluble gp120, is allowed to bind to cellular receptor CCR5. This system can be used to screen for HIV entry inhibitors. One of the problems with this approach is the availability and expense of purified gp120. This reagent can readily be prepared in crude broths but very pure samples are difficult to obtain. A practical question, then, is to what extent would uncertainty in the concentration of gp120 affect an assay that examines the binding of a complex of radioactive CD4 and gp120 with the CCR5 receptor in the presence of potential drugs that block the complex? It can be shown in this case that the model of interaction predicts the following equation for the relationship between the concentrations of radioactive CD4 [CD], crude gp120 [gp], [CCR5], and the ratio of the observed potency of a displacing ligand [B] to its true potency (i.e., to what extent errors in the potency estimation will be made with errors in the true concentration of gp120; see Section 3.14.2):

$$K_4 = \frac{[IC_{50}]}{([CD]/K_1)([gp]/K_2) + 1}$$

(3.5)

where K_4, K_1, and K_2 are the equilibrium dissociation constants of the ligand [B], CD4, and gp120 and the site of interaction with CCR5/CD4/gp120. The relationship between the concentration of radioligand used in the assay and the ratio of the observed potency of the ligand in blocking the binding to the true potency is shown in Figure 3.4. The gray lines indicate this ratio with a 50% error in the concentration of gp120 (crude gp120 preparation). It can be seen from this figure that as long as the concentration of radioligand is kept below

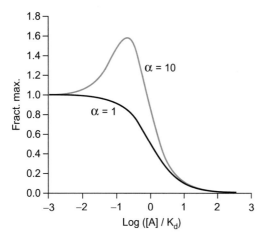

FIGURE 3.3 Displacement of prebound radioligand [A*] by nonradioactive concentrations of [A]. Curve for $\alpha = 1$ denotes no cooperativity in binding (i.e., formation of the receptor dimer does not lead to a change in the affinity of the receptor for either [A] or [A*]). The curve $\alpha = 10$ indicates a system whereby formation of the receptor dimer leads to a tenfold increase in the affinity for both [A*] and [A]. In this case, it can be seen that addition of the nonradioactive ligand [A] actually leads to an increase in the amount of radioligand [A*] bound before a decrease at higher concentrations of [A]. For this simulation [A*]/K_d = 0.1.

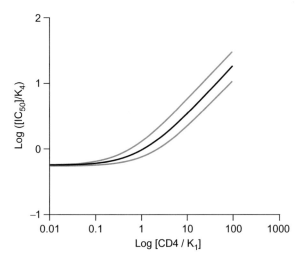

FIGURE 3.4 Errors in the estimation of ligand potency for displacement of radioactive CD4–gp120 complex (surrogate for HIV binding) as a function of the concentration of radioactive CD4 (expressed as a fraction of the equilibrium dissociation constant of the CD4 for its binding site). Gray lines indicate a 50% error in the concentration of gp120. It can be seen that very little error in the potency estimation of a displacing ligand is incurred at low concentrations of radioligand but that this error increases as the concentration of CD4 is increased.

$[CD_4]/K_1 = 0.1$, differences between the assumed concentration of gp120 in the assay and true concentrations make little difference to the estimation of ligand potency. In this case, the model delineates experimental parameters for the optimal performance of the assay.

3.5 CLASSICAL MODEL OF RECEPTOR FUNCTION

The binding of a ligand [A] to a receptor R is assumed to follow mass action according to the Langmuir adsorption isotherm (see Equation 1.4), as defined by Clark [1,4]. No provision for different drugs of differing propensities to stimulate receptors was made until E. J. Ariens [6,7] introduced a proportionality factor (termed *intrinsic activity* and denoted α in his terminology) to the binding function [5]. Intrinsic activity is the maximal response to an agonist expressed as a fraction of the maximal response for the entire system (i.e., $\alpha = 1$ indicates that the agonist produces the maximal response, $\alpha = 0.5$ indicates half the maximal response, and so on). An intrinsic activity of zero indicates no agonism. Within this framework, the equation for response is thus:

$$\text{Response} = \frac{[A]\alpha}{[A] + K_A} \qquad (3.6)$$

where K_A is the equilibrium dissociation of the agonist-receptor complex. Note how in this scheme, response is assumed to be a direct linear function of receptor occupancy multiplied by a constant. This latter requirement

was seen to be a shortcoming of this approach since it was known that many nonlinear relationships between receptor occupancy and tissue response existed. This was rectified by Stephenson [5], who revolutionized receptor theory by introducing the abstract concept of *stimulus*. This is the amount of activation given to the receptor upon agonist binding. Stimulus is processed by the tissue to yield response. The magnitude of the stimulus is a function (denoted f in Equation 3.7) of another abstract quantity, referred to as *efficacy* (denoted e in Equation 3.7). Stephenson also assumed that the tissue response was some function (not direct) of stimulus. Thus, tissue response was given by:

$$\text{Response} = f(\text{Stimulus}) = f\left[\frac{[A]e}{[A] + K_A}\right]. \qquad (3.7)$$

It can be seen that efficacy in this model is both an agonist and a tissue-specific term. Furchgott [9] separated the tissue and agonist components of efficacy by defining a term *intrinsic efficacy* (denoted ε), which is a strictly agonist-specific term (i.e., this term defines the quantum stimulus given to a single receptor by the agonist). The product of receptor number ($[R_t]$) and intrinsic efficacy is then considered to be the agonist- and tissue-dependent element of agonism:

$$\text{Response} = f\left[\frac{[A] \cdot \varepsilon \cdot [R_t]}{[A] + K_A}\right]. \qquad (3.8)$$

The function f is usually hyperbolic, which introduces the nonlinearity between receptor occupancy and response. A common experimentally observed relationship between receptor stimulus and response is a rectangular hyperbola (see Chapter 2). Thus, response can be thought of as a hyperbolic function of stimulus:

$$\text{Response} = \frac{\text{Stimulus}}{\text{Stimulus} + \beta}, \qquad (3.9)$$

where β is a fitting factor representing the efficiency of coupling between stimulus and response. Substituting for stimulus from Equation 3.7 and rearranging, response in classical theory is given as:

$$\text{Response} = f\left[\frac{[A][R_t]\varepsilon/\beta}{[A](([R_t]\varepsilon/\beta) +) + K_A}\right]. \qquad (3.10)$$

The various components of classical theory relating receptor occupancy to tissue response are shown schematically in Figure 3.5. It will be seen that this formally is identical to the equation for response derived in the operational model (see material following), where $\tau = [R_t]\varepsilon/\beta$.

It is worth exploring the effects of the various parameters on agonist response in terms of classical receptor theory. Figure 3.6 shows the effect of changing efficacy. It can be seen that increasing efficacy causes an increased maximal response with little shift to the left of the

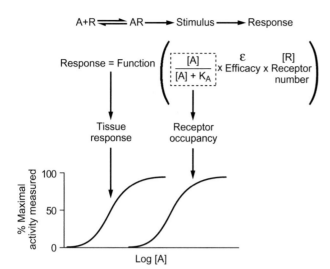

FIGURE 3.5 Major components of classical receptor theory. Stimulus is the product of intrinsic efficacy (ε), receptor number [R], and fractional occupancy as given by the Langmuir adsorption isotherm. A stimulus-response transduction function f translates this stimulus into tissue response. The curves defining receptor occupancy and response are translocated from each other by the stimulus-response function and intrinsic efficacy.

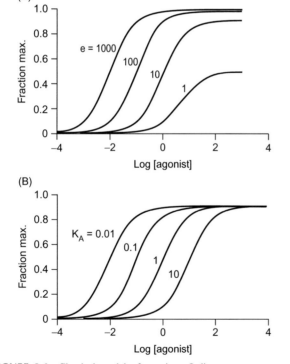

FIGURE 3.6 Classical model of agonism. Ordinates: response as a fraction of the system maximal response. Abscissae: logarithms of molar concentrations of agonist. (A) Effect of changing efficacy as defined by Stephenson [5]. Stimulus-response coupling defined by hyperbolic function Response = stimulus/(stimulus + 0.1). (B) Dose-response curves for agonist of e = 1 and various values for K_A.

dose-response curves until the system maximal response is achieved. Once this occurs (i.e., the agonist is a full agonist in the system), increasing efficacy has no further

effect on the maximal response, but rather causes shifts to the left of the dose-response curves (Figure 3.6A). In contrast, changing K_A, the equilibrium dissociation constant of the agonist-receptor complex, has no effect on maximal response but only shifts the curves along the concentration axis (Figure 3.6B).

3.6 THE OPERATIONAL MODEL OF RECEPTOR FUNCTION

Black and Leff [11] presented a model, termed the *operational model*, which avoids the inclusion of ad hoc terms for efficacy. Since its publication in 1983, the operational model has become the pre-eminent model for describing and quantifying agonism. This model is based on the experimental observation that the relationship between agonist concentration and tissue response is most often hyperbolic. This allows for response to be expressed in terms of receptor and tissue parameters (see Section 3.14.3):

$$\text{Response} = \frac{[A] \cdot \tau \cdot E_{\max}}{[A](\tau + 1) + K_A}, \qquad (3.11)$$

where the maximal response of the system is $E_{\max}$, the equilibrium dissociation constant of the agonist-receptor complex is K_A, and τ is the term that quantifies the power of the agonist to produce response (efficacy) and the ability of the system to process receptor stimulus into response. Specifically, τ is the ratio $[R_t]/K_E$, which is the receptor density divided by a transducer function expressing the ability of the system to convert agonist-receptor complex to response and the efficacy of the agonist. In this sense, K_E resembles Stephenson's efficacy term, except that it emanates from an experimental and pharmacological rationale (see Section 3.14.3). The essential elements of the operational model can be summarized graphically. In Figure 3.7, the relationship between agonist concentration and receptor binding (plane 1), the amount of agonist-receptor complex and response (plane 2), and agonist concentration and response (plane 3) can be seen. Early iterations of the operational model were, in fact, referred to as the "shoe-box" model, and the three planes were depicted as a box to show the interrelationship of response, transduction, and occupancy. The operational model furnishes a unified view of receptor occupancy, stimulation, and production of response through cellular processing. Figure 3.8A shows the effects of changing τ on dose-response curves. It can be seen that the effects are identical to changes in efficacy in the classical model; namely, an increased maximal response of partial agonism until the system maximal response is attained followed by sinistral displacements of the curves. As with the classical model, changes in K_A cause only

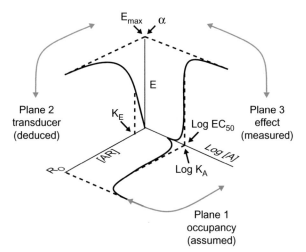

FIGURE 3.7 Principal components of the operational model. The 3-D array defines processes of receptor occupation (plane 1), the transduction of the agonist occupancy into response (plane 2) in defining the relationship between agonist concentration, and tissue response (plane 3). The term α refers to the intrinsic activity of the agonist.

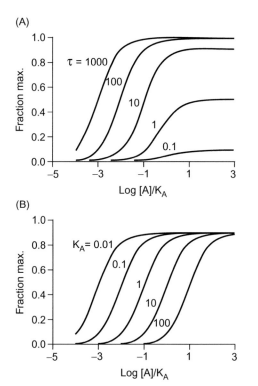

FIGURE 3.8 Operational model of agonism. Ordinates: response as a fraction of the system maximal response. Abscissae: logarithms of molar concentrations of agonist. (A) Effect of changing τ values. (B) Effect of changing K_A.

changes in the location parameter of the curve along the concentration axis (Figure 3.8B).

The operational model, as presented, shows dose-response curves with slopes of unity. This pertains specifically only to stimulus-response cascades where there is no cooperativity and the relationship between stimulus

([AR] complex) and overall response is controlled by a hyperbolic function with slope = 1. In practice, it is known that there are experimental dose-response curves with slopes that are not equal to unity and there is no *a priori* reason for there not to be cooperativity in the stimulus-response process. To accommodate the fitting of real data (with slopes not equal to unity) and the occurrence of stimulus-response cooperativity, a form of the operational model equation can be used with a variable slope (see Section 3.14.4):

$$E = \frac{E_{max}\tau^n[A]^n}{([A]+K_A)^n + \tau^n[A]^n}. \tag{3.12}$$

The operational model is used throughout this book for the determination of drug parameters in functional systems.

3.7 TWO-STATE THEORY

Two-state theory was originally formulated for ion channels. The earliest form, proposed by Del Castillo and Katz [15], was composed of a channel that when bound to an agonist changed from a closed to an open state. In the absence of agonist, all the channels are closed:

$$A + R \rightleftarrows AR_{closed} \rightleftarrows AR_{open}. \tag{3.13}$$

From theories on cooperative enzymes proposed by Monod and coworkers [16] came the idea that channels could coexist in both open and closed states:

$$
\begin{array}{ccc}
AR_{closed} & \xrightarrow{\alpha L} & AR_{open} \\
K \Updownarrow & & \Updownarrow \alpha K \\
R_{closed} & \xrightarrow{L} & R_{open} \\
+ & & + \\
A & & A
\end{array}
\tag{3.14}
$$

The number of channels open, as a fraction of the total number of channels, in the presence of a ligand [A] is given as (see Section 3.14.5):

$$\rho_{open} = \frac{\alpha L[A]/K_A + L}{[A]/K_A(1+\alpha L) + L + 1}. \tag{3.15}$$

There are some features of this type of system of note. First, it can be seen that there can be a fraction of the channels open in the absence of agonist. Specifically, Equation 3.15 predicts that in the absence of agonist ([A] = 0) the fraction of channels open is equal to $\rho_{open} = L/(1+L)$. For non-zero values of L this indicates that ρ_{open} will be >1. Second, ligands with preferred affinity for the open channel ($\alpha > 1$) will cause opening of the channel (they will be agonists). This can be seen from the ratio of channels open in the absence and presence of a saturating concentration of ligand [$\rho_\infty/\rho_0 = \alpha(1 + L)/(1 + \alpha L)$]. This equation reduces to:

$$\frac{\rho_\infty}{\rho_0} = \frac{1 + L}{(1/\alpha) + L}. \qquad (3.16)$$

It can be seen that for values $\alpha > 1$, the value $(1/\alpha) < 1$, and the denominator in Equation 3.16 will be less than the numerator. The ratio with the result that ρ_∞/ρ_0 will be > 1 (increased channel opening; i.e., agonism). Also, the potency of the agonist will be greater as the spontaneous channel opening is greater. This is because the observed EC_{50} of the agonist is:

$$EC_{50} = \frac{K_A(1 + L)}{(1 + \alpha L)}. \qquad (3.17)$$

This equation shows that the numerator will always be less than the denominator for $\alpha > 1$ (therefore, the $EC_{50} < K_A$, indicating increased potency over affinity), and that this differential gets larger with increasing values of L (increased spontaneous channel opening). The effects of an agonist with a tenfold greater affinity for the open channel, in systems of different ratios of spontaneously open channels, are shown in Figure 3.9. It can be seen that the maximal agonist activity, the elevated basal activity, and the agonist potency are increased with increasing values of L. Two-state theory has been applied to receptors [17−19], and was required to explain the experimental findings relating to constitutive activity in the late 1980s. Specifically, the ability of channels to spontaneously open with no ligand present was adapted for the model of receptors that could spontaneously form an activated state (in the absence of an agonist *vide infra*).

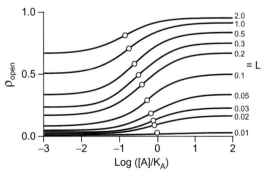

FIGURE 3.9 Dose-response curves to an agonist in a two-state ion-channel system. Ordinates: fraction of open channels. Abscissae: logarithms of molar concentrations of agonist. Numbers next to the curves refer to values of L (ratio of spontaneously open channels to closed channels). Curve calculated for an agonist with a tenfold higher affinity for the open channel ($\alpha = 10$). Open circles show EC_{50} values for the dose-response curves showing the increased potency to the agonist with increasing spontaneously open channels (increasing values of L).

3.8 THE TERNARY COMPLEX MODEL

Numerous lines of evidence in the study of G-protein-coupled receptors indicate that these receptors become activated, translocate in the cell membrane, and subsequently bind with other membrane-bound proteins. It was first realized that guanine nucleotides could affect the affinity of agonists but not antagonists, suggesting the two-stage binding of ligand to receptor and subsequently the complex to a G-protein [20−22]. The model describing such a system, first described by DeLean and colleagues [13], is termed the *ternary complex model*. Schematically, the process is:

$$A + R \rightleftarrows AR + G \rightleftarrows ARG, \qquad (3.18)$$

where the ligand is A, the receptor R, and the G-protein G. For a number of years this model was used to describe pharmacological receptor effects until new experimental evidence forced the modification of the original concept. Specifically, the fact that recombinant G-protein-coupled receptor systems demonstrate constitutive activity shows that receptors spontaneously form activated states capable of producing response through G-proteins in the absence of agonists. This necessitated modification of the ternary complex model.

3.9 THE EXTENDED TERNARY COMPLEX MODEL

The resulting modification is called the *extended ternary complex model* [3], which describes the spontaneous formation of active state receptor ([R_a]) from an inactive state receptor ([R_i]) according to an allosteric constant ($L = [R_a]/[R_i]$). The active state receptor can form a complex with G-protein ([G]) spontaneously to form R_aG, or agonist activation can induce formation of a ternary complex AR_aG:

$$(3.19)$$

As described in Section 3.14.6, the fraction ρ of G-protein-activating species (producing response) − namely, [R_aG] and [AR_aG] − as a fraction of the total number of receptor species [R_{tot}] is given by:

$$\rho = \frac{L[G]/K_G(1 + \alpha\gamma\,[A]/K_A)}{[A]/K_A(1 + \alpha L(1 + \gamma\,[G]/K_G)) + L(1 + [G]/K_G) + 1}, \qquad (3.20)$$

where the ligand is [A] and K_A and K_G are the equilibrium dissociation constants of the ligand-receptor and

G-protein receptor complexes, respectively. The term α refers to the multiple differences in affinity of the ligand for R_a over R_i (i.e., for $\alpha = 10$ the ligand has a tenfold greater affinity for R_a over R_i). Similarly, the term γ defines the multiple difference in affinity of the receptor for G-protein when the receptor is bound to the ligand. Thus, $\gamma = 10$ means that the ligand-bound receptor has a tenfold greater affinity for the G-protein than the ligand-unbound receptor.

It can be seen that the constants α and γ, insofar as they quantify the ability of the ligand to selectively cause the receptor to couple to G-proteins, become the manifestation of efficacy. Therefore, if a ligand produces a bias of the system toward more active receptor species (positive α) and/or enables the ligand-occupied receptor to bind to G-proteins with a higher affinity (positive γ), then it will be an agonist with positive efficacy. In addition, if a ligand selectively stabilizes the inactive state of the receptor ($\alpha < 1$) or reduces the affinity of the receptor for G-proteins ($\gamma < 1$), then it will have negative efficacy and subsequently will reverse elevated basal receptor activity. This will be observed as *inverse agonism*, but only in systems that demonstrate *constitutive receptor activity*.

3.10 CONSTITUTIVE RECEPTOR ACTIVITY AND INVERSE AGONISM

The extended ternary complex model can take into account the phenomenon of constitutive receptor activity. In genetically engineered systems where receptors can be expressed in high density, Costa and Herz [2] noted that high levels of receptor expression uncovered the existence of a population of spontaneously active receptors and that these receptors produce an elevated basal response in the system. The relevant factor is the ratio of receptors and G-proteins (i.e., elevated levels of receptor cannot yield constitutive activity in the absence of adequate amounts of G-protein, and vice versa). Constitutive activity (due to the $[R_aG]$ species) in the absence of ligand ($[A] = 0$) is expressed as:

$$\text{Constitutive Activity} = \frac{L[G]/K_G}{L(1 + [G]/K_G) + 1}. \quad (3.21)$$

From this equation it can be seen that for a given receptor density systems can spontaneously produce physiological response and that this response is facilitated by high G-protein concentration, high-affinity receptor/G-protein coupling (low value of K_G), and/or a natural tendency for the receptor to spontaneously form the active state. This latter property is described by the magnitude of L, a thermodynamic constant unique for every receptor.

Constitutive receptor activity is extremely important because it allows the discovery of ligands with negative efficacy. Before the discovery of constitutive GPCR activity, efficacy was considered only as a positive vector

(i.e., producing an increased receptor activity, and only ligand-mediated activation of receptors was thought to induce G-protein activity). With the discovery of spontaneous activation of G-proteins by unliganded receptors came the prospect of ligands that selectively inhibit this spontaneous activation, specifically inverse agonism.

Constitutive activity can be produced in a recombinant system by increasing the level of receptors expressed on the cell membrane. The formation of the constitutively active species ($[R_aG]$) is shown as:

$$R_i \underset{}{\overset{L}{\rightleftharpoons}} R_a \underset{\underset{G}{\nearrow K_g}}{\rightleftharpoons} R_aG \quad (3.22)$$

The dependence of constitutive activity on $[R_i]$ is given by (see Section 3.14.7):

$$\frac{[R_aG]}{[G_{tot}]} = \frac{[R_i]}{[R_i] + (K_G/L)}, \quad (3.23)$$

where $[R_i]$ is the receptor density, L is the allosteric constant describing the propensity of the receptor to spontaneously adopt the active state, and K_G is the equilibrium dissociation constant for the activated receptor/G-protein complex. It can be seen from Equation 3.23 that a hyperbolic relationship is predicted between constitutive activity and receptor concentration. Constitutive activity is favored by a large value of L (low-energy barrier to spontaneous formation of the active state) and/or a tight coupling between the receptor and the G-protein (low value for K_G). This provides a practical method of engineering constitutively active receptor systems; namely, through the induction of high levels of receptor expression. For example, in a system containing 1000 receptors with a native K_G/L value of 10^5 M, 0.9% of the G-proteins (i.e., nine G-proteins) will be activated. If this same system were to be subjected to an engineered receptor expression (through genetic means) of 100,000 receptors, then the number of activated G-proteins would rise to 50% (50,000 G-proteins). At some point, the threshold for observation of visibly elevated basal response in the cell will be exceeded, and the increased G-protein activation will result in an observable constitutive receptor activity.

Constitutive receptor systems are valuable in that they are capable of detecting inverse agonism and negative efficacy. Ligands that destabilize the spontaneous formation of activated receptor/G-protein complexes will reduce constitutive activity and function as inverse agonists in constitutively active receptor systems. The therapeutic relevance of inverse agonism is still unknown but it is clear that inverse agonists differ from conventional competitive antagonists. As more therapeutic experience is gained with these two types of antagonists, the importance of negative efficacy in the therapeutic arena will become clear. At this point it is important to note if a given antagonist possesses a property for retrospective evaluation of its effects.

The most probable mechanism for inverse agonism is the same one operable for positive agonism; namely, selective receptor state affinity. However, unlike agonists that have a selectively higher affinity for the receptor active state (to induce G-protein activation and subsequent physiological response), inverse agonists have a selectively higher affinity for the inactive receptor state and thus uncouple already spontaneously coupled [R_aG] species in the system.

It can be seen from Equation 3.23 that the magnitude of the allosteric constant L and/or the magnitude of the receptor/G-protein ratio determines the amount of constitutive activity in any receptor system. In binding studies, low levels of [R_aG] complex (with concomitant activation of G-protein) may be insignificant in comparison to the levels of total ligand-bound receptor species (i.e., [AR_aG] and [AR]). However, in highly coupled functional receptor systems a low level of spontaneous receptor interaction may result in a considerable observable response (due to stimulus-response amplification of stimulus; see Chapter 2). Thus, the observed constitutive activity in a functional system (due to high receptor density) can be much greater than expected from the amounts of active receptor species generated (see Figure 3.10). This suggests that for optimal observation of constitutive receptor activity and detection of inverse agonism, functional, rather than radioligand binding, systems should be used.

A practical approach to constructing constitutively active receptor systems, as defined by Equation 3.23, is through receptor over-expression. Thus, exposure of surrogate cells to high concentrations of cDNA for receptors yields increasing cellular expression of receptors. This in turn, can lead to elevated basal response due to

spontaneous receptor activation. Figure 3.11 shows the development of constitutive receptor activity in melanophore cells transfected with cDNA for human calcitonin receptor. Melanophores are especially well suited for experiments with constitutive activity, as the effects can be seen in real time with visible light. Figures 3.11A and B show the difference in the dispersion of melanin (response to G_s-protein activation due to constitutive calcitonin receptor activity) upon transfection with cDNA for the receptor. Figure 3.11C shows the dose-response relationship between the cDNA added and the constitutive activity as predicted by Equation 3.23.

As described by the extended ternary complex model, the extent of constitutive activity observed will vary with the receptor according to the magnitude of L for each receptor. This is shown in Figure 3.12, where the constitutive activity as a function of cDNA concentration is shown for a number of receptors. It can be seen from this figure that increasing receptor expression (assumed to result from the exposure to increasing concentrations of receptor cDNA) causes elevation of basal cellular response. It can also be seen that the threshold and maximal asymptotic value for this effect varies with receptor type, thereby reflecting the different propensity of receptors to spontaneously form the active state (varying magnitudes of L).

The term 'inverse agonist' is in some ways a misnomer, as these ligands really are simply antagonists with an added feature that allows them to reduce elevated basal activity. Thus, in the absence of constitutive activity, inverse agonists function like competitive antagonists. However, the fact that reversal of elevated basal activity produces a concentration-response curve indicative of a type of agonism leads to behaviors for these molecules that parallel some behaviors of normal positive agonists. Inverse agonism can be modeled with the Black-Leff

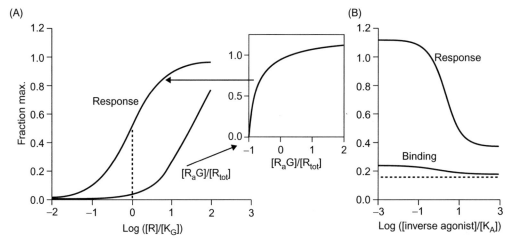

FIGURE 3.10 Constitutive activity due to receptor over-expression: visualization through binding and function. (A) Constitutive activity observed as receptor species ([R_aG]/[R_{tot}]) and cellular function ([R_aG]/([R_aG] + β), where $\beta = 0.03$. Stimulus-response function ([R_aG]/([R_aG] + β)) shown in inset. The output of the [R_aG] function becomes the input for the response function. Dotted line shows relative amounts of elevated receptor species and functional response at [R]/K_G = 1. (B) Effects of an inverse agonist in a system with [R]/K_G = 1 (see panel A) as observed through receptor binding and cellular function.

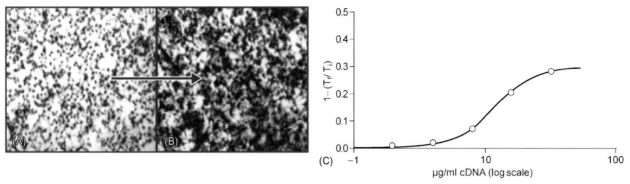

FIGURE 3.11 Constitutive activity in melanophores expressing hCTR2 receptor. (A) Basal melanophore activity. (B) Effect of transfection with human cDNA for human calcitonin receptors (16 μg/ml). (C) Concentration-response curve for cDNA for human calcitonin receptors (abscissae as log scale) and constitutive activity. Data redrawn from [26].

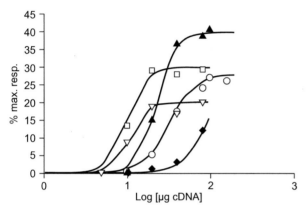

FIGURE 3.12 Dependence of constitutive receptor activity as ordinates (expressed as a percent of the maximal response to a full agonist for each receptor) versus magnitude of receptor expression (expressed as the amount of human cDNA used for transient transfection, logarithmic scale) in *Xenopus laevis* melanophores. Data shown for human chemokine CCR5 receptors (open circles), chemokine CXCR receptors (filled triangles), neuropeptide Y type 1 receptors (filled diamonds), neuropeptide Y type 2 receptors (open squares), and neuropeptide Y type 4 receptors (open inverted triangles). Data recalculated and redrawn from [26].

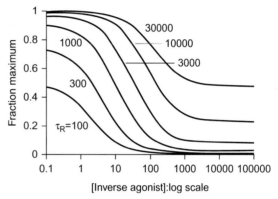

FIGURE 3.13 Inverse agonism as calculated by equation 3.24. Shown are curves for $\tau_R = 100$, 300, 1000, 3000 and 10000 in a system of $L = 10^{-3}$[G]/$K_G = 10$. The inverse agonist has $\alpha = 0.03$ and $\gamma = 0.1$.

operational model by utilizing the expression for active receptor species given by the extended ternary complex model (Equation 3.20), multiplying this by receptor density [R_{tot}] and inserting the result into the base expression for the Black-Leff model (Equation 3.54) to yield:

$$\text{Response} = \frac{L[G]/K_G(1 + \alpha\gamma\,[A]/K_A)\tau_R}{\begin{array}{c}[A]/K_A(1 + \alpha L(1 + \gamma\,[G]/K_G(1 + \tau_R))) \\ + L[G]/K_G(1 + \tau_R)L + 1\end{array}}$$

(3.24)

The efficacy term τ_R is the efficacy of the spontaneously formed active state of the receptor. Figure 3.13 shows the effect of increasing receptor density on the concentration-response curve to an inverse agonist ($\alpha = 0.03$, $\gamma = 0.1$). Thus, as there is a greater receptor reserve in the system (increasing τ_R), concentration-response curves shift to the right and the maximal inverse effect decreases. Thus, in a very sensitive system, partial inverse agonism can result.

3.11 THE CUBIC TERNARY COMPLEX MODEL

While the extended ternary complex model accounts for the presence of constitutive receptor activity in the absence of ligands, it is thermodynamically incomplete from the standpoint of the interaction of receptor and G-protein species. Specifically, it must be possible from a thermodynamic point of view for the inactive state receptor (ligand bound and unbound) to interact with G-proteins. The cubic ternary complex model accommodates this possibility [23−25]. From a practical point of view, it allows for the potential of receptors (whether unbound or bound by inverse agonists) to sequester G-proteins into a non-signaling state.

A schematic representation of receptor systems in terms of the cubic ternary complex model is shown in Figure 3.14. The amount of signaling species (as a fraction of total receptor) as defined by the cubic ternary complex model (see Section 3.13.8) predicts that the constitutive activity of receptor systems can reach a maximal asymptote which is below the system maximum (partial constitutive activity). This is because the cubic ternary

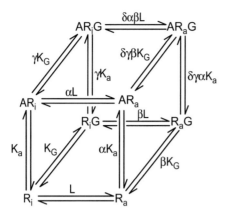

FIGURE 3.14 Major components of the cubic ternary complex model [23–25]. The major difference between this model and the extended ternary complex model is the potential for formation of the [AR$_i$G] complex and the [R$_i$G] complex, both receptor/G-protein complexes that do not induce dissociation of G-protein subunits and subsequent response. Efficacy terms in this model are α, γ, and δ.

complex model predicts the maximal constitutive activity, as given by Equation 3.25:

$$\rho = \frac{\beta L[G]/K_G(1 + \alpha\gamma\delta[A]/K_A)}{[A]/K_A(1 + \alpha L + \gamma[G]/K_G(1 + \alpha\gamma\beta\delta L)) + [G]/K_G(1 + \beta L) + L + 1} \quad (3.25)$$

There are some specific differences between the cubic and extended ternary complex models in terms of their predictions of system and drug behavior. The first is that the receptor, either ligand bound or not bound, can form a complex with the G-protein and that this complex need not signal (i.e., [AR$_i$G] and [R$_i$G]). Under these circumstances, an inverse agonist (one that stabilizes the inactive state of the receptor) theoretically can form inactive ternary complexes and thus sequester G-proteins away from signaling pathways. There is evidence that this can occur with cannabinoid receptors [27]. The cubic ternary complex model also where [A] = 0 and [G] → ∞ predicts:

Maximal Constitutive Activity = $\beta L/(1 + \beta L)$.   (3.26)

It can be seen from this equation that maximal constitutive activity need not reach a maximal asymptote of unity. Submaximal constitutive activity has been observed with some receptors with maximal receptor expression [26]. While there is scattered evidence that the cubic ternary complex is operative in some receptor systems, and while it is thermodynamically more complete, it also is heuristic in that it includes more individually nonverifiable constants than other models. This makes this model limited in practical application.

3.12 MULTISTATE RECEPTOR MODELS AND PROBABILISTIC THEORY

The previously discussed models fall under the category of "linkage models," in that the protein species are all identified and linked together with the energies for their formation controlling their relative prevalence. These models work well as approximations, but fall short for descriptions of true protein thermodynamics where multiple conformations of unknown identity can coexist. Linkage model approximations can be used to define the relationship between general protein species (i.e., ligand bound and unbound) but cannot accommodate complex multistate receptor systems. However, sometimes such multistate models are required to describe nuances of receptor signaling and ligand functional selectivity. While multistate models do not define actual receptor species, they can estimate the probability of their formation. To describe a multistate model quantitatively, it is simplest to arbitrarily begin with one receptor state (referred to as [R$_o$]e) and define the affinity of a ligand [A] and a G-protein [G] for that state as [28,29]:

$$^A K_o = [AR_o]/[R_o][A] \quad (3.27)$$

and:

$$^G K_o = [GR_o]/[R_o][G], \quad (3.28)$$

respectively. It is useful to define a series of probabilities en route to the presentation of Equations 3.29 to 3.32. The probability of the receptor being in that form is denoted p$_o$ while the probability of the receptor forming another conformation [R$_1$] is defined as p$_1$. The ratio of the probabilities for forming state R$_1$ versus R$_o$ is given as j$_1$ where j$_1$ = p$_{1/}$p$_o$; the value j controls the energy of transition between the states. The relative probability of forming state [R$_1$] with ligand binding is denoted ^{A}j$_1$ = ^{A}p$_1$/^{A}p$_o$ and with G-protein binding as ^{G}j$_1$ = ^{G}p$_1$/^{G}p$_o$. An important vector operating on this system is defined as b, where b refers to the fractional stabilization of a state with binding of either ligand (defined ^{A}b$_1$ = ^{A}j$_1$/j$_i$) or G-protein (^{G}b$_1$ = ^{G}j$_1$/j$_i$). Every ligand and G-protein has characteristic values of b for each receptor state and it is these b vectors that constitute ligand affinity and efficacy. With these probabilities and vectors, the following operators are defined:

$$\Omega = 1 + \Sigma j_i \quad (3.29)$$

$$\Omega_A = 1 + \Omega\Sigma^A b_i p_i \quad (3.30)$$

$$\Omega_G = 1 + \Omega\Sigma^G b_i p_i \quad (3.31)$$

$$\Omega_{AG} = 1 + \Omega\Sigma^A b_i{}^G b_i p_i, \quad (3.32)$$

where i refers to the specific conformational state and the superscripts G and A refer to the G-protein and ligand-bound forms, respectively. With these functions defined, it can be shown that macroaffinity is given by:

$$\text{Macroaffinity } (K) = {}^A k_0 \Omega_A (\Omega)^{-1}, \quad (3.33)$$

where k$_0$ is related to the interaction free energy between ligand and a reference microstate of the receptor. A measure of efficacy is given by:

$$\text{Efficacy } (\alpha) = (\Omega\Omega_{AG})(\Omega_A\Omega_G)^{-1} \quad (3.34)$$

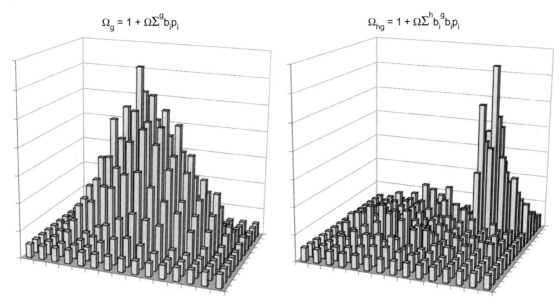

$$\Omega_g = 1 + \Omega\Sigma^g b_i p_i \qquad\qquad \Omega_{hg} = 1 + \Omega\Sigma^h b_i{}^g b_i p_i$$

FIGURE 3.15 Relative abundance of different receptor conformations shown as histograms. Left panel shows receptor at rest and right panel the ensemble of conformations when bound by a ligand. In the right panel, the conformations for which the ligand has high affinity are stabilized and enriched at the expense of other conformations. The composition of the new collection of conformations depends upon the molecular structure of the agonist allowing for ligand-specific pharmacological effect.

With this model, the effects of ligand binding on collections of receptor conformations (ensembles) can be simulated (see Figure 3.15). The unique feature of this model is that it allows the simulation of collections of conformations that may have differing pharmacological effects. This is extremely useful in the description of agonist functional selectivity where different agonists activate different portions of stimulus-response cascades through activation of the same receptor (see [30]).

3.13 CHAPTER SUMMARY AND CONCLUSIONS

- Models are constructed from samples of data and can be used to predict the behavior of the system for all conditions (the population of data).
- Preferred models have parameters that have some physiological or pharmacological rationale. In general, the behavior of these parameters can be likened to changes in potency and/or efficacy of drugs.
- Models can resolve apparent conflicts in observed data and be used to optimally design experiments.
- From the time of A. J. Clark until the late 1970s, receptor models have been refined to describe drug affinity and efficacy. These ideas are collectively referred to as "classical" receptor theory.
- A major modification in the description of drug function is termed the *operational model*. This model is theoretically more sound than classical theory and extremely versatile for estimating drug parameters in functional systems.

- The observation that receptors can demonstrate spontaneous activity necessitated elements of ion two-state theory to be incorporated into receptor theory.
- The ternary complex model followed by the extended ternary complex model was devised to describe the action of drugs on G-protein-coupled receptors.
- The discovery of constitutive receptor activity uncovered a major new idea in receptor pharmacology; namely, the concept of negative efficacy and inverse agonism.
- The cubic ternary complex model considers receptors and G-proteins as a synoptic system with some interactions that do not lead to visible activation.

3.14 DERIVATIONS

- Radioligand binding to receptor dimers demonstrating cooperative behavior (3.14.1).
- Effect of variation in an HIV-1 binding model (3.14.2).
- Derivation of the operational model (3.14.3).
- Operational model forcing function for variable slope (3.14.4).
- Derivation of two-state theory (3.14.5).
- Derivation of the extended ternary complex model (3.14.6).
- Dependence of constitutive activity on receptor density (3.14.7).
- Derivation of the cubic ternary complex model (3.14.8).

3.14.1 Radioligand Binding to Receptor Dimers Demonstrating Cooperative Behavior

It is assumed that receptor dimers can form in the cell membrane (two [R] species to form one [R-R] species). Radioligand [A*] can bind to the receptor [R] to form radioactive complexes [A*R], [A*R - AR], and [A*R-A*R]. It is also assumed that there is an allosteric interaction between the receptors when they dimerize. Therefore, the affinity of the receptor(s) changes with dimerization:

$$
\begin{array}{c}
A \\
+ \\
A \qquad R \\
+ \qquad + \\
A^* + R \underset{}{\overset{K}{\rightleftharpoons}} A^*R + A^* + R \underset{}{\overset{\alpha K}{\rightleftharpoons}} A^*R\text{-}RA^* \\
\Big\updownarrow K \qquad \Big\updownarrow \alpha K \\
A^* + R + AR \underset{\alpha K}{\longrightarrow} A^*R\text{-}RA^* \\
+ \\
A \\
+ \\
R \\
\Big\updownarrow \alpha K \\
AR\text{-}RA
\end{array}
$$

$$(3.35)$$

The conservation equation for the total receptor species is given as:

$$
\begin{aligned}
[R_{tot}] = {} & [R] + [AR] + [A^*R] + [A^*R\text{-}AR] \\
& + [AR\text{-}AR] + [A^*R\text{-}A^*R].
\end{aligned}
$$

$$(3.36)$$

The radioactive signal (denoted ρ) is produced from the receptor species bound to radioligand [A*]:

$$
\rho = \frac{[A^*R] + [A^*R\text{-}AR] + 2[A^*R\text{-}A^*R]}{[R_{tot}]}. \tag{3.37}
$$

Using the equilibrium equations for the system, this equation becomes:

$$
\rho = \frac{[A^*]K + \alpha[A^*][A]K^2 + 2\alpha[A^*]^2K^2}{1 + [A]K + [A^*]K + \alpha[A^*][A]K^2 + \alpha[A]^2K^2 + a[A^*]^2K^2}, \tag{3.38}
$$

where K is the association constant. Assume that a fixed concentration of radioligand [A*] is bound to the receptor, yielding a fixed radioactive signal. In the presence of a range of concentrations of a nonradioactive version of ligand [A], the signal from a fixed concentration of radioactive ligand ([A*]) (denoted ω) can be calculated

from the ratio of Equation 3.38 with [A] = 0 and [A*] fixed over the equations evaluated with [A*] fixed:

$$
\omega = \frac{([A^*]/K_d) + \alpha[A^*]K_d^2 + 2\alpha([A^*]/K_d)^2}{\begin{array}{c}(1 + [A^*]/K_d) + \alpha([A^*]/K_d)^2\end{array}}{\begin{array}{c}(1 + [A]/K_d + [A^*]/K_d + \alpha([A^*][A]/K_d^2) + \alpha([A^*]/K_d)^2 \\ + \alpha([A]/K_d)^2)([A^*]/K_d) + 2\alpha([A^*]/K_d)^2)\end{array}}
$$

$$(3.39)$$

where $K_d = 1/K$. Using Equation 3.39, displacement curves for this system can be calculated. If the binding of one ligand is positively cooperative with respect to the binding of the other ($\alpha > 1$) (binding of one [A] and subsequent dimerization with another receptor increases the affinity for the second [A]), then an apparently paradoxical *increase* in the radioactive signal is observed from addition of nonradioactive ligand if low concentrations of radioligand are used.

3.14.2 Effect of Variation in an HIV-1 Binding Model

Assuming that all interactions of the species are possible, the system consists of the receptor CCR5 [R], radioligand CD4 [CD], viral coat protein gp120 [gp], and potential displacing ligand [B]:

$$
\begin{array}{c}
B \\
gp \qquad + \qquad CD \\
+ \qquad\qquad + \\
gp + CD \underset{}{\overset{K_1'}{\rightleftharpoons}} gp\text{-}CD + R \underset{}{\overset{K_2'}{\rightleftharpoons}} gpCD \\
{}^{K_5'}\diagdown \quad \Big\updownarrow K_4' \quad \diagup {}^{K_3'} \\
CD\text{-}R \qquad\quad gp\text{-}R \\
B\text{-}R
\end{array}
$$

$$(3.40)$$

The CCR5 receptor conservation equation is given as:

$$
[R_{total}] = [R] + [CDR] + [gpCDR] + [gpR] + [BR], \tag{3.41}
$$

where the concentration of the complex between viral coat protein gp120 and receptor is [gpR], concentration of complex between the receptor and complex between gp120 and CD4 is [gpCDR], membrane protein CD4 receptor complex density is [CDR], and foreign ligand B receptor complex is [BR]. The signal is generated by radioactive CD4 resulting from the two receptor-bound species [gpCDR] and [CDR]. It is assumed that [gp] > [CD] > [R] (as is common in experimental systems). The signal, as a fraction of the total receptor concentration, is given by:

$$
\text{Fractional signal} = \rho = \frac{[gpCDR] + [CDR]}{[R_{total}]}. \tag{3.42}
$$

From the equilibrium equations, expressions for the various receptor species can be derived and substituted into Equation 3.42. With conversion of all equilibrium association constants to equilibrium dissociation constants, a general binding expression results for radioactive CD4 binding to CCR5 with gp120 as a cofactor [14]:

$$\rho = \frac{([CD]/K_1)([gp]K_2) + [CD]/K_5}{[CDK_1]([gp]/K_2 + K_1/K_5) + [gp]/K_3 + [B]/K_4 + 1}$$

(3.43)

where the equilibrium dissociation constants are denoted K_1 (gp/CD4), K_2 (gp-CD4 complex/receptor), K_3 (gp/receptor), K_4 (ligand B/receptor), and K_5 (CD4/receptor). The observed affinity of the radiolabel CD4 is given by the expression:

$$K_{obs} = \frac{K_1(([gp]/K_3) + [B]/K_4 + 1)}{[gp]/K_2 + K_1/K_5}.$$

(3.44)

Solving Equation 3.44 for $[B] = 0$ and variable $[B]$ yields the equation defining the IC_{50} of a nonradioactive ligand inhibitor (defined as the molar concentration of ligand $[B]$ that blocks the radioactive binding signal by 50%). This yields the equation for the concentration of $[B]$ that produces 50% inhibition of radioactive CD4 binding:

$$IC_{50} = K_4([CD]/K_1([gp]/K_2 + K_1/K_5) + [gp]/K_3 + 1).$$

(3.45)

From Equation 3.45 it can be seen that the system-independent measure of affinity (K_4) is given by:

$$K_4 = \frac{[IC_{50}]}{([CD]/K_1([gp]/K_2 + K_1/K_5) + [gp]/K_3 + 1)}.$$

(3.46)

The assay returns the IC_{50}, the concentration of $[B]$ that blocks the binding by 50%. The desired estimate is K_4, the system-independent estimate of the affinity of $[B]$ for the interactants of the system. This model addresses the following question: What is the effect of variation in [gp120] on the IC_{50} and hence the estimate of K_4? At this point it is useful to define two ratios. The first is the ratio of the differential affinity of the gp/CD4 complex versus the affinity of gp120 for the receptor alone. This is defined as $\theta = K_3/K_2$. Large values of θ indicate that the preformed complex gp/CD4 is the principal binding species to the receptor and that the affinity of gp for the receptor is relatively unimportant. In experimental systems, this is found to be true. The second useful ratio is the differential affinity of CD4 for gp120 over the receptor. This is defined as $\psi = K_5/K_1$. High values of ψ indicate that CD4 prefers to form the CD4/gp120 complex over binding to the receptor, and this agrees with the known physiology of HIV entry into cells via this mechanism:

$$K_4 = \frac{[IC_{50}]}{([CD]/K_1([gp]/K_2 + 1/\psi) + [gp]/\theta K_2 + 1)}.$$

(3.47)

Consistent with the known physiology, the values of both θ and ψ are high. Therefore, $1/\theta$ and $1/\psi \rightarrow 0$ and Equation 3.47 leads to a relation of the form:

$$K_4 = \frac{[IC_{50}]}{([CD]/K_1)([gp]/K_2) + 1}.$$

(3.48)

It can be seen from Equation 3.48 that unknown variation in gp120 levels can lead to differences in the correction factor between the experimentally observed IC_{50} and the desired quantity K_4. However, this variation is minimal if low levels of control signal are used for screening (i.e., minimal concentration of CD4 is used to gain an acceptable signal-to-noise ratio).

3.14.3 Derivation of the Operational Model

The basis of this model is the experimental fact that most agonist dose-response curves are hyperbolic in nature. The reasoning for making this assumption is as follows. If agonist binding is governed by mass action, then the relationship between the agonist-receptor complex and response must be either linear or hyperbolic as well. Response is thus defined as:

$$Response = \frac{[A] \cdot E_{max}}{[A] + v}$$

(3.49)

where the concentration of agonist is $[A]$, E_{max} is the maximal response of the system, and v is a fitting parameter determining the sensitivity of the system to $[A]$. This expresses the agonist concentration as:

$$[A] = \frac{Response \cdot v}{E_{max}[A] - Response}$$

(3.50)

Also, mass action defines the concentration of agonist-receptor complex as:

$$[AR] = \frac{[A] \cdot [R_t]}{[A] + K_A}$$

(3.51)

where $[R_t]$ is the receptor density and K_A is the equilibrium dissociation constant of the agonist-receptor complex. This yields a function for $[A]$ as well:

$$[A] = \frac{[AR] \cdot K_A}{[R_t] - [AR]}$$

(3.52)

Equating Equations 3.49 and 3.51 and rearranging yields:

$$Response = \frac{[AR] \cdot E_{max} \cdot K_A}{[AR](K_A - v) + [R_t]v}$$

(3.53)

It can be seen that if $K_A < v$ then negative and/or infinite values for response are allowed. No physiological counterpart to such behavior exists. This leaves a linear relationship between agonist concentration and response (where $K_A = v$) or a hyperbolic one ($K_A > v$). There are few if any cases of truly linear relationships between agonist concentration and tissue response. Therefore, the default for the relationship is a hyperbolic one.

Assuming a hyperbolic relationship between response and the amount of agonist-receptor complex, response is defined as:

$$\frac{\text{Response}}{E_{max}} = \frac{[AR]}{[AR] + K_E}, \quad (3.54)$$

where K_E is the fitting parameter for the hyperbolic response. However, K_E also has a pharmacological meaning, in that it is the concentration of [AR] complex that produces half the maximal response. It also defines the ease with which the agonist produces response (i.e., it is a transduction constant). The more efficient the process from production to [AR] to response, the smaller is K_E. Combining Equations 3.52 and 3.53 yields the quintessential equation for the operational model:

$$\text{Response} = \frac{[A] \cdot [R_t] \cdot E_{max}}{[A]([R_t] + K_E) + K_A \cdot K_E} \quad (3.55)$$

A very useful constant used to characterize the propensity of a given system and a given agonist to yield response is the ratio $[R_t]/K_E$. This is denoted τ. Substituting for τ yields the working equation for the operational model:

$$\text{Response} = \frac{[A] \cdot \tau \cdot E_{max}}{[A](\tau + 1) + K_A} \quad (3.56)$$

This model also can accommodate a dose-response curve having Hill coefficients different from unity (see next section). This can occur if the stimulus-response coupling mechanism has inherent cooperativity. A general procedure can be used to change any receptor model into a variable slope operational function. This is done by passing the receptor stimulus through a forcing function.

3.14.4 Operational Model Forcing Function for Variable Slope

The operational model allows the simulation of cellular response from receptor activation. In some cases, there may be cooperative effects in the stimulus-response cascades translating activation of receptor-to-tissue response. This can cause the resulting concentration-response curve to have a Hill coefficient different from unity. In general, there is a standard method for doing this; namely, re-expressing the receptor occupancy and/or activation expression (defined by the particular molecular model of receptor function) in terms of the operational model with Hill coefficient not equal to unity. The operational model utilizes the concentration of response-producing receptor as the substrate for a Michaelis–Menten type of reaction, given as:

$$\text{Response} = \frac{[\text{Activated Receptor}]E_{max}}{[\text{Activated Receptor}] + K_E}, \quad (3.57)$$

where K_E is the concentration of activated receptor species that produces half maximal response in the cell and E_{max} is the maximal capability of response production by the cell. If the system exhibits cooperativity at the cellular level, then Equation 3.57 can be rewritten as:

$$\text{Response} = \frac{[\text{Activated Receptor}]^n E_{max}}{[\text{Activated Receptor}]^n + K_E^n} \quad (3.58)$$

where n is the slope of the concentration-response curve. The quantity of activated receptor is given by $\rho_{AR} \times [R_t]$, where ρ_{AR} is the fraction of total receptor in the activated form and $[R_t]$ is the total receptor density of the preparation. Substituting into Equation 3.58 and defining $\tau = [R_t]/K_E$ yields:

$$\text{Response} = \frac{\rho_{AR}^n \tau^n E_{max}}{\rho_{AR}^n \tau^n + 1}. \quad (3.59)$$

The fractional receptor species ρ_{AR} is generally given by:

$$\rho_{AR^n} = \frac{[\text{Active Receptor Species}]^n}{[\text{Total Receptor Species}]^n}, \quad (3.60)$$

where the active receptor species are the ones producing response and the total receptor species given by the receptor conservation equation for the particular system $\rho_{AR} = \text{numerator/denominator}$). It follows that:

$$\text{Response} = \frac{(\text{Active Receptor})^n \tau^n E_{max}}{(\text{Active Receptor})^n \tau^n + (\text{Total Receptor})^n} \quad (3.61)$$

Therefore, the operational model for agonism can be rewritten for variable slope by passing the stimulus equation through the forcing function (Equation 3.61) to yield:

$$\text{Response} = \frac{\tau^n \cdot [A]^n \cdot E_{max}}{([A] + K_A)^n + \tau^n [A]^n} \quad (3.62)$$

3.14.5 Derivation of Two-State Theory

A channel exists in two states: open (R_{open}) and closed (R_{closed}). A ligand [A] binds to both with an equilibrium association constant K for the closed channel and αK for the open channel:

$$\begin{array}{ccc} AR_{closed} & \xrightarrow{\alpha L} & AR_{open} \\ K \Updownarrow & & \Updownarrow \alpha K \\ R_{closed} & \xrightarrow{L} & R_{open} \\ + & & + \\ A & & A \end{array} \quad (3.63)$$

The equilibrium equations for the various species are:

$$[AR_{closed}] = [AR_{open}]/\alpha L, \quad (3.64)$$

$$[R_{closed}] = [AR_{open}]/\alpha L[A]K, \qquad (3.65)$$

and:

$$[R_{closed}] = [AR_{open}]/\alpha[A]K. \qquad (3.66)$$

The conservation equation for channel species is:

$$[R_{total}] = [AR_{open}] + [AR_{closed}] + [R_{open}] + [R_{closed}]. \quad (3.67)$$

The amount of open channel, expressed as a fraction of total channel $\rho_{open} = ([AR_{open}] + [R_{open}])/[R_{total}])$, is:

$$\rho_{open} = \frac{\alpha L[A]/K_A + L}{[A]/K_A(1 + \alpha L) + L + 1}, \qquad (3.68)$$

where K_A is the equilibrium dissociation constant of the ligand-channel complex.

3.14.6 Derivation of the Extended Ternary Complex Model

The extended ternary complex model [3] was conceived after it was clear that receptors could spontaneously activate G-proteins in the absence of agonist. It is an amalgam of the ternary complex model [13] and two-state theory which allows proteins to spontaneously exist in two conformations, each having different properties with respect to other proteins and to ligands. Thus, two receptor species are described: $[R_a]$ (active state receptor able to activate G-proteins) and $[R_i]$ (inactive state receptors). These coexist according to an allosteric constant ($L = [R_a]/[R_i]$):

$$
\begin{array}{ccccc}
 & \overset{\alpha L}{\underset{}{\rightleftharpoons}} & & \overset{\gamma K_g}{\underset{}{\rightleftharpoons}} & \\
AR_i & & AR_a & & AR_aG \\
K_a \updownarrow & & \alpha K_a \updownarrow & & \updownarrow \alpha\gamma K_a \\
R_i & \overset{L}{\underset{}{\rightleftharpoons}} & R_a & \underset{K_g}{\overset{}{\rightleftharpoons}} & R_aG \\
& & & G &
\end{array}
\qquad (3.69)
$$

The equilibrium equations for the various species are:

$$[AR_i] = [AR_aG]/\alpha\gamma L[G]K_g, \qquad (3.70)$$

$$[AR_a] = [AR_aG]/\gamma[G]K_g, \qquad (3.71)$$

$$[R_a] = [AR_aG]/\alpha\gamma[G]K_g[A]K_a, \qquad (3.72)$$

$$[R_i] = [AR_aG]/\alpha\gamma L[G]K_g[A]K_a, \qquad (3.73)$$

and:

$$[R_aG] = [AR_aG]/\alpha\gamma[A]K_a. \qquad (3.74)$$

The conservation equation for receptor species is:

$$[R_{tot}] = [AR_aG] + [R_aG] + [AR_a] + [AR_i] + [R_a] + [R_i]. \qquad (3.75)$$

It is assumed that the receptor species leading to G-protein activation (and therefore physiological response) are complexes between the activated receptor ($[R_a]$) and the G-protein; namely, $[AR_aG] + [R_aG]$. The fraction of the response-producing species of the total receptor species $(([AR_aG] + [R_aG])/R_{tot})$ is denoted ρ and given by:

$$\rho = \frac{L[G]/K_G(1 + \alpha\gamma[A]/K_A)}{[A]/K_A(1 + \alpha L(1 + \gamma[G]/K_G)) + L(1 + [G]/K_G) + 1}. \qquad (3.76)$$

3.14.7 Dependence of Constitutive Activity on Receptor Density

The production of signaling species ($[R_aG]$) by spontaneous coupling of the active state receptor species ($[R_a]$) to G-protein ($[G]$) is shown as:

$$
R_i \overset{L}{\underset{}{\rightleftharpoons}} R_a \underset{K_g \atop G}{\overset{}{\rightleftharpoons}} R_aG
\qquad (3.77)
$$

The equilibrium equations are:

$$L = [R_a]/[R_i] \qquad (3.78)$$

and:

$$K_G = [R_aG]/[R_a][G]. \qquad (3.79)$$

The conservation equation for G-protein is $[G_{tot}] = [G] + [R_aG]$. The amount of receptor-activated G-protein expressed as a fraction of total G-protein ($[R_aG]/[G_{tot}]$) is:

$$\frac{[R_aG]}{[G_{tot}]} = \frac{[R_i]}{[R_i] + (K_G/L)}, \qquad (3.80)$$

where L is the allosteric constant and $[R_i]$ is the amount of transfected receptor in the inactive state.

3.14.8 Derivation of the Cubic Ternary Complex Model

The cubic ternary complex model takes into account the fact that both the active and inactive receptor species must have a finite affinity for G-proteins [23–25]. The two receptor species are denoted $[R_a]$ (active state receptor able to activate G-proteins) and $[R_i]$ (inactive state receptors). These can form species $[R_iG]$ and $[R_aG]$ spontaneously, and species $[AR_iG]$ and $[AR_aG]$ in the presence of ligand.

This forms eight vertices of a cube (see Figure 3.13). The equilibrium equations for the various species are:

$$[AR_i] = [AR_aG]/\alpha\gamma\delta\beta L[G]K_g, \qquad (3.81)$$

$$[AR_a] = [AR_aG]/\gamma\beta\delta[G]K_g, \qquad (3.82)$$

$$[R_a] = [AR_aG]/\alpha\gamma\delta\beta[G]K_g[A]K_a, \quad (3.83)$$

$$[R_i] = [AR_aG]/\alpha\gamma\delta\beta L[G]K_g[A]K_a, \quad (3.84)$$

$$[R_aG] = [AR_aG]/\alpha\gamma\delta[A]K_a, \quad (3.85)$$

$$[R_iG] = [AR_aG]/\alpha\gamma\delta\beta L[A]K_a, \quad (3.86)$$

and:

$$[AR_iG] = [AR_aG]/\alpha\delta\beta L. \quad (3.87)$$

The conservation equation for receptor species is:

$$[R_{tot}] = [AR_aG] + [AR_iG] + [R_iG] \\ + [R_aG] + [AR_a] + [AR_i] + [R_a] + [R_i]. \quad (3.88)$$

It is assumed that the receptor species leading to G-protein activation (and therefore physiological response) are complexes between the activated receptor ($[R_a]$) and the G-protein; namely, $[AR_aG] + [R_aG]$. The fraction of the response-producing species of the total receptor species — $([AR_aG] + [R_aG])/R_{tot}$ — is denoted ρ and is given by:

$$\rho = \frac{\beta L[G]/K_G(1 + \alpha\gamma\delta[A]/K_A)}{[A]/K_A(1 + \alpha L + \gamma[G]/K_G(1 + \alpha\gamma\beta L)) + [G]/K_G(1 + \beta L) + L + 1}. \quad (3.89)$$

REFERENCES

[1] Clark AJ. The mode of action of drugs on cells. London: Edward Arnold; 1933.
[2] Costa T, Herz A. Antagonists with negative intrinsic activity at δ-opioid receptors coupled to GTP-binding proteins. Proc Natl Acad Sci USA 1989;86:7321–5.
[3] Samama P, Cotecchia S, Costa T, Lefkowitz RJ. A mutation-induced activated state of the β2-adrenergic receptor: extending the ternary complex model. J Biol Chem 1993;268:4625–36.
[4] Clark AJ. General pharmacology. In: Heffter A, editor. Handbuch der Experimentellen Pharmakologie, 4. Berlin: Springer; 1937165–176. *Ergansungsweerk band.*
[5] Stephenson RP. A modification of receptor theory. Br J Pharmacol 1956;11:379–93.
[6] Ariens EJ. Affinity and intrinsic activity in the theory of competitive inhibition. Arch Int Pharmacodyn Ther 1954;99:32–49.
[7] Ariens EJ. Molecular pharmacology, Vol. 1. New York: Academic Press; 1964.
[8] MacKay D. A critical survey of receptor theories of drug action. In: Van Rossum JM, editor. Kinetics of drug action. Berlin: Springer-Verlag; 1977. p. 255–322.
[9] Furchgott RF. The use of β-haloalkylamines in the differentiation of receptors and in the determination of dissociation constants of receptor-agonist complexes. In: Harper NJ, Simmonds AB, editors. Advances in drug research. New York: Academic Press; 1966. p. 21–55.
[10] Furchgott RF. The classification of adrenoreceptors (adrenergic receptors): an evaluation from the standpoint of receptor theory. In: Blaschko H, Muscholl E, editors. Handbook of experimental pharmacology, catecholamines, Vol. 33. Berlin: Springer-Verlag; 1972. p. 283–335.
[11] Black JW, Leff P. Operational models of pharmacological agonist. Proc R Soc Lond [Biol] 1983;220:141.
[12] Cuatrecasas P. Membrane receptors. Ann Rev Biochem 1974;43:169–214.
[13] DeLean A, Stadel JM, Lefkowitz RJ. A ternary complex model explains the agonist-specific binding properties of adenylate cyclase coupled β-adrenergic receptor. J Biol Chem 1980;255:7108–17.
[14] Kenakin TP. The pharmacologic consequences of modeling synoptic receptor systems. In: Christopoulos A, editor. Biomedical applications of computer modeling. Boca Raton: CRC Press; 2000. p. 1–20.
[15] Del Castillo J, Katz B. Interaction at end-plate receptors between different choline derivatives. Proc R Soc London, B 1957;146:369–81.
[16] Monod J, Wyman J, Changeux JP. On the nature of allosteric transition. J Mol Biol 1965;12:306–29.
[17] Colquhoun D. The relationship between classical and cooperative models for drug action. In: Rang HP, editor. A symposium on drug receptors. Baltimore: University Park Press; 1973. p. 149–82.
[18] Karlin A. On the application of 'a plausible model' of allosteric proteins to the receptor for acetylcholine. J Theoret Biol 1967;16:306–20.
[19] Thron CD. On the analysis of pharmacological experiments in terms of an allosteric receptor model. Mol Pharmacol 1973;9:1–9.
[20] Hulme EC, Birdsall NJM, Burgen ASV, Metha P. The binding of antagonists to brain muscarinic receptors. Mol Pharmacol 1978;14:737–50.
[21] Lefkowitz RJ, Mullikin D, Caron MG. Regulation of β-adrenergic receptors by guanyl-5'-yl imidodiphosphate and other purine nucleotides. J Biol Chem 1976;251:4686–92.
[22] MaGuire ME, Van Arsdale PM, Gilman AG. An agonist-specific effect of guanine nucleotides on the binding of the beta adrenergic receptor. Mol Pharmacol 1976;12:335–9.
[23] Weiss JM, Morgan PH, Lutz MW, Kenakin TP. The cubic ternary complex receptor-occupancy model. I Model description J Theroet Biol 1996;178:151–67.
[24] Weiss JM, Morgan PH, Lutz MW, Kenakin TP. The cubic ternary complex receptor-occupancy model. *II. Understanding apparent affinity.* J Theroet Biol 1996;178:169–82.
[25] Weiss JM, Morgan PH, Lutz MW, Kenakin TP. The cubic ternary complex receptor-occupancy model. *III. Resurrecting efficacy.* J Theoret Biol 1996;181:381–97.
[26] Chen G, Way J, Armour S, Watson C, Queen K, Jayawrickreme C, et al. Use of constitutive G-protein-coupled receptor activity for drug discovery. Mol Pharmacol 1999;57:125–34.
[27] Bouaboula M, Perrachon S, Milligan L, Canatt X, Rinaldi-Carmona M, Portier M, et al. A selective inverse agonist for central cannabinoid receptor inhibits mitogen-activated protein kinase activation stimulated by insulin or insulin-like growth factor. J Biol Chem 1997;272:22330–9.
[28] Onaran HO, Costa T. Agonist efficacy and allosteric models of receptor action. Ann N Y Acad Sci 1997;812:98–115.
[29] Onaran HO, Scheer A, Cotecchia S, Costa T. A look at receptor efficacy. In: Kenakin TP, Angus JA, editors. From the signaling network of the cell to the intramolecular motion of the receptor The pharmacology of functional, biochemical, and recombinant systems handbook of experimental pharmacology, Vol. 148. Heidelberg: Springer; 2000. p. 217–80.
[30] Kenakin TP. Collateral efficacy as pharmacological problem applied to new drug discovery. Expert Opin Drug Disc 2006;1:635–52.

Pharmacological Assay Formats: Binding

The yeoman work in any science ... is done by the experimentalist who must keep the theoreticians honest.

— Michio Kaku (1995)

4.1 The Structure of This Chapter
4.2 Binding Theory and Experiment
4.3 Complex Binding Phenomena:
    Agonist Affinity from
    Binding Curves

4.4 Experimental Prerequisites for
    Correct Application of Binding
    Techniques
4.5 Chapter Summary and
    Conclusions

4.6 Derivations
References

4.1 THE STRUCTURE OF THIS CHAPTER

This chapter discusses the application of binding techniques to the study of drug-receptor interaction. It will be seen that the theory of binding and the methods used to quantify drug effect are discussed before the experimental prerequisites for good binding experiments are given. This may appear to be placing the cart before the horse in concept. However, the methods used to detect and rectify non-equilibrium experimental conditions utilize the very methods used to quantify drug effect. Therefore, they must be understood before their application to optimize experimental conditions can be discussed. This chapter first presents what the experiments strive to achieve, and then explores the possible pitfalls of experimental design that may cause the execution to fall short of the intent.

4.2 BINDING THEORY AND EXPERIMENT

A direct measure of the binding of a molecule to a protein target can be made if there is some means to distinguish the bound molecule from the unbound, and a means to quantify the amount bound. Historically, the first widely used technique to do this was radioligand binding. Radioactive molecules can be detected by observation of radioactive decay, and their amount quantified through calibration curves relating the amount of molecule to the amount of radioactivity detected. An essential part of this process is the ability to separate the bound from the unbound molecule. This can be done by taking advantage of the size of the protein versus the soluble small molecule. The protein can be separated by centrifugation, equilibrium dialysis, or filtration. Alternatively, the physical proximity of the molecule to the protein can be used. For example, in scintillation proximity assays, the receptor protein adheres to a bead containing scintillant, a chemical that produces light when close to radioactivity. Thus, when radioactive molecules are bound to the receptor (and therefore are near the scintillant) a light signal is produced, heralding the binding of the molecule. Other methods of detecting molecules such as fluorescence are increasingly being utilized in binding experiments. For example, molecules that produce different qualities of fluorescence, depending on their proximity to protein, can be used to quantify binding. Similarly, in fluorescence polarization experiments, fluorescent ligands (when not bound to protein) reduce the degree of light polarization of light passing through the medium through free rotation. When these same ligands are bound, their rotation is reduced, thereby concomitantly reducing the effect on polarization. Thus, binding can be quantified in terms of the degree of light polarization in the medium.

In general, there are emerging technologies available to discern bound from unbound molecules, and many of these can be applied to receptor studies. It will be assumed from

T. P. Kenakin: A Pharmacology Primer, Fourth edition. DOI: http://dx.doi.org/10.1016/B978-0-12-407663-1.00004-1
© 2014 Elsevier Inc. All rights reserved.

this point that the technological problems associated with determining bound species are not an experimental factor, and subsequent discussions will focus on the interpretation of the resulting binding data. Several excellent sources of information on the technology and practical aspects of binding are available [1−3].

Binding experiments can be done in three modes: saturation, displacement, and kinetic. Saturation binding directly observes the binding of a tracer ligand (radioactive, fluorescent, or otherwise detectable) to the receptor. The method quantifies the maximal number of binding sites and the affinity of the ligand for the site (equilibrium dissociation constant of the ligand-receptor complex). This is a direct measure of binding using the Langmuir adsorption isotherm model. A major limitation of this technique is the obvious need for the ligand to be traceable (i.e., it can be done only for radioactive or fluorescent molecules). Displacement studies overcome this limitation by allowing measurement of the affinity of non-traceable ligands through their interference with the binding of tracer ligands. Thus, molecules are used to displace or otherwise prevent the binding of tracer ligands and the reduction in signal is used to quantify the affinity of the displacing ligands. Finally, kinetic studies follow the binding of a tracer ligand with time. This can yield first-order rate constants for the onset and offset of binding, which can be used to calculate equilibrium binding constants to assess the temporal approach to equilibrium or to determine binding reversibility or to detect allosteric interactions. Each of these is considered separately. The first step is to discuss some methodological points common to all these types of binding experiments.

The aim of a binding experiment is to define and quantify the relationship between the concentration of ligand in the receptor compartment and the portion of the concentration that is bound to the receptor at any one instant. A first prerequisite is to know that the amount of bound ligand that is measured is bound only to the receptor and not to other sites in the sample tube or well (i.e., cell membrane, wall of the vessel containing the experimental solution, and so on). The amount of ligand bound to these auxiliary sites but not specifically to the target is referred to as *non-specific binding* (denoted *nsb*). The amount bound only to the pharmacological target of interest is termed the *specific binding*. The amount of specific binding is defined operationally as the bound ligand that can be displaced by an excess concentration of a specific antagonist for the receptor that is not radioactive (or otherwise does not interfere with the signals). Therefore, another prerequisite of binding experiments is the availability of a non-tracer ligand (for the specific target defined as one that does not interfere with the signal, whether it be radioactivity, fluorescence, or polarized light). Optimally, the chemical structure of the ligand used to define nsb should be different from the binding tracer ligand. This is because

the tracer may bind to non-receptor sites (i.e., adsorption sites, other non-specific proteins), and if a non-radioactive version of the same molecular structure is used to define specific binding, it may protect those very same non-specific sites (which erroneously define specific binding). A ligand with different chemical structure may not bind to the same non-specific sites and thus lessen the potential of defining nsb sites as biologically relevant receptors.

The non-specific binding of low concentrations of biologically active ligands is essentially linear and non-saturable within the ranges used in pharmacological binding experiments. For a traceable ligand (radioactive, fluorescent, and so on), non-specific binding is given as:

$$nsb = k \cdot [A^*] \qquad (4.1)$$

where k is a constant defining the concentration relationship for non-specific binding and $[A^*]$ is the concentration of the traceable molecule. The specific binding is saturable and defined by the Langmuir adsorption isotherm:

$$\text{Specific binding} = \frac{[A^*]}{[A^*] + K_d} \qquad (4.2)$$

where K_d is the equilibrium dissociation constant of the ligand-receptor complex. The total binding is the sum of these and is given as:

$$\text{Total binding} = \frac{[A^*] \cdot B_{max}}{[A^*] + K_d} + k \cdot [A^*] \qquad (4.3)$$

The two experimentally derived variables are nsb and total binding. These can be obtained by measuring the relationship between the ligand concentration and the amount of ligand bound (total binding) and the amount bound in the presence of a protecting concentration of receptor-specific antagonist. This latter procedure defines the nsb. Theoretically, specific binding can be obtained by subtracting these values for each concentration of ligand, but a more powerful method is to fit the two data sets (total binding and nsb) to Equations 4.1 and 4.3 simultaneously. One reason that this is preferable is that more data points are used to define specific binding. A second reason is that a better estimate of the maximal binding (B_{max}) can be made by simultaneously fitting two functions. Since B_{max} is defined at theoretically infinite ligand concentrations, it is difficult to obtain data in this concentration region. When there is a paucity of data points, non-linear fitting procedures tend to overestimate the maximal asymptote. The additional experimental data (total plus non-specific binding) reduces this effect and yields more accurate B_{max} estimates.

In binding, a good first experiment is to determine the time required for the binding reaction to come to equilibrium with the receptor. This is essential to know, since most binding reactions are made in stop-time mode, and real-time observation of the approach to equilibrium is not possible (this is not true of more recent fluorescent

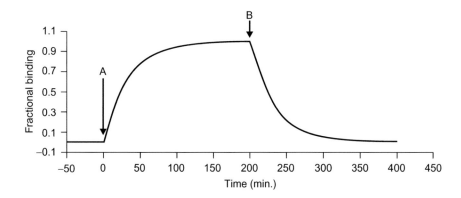

FIGURE 4.1 **Time course for the onset of a radioligand onto the receptor and the reversal of radioligand binding upon addition of a high concentration of a non-radioactive antagonist ligand.** The object of the experiment is to determine the times required for steady-state receptor occupation by the radioligand and confirmation of reversibility of binding. The radioligand is added at point A, and an excess competitive antagonist of the receptor at point B.

techniques where visualization of binding in real time can be achieved). A useful experiment is to observe the approach to equilibrium of a given concentration of tracer ligand and then to observe reversal of binding by addition of a competitive antagonist of the receptor. An example of this experiment is shown in Figure 4.1. Valuable data are obtained with this approach, since it indicates the time needed to reach equilibrium, and confirms the fact that the binding is reversible. Reversibility is essential to the attainment of steady states and equilibria (i.e., irreversible binding reactions do not come to equilibrium).

4.2.1 Saturation Binding

A saturation binding experiment consists of the equilibration of the receptor with a range of concentrations of traceable ligand in the absence (total binding) and presence of a high concentration (approximately $100 \times K_d$) of antagonist to protect the receptors (and thus determine the nsb). Simultaneous fitting of the total binding curve (Equation 4.3) and nsb line (Equation 4.1) yields the specific binding with parameters of maximal number of binding sites (B_{max}) and equilibrium dissociation constant of the ligand-receptor complex (K_d) (see Equation 4.2). An example of this procedure for the human calcitonin receptor is shown in Figure 4.2. Before the widespread use of non-linear fitting programs, the Langmuir equation was linearized for ease of fitting graphically. Thus, specific binding ([A*R]) according to mass action, represented as:

$$\frac{[A^*R]}{B_{max}} = \frac{[A^*]}{[A^*] + K_d} \qquad (4.4)$$

yields a straight line with the transforms:

$$\frac{[A^*R]}{[A^*]} = \frac{B_{max}}{K_d} - \frac{[A^*R]}{K_d} \qquad (4.5)$$

referred to alternatively as a Scatchard, Eadie, or Eadie–Hofstee plot. From this linear plot, $K_d = -1/\text{slope}$ and the x intercept equals B_{max}.

Alternatively, another method of linearizing the data points is by using:

$$\frac{1}{[A^*R]} = \frac{1}{[A^*]} \cdot \frac{K_d}{B_{max}} + \frac{1}{B_{max}} \qquad (4.6)$$

This is referred to as a *double reciprocal* or *lineweaver Burk plot.* From this linear plot, $K_d = \text{slope/intercept}$ and the $1/\text{intercept} = B_{max}$. Finally, a linear plot can be achieved with:

$$\frac{[A^*]}{[A^*R]} = \frac{[A^*]}{B_{max}} + \frac{K_d}{B_{max}} \qquad (4.7)$$

This is referred to as a Hanes, Hildebrand–Benesi, or Scott plot. From this linear plot, $K_d = \text{intercept/slope}$ and $1/\text{slope} = B_{max}$.

Examples of these are shown for the saturation data in Figure 4.2. At first glance, these transformations may seem like ideal methods for analyzing saturation data. However, transformation of binding data is not generally recommended. This is because transformed plots can distort experimental uncertainty, produce compression of data, and cause large differences in data placement. Also, these transformations violate the assumptions of linear regression and can be curvilinear simply because of statistical factors (for example, Scatchard plots combine dependent and independent variables). These transformations are valid only for ideal data and are extremely sensitive to different types of experimental errors. They should not be used for estimation of binding parameters. Scatchard plots compress data to the point where a linear plot can be obtained. Figure 4.3 shows a curve with an estimate of B_{max} that falls far short of being able to furnish an experimental estimate of the B_{max}, yet the Scatchard plot is linear with an apparently valid estimate from the abscissal intercept.

In general, non-linear fitting of the data is essential for parameter estimation. Linear transformations, however, are useful for visualization of trends in data. Variances from a straight edge are more discernible to the human eye than are differences from curvilinear shapes, so linear transforms can be a useful diagnostic tool.

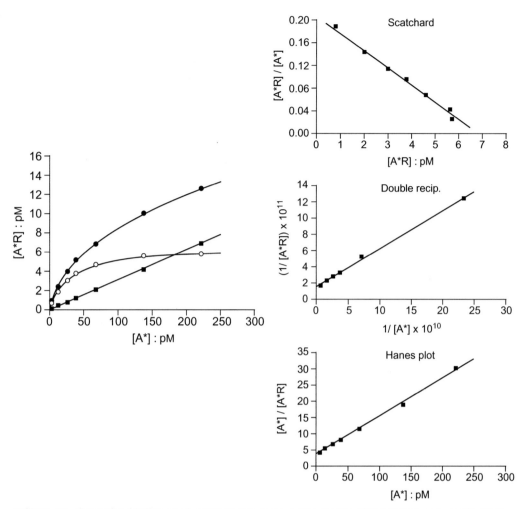

FIGURE 4.2 Saturation binding. Left panel: Curves showing total binding (filled circles), non-specific binding (filled squares), and specific binding (open circles) of the calcitonin receptor antagonist radiolabel ^{125}I AC512 ($B_{max} = 6.63$ pM; $K_d = 26.8$ pM). Data redrawn from [1]. Panels to the right show linear variants of the specific binding curve: Scatchard (Equation 4.5), double reciprocal (Equation 4.6), and Hanes plots (Equation 4.7) cause distortion and compression of data. Non-linear curve-fitting techniques are preferred.

FIGURE 4.3 Erroneous estimation of maximal binding with Scatchard plots. The saturation binding curve shown to the left has no data points available to estimate the true B_{max}. The Scatchard transformation to the right linearizes the existing points, allowing an estimate of the maximum to be made from the x-axis intercept. However, this intercept in no way estimates the true B_{max} since there are no data to define this parameter.

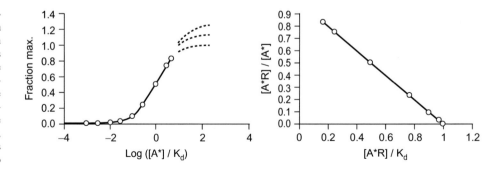

An example of where the Scatchard transformation shows significant deviation from a rectangular hyperbola is shown in Figure 4.4. The direct presentation of the data shows little deviation from the saturation binding curve as defined by the Langmuir adsorption isotherm. The data at 10 and 30 nM yield slightly underestimated levels of binding, a common finding if slightly too much protein is used in the binding assay (see Section 4.4.1). While this difference is nearly undetectable when the data are presented as a direct binding curve, it does produce a deviation from linearity in the Scatchard curve (see Figure 4.4B).

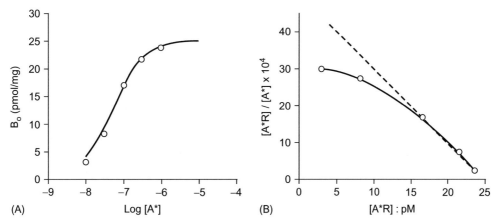

FIGURE 4.4 Saturation binding expressed directly and with a Scatchard plot. (A) Direct representation of a saturation binding plot (B_{max} = 25 pmol/mg, K_d = 50 nM). Data points are slightly deviated from ideal behavior (lower two concentrations yield slightly lower values for binding, as is common when slightly too much receptor protein is used in the assay, *vide infra*). (B) Scatchard plot of the data shown in panel A. It can be seen that the slight deviations in the data lead to considerable deviations from linearity on the Scatchard plot.

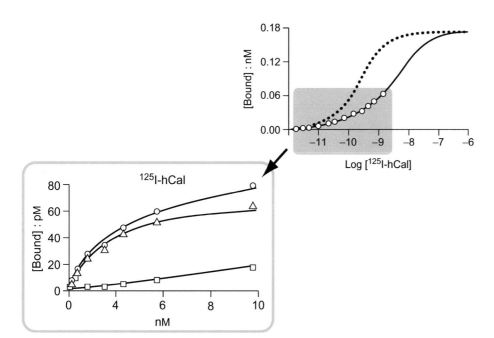

FIGURE 4.5 Saturation binding of the radioligand human ^{125}I-human calcitonin to human calcitonin receptors in a recombinant cell system in human embryonic kidney cells. Left-hand panel shows total binding (open circles), nonspecific binding (open squares), and specific receptor binding (open triangles). The specific binding appears to reach a maximal asymptotic value. The specific binding is plotted on a semi-logarithmic scale (shown in the right-hand panel). The solid line on this curve indicates an estimate of the maximal receptor binding. The data points (open circles) on this curve show that the data define less than half the computer-estimated total saturation curve. Data redrawn from [4].

Estimating the B_{max} value is technically difficult since it basically is an exercise in estimating an effect at infinite drug concentration. Therefore, the accuracy of the estimate of B_{max} is proportional to the maximal levels of radioligand that can be used in the experiment. The attainment of saturation binding can be deceiving when the ordinates are plotted on a linear scale, as they are in Figure 4.2. Figure 4.5 shows a saturation curve for calcitonin binding that appears to reach a maximal asymptote on a linear scale. However, replotting the graph on a semi-logarithmic scale illustrates the illusion of maximal binding on the linear scale and, in this case, how far short of true maxima a linear scale can present

a saturation binding curve. An example of how to measure the affinity of a radioligand and obtain an estimate of B_{max} (maximal number of binding sites for that radioligand) is given in Section 13.1.1.

4.2.2 Displacement Binding

In practice, there will be a limited number of ligands available that are chemically traceable (i.e., radioactive, fluorescent). Therefore, the bulk of radioligand experiments designed to quantify ligand affinity are done in a displacement mode whereby a ligand is used to displace or otherwise affect the binding of a traceable ligand. In general, an inverse sigmoidal curve is obtained with reduction in radioligand binding upon addition of non-radioactive antagonist. An example of how to measure the affinity of a displacing ligand is given in Section 13.1.2.

The equations describing the amount of bound radioligand observed in the presence of a range of concentrations of non-traceable ligand vary with the model used for the molecular antagonism. These are provided in material following, with brief descriptions. More detailed discussions of these mechanisms can be found in Chapter 6. If the binding is competitive (both ligands compete for the same binding domain on the receptor), the amount of tracer ligand-receptor complex (ρ^*) is given as (see Section 4.6.1):

$$\rho^* = \frac{[A^*]/K_d}{[A^*]/K_d + [B]/K_B + 1} \qquad (4.8)$$

where the concentration of tracer ligand is $[A^*]$, the non-traceable displacing ligand is $[B]$, and K_d and K_B are respective equilibrium dissociation constants. If the binding is non-competitive (binding of the antagonist precludes the binding of the tracer ligand), the signal is given by (see Section 4.6.2):

$$\rho^* = \frac{[A^*]/K_d}{[A^*]/K_d([B]/K_B + 1) + [B]/K_B + 1} \qquad (4.9)$$

If the ligand allosterically affects the affinity of the receptor (antagonist binds to a site separate from that for the tracer ligand) to produce a change in receptor conformation to affect the affinity of the tracer (*vide infra*) for the tracer ligand (see Chapter 7 for more detail), the displacement curve is given by (see Section 4.6.3):

$$\rho^* = \frac{[A^*]/K_d(1 + \alpha[B]/K_B)}{[A^*]/K_d(1 + \alpha[B]/K_B) + [B]/K_B + 1} \qquad (4.10)$$

where α is the multiple factor by which the non-tracer ligand affects the affinity of the tracer ligand (i.e., $\alpha = 0.1$

indicates that the allosteric displacing ligand produces a tenfold decrease in the affinity of the receptor for the tracer ligand).

As noted previously, in all cases these various functions describe an inverse sigmoidal curve between the displacing ligand and the signal. Therefore, the mechanism of interaction cannot be determined from a single displacement curve. However, observation of a *pattern* of such curves obtained at different tracer ligand concentrations (range of $[A^*]$ values) may indicate whether the displacements are due to a competitive, non-competitive, or allosteric mechanism.

Competitive displacement for a range of $[A^*]$ values (Equation 4.8) yields the pattern of curves shown in Figure 4.6A. A useful way to quantify the displacement is to determine the concentration of displacing ligand that produces a diminution of the signal to 50% of the original value. This concentration of displacing ligand will be referred to as the IC_{50} (inhibitory concentration for 50% decrease). For competitive antagonists, it can be shown that the IC_{50} is related to the concentration of tracer ligand $[A^*]$ by (see Section 4.6.4):

$$IC_{50} = K_B \cdot ([A^*]/K_d + 1) \qquad (4.11)$$

This is a linear relation often referred to as the Cheng–Prusoff relationship [5]. It is characteristic of competitive ligand-receptor interactions. An example is shown in Figure 4.6B.

In most conventional biochemical binding studies, the concentration of receptor protein is well below that of the ligands and thus the binding process does not significantly deplete the ligands. However, there are certain procedures such as fluorescent binding assays which require high concentrations of receptor to maximize the window for observing a response. Under these circumstances the fluorescent probe concentration is kept below the K_d value (where K_d is the equilibrium dissociation constant of the fluorescent probe-receptor complex) and the receptor concentration is maximized (above the K_d value) [6].

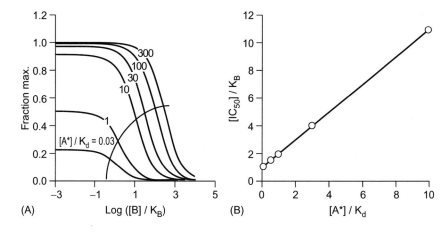

FIGURE 4.6 Displacement of a radioligand by a competitive non-radioactive ligand. (A) Displacement of radioactivity (ordinate scale) as curves shown for a range of concentrations of displacing ligand (abscissae as log scale). Curves shown for a range of radioligand concentrations denoted on the graph in units of $[A^*]/K_d$. Curved line shows the path of the IC_{50} for the displacement curves along the antagonist concentration axis. (B) Multiple values of the K_i for the competitive displacing ligand (ordinate scale) as a function of the concentration of radioligand being displaced (abscissae as linear scale). Linear relationship shows the increase in observed IC_{50} of the antagonist with increasing concentrations of radioligand to be displaced (according to Equation 4.11).

In these types of assays, the standard correction for IC_{50} to K_i values is not valid and a revised procedure utilizing the following equation must be used [6]:

$$K_i = \frac{[I]_{50}}{[A^*]_{50}/K_d + [R]_0/K_d + 1} \quad (4.12)$$

where $[I]_{50}$ is the free antagonist concentration at 50% inhibition, K_d is the equilibrium dissociation constant of the fluorescent probe-receptor complex, $[A^*]_{50}$ is the free concentration of fluorescent probe at 50% inhibition and $[R]_0$ is the free concentration of receptor at 0% inhibition. The practical application of this equation is discussed in detail in Section 4.6.4.

The displacement of a tracer ligand, for a range of tracer ligand concentrations, by a non-competitive antagonist is shown in Figure 4.7. In contrast to the pattern shown for competitive antagonists, the IC_{50} for inhibition of tracer binding does not change with increasing tracer ligand concentrations. In fact, it can be shown that the IC_{50} for inhibition is equal to the equilibrium dissociation

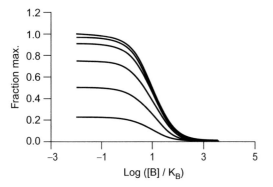

FIGURE 4.7 **Displacement curves for a non-competitive antagonist.** Displacement curve according to Equation 4.9 for values of radioligand $[A^*]/K_d = 0.3$ (curve with lowest ordinate scale beginning at 0.25), 1, 3, 10, 30, and 100. While the ordinate scale on these curves increases with increasing $[A^*]/K_d$ values, the location parameter along the x-axis does not change.

constant of the non-competitive antagonist-receptor complex (see Section 4.6.2).

Allosteric antagonist effects can be an amalgam of competitive and non-competitive profiles in terms of the relationship between IC_{50} and $[A^*]$. This relates to the magnitude of the term α, specifically the multiple ratio of the affinity of the receptor for $[A^*]$ imposed by the binding of the allosteric antagonist. A hallmark of allosteric inhibition is that it is saturable (i.e., the antagonism maximizes upon saturation of the allosteric binding site). Therefore, if a given antagonist has a value of α of 0.1, this means that the saturation binding curve will shift to the right by a factor of ten in the presence of an infinite concentration of allosteric antagonist. Depending on the initial concentration of radioligand, this may cause the displacement binding curve to fail to reach nsb levels. This effect is illustrated in Figure 4.8. Therefore, in contrast to competitive antagonists, where displacement curves all take binding of the radioligand to nsb values, an allosteric ligand will displace only to a maximum value determined by the initial concentration of radioligand and the value of α for the allosteric antagonist. In fact, if a displacement curve is observed where the radioligand binding is not displaced to nsb values, this is presumptive evidence that the antagonist is operating through an allosteric mechanism. The maximum displacement of a given concentration of radioligand $[A^*]$ by an allosteric antagonist with given values of α is (see Section 4.6.5):

$$\text{Maximal Fractional Inhibition} = \frac{[A^*]K_d + 1}{[A^*]/K_d + 1/\alpha} \quad (4.13)$$

where K_d is the equilibrium dissociation constant of the radioligand-receptor complex (obtained from saturation binding studies). The observed displacement for a range of allosteric antagonists for two concentrations of radioligands is shown in Figure 4.9. The effects shown in Figure 4.9 indicate a practical test for the detection of allosteric versus competitive antagonism in displacement

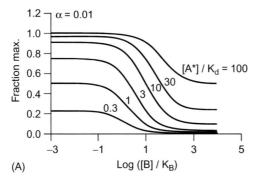
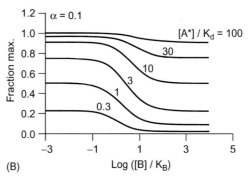

FIGURE 4.8 Displacement curves according to Equation 4.10 for an allosteric antagonist with different cooperativity factors (panel A, $\alpha = 0.01$; panel B, $\alpha = 0.1$). Curves shown for varying values of radioligand ($[A^*]/K_d$). It can be seen that the curves do not reach nsb values for high values of radioligand and that this effect occurs at lower concentrations of radioligand for antagonists of higher values of α.

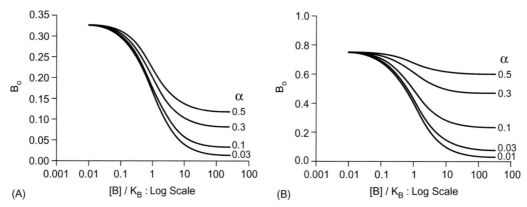

FIGURE 4.9 Displacement curves for allosteric antagonists with varying values of α (shown on figure). Ordinates: bound radioligand. (A) Concentration of radioligand $[A^*]/K_d = 0.1$. (B) Displacement of higher concentration of radioligand $[A^*]/K_d = 3$.

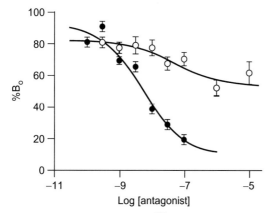

FIGURE 4.10 Displacement of bound ^{125}I-MIP-1α from chemokine C receptors type 1 (CCR1) by MIP-1α (filled circles) and the allosteric ligand UCB35625 (open circles). Note how the displacement by the allosteric ligand is incomplete. Data redrawn from [7].

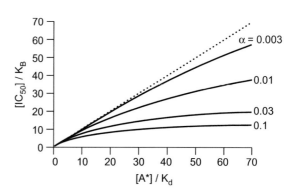

FIGURE 4.11 Relationship between the observed IC$_{50}$ for allosteric antagonists and the amount of radioligand present in the assay according to Equation 4.14. Dotted line shows relationship for a competitive antagonist.

binding studies. If the value of the maximal displacement varies with different concentrations of radioligand, this would suggest that an allosteric mechanism is operative. Figure 4.10 shows the displacement of the radioactive peptide ligand ^{125}I-MIP-1α from chemokine CCR1 receptors by non-radioactive peptide MIP-1α and by the allosteric small molecule modulator UCB35625. Clearly, the non-peptide ligand does not reduce binding to nsb levels, indicating an allosteric mechanism for this effect [7].

Another, more rigorous, method to detect allosteric mechanisms (and one that may furnish a value of α for the antagonist) is to formally observe the relationship between the concentration of radioligand and the observed antagonism by displacement with the IC$_{50}$ of the antagonist. As shown with Equation 4.11, for a competitive antagonist this relationship is linear (Cheng–Prusoff correction). For

an allosteric antagonist, the relationship is hyperbolic and given by (see Section 4.6.6):

$$IC_{50} = K_B \frac{(1 + ([A^*]/K_d))}{(1 + \alpha([A^*]/K_d)} \tag{4.14}$$

It can be seen from this equation that the maximum of the hyperbola defined by a given antagonist (with ordinate values expressed as the ratio of IC$_{50}$ to K_B) will have a maximum asymptote of $1/\alpha$. Therefore, observation of a range of IC$_{50}$ values needed to block a range of radioligand concentrations can be used to estimate the value of α for a given allosteric antagonist. Figure 4.11 shows the relationship between the IC$_{50}$ for allosteric antagonism and the concentration of radioligand used in the assay, as a function of α. It can be seen that, unlike the linear relationship predicted by Equation 4.11 (see Figure 4.6B), the curves are hyperbolic in nature. This is

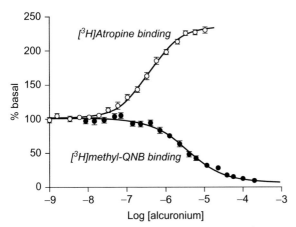

FIGURE 4.12 Effect of alcuronium on the binding of [³H]-methyl-QNB (filled circles) and [3H]-atropine (open circles) on muscarinic receptors. Ordinates are percentage of initial radioligand binding. Alcuronium decreases the binding of [³H]-methyl-QNB and increases the binding of [3H]-atropine. Data redrawn from [8].

TABLE 4.1 Differential Effects of the Allosteric Modulator Alcuronium on Various Probes for the m2 Muscarinic Receptor

Agonists[a]	(1/α)
Arecoline	1.7
Acetylcholine	10
Bethanechol	10
Carbachol	9.5
Furmethide	8.4
Methylfurmethide	7.3
Antagonists	
Atropineb	0.26
Methyl-N-piperidinyl benzilate[b]	0.54
Methyl-N-quinuclidinyl benzilate[c]	63
Methyl-N-scopolamine	0.24

[a]From [10].
[b]From [11].
[c]From [8].

another hallmark of allosteric versus simple competitive antagonist behavior.

An allosteric ligand changes the shape of the receptor, and in so doing will necessarily alter the rate of association and dissociation of some trace ligands. This means that allosterism is tracer dependent (i.e., an allosteric change detected by one radioligand may not be detected in the same way, or even detected at all, by another). For example, Figure 4.12 shows the displacement binding of two radioligand antagonists, [³H]-methyl-QNB and [³H]-atropine, on muscarinic receptors by the allosteric ligand alcuronium. It can be seen that quite different effects are observed. In the case of [³H]-methyl-QNB, the allosteric ligand displaces the radioligand and reduces binding to the nsb level. In the case of [³H]-atropine, the allosteric ligand actually enhances binding of the radioligand [8]. There are numerous cases of probe dependence for allosteric effects. For example, the allosteric ligand strychnine has little effect on the affinity of the agonist methylfurmethide (twofold enhanced binding) but a much greater effect on the agonist bethanechol (49-fold enhancement of binding [9]). An example of the striking variation of allosteric effects on different probes by the allosteric modulator alcuronium is shown in Table 4.1 [8,10,11].

4.2.3 Kinetic Binding Studies

A more sensitive and rigorous method of detecting and quantifying allosteric effects is through observation of the kinetics of binding.

In general, the kinetics of most allosteric modulators have been shown to be faster than the kinetics of binding

of the tracer ligand. This is an initial assumption for this experimental approach. Under these circumstances, the rate of dissociation of the tracer ligand (ρ_{A^*t}) in the presence of the allosteric ligand is given by [12,13]:

$$\rho_{A^*t} = \rho_{A^*} \cdot e^{-k_{off-obs} \cdot t} \qquad (4.15)$$

where ρ_A^* is the tracer ligand receptor occupancy at equilibrium and $k_{off-obs}$ is given by:

$$k_{off-obs} = \frac{\alpha[B]k_{off-A^*B}/K_B + k_{off-A^*}}{1 + \alpha[B]/K_B} \qquad (4.16)$$

Therefore, the rate of offset of the tracer ligand in the presence of various concentrations of allosteric ligand can be used to detect allosterism (change in rates with allosteric ligand presence) and to quantify both the affinity ($1/K_B$) and α value for the allosteric ligand. Allosteric modulators (antagonists) will generally decrease the rate of association and/or increase the rate of dissociation of the tracer ligand. Figure 4.13 shows the effect of the allosteric ligand 5-(N-ethyl-N-isopropyl)-amyloride (EPA) on the kinetics of binding (rate of offset) of the tracer ligand [³H]-yohimbine to α₂-adrenoceptors. It can be seen from this figure that EPA produces a concentration-dependent increase in the rate of offset of the tracer ligand, thereby indicating an allosteric effect on the receptor.

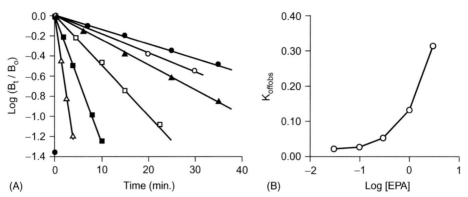

FIGURE 4.13 Effect of the allosteric modulator 5-(N-ethyl-N-isopropyl)-amyloride (EPA) on the kinetics dissociation of [^{3}H] yohimbine from α_2-adrenoceptors. (A) Receptor occupancy of [^{3}H] yohimbine with time in the absence (filled circles) and presence (open circles) of EPA 0.03 mM, 0.1 mM (filled triangles), 0.3 mM (open squares), 1 mM (filled squares), and 3 mM (open triangles). (B) Regression of observed rate constant for offset of concentration of [^{3}H] yohimbine in the presence of various concentrations of EPA on concentrations of EPA (abscissae in mM on a logarithmic scale). Data redrawn from [13].

4.3 COMPLEX BINDING PHENOMENA: AGONIST AFFINITY FROM BINDING CURVES

The foregoing discussion has been restricted to the simple Langmuirian system of the binding of a ligand to a receptor. The assumption is that this process produces no change in the receptor (i.e., analogous to Langmuir's binding of molecules to an inert surface). The conclusions drawn from a system where the binding of the ligand changes the receptor are different. One such process is agonist binding, in which, due to the molecular property of efficacy, the agonist produces a change in the receptor upon binding to elicit a response. Under these circumstances, the simple schemes for binding discussed for antagonists may not apply. Specifically, if the binding of the ligand changes the receptor (produces an isomerization to another form) the system can be described as:

$$A + R \underset{}{\overset{K_a}{\rightleftharpoons}} AR \underset{\sigma}{\overset{\chi}{\rightleftharpoons}} AR^* \qquad (4.17)$$

Under these circumstances, the observed affinity of the ligand for the receptor will not be described by K_A (where $K_A = 1/K_a$) but rather by that microaffinity modified by a term describing the avidity of the isomerization reaction. The observed affinity will be given by (see Section 4.6.7):

$$K_{obs} = \frac{K_A \cdot \chi/\sigma}{1 + \chi/\sigma} \qquad (4.18)$$

One target type for which the molecular mechanism of efficacy has been partly elucidated is the G-protein-coupled receptor (GPCR). It is known that activation of GPCRs leads to an interaction of the receptor with separate membrane G-proteins to cause dissociation of

the G-protein subunits and subsequent activation of effectors (see Chapter 2). For the purposes of binding, this process can lead to an aberration in the binding reaction as perceived in experimental binding studies. Specifically, the activation of the receptor with subsequent binding of that receptor to another protein (to form a ternary complex of receptor, ligand, and G-protein) can lead to the apparent observation of a "high-affinity" site — a ghost site that has no physical counterpart but appears to be a separate binding site on the receptor. This is caused by two-stage binding reactions, represented as:

$$A + R \overset{K_a}{\rightleftharpoons} AR + [G] \overset{K_g}{\rightleftharpoons} ARG \qquad (4.19)$$

In the absence of two-stage binding, the relative quantities of [AR] and [R] are controlled by the magnitude of K_a in the presence of ligand [A]. This, in turn, defines the affinity of the ligand for R (affinity = [AR]/([A] [R])). Therefore, if an outside influence alters the quantity of [AR], the observed affinity of the ligand for the receptor R will change. If a ligand predisposes the receptor to bind to G-protein, then the presence of G-protein will drive the binding reaction to the right (i.e., [AR] complex will be removed from the equilibrium defined by K_a). Under these circumstances, more [AR] complex will be produced than that governed by K_a. The observed affinity will be higher than it would be in the absence of G-protein. Therefore, the property of the ligand that causes the formation of the ternary ligand/receptor/G-protein complex (in this case, efficacy) will cause the ligand to have a higher affinity than it would have if the receptor were present in isolation (no G-protein present). Figure 4.14 shows the effect of adding a G-protein to a receptor system on the affinity of an agonist. As shown in this figure, the muscarinic agonist oxotremorine has a receptor equilibrium dissociation constant of 6 μM in a reconstituted phospholipid vesicle devoid of G-proteins. However, upon addition of G$_0$ protein, the affinity increases by a factor of 600 (10 nM).

This effect can actually be used to estimate the efficacy of an agonist (i.e., the propensity of a ligand to demonstrate high affinity in the presence of G-protein, *vide infra*). The observed affinity of such a ligand is given by (see Section 4.6.8):

$$K_{obs} = \frac{K_A}{1 + [G]/K_G} \qquad (4.20)$$

where K$_G$ is the equilibrium dissociation constant of the receptor/G-protein complex. A low value for K$_G$ indicates tight binding between receptors and G-proteins (i.e., high efficacy). It can be seen that the observed affinity of the ligand will be increased (decrease in the equilibrium dissociation constant of the ligand-receptor complex) with increasing quantities of G-protein [G] and/or very efficient binding of the ligand-bound receptor to the G-protein (low

value of K$_G$, the equilibrium dissociation constant for the ternary complex of ligand/receptor/G-protein). The effects of various concentrations of G-protein on the binding saturation curve to an agonist ligand are shown in Figure 4.15A. It can be seen from this figure that increasing concentrations of G-protein in this system cause a progressive shift to the left of the saturation dose-response curve. Similarly, the same effect is observed in displacement experiments. Figure 4.15B shows the effect of different concentrations of G-protein on the displacement of a radioligand by a non-radioactive agonist.

The previous discussion assumes that there is no limitation on the stoichiometry relating receptors and G-proteins. In recombinant systems, where receptors are expressed in surrogate cells (often in large quantities), it is possible that there may be limited quantities of G-protein available for complexation with receptors. Under these circumstances, complcx saturation and/or displacement curves can be observed in binding studies. Figure 4.16A shows the effect of different submaximal effects of G-protein on the saturation binding curve to an agonist radioligand. It can be seen that clear two-phase curves can be obtained. Similarly, two-phase displacement curves also can be seen with agonist ligands displacing a radioligand in binding experiments with subsaturating quantities of G-protein (Figure 4.16B). Figure 4.17 shows an experimental displacement curve of the antagonist radioligand for human calcitonin receptors [^{125}I]-AC512 by the agonist amylin in a recombinant system where the number of receptors exceeds the amount of G-protein available for complexation to the ternary complex state. It can be seen that the displacement curve has two distinct phases: a high-affinity (presumably due to coupling to G-protein) binding process followed by a lower-affinity binding (no benefit of G-protein coupling).

While high-affinity binding due to ternary complex formation (ligand binding to the receptor followed by binding to a G-protein) can be observed in isolated systems where

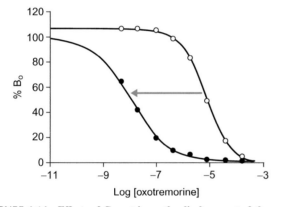

FIGURE 4.14 **Effects of G-protein on the displacement of the muscarinic antagonist radioligand [^{3}H]-L-quinuclidinyl benzylate by the agonist oxotremorine.** Displacement in reconstituted phospholipid vesicles (devoid of G-protein sububits) shown in open circles. Addition of G-protein (G$_0$ 5.9 nM βγ-subunit/3.4 nM α$_0$-IDP subunit) shifts the displacement curve to the left (higher affinity; see filled circles) by a factor of 600. Data redrawn from [14].

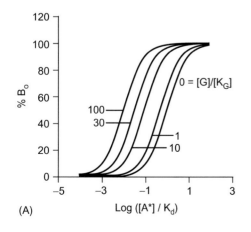

(A)

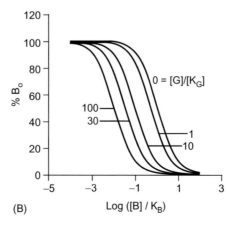

(B)

FIGURE 4.15 **Complex binding curves for agonists in G-protein unlimited receptor systems.** (A) Saturation binding curves for an agonist where there is high-affinity binding due to G-protein complexation. Numbers next to curves refer to the amount of G-protein in the system. (B) Displacement of antagonist radioligand by same agonist in G-protein unlimited system.

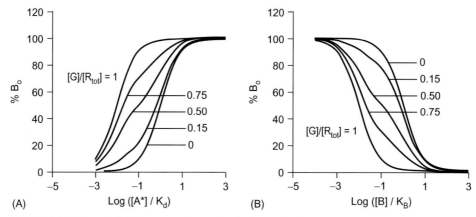

FIGURE 4.16 Complex binding curves for agonists in G-protein limited receptor systems. (A) Saturation binding curves for an agonist where the high-affinity binding due to G-protein complexation $= 100 \times K_d$ (i.e., Kobs $= K_d/100$). Numbers next to curves refer to ratio of G-protein to receptor. (B) Displacement of antagonist radioligand by same agonist in G-protein limited system.

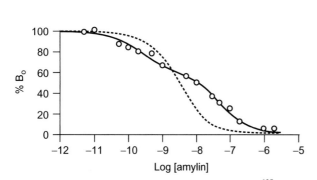

FIGURE 4.17 Displacement of antagonist radioligand ^{125}I-AC512 by the agonist amylin. Ordinates: percentage of initial binding value for AC512. Abscissae: logarithms of molar concentrations of rat amylin. Open circles are data points, solid line fit to two-site model for binding. Dotted line indicates a single phase displacement binding curve with a slope of unity. Data redrawn from [4].

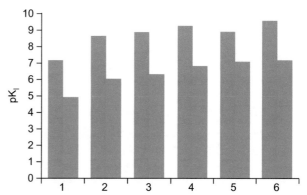

FIGURE 4.18 Affinity of adenosine receptor agonists in whole cells (red bars) and membranes (blue bars, high-affinity binding site). Data shown for (1) 2-phenylaminoadenosine, (2) 2-chloroadenosine, (3) 5'-N-ethylcarboxamidoadenosine, (4) N6-cyclohexyladenosine, (5) (-)-(R)-N6-phenylisopropyladenosine, and (6) N6-cyclopentyladenosine. Data redrawn from [15].

the ternary complex can accumulate and be quantified, this effect is cancelled in systems where the ternary complex is not allowed to accumulate. Specifically, in the presence of high concentrations of GTP (or a chemically stable analog of GTP such as GTPγS), the formation of the ternary complex [ARG] is followed immediately by hydrolysis of GTP and the G-protein and dissociation of the G-protein into α- and $\gamma\beta$-subunits (see Chapter 2 for further details). This causes subsequent dissolution of the ternary complex. Under these conditions, the G-protein complex does not accumulate, and the coupling reaction promoted by agonists is essentially nullified (with respect to the observable radioactive species in the binding reaction). When this occurs, the high-affinity state is not observed in the binding experiment. This has a practical consequence in binding experiments. In broken-cell preparations for binding, the

concentration of GTP can be depleted and thus the two-stage binding reaction is observed (i.e., the ternary complex accumulates). However, in whole-cell experiments, the intracellular concentration of GTP is high and the ternary complex [ARG] species does not accumulate. Under these circumstances, the high-affinity binding of agonists is not observed, only the so-called "low-affinity" state of agonist binding to the receptor. Figure 4.18 shows the binding (by displacement experiments) of a series of adenosine receptor agonists to a broken-cell membrane preparation (where high-affinity binding can be observed) and the same agonists in a whole-cell preparation (where the results of G-protein coupling are not observed). It can be seen from this figure that a phase shift for the affinity of the agonists under these two binding experiment conditions is observed. The broken-cell preparation reveals the

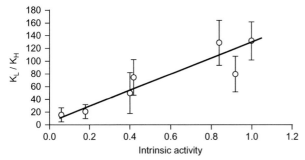

FIGURE 4.19 Correlation of the GTP shift for β-adrenoceptor agonists in turkey erythrocytes (ordinates) and intrinsic activity of the agonists in functional studies (abscissae). Data redrawn from [16].

TABLE 4.2 Criteria for Binding Experiments

Minimal criteria and optimal conditions for binding experiments: The means of making the ligand chemically detectable (i.e., addition of radioisotope label, fluorescent probe) does not significantly alter the receptor biology of the molecule.

- The binding is saturable.
- The binding is reversible and able to be displaced by other ligands.
- There is a ligand available to determine non-specific binding.
- There is sufficient biological binding material to yield a good signal-to-noise ratio but not too much so as to cause depletion of the tracer ligand.
- For optimum binding experiments, the following conditions should be met: There is a high degree of specific binding and a concomitantly low degree of non-specific binding.
- Agonist and antagonist tracer ligands are available.
- The kinetics of binding are rapid.
- The ligand used for determination of non-specific binding has a different molecular structure from the tracer ligand.

---

effects of the ability of the agonists to promote G-protein coupling of the receptor. This latter property, in effect, is the efficacy of the agonist. Thus, ligands that have a high observed affinity in broken-cell systems often have a high efficacy. A measure of this efficacy can be obtained by observing the magnitude of the phase shift of the affinities measured in broken-cell and whole-cell systems.

A more controlled experiment to measure the ability of agonists to induce the high-affinity state, in effect a measure of efficacy, can be done in broken-cell preparations in the presence and absence of saturating concentrations of GTP (or GTPγS). Thus, the ratio of the affinity in the absence and presence of GTP (ratio of the high-affinity and low-affinity states) yields an estimate of the efficacy of the agonist. This type of experiment is termed the "GTP shift" after the shift to the right of the displacement curve for agonist ligands after cancellation of G-protein coupling. Figure 4.19 shows the effects of saturating concentrations of GTPγS on the affinity of β-adrenoceptor agonists in turkey erythrocytes. As can be seen from this figure, a correlation of the magnitude of GTP shifts for a series of agonists and their intrinsic activities as measured in functional studies (a more direct measure of agonist efficacy; see Chapter 5). The GTP shift experiment is a method to estimate the efficacy of an agonist in binding studies.

The previous discussions indicate how binding experiments can be useful in characterizing and quantifying the activity of drugs (provided the effects are detectable as changes in ligand affinity). As for any experimental procedure, there are certain prerequisite conditions that must be attained for the correct application of this technique to the study of drugs and receptors. A short list of required and optimal experimental conditions for successful binding experiments is given in Table 4.2. Some special experimental procedures for determining equilibrium conditions involve the adjustment of biological material (i.e., membrane or cells) for maximal signal-to-noise ratios and/or temporal approach to equilibrium. These are outlined in the material following.

4.4 EXPERIMENTAL PREREQUISITES FOR CORRECT APPLICATION OF BINDING TECHNIQUES

4.4.1 The Effect of Protein Concentration on Binding Curves

In the quest for optimal conditions for binding experiments, there are two mutually exclusive factors with regard to the amount of receptor used for the binding reaction. On the one hand, increasing receptor (B_{max}) also increases the signal strength and usually the signal-to-noise ratio. This is a useful variable to manipulate. On the other hand, a very important prerequisite to the use of the Langmuirian type kinetics for binding curves is that the binding reaction does not change the concentration of tracer ligand being bound. If this is violated (i.e., if the binding is high enough to deplete the ligand), then distortion of the binding curves will result. The amount of tracer ligand-receptor complex as a function of the amount of receptor protein present is given as (see Section 4.6.9):

$$[A^*R] = \frac{1}{2}\Big\{\big[A_T^*\big] + K_d + B_{max}$$
$$- \sqrt{([A_T^*] + K_d + B_{max})^2 - 4[A_T^*]B_{max}}\Big\} \quad (4.21)$$

where the radioligand-receptor complex is $[A^*R]$ and $[A_T^*]$ is the total concentration of radioligand. Ideally, the amount of receptor (magnitude of B_{max}) should not limit the amount of $[A^*R]$ complex formed and there

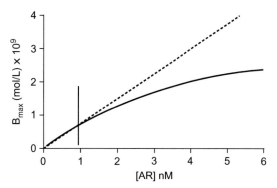

FIGURE 4.20 Effect of increasing protein concentration on the binding of a tracer ligand present at a concentration of $3 \times K_d$. Ordinates: [A*R] in moles/L calculated with Equation 4.21. Abscissae: B_{max} in moles/L $\times 10^9$. Values of B_{max} greater than the vertical solid line indicate region where the relationship between B_{max} and [A*R] begins to be non-linear and where aberrations in the binding curves will be expected to occur.

should be a linear relationship between [A*R] and B_{max}. However, Equation 4.21 indicates that the amount of [A*R] complex formed for a given [A*] indeed can be limited by the amount of receptor present (magnitude of B_{max}) as B_{max} values exceed K_d. A graph of [A*R] for a concentration of [A*] = $3 \times K_d$ as a function of B_{max} is shown in Figure 4.20. It can be seen that as B_{max} increases, the relationship changes from linear to curvilinear as the receptor begins to deplete the tracer ligand. The degree of curvature varies with the initial amount of [A*] present. Lower concentrations are affected at lower B_{max} values than are higher concentrations. The relationship between [AR] and B_{max} for a range of concentrations of [A*] is shown in Figure 4.21A. When B_{max} levels are exceeded (beyond the linear range), saturation curves shift to the right and do not come to an observable maximal asymptotic value. The effect of excess receptor concentrations on a saturation curve is shown in Figure 4.21B.

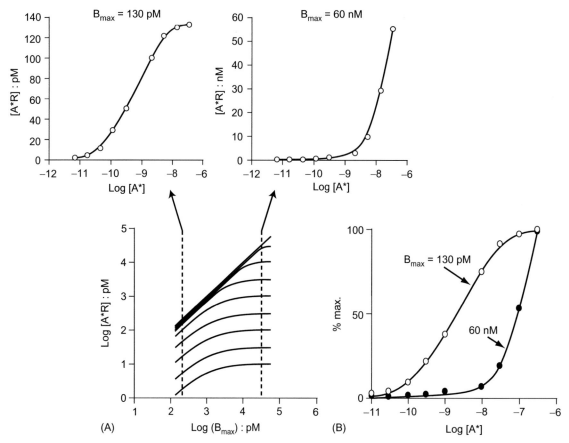

FIGURE 4.21 Effects of excess protein on saturation curves. (A) Bound ligand for a range of concentrations of radioligand, as a function of pM of receptor (Figure 4.20 is one example of these types of curves). The binding of the range of concentrations of radioligands are taken at two values of B_{max} (shown by the dotted lines; namely, 130 pM and 60 nM) and plotted as saturation curves for both B_{max} values on the top panels (note the difference in the ordinate scales). (B) The saturation curves shown on the top panels are replotted as a percentage of the maximal binding for each level of B_{max}. These comparable scales allow comparison of the saturation curves and show the dextral displacement of the curves with increasing protein concentration.

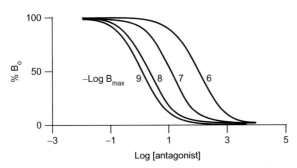

FIGURE 4.22 **Effect of excess protein concentration on displacement curves (as predicted by Equation 4.22).** As the B_{max} increases ($-\log B_{max}$ values shown next to curves) the displacement curves shift to the right.

For displacement curves, a similar error occurs with excess protein concentrations. The concentration of $[A^*R]$ in the presence of a non-tracer-displacing ligand $[B]$ as a function of B_{max} is given by (see Section 4.6.10):

$$[A^*R] = \frac{1}{2}\Big\{[A_T^*] + K_d(1 + [B]/K_B) + B_{max}$$
$$- \sqrt{([A_T^*] + K_d(1+[B]/K_B) + B_{max})^2 - 4[A_T^*]B_{max}}\Big\}$$

$$(4.22)$$

where the concentration of the displacing ligand is $[B]$ and K_B is the equilibrium dissociation constant of the displacing ligand-receptor complex. A shift to the right of displacement curves, with a resulting error in the IC_{50} values, occurs with excess protein concentration (see Figure 4.22).

4.4.2 The Importance of Equilibration Time for Equilibrium between Two Ligands

In terms of ensuring that adequate time is allowed for the attainment of equilibrium between a single ligand and receptors, the experiment shown in Figure 4.1 is useful. However, in displacement experiments there are two ligands (tracer and non-traceable ligand) present and they must compete for the receptor. This competition can take considerably longer than the time required for just a single ligand. This is because the free ligands can bind only to free unbound receptors (except in the case of allosteric mechanisms, *vide infra*). Therefore, the likelihood of a receptor being free to accept a ligand depends on the reversibility of the other ligand, and vice versa. Assuming mass action kinetics describe the binding of the radioligand $[A^*]$ and competitive antagonist $[B]$:

$$A^* + R \underset{k_2}{\overset{k_1}{\rightleftharpoons}} A^*R \qquad (4.23)$$

where $[A]$ is the radioligand and k_1 and k_2 the respective rates of onset and offset from the receptor.

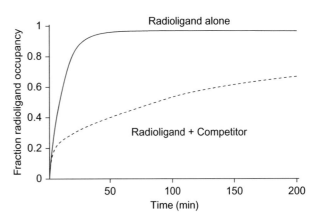

FIGURE 4.23 Binding kinetics of a radioligand with: $k_1 = 3.0 \times 10^5\ min^{-1}\ mol^{-1}$, $k_2 = 3.0 \times 10^{-3}\ min^{-1}$, $[A]/K_A = 3.0$ in the absence (solid line) and presence (dotted line) of a competitor for receptor binding ($k_3 = 10^6\ min^{-1}\ mol^{-1}$, $k_4 = 0.03\ min^{-1}$, $[B]/K_B = 10$).

$$B + R \underset{k_4}{\overset{k_3}{\rightleftharpoons}} BR \qquad (4.24)$$

where $[B]$ is the competitor and k_3 and k_4 the respective rates of onset and offset from the receptor. As described by Motulsky and Mahan [18], the following differential equations describe the binding of the radioligand and competitor with time:

$$d[A^*R]/dt = [A^*][R]k_1 - [AR]k_2 \qquad (4.25)$$

$$d[BR]/dt = [B][R]k_3 - [BR]k_4 \qquad (4.26)$$

The solution to the differential equations leads to an expression that describes the amount of radioligand bound to receptors with time in the presence of the competitor:

$$\rho_{A^*t} = \frac{k_1[A^*]}{\Omega - \psi}\left[\frac{k_4(\Omega - \Psi)}{\Omega\Psi} + \frac{(k_4 - \Omega)}{\Omega}e^{-\Omega t} - \frac{(k_4 - \Psi)}{\Psi}e^{-\Psi t}\right]$$

$$(4.27)$$

where:

$$\Omega = \tfrac{1}{2}[k_3[B] + k_4 + k_1[A^*] + k_2$$
$$+ ((k_3[B] + k_4 - k_1[A^*] - k_2)^2 + 4k_3k_1[A^*][B])^{1/2}]$$

and:

$$\Psi = \tfrac{1}{2}[k_3[B] + k_4 + k_1[A^*] + k_2$$
$$- ((k_3[B] + k_4 - k_1[A^*] - k_2)^2 + 4k_3k_1[A^*][B])^{1/2}]$$

Figure 4.23 shows the kinetics of binding of a radioligand in the absence and presence of a competitor with comparatively rapid binding kinetics; it can be seen that it takes longer to reach equilibrium for the radioligand in the presence of the competitor. This should be considered

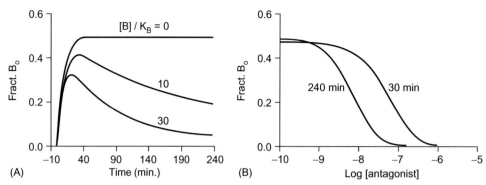

FIGURE 4.24   Time course for equilibration of two ligands for a single receptor.   (A) Time course for displacement of a radioligand present at a concentration of $[A^*]/K_d = 1$. Kinetic parameter for the radioligand $k_1 = 105 \ s^{-1} \ mol^{-1}$, $k_2 = 0.05 \ s^{-1}$. Equilibrium is attained within 30 minutes in the absence of a second ligand ($[B]/K_B = 0$). Addition of an antagonist (kinetic parameters = $k_1 = 106 \ s^{-1} \ mol^{-1}$, $k_2 = 0.001 \ s^{-1}$) at concentrations of $[B]/K_B = 10$ and 30, as shown in panel A. (B) Displacement of radioligand $[A^*]$ by the antagonist B measured at 30 minutes and at 240 minutes. It can be seen that a tenfold error in the potency of the displacing ligand [B] is introduced into the experiment by inadequate equilibration time.

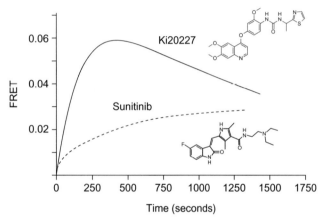

FIGURE 4.25   Fluorescence Resonance Energy Transfer (FRET) signal for a labeled antibody for colony-stimulating factor 1 receptors and small molecule kinase inhibitor tracer conjugated to a label. Antibody, tracer and antagonist were added simultaneously and the FRET signal monitored in real time; data shown for Ki20227 (316 nM, $t_{1/2} = 330$ min) and sunitinib (316 nM, $t_{1/2} = 1$ min). Data redrawn from [20].

when designing binding experiments, i.e., measurement of radioligand kinetics to determine when the experiment should be terminated and measurements taken by observation of radioligand binding alone may underestimate the time needed for attainment of equilibrium.

Radioligand binding experiments are usually initiated by addition of the membrane to a premade mixture of radioactive and non-radioactive ligand. After a period of time thought adequate to achieve equilibrium (guided by experiments like that shown in Figure 4.1), the binding reaction is halted and the amount of bound radioligand is quantified. Figure 4.24 shows the potential hazard of using kinetics observed for a single ligand (i.e., the radioligand) as being indicative of a two-ligand system. In the absence of another ligand, Figure 4.23A shows that the radioligand comes to equilibrium binding within 30 minutes. However, in the

presence of a receptor antagonist (at two concentrations $[B]/K_B = 10$ and 30), a clearly biphasic receptor occupancy pattern by the radioligand can be observed, in which the radioligand binds to free receptors quickly (before occupancy by the slower acting antagonist) and then a re-equilibration occurs as the radioligand and antagonist redistribute according to the rate constants for receptor occupancy of each. The equilibrium for the two ligands does not occur until > 240 minutes. Figure 4.23B shows the difference in the measured affinity of the antagonist at times of 30 and 240 minutes. Figure 4.25 shows this effect with Fluorescence Resonance Energy Transfer (FRET) binding where the tracer and antagonist are added simultaneously and the FRET signal is monitored in real time. This figure shows that a biphasic binding curve is seen for the slowly dissociating antagonist Ki20227 and not for the rapidly dissociating antagonist sunitinib [20]. It can also be seen from these data that the times thought adequate from the observation of a single ligand to the receptor (as that shown in Figure 4.1) may be quite inadequate compared to the time needed for two ligands to come to temporal equilibrium with the receptor. Therefore, in the case of displacement experiments utilizing more than one ligand, temporal experiments should be carried out to ensure that adequate times are allowed for complete equilibrium to be achieved for two ligands.

4.5 CHAPTER SUMMARY AND CONCLUSIONS

- If there is a means to detect (i.e., radioactivity, fluorescence) and differentiate between protein-bound and free ligand in solution, then binding can directly quantify the interaction between ligands and receptors.

- Binding experiments are done in three general modes: saturation, displacement, and kinetic binding.
- Saturation binding requires a traceable ligand but directly measures the interaction between a ligand and a receptor.
- Displacement binding can be done with any molecule and measures the interference of the molecule with a bound tracer.
- Displacement experiments yield an inverse sigmoidal curve for nearly all modes of antagonism. Competitive, non-competitive, and allosteric antagonism can be discerned from the pattern of multiple displacement curves.
- Allosteric antagonism is characterized by the fact that it attains a maximal value. A sensitive method for the detection of allosteric effects is through studying the kinetics of binding.
- Kinetic experiments are also useful to determine the time needed for attainment of equilibria and to confirm reversibility of binding.
- Agonists can produce complex binding profiles due to the formation of different protein species (i.e., ternary complexes with G-proteins). The extent of this phenomenon is related to the magnitude of agonist efficacy and can be used to quantify efficacy.
- While the signal-to-noise ratio can be improved with increasing the amount of membrane used in binding studies, too much membrane can lead to depletion of radioligand with a concomitant introduction of errors in the estimates of ligand affinity.
- The time to reach equilibrium for two ligands and a receptor can be much greater than that required for a single receptor and a single ligand.

4.6 DERIVATIONS

- Displacement binding: competitive interaction (4.6.1).
- Displacement binding: non-competitive interaction (4.6.2).
- Displacement of a radioligand by an allosteric antagonist (4.6.3).
- Relationship between IC_{50} and K_I for competitive antagonists (4.6.4).
- Maximal inhibition of binding by an allosteric antagonist (4.6.5).
- Relationship between IC_{50} and K_I for allosteric antagonists (4.6.6).
- Two-stage binding reactions (4.6.7).
- Effect of G-protein coupling on observed agonist affinity (4.6.8).
- Effect of excess receptor in binding experiments: saturation binding curve (4.6.9).
- Effect of excess receptor in binding experiments: displacement experiments (4.6.10).

4.6.1 Displacement Binding: Competitive Interaction

The effect of a non-radioactive ligand [B] displacing a radioligand [A*] by a competitive interaction is shown schematically as:

$$
\begin{array}{c}
B \\
+ \\
A + R \xrightleftharpoons{K_a} AR, \\
K_b \updownarrow \\
BR
\end{array} \qquad (4.28)
$$

where K_a and K_b are the respective ligand-receptor association constants for radioligand and non-radioactive ligand. The following equilibrium constants are defined:

$$[R] = \frac{[A^*R]}{[A^*]K_a} \qquad (4.29)$$

$$[BR] = K_b[B][R] = \frac{K_b[B][A^*R]}{[A^*]K_a} \qquad (4.30)$$

Total receptor concentration $[R_{tot}] = [R] + [A^*R] + [BR]$ (4.31)

This leads to the expression for the radioactive species $[A^*R]/[R_{tot}]$ (denoted as ρ^*):

$$\rho^* = \frac{[A^*]K_a}{[A^*]K_a + [B]K_b + 1} \qquad (4.32)$$

Converting to equilibrium dissociation constants (i.e., $K_d = 1/K_a$) leads to the equation:

$$\rho^* = \frac{[A^*]/K_d}{[A^*]/K_d + [B]/K_B + 1} \qquad (4.33)$$

4.6.2 Displacement Binding: Non-competitive Interaction

It is assumed that mass action defines the binding of the radioligand to the receptor and that the non-radioactive ligand precludes binding of the radioligand [A*] to receptor. There is no interaction between the radioligand and displacing ligand. Therefore, the receptor occupancy by the radioligand is defined by mass action times the fraction q of receptor not occupied by non-competitive antagonist:

$$\rho^* = \frac{[A^*]/K_d}{[A^*]/K_d + 1} \cdot q \qquad (4.34)$$

where K_d is the equilibrium dissociation constant of the radioligand-receptor complex. The fraction of receptor bound by the non-competitive antagonist is given as $(1 - q)$. This yields the following expression for q:

$$q = (1 + [B]/K_B)^{-1} \qquad (4.35)$$

Combining Equations 4.34 and 4.35 and rearranging yield the following expression for radioligand bound in the presence of a non-competititve antagonist:

$$\rho^* = \frac{[A^*]/K_d}{[A^*]/K_d([B]/K_B + 1) + [B]/K_B + 1} \qquad (4.36)$$

The concentration that reduces binding by 50% is denoted as the IC_{50}. The following relation can be defined:

$$\frac{[A^*]/K_d}{[A^*]/K_d(IC_{50}/K_B + 1) + IC_{50}/K_B + 1} = \frac{0.5[A^*]/K_d}{[A^*]/K_d + 1} \qquad (4.37)$$

It can be seen that the equality defined in Equation 4.37 is true only when $IC_{50} = K_B$ (i.e., the concentration of a non-competitive antagonist that reduces the binding of a tracer ligand by 50% is equal to the equilibrium dissociation constant of the antagonist-receptor complex).

4.6.3 Displacement of a Radioligand by an Allosteric Antagonist

It is assumed that the radioligand $[A^*]$ binds to a site separate from the one binding an allosteric antagonist $[B]$. Both ligands have equilibrium association constants for receptor complexes of K_a and K_b, respectively. The binding of either ligand to the receptor modifies the affinity of the receptor for the other ligand by a factor α. There can be three ligand-bound receptor species; namely, $[A^*R]$, $[BR]$, and $[BA^*R]$:

$$
\begin{array}{ccc}
B & & B \\
+ & & + \\
A^* + R & \xrightleftharpoons{K_a} & A^*R \\
K_b \big\downarrow\big\uparrow & & \big\downarrow\big\uparrow \alpha K_b \\
A^* + BR & \xrightleftharpoons{\alpha K_a} & A^*RB
\end{array}
\qquad (4.38)
$$

The resulting equilibrium equations are:

$$K_a = [A^*R]/[A^*][R] \qquad (4.39)$$

$$K_b = [BR]/[B][R] \qquad (4.40)$$

$$\alpha K_a = [A^*RB]/[BR][A^*] \qquad (4.41)$$

$$\alpha K_b = [A^*RB]/[A^*R][B] \qquad (4.42)$$

Solving for the radioligand-bound receptor species $[A^*R]$ and $[A^*RB]$ as a function of the total receptor species:

$([R_{tot}] = [R] + [A^*R] + [BR] + [A^*RB])$ yields

$$
\frac{[A^*R] + [A^*RB]}{[R_{tot}]}
$$

$$
= \frac{((1/\alpha[B]K_b) + 1)}{((1/\alpha[B]K_b) + (1/\alpha K_a) + (1/\alpha[A^*]K_aK_b) + 1)}
$$

$$(4.43)$$

Simplifying and changing association to dissociation constants (i.e., $K_d = 1/K_a$) yield (as defined by Ehlert, [19]):

$$\rho^* = \frac{[A^*]/K_d(1 + \alpha[B]/K_B)}{[A^*]/K_d(1 + \alpha[B]/K_B) + [B]/K_B + 1} \qquad (4.44)$$

4.6.4 Relationship between IC_{50} and K_I for Competitive Antagonists

A concentration of displacing ligand that produces a 50% decrease in ρ^* is defined as the IC_{50}. The following relation can be defined:

$$\frac{[A^*]/K_d}{[A^*]/K_d + 1} = \frac{0.5[A^*]/K_d}{[A^*]/K_d + IC_{50}/K_B + 1} \qquad (4.45)$$

From this, the relationship between the IC_{50} and the amount of tracer ligand $[A^*]$ is defined as [2]:

$$IC_{50} = K_B \cdot ([A^*]/K_d + 1) \qquad (4.46)$$

If it cannot be assumed that the free concentration of binding probe molecule (in most cases a fluorescent) and/or competing ligand does not change with receptor binding, then the calculation of K_i values from IC_{50} values requires a different procedure [6]. The base equation for the conversion is:

$$K_i = \frac{[I]_{50}}{[A^*]_{50}/k_d + [R]_0/K_d + 1} \qquad (4.47)$$

where $[I]_{50}$ is the free antagonist concentration at 50% inhibition, K_d is the equilibrium dissociation constant of the fluorescent probe-receptor complex, $[A^*]_{50}$ is the free concentration of fluorescent probe at 50% inhibition and $[R]_0$ is the free concentration of receptor at 0% inhibition.

The value for $[R]_0$ is obtained from calculating the positive root of:

$$[R]_0{}^2 + [R]_0(K_d + [A^*]_T) - [R]_T = 0 \quad (4.48)$$

where $[A^*]_T$ and $[R]_T$ are the total concentration of fluorescent probe and receptor respectively. The positive root of Equation 4.48 is:

$$[R]_0 = 0.5\left[\sqrt{(K_d + [A^*]_T)^2 + 4[R]_T} - K_d - [A^*]_T\right] \quad (4.49)$$

The conservation equation for total receptor in the absence of antagonist [B] is:

$$[R]_T = [R]_0 + [A^*R]_0 \quad (4.50)$$

A value for $[A^*R]_0$ can be calculated. For the total fluorescent probe concentration, the following relation holds:

$$[A^*]_T = [A^*]_0 + [A^*R]_0 \quad (4.51)$$

From Equation 4.51 and obtaining $[A^*R]_0$ from Equation 4.50, a value for $[A^*]_0$ is obtained. A value of $[A^*R]_{50}$ is then defined as the concentration of tracer-receptor complex present at 50% inhibition of binding ($[A^*R]_{50} = [A^*R]_0/2$). By analogy to Equation 4.51, $[A^*]_{50} = [A^*R]_T - [A^*R]_{50} = [A^*]_T - [A^*R]_0/2$. The conservation equation for receptor in the presence of a concentration of antagonist that produces 50% reduction in binding is:

$$[R]_T = [R]_{50} + [A^*R]_{50} + [BR]_{50} \quad (4.52)$$

The value for free receptor at the 50% inhibition point (defined as $[R]_{50}$) is given by the mass action equation for free tracer ligand concentration at 50% inhibition:

$$K_d = ([R]_{50}[A^*]_{50})/[A^*]_{50} \quad (4.53)$$

By analogy to Equation 4.51:

$$I_{50} = IC_{50} - [BR]_{50} \quad (4.54)$$

where IC_{50} is the concentration of antagonist found to reduce the binding by 50% under experimental conditions. Substituting for $[BR]_{50}$ from Equation 4.52 with $[A^*R]_{50}$ as $[A^*R]_0/2$ from Equation 4.53 yields:

$$[I]_{50} = IC_{50} - [R]_T + \left((K_d[A^*R]_{50})/[A^*]_{50}\right) + [A^*R]_{50} \quad (4.55)$$

Thus the procedure begins with the determination of $[R]_0$ (Equation 4.49), then $[A^*R]_0$ (Equation 4.50), and obtaining $[A^*]_0$ (Equation 4.51). This is followed by dividing $[A^*R]_0$ by 2 to yield $[A^*R]_{50}$, calculating $[R]_{50}$ (Equation 4.53) which then allows calculation of $[BR]_{50}$ (Equation 4.52). The I_{50} value then is calculated (Equation 4.54) Substituting for I_{50}, $[A^*]_{50}$ and $[R]_0$ into Equation 4.47 allows calculation of the true K_i value for the antagonist.

4.6.5 Maximal Inhibition of Binding by an Allosteric Antagonist

From Equation 4.39, the ratio of bound radioligand $[A^*]$ in the absence and presence of an allosteric antagonist [B], denoted by ρ_{A^*}/ρ_{A^*B}, is given by:

$$\frac{\rho_{A^*B}}{\rho_{A^*}} = \frac{[A^*]/K_d(1 + \alpha[B]/K_B) + [B]/K_B + 1}{([A^*]/K_d + 1)\cdot(1 + \alpha[B]/K_B)} \quad (4.56)$$

The fractional inhibition is the reciprocal; namely, ρ_{A^*}/ρ_{A^*B}. The maximal fractional inhibition occurs as $[B]/K_B \to \infty$. Under these circumstances, maximal inhibition is given by:

$$\text{Maximal Inhibition} = \frac{[A^*]/K_d + 1}{[A^*]/K_d + 1/\alpha} \quad (4.57)$$

4.6.6 Relationship between IC_{50} and K_I for Allosteric Antagonists

The concentration of allosteric antagonist [B] that reduces a signal from a bound amount $[A^*]$ of radioligand by 50% is defined as the IC_{50}:

$$\frac{(1 + [A^*]/K_d)}{[A^*]/K_d(1 + \alpha IC_{50}/K_B) + IC_{50}/K_B + 1} = 0.5 \quad (4.58)$$

This equation reduces to:

$$IC_{50} = K_B \frac{(1 + ([A^*]/K_d))}{(1 + \alpha([A^*]/K_d))} \quad (4.59)$$

4.6.7 Two-Stage Binding Reactions

Assume that the ligand [A] binds to receptor [R] to produce a complex [AR], and by that reaction changes the receptor from [R] to $[R^*]$:

$$A + R \underset{}{\overset{K_a}{\rightleftharpoons}} AR \underset{\sigma}{\overset{\chi}{\rightleftharpoons}} AR^* \quad (4.60)$$

The equilibrium equations are:

$$K_a = [A][R]/[AR] \quad (4.61)$$

$$\chi/\sigma = [AR]/[AR^*] \quad (4.62)$$

The receptor conservation equation is:

$$[R_{tot}] = [R] + [AR] + [AR^*] \quad (4.63)$$

Therefore, the quantity of end product $[AR^*]$ formed for various concentrations of [A] is given as:

$$\frac{[AR^*]}{[R_{tot}]} = \frac{[A]/K_A}{[A]/K_A(1 + \chi/\sigma) + \chi/\sigma} \quad (4.64)$$

where $K_A = 1/K_a$. The observed equilibrium dissociation constant (K_{obs}) of the complete two-stage process is given as:

$$K_{obs} = \frac{K_A \cdot \chi/\sigma}{1 + \chi/\sigma} \quad (4.65)$$

It can be seen that for non-zero positive values of χ/σ; (binding promotes formation of R*), $K_{obs} < K_A$.

4.6.8 Effect of G-protein Coupling on Observed Agonist Affinity

Receptor [R] binds to agonist [A] and goes on to form a ternary complex with G-protein [G]:

$$A + R \underset{K_a}{\rightleftharpoons} AR + [G] \underset{K_g}{\rightleftharpoons} ARG \quad (4.66)$$

The equilibrium equations are:

$$K_a = [A][R]/[AR] \quad (4.67)$$

$$K_g = [AR][G]/[ARG] \quad (4.68)$$

The receptor conservation equation is:

$$[R_{tot}] = [R] + [AR] + [ARG] \quad (4.69)$$

Converting association to dissociation constants (i.e., $1/K_a = K_A$):

$$\frac{[ARG]}{[R_{tot}]} = \frac{([A]/K_A)([G]/K_G)}{[A]/K_A(1 + [G]/K_G) + 1} \quad (4.70)$$

The observed affinity according to Equation 4.70 is:

$$K_{obs} = \frac{K_A}{1 + ([G]/K_G)} \quad (4.71)$$

4.6.9 Effect of Excess Receptor in Binding Experiments: Saturation Binding Curve

The Langmuir adsorption isotherm for radioligand binding [A*] to a receptor to form a radioligand-receptor complex [A*R] can be rewritten in terms of one where it is not assumed that receptor binding produces a negligible effect on the free concentration of ligand

$$[A*R] = \frac{([A_T^*] - [A*R])B_{max}}{[A_T^*] - [A*R] + K_d} \quad (4.72)$$

where B_{max} reflects the maximal binding (in this case, the maximal amount of radioligand-receptor complex). Under these circumstances, analogous to the derivation shown in Section 2.11.4, the concentration of radioligand bound is:

$$[A*R]^2 - [A*R](B_{max} + [A_T^*] + K_d) + [A_T^*]B_{max} = 0 \quad (4.73)$$

One solution to Equation 4.73 is:

$$[A*R] = \frac{1}{2}\left\{ [A_T^*] + K_d + B_{max} - \sqrt{([A_T^*] + K_d + B_{max})^2 - 4[A_T^*]B_{max}} \right\} \quad (4.74)$$

4.6.10 Effect of Excess Receptor in Binding Experiments: Displacement Experiments

The equation for the displacement of a radioligand [A*] by a non-radioactive ligand [B] can be rewritten in terms of one where binding does deplete the amount of radioligand in the medium (no change in [A*_{free}]):

$$[A*R] = \frac{([A_T^*] - [A*R])B_{max}}{[A_T^*] - [A*R] + K_d + [B]/K_B} \quad (4.75)$$

where B_{max} reflects the maximal formation of radioligand-receptor complex. Under these circumstances, the concentration of radioligand bound in the presence of a non-radioactive ligand displacement is:

$$[A*R]^2 - [A*R](Bmax + [A_T^*] + K_d(1 + [B]/KB)) + [A_T^*]B_{max} = 0. \quad (4.76)$$

One solution to Equation 4.76 is:

$$[A*R] = \frac{1}{2}\left\{ [A_T^*] + K_d(1 + [B]/K_B) + B_{max} - \sqrt{([A_T^*] + K_d(1+[B]K_B) + B_{max})^2 - 4[A_T^*]B_{max}} \right\} \quad (4.77)$$

REFERENCES

[1] Hulme EC. Receptor biochemistry: A practical approach. Oxford: Oxford University Press; 1990.
[2] Klotz IM. Ligand-receptor energetics: A guide for the perplexed. New York: John Wiley and Sons; 1997.
[3] Limbird LE. Cell surface receptors: A short course on theory and methods. Boston: Martinus Nihjoff; 1995.
[4] Chen W-J, Armour S, Way J, Chen G, Watson C, Irving P, et al. Expression cloning and receptor pharmacology of human calcitonin receptors from MCF-7 cells and their relationship to amylin receptors. Mol Pharmacol 1997;52:1164–75.
[5] Cheng YC, Prusoff WH. Relationship between the inhibition constant (Ki) and the concentration of inhibitor which causes 50 percent inhibition (I50) of an enzymatic reaction. Biochem Pharmacol 1973;22:3099–108.

[6] Nikolovska-Coleska Z, Wang R, X. fang, Pan H, Tomita Y, Li P, et al. Development and optimization of a binding assay for the XIAP BIR3 domain using fluorescence polarization. Analyt Biochem 2004;332:261−73.

[7] Sabroe I, Peck MJ, Van Keulen BJ, Jorritsma A, Simmons G, Clapham PR, et al. A small molecule antagonist of chemokine receptors CCR1 and CCR3. J Biol Chem 2000;275:25985−92.

[8] Hejnova L, Tucek S, El-Fakahany EE. Positive and negative allosteric interactions on muscarinic receptors. Eur J Pharmacol 1995;291:427−30.

[9] Jakubic J, El-Fakahany EE. Positive cooperativity of acetylcholine and other agonists with allosteric ligands on muscarinic acetylcholine receptors. Mol Pharmacol 1997;52:172−7.

[10] Jakubic J, Bacakova L, El-Fakahany EE, Tucek S. Positive cooperativity of acetylcholine and other agonists with allosteric ligands on muscarinic acetylcholine receptors. Mol Pharmacol 1997;52:172−9.

[11] Proska J, Tucek S. Mechanisms of steric and cooperative interactions of alcuronium on cardiac muscarinic acetylcholine receptors. Mol Pharmacol 1994;45:709−17.

[12] Christopoulos A. Quantification of allosteric interactions at G-protein coupled receptors using radioligand assays. In: Enna SJ, editor. Current protocol in pharmacology. New York: Wiley and Sons; 2000. p. 1.22.21−1.22.40.

[13] Lazareno S, Birdsall NJM. Detection, quantitation, and verification of allosteric interactions of agents with labeled and unlabeled ligands at G protein-coupled receptors: interactions of strychnine and acetylcholine at muscarinic receptors. Mol Pharmacol 1995;48:362−78.

[14] Leppick RA, Lazareno S, Mynett A, Birdsall NJ. Characterization of the allosteric interactions between antagonists and amiloride at the human α2A-adrenergic receptor. Mol Pharmacol 1998;53:916−25.

[15] Florio VA, Sternweis PC. Mechanism of muscarinic receptor action on Go in reconstituted phospholipid vesicles. J Biol Chem 1989;264:3909−15.

[16] Gerwins P, Nordstedt C, Fredholm BB. Characterization of adenosine A1 receptors in intact DDT1 MF-2 smooth muscle cells. Mol Pharmacol 1990;38:660−6.

[17] Lefkowitz RJ, Caron MG, Michel T, Stadel JM. Mechanisms of hormone-effector coupling: the β-adrenergic receptor and adenylate cyclase. Fed Proc 1982;41:2664−70.

[18] Motulsky HJ, Mahan LC. The kinetics of competitive radioligand binding predicted by the law of mass action. Mol Pharmacol 1984;25:1−9.

[19] Ehlert FJ. The relationship between muscarinic receptor occupancy and adenylate cyclase inhibition in the rabbit myocardium. Mol Pharmacol 1985;28:410−21.

[20] Uitdhaag CM, Sunnen CM, van Doornmalen AM, de Rouw N, Oubrie A, Azevedo R, et al. Multidimensional profiling of CSF1R screening hits and inhibitors: assessing cellular activity, target residence time, and selectivity in a higher throughput way. J Biomolec Screen 2011;16:1007−17.

Chapter 5

Agonists: The Measurement of Affinity and Efficacy in Functional Assays

5.1 Functional Pharmacological Experiments

5.2 The Choice of Functional Assays

5.3 Recombinant Functional Systems

5.4 Functional Experiments: Dissimulation in Time

5.5 Experiments in Real Time Versus Stop-Time

5.6 Quantifying Agonism: The Black-Leff Operational Model of Agonism

5.7 Biased Signaling

5.8 Null Analyses of Agonism

5.9 Chapter Summary and Conclusions

5.10 Derivations References

Cells let us walk, talk, think, make love, and realize the bath water is cold.

— Lorraine Lee Cudmore, "The Center of Life" (1977)

5.1 FUNCTIONAL PHARMACOLOGICAL EXPERIMENTS

Another major approach to the testing of drug activity is the use of functional assays. These are composed of any biological system that yields a biochemical product or physiological response to drug stimulation. Such assays detect molecules which produce a biological response or those that block the production of a physiological response. These can be whole tissues, cells in culture, or membrane preparations. Like biochemical binding studies, the pharmacological output can be tailored by using selective stimulation. Whereas in binding studies the output can be selected by the choice of radioligand or other traceable probe, in functional studies the output can be selected by choice of agonist. When necessary, selective antagonists can be used to obviate unwanted functional responses and isolate the receptor of interest. This practice was more prevalent in isolated tissue studies, where the tissue was chosen for the presence of the target receptor, and in some cases this came with concomitant presence of other related and obfuscating receptor responses.

In recombinant systems, a surrogate host cell line with a blank cellular background can often be chosen. This results in much more selective systems and less need for selective agonist probes.

There are two main differences between binding and functional experiments. The first is that functional responses are usually highly amplified translations of receptor stimulus (see Chapter 2). Therefore, while binding signals emanate from complete receptor populations, functional readouts often utilize only a small fraction of the receptor population in the preparation. This can lead to a greatly increased sensitivity to drugs that possess efficacy. No differences should be seen for antagonists. This amplification can be especially important for the detection of agonism, since potency may be more a function of ligand efficacy than affinity. Thus, a highly efficacious agonist may produce detectable responses at 100 to 1000 times lower concentrations than those that produce measurable amounts of displacement of a tracer in binding studies. The complex interplay between affinity and efficacy can be misleading in structure activity studies for agonists. For example, Figure 5.1 shows the lack of correlation of relative agonist potency for two dopamine-receptor subtypes and the binding affinity on those receptor subtypes for a series of dopamine agonists. These data show that, for these molecules, changes in chemical structure lead to changes in relative efficacy that are not reflected in the affinity measurement. The relevant activity is relative agonist potency. Therefore, the affinity data

T. P. Kenakin: A Pharmacology Primer, Fourth edition. DOI: http://dx.doi.org/10.1016/B978-0-12-407663-1.00005-3
© 2014 Elsevier Inc. All rights reserved.

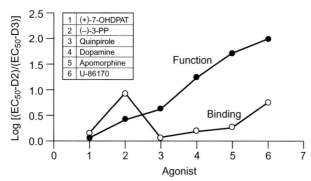

FIGURE 5.1 Ratio of affinity (open circles) and agonist potency (filled circles) for dopamine agonists on dopamine D2 versus D3 receptors. Abscissae: numbers referring to agonist key on right. Data calculated from [1].

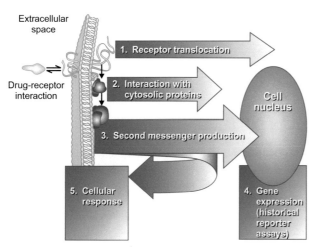

FIGURE 5.2 Different types of functional readouts of agonism. Receptors need not mediate cellular response but may demonstrate behaviors such as internalization into the cytoplasm of the cell (mechanism 1). Receptors can also interact with membrane proteins such as G-proteins (mechanism 2) and produce cytosolic messenger molecules (mechanism 3), which can go on to mediate gene expression (mechanism 4). Receptors can also mediate changes in cellular metabolism (mechanism 5).

are misleading. In this case, a functional assay is the correct approach for optimization of these molecules.

Functional assays give flexibility in terms of the biochemical functional response which can be monitored for drug activity. Figure 5.2 shows some of the possibilities. In some cases, the immediate receptor stimulus can be observed, such as the activation of G-proteins by agonist-activated receptor. Specifically, this is in the observation of an increased rate of exchange of guanosine diphosphate (GDP) to guanosine triphosphate (GTP) on the G-protein α-subunit. Following G-protein activation comes initiation of effector mechanisms. For example, this can include activation of the enzyme adenylyl cyclase to produce the second messenger cyclic AMP. This and other second messengers go on to activate enzymatic

biochemical cascades within the cell. A second layer of response observation is the measurement of the quantity of these second messengers. Yet another layer of response is the observation of the effects of the second messengers. Thus, activation of enzymes such as MAP kinase can be used to monitor drug activity.

A second difference between binding and function is the quality of drug effect that can be observed. Specifically, functional studies reveal interactions between receptors and cellular components which may not be observed in binding studies, such as some allosteric effects or other responses in a receptor's pharmacological repertoire (i.e., receptor internalization). For example, the cholecystokinin (CCK) receptor antagonist D-Tyr-Gly-[(Nle28,31,D-Trp30)cholecystokinin-26-32]-phenethyl ester is a receptor antagonist and does not produce receptor stimulation. While ostensibly this may appear to indicate a lack of efficacy, this ligand does produce profound receptor internalization [2]. Therefore, a different kind of efficacy is revealed in functional studies, which would not have been evident in binding.

A practical consideration is the need for a radioactive ligand in binding studies. There are instances where there is no such traceable probe or it is too expensive to be a viable approach. Functional studies require only that an endogenous agonist be available. As with binding studies, dissimulations in the value of the independent variable (namely, drug concentration) lead to corresponding errors in the observed value of the dependent variable (in the case of functional experiments, cellular response). The factors involved (namely, drug solubility and adsorption; see Chapter 2) are equally important in functional experiments. However, there are some additional factors unique to functional studies that should be considered. These are dealt with in Section 5.4.

5.2 THE CHOICE OF FUNCTIONAL ASSAYS

There are a number of assay formats that are available to test drugs in a functional mode. As discussed in Chapter 2, a main theme throughout the various stimulus-response cascades found in cells is the amplification of receptor stimulus occurring as a function of the distance, in biochemical steps and reactions, away from the initial receptor event. Specifically, the farther down the stimulus-response pathway the agonism is observed, the more amplified the signal. Figure 5.3 illustrates the effects of three agonists at different points along the stimulus-response cascade of a hypothetical cell. At the initial step (i.e., G-protein activation, ion channel opening), all are partial agonists, and it can be seen that the order of potency is $2 > 1 > 3$ and the order of efficacy is $3 > 2 > 1$. If the effects of these agonists were to be

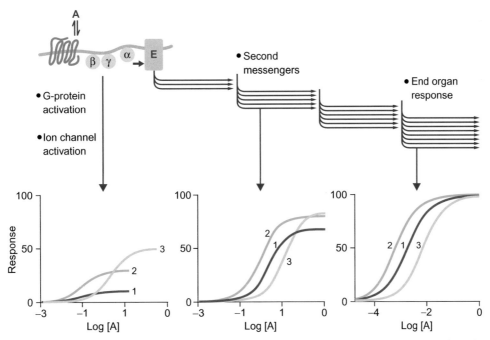

FIGURE 5.3 Amplification inherent in different vantage points along the stimulus-response pathway in cells. Agonists have a rank order of efficacy of $3 > 2 > 1$ and a rank order of potency of $2 > 1 > 3$. Assays proximal to the agonist-receptor interaction have the least amplification. The product of the initial interaction goes on to activate other processes in the cell. The signal is generally amplified. As this continues, texture with respect to differences in efficacy is lost and the agonists all demonstrate full agonism.

observed at a step further in the stimulus-response cascade (i.e., production of second messenger), it can be seen that agonists 2 and 3 are full agonists, while agonist 1 is a partial agonist. Their rank order of potency does not change but now there is no distinction between the relative efficacies of agonists 2 and 3. At yet another step in the cascade (namely, end organ response), all are full agonists with the same rank order of potency. The point of this simulation is to note the differences, in terms of the characterization of the agonists (full versus partial agonists, relative orders of efficacy), which occur by simply viewing their effects at different points along the stimulus-response pathway.

Historically, isolated tissues have been used as the primary form of functional assay, but since these usually come from animals, the species differences, coupled with the fact that human recombinant systems can now be used, have made this approach obsolete. Functional assays in whole-cell formats, where end organ response is observed (these will be referred to as group I assays), can be found as specialized cells such as melanophores, yeast cells, or microphysiometry assays. Group II assays record the product of a pharmacological stimulation (for example, an induction of a gene that goes on to produce a traceable product such as a light-sensitive protein). Second messengers (such as cyclic AMP, calcium, and inositol triphosphate) can also be monitored directly either in whole-cell or broken-cell formats (group III

assays). Finally, membrane assays such as the observation of binding of GTPγS to G-proteins can be used. While this is an assay carried out in binding mode, it measures the ability of agonists to induce a response, and thus may also be considered a functional assay. It is worth considering the strengths and shortcomings of all these approaches.

Group I assays (end organ response) are the most highly amplified and therefore most sensitive assays. This is an advantage in screening for weakly efficacious agonists, but has the disadvantage of showing all agonists above a given level of efficacy to be full agonists. Under these circumstances, information about efficacy cannot be discerned from the assay, since at least for all the agonists that produce maximal system response, no information regarding relative efficacy can be obtained. There are cell culture group I assays. One such approach uses microphysiometry. All cells respond to changes in metabolism by adjusting the internal hydrogen ion concentration. This process is tightly controlled by hydrogen ion pumps that extrude hydrogen ions into the medium surrounding the cell. Therefore, with extremely sensitive monitoring of the pH surrounding cells in culture, a sensitive indicator of cellular function can be obtained. Microphysiometry measures the hydrogen ion extrusion of cells to yield a generic readout of cellular function. Agonists can perturb this control of hydrogen ion output. One of the major advantages of this format is that it is generic (i.e., the

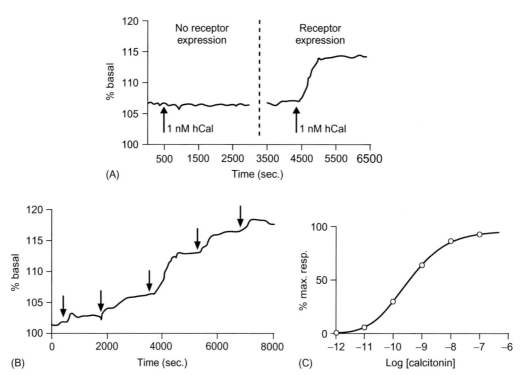

FIGURE 5.4 Microphysiometry responses of HEK 293 cells transfected with human calcitonin receptor. (A) Use of microphysiometry to detect receptor expression. Before transfection with human calcitonin receptor cDNA, HEK cells do not respond to human calcitonin. After transfection, calcitonin produces a metabolic response, thereby indicating successful membrane expression of receptors. (B) Cumulative concentration-response curve to human calcitonin shown in real time. Calcitonin added at the arrows in concentrations of 0.01, 0.1, 1.10, and 100 nM. (C) Dose-response curve for the effects seen in panel B.

observed pH does not depend on the nature of the biochemical coupling mechanisms in the cytosol of the cell). For example, the success of cell transfection experiments can be monitored with microphysiometry. Unless receptors are biochemically tagged, it may be difficult to determine whether the transfection of cDNA for a receptor into a cell actually results in membrane expression of the receptor. On occasion, the cell is unable to process the cDNA to form the complete receptor and it is not expressed on the cell surface. Figure 5.4A shows microphysiometry responses to calcitonin (an agonist for the human calcitonin receptor) before and after transfection of the cells with cDNA for the human calcitonin receptor. The appearance of the calcitonin response indicates that successful membrane expression of the receptor occurred. Another positive feature of this format is the fact that responses can be observed in real time. This allows the observation of steady states and the possibility of obtaining cumulative dose-response curves to agonists (see Figure 5.4B and C).

A specialized cell type that is extremely valuable in drug discovery is the *Xenopus laevis* melanophore. This is a cell derived from the skin of frogs that controls the dispersion of pigment in response to receptor stimulation. Thus, activation of G_i protein causes the formation of small granules of pigment in the cell, rendering them

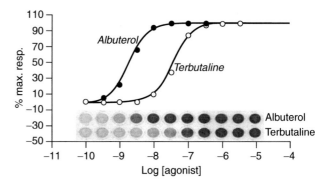

FIGURE 5.5 Melanophores, transfected with human β-adrenoceptors, disperse melanin to become opaque when stimulated with β-adrenoceptor agonists such as albuterol and terbutaline. Inset shows light transmission through a melanophore cell monolayer with increasing concentration of agonist. Light transmission is quantified and can be used to calculate graded responses to the agonists.

transparent to visible light. In contrast, activation of G_s and G_q protein causes dispersion of the melanin, resulting in an opaque cell (loss of transmittance of visible light). Therefore, the activation of receptors can be observed in real time through changes in the transmittance of visible light through a cell monolayer. Figure 5.5 shows the activation of human β-adrenoceptors in melanophores by β-adrenoceptor agonists. It can be seen that activation of

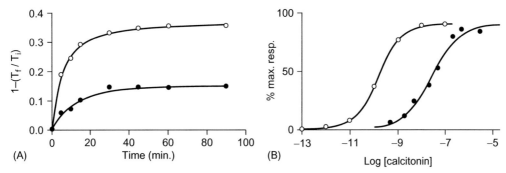

FIGURE 5.6 Calcitonin receptor responses. (A) Real-time melanin dispersion (reduced light transmittance) caused by agonist activation (with human calcitonin) of transfected human calcitonin receptors type II in melanophores. Responses to 0.1 nM (filled circles) and 10 nM (open circles) human calcitonin. (B) Dose-response curves to calcitonin in melanophores (open circles) and HEK 293 cells, indicating calcium transient responses (filled circles).

G_s protein by the activated β-adrenoceptor leads to an increase in pigmentation of the melanophore. This, in turn, is quantified as a reduced transmittance of visible light to yield graded responses to the agonists. One of the key features of this format is that the responses can be observed in real time. Figure 5.6A shows the reduced transmittance to visible light of melanophores transfected with human calcitonin receptors activated with the agonist human calcitonin. Another feature of this format is that the transfected receptors are very efficiently coupled (i.e., agonists are extremely potent in these systems). Figure 5.6B shows the dose-response curve for human calcitonin in transfected melanophores compared to the less efficiently coupled calcium fluorescence assay in human embryonic kidney cells for this same receptor.

Another specialized cell line that has been utilized for functional drug screening is derived from yeast cells. A major advantage of this format is that there are few endogenous receptors and G-proteins, leading to a very low background signal (i.e., the major signal is the transfected receptor of interest). Yeast can be genetically altered to fail to grow in a medium lacking histidine unless a previously transfected receptor is present. Coupled with the low maintenance and high growth rate, yeast cells are a viable system of high-throughput screening and secondary testing of drugs.

Group II assays consist of those which monitor cellular second messengers. Thus, activation of receptors to cause G_s protein activation of adenylate cyclase will lead to elevation of cytosolic or extracellularly secreted cyclic AMP. This second messenger phosphorylates numerous cyclic AMP-dependent protein kinases, which go on to phosphorylate metabolic enzymes, and transport and regulatory proteins (see Chapter 2). Cyclic AMP can be detected either radiometrically or by fluorescent probe technology.

Another major second messenger in cells is the calcium ion. Virtually any mammalian cell line can be used to measure transient calcium currents by fluorescence

assays when cells are preloaded with an indicator dye that allows monitoring of changes in cytosolic calcium concentration. These responses can be observed in real time, but one of their characteristic is that they are transient. This may lead to problems with hemi-equilibria in antagonist studies, whereby the maximal responses to agonists may be depressed in the presence of antagonists. These effects are discussed more fully in Chapter 6.

Another approach to the measurement of functional cellular responses is through the use of reporter assays (group III). Reporter assays yield the amount of cellular product made in response to stimulation of the cell. For example, elevation of cyclic AMP causes activation of protein kinase A. The activated subunits resulting from protein kinase A activation bind to cyclic AMP response element binding (CREB) protein, which then binds to a promoter region of cyclic AMP-inducible genes. If the cell is previously stably transfected with genes for the transcription of luciferase in the nucleus of the cell, elevation of cyclic AMP will induce the transcription of this protein. Luciferase produces visible light when brought into contact with the substrate LucLite, and the amount of light produced is proportional to the amount of cyclic AMP produced. Therefore, the cyclic AMP produced through receptor stimulation leads to a measurable increase in the observed light produced upon lysis of the cell. There are numerous other reporter systems for cyclic AMP and inositol triphosphate, which are two prevalent second messengers in cells (see Chapter 2). It can be seen that such a transcription system has the potential for great sensitivity, since the time of exposure can be somewhat tailored to amplify the observed response. However, this very advantage can also be a disadvantage, since the time of exposure to possible toxic effects of drugs is also increased. One advantage of real-time assays such as melanophores and microphysiometry is their ability to obtain responses in a short period of time, and thereby possibly reduce toxic effects that require longer periods of time to become manifest. Reporter responses are

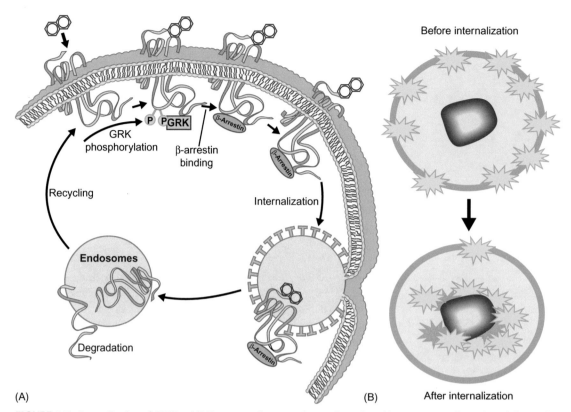

(A)   (B)   After internalization

FIGURE 5.7   Internalization of GPCRs. (A) Receptors adopt an active conformation either spontaneously or through interaction with a ligand and become phosphorylated. This promotes β-arrestin binding, which precedes internalization of the receptor into clatherin pits. Receptors then are either degraded in endosomes or recycled to the cell surface. (B) A fluorescent analog of β-arrestin can be visualized and tracked according to location either at the cell membrane (receptors not internalized) or near the cell nucleus (internalized receptors). This enables detection of changes in GPCRs.

routinely measured after a 24-hour incubation (to give sufficient time for gene transcription). Therefore, the exposure time to drug is increased with a concomitant possible increase in toxic effects.

Finally, receptor stimulus can be measured through membrane assays directly monitoring G-protein activation (group IV assays). In these assays, radiolabeled GTP (in a stable form; for example, GTPγS) is present in the medium. As receptor activation takes place, the GDP previously bound to the inactive state of the G-protein is released and the radiolabeled GTPγS binds to the G-protein. This is quantified to yield a measure of the rate of GDP/GTPγS exchange, and hence receptor stimulus.

The majority of functional assays involve primary signaling. In the case of G-protein-coupled receptors (GPCRs), this involves activation of G-proteins. However, receptors have other behaviors − some of which can be monitored to detect ligand activity. For example, upon stimulation many receptors are desensitized through phosphorylation and subsequently taken into the cell and either recycled back to the cell surface or digested. This process can be monitored by observing ligand-mediated receptor internalization. For many receptors this involves the migration of a cytosolic protein called β-arrestin. Therefore, the transfection of

fluorescent β-arrestin to cells furnishes a method for tracking the movement of the fluorescent β-arrestin from the cytosol to the inner membrane surface as receptors are activated (Figure 5.7). Alternative approaches to detecting internalization of GPCRs involve pH-sensitive cyanine dyes such as CypHer-5, which fluoresce when irradiated with red laser light, but only in an acidic environment. Therefore, epitope tagging of GPCRs allows binding of antibodies labeled with CypHer-5 to allow detection of internalized receptors (those that are in the acidic internal environment of the cell and thus fluoresce in laser light) [3]. A general list of minimal and optimal conditions for functional assays is given in Table 5.1.

5.3 RECOMBINANT FUNCTIONAL SYSTEMS

The advent of molecular biology and the ability to express transfected genes (through transfection with cDNA) into surrogate cells to create functional recombinant systems has brought a revolution in pharmacology. Previously, pharmacologists were constrained to the prewired sensitivity of isolated tissues for the study of agonists. As discussed

TABLE 5.1 Minimal and Optimal Criteria for Experiments Utilizing Cellular Function

Minimal

- An agonist and antagonist to define the response on the target are available.
- The agonist is reversible (after washing with drug-free medium).

Optimal

- The response should be sustained and not transient. No significant desensitization of the response occurs within the time span of the experiment.
- The response production should be rapid.
- The responses can be visualized in real time.
- There are independent methods to either modulate or potentiate functional responses.
- There is a capability to alter the receptor density (or cells available with a range of receptor densities).

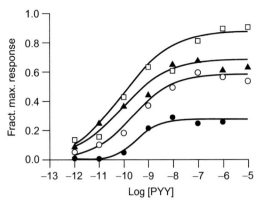

FIGURE 5.8 Dose-response curves to peptide PYY (YPAKPEAPGEDASPEELSRYYASLRHYLNLVTRQRY$_{NH2}$) in melanophores. Ordinates: minus values for $1 - T_f/T_i$ reflecting increases in light transmission. Abscissae: logarithms of molar concentrations of PYY. Cells transiently transfected with cDNA for the human NPY1 receptor. Levels of cDNA = $10\,\mu g$ (filled circles), $20\,\mu g$ (open circles), $40\,\mu g$ (filled triangles), and $80\,\mu g$ (open squares). Data redrawn from [4].

in Chapter 2, different tissues possess different densities of receptors, different receptor co-proteins in the membranes, and different efficiencies of stimulus-response mechanisms. Judicious choice of tissue type could yield uniquely useful pharmacologic systems (i.e., sensitive screening tissues). However, before the availability of recombinant systems these choices were limited. With the ability to express different densities of human target proteins such as receptors has come a transformation in drug discovery. Recombinant cellular systems can now be made with a range of sensitivities to agonists. The techniques involved in the construction of recombinant receptor systems are beyond the scope of this chapter, but some general ideas are useful in that they can be used for the creation of optimal systems for drug discovery.

The first idea to consider is the effect of receptor density on the sensitivity of a functional system to agonists. Clearly, if quanta of stimulus are delivered to the stimulus-response mechanism of a cell per activated receptor, the amount of the total stimulus will be directly proportional to the number of receptors activated. Figure 5.8 shows G_i-protein-mediated responses of melanophores transiently transfected with cDNA for human neuropeptide Y-1 receptors. As can be seen from this figure, increasing receptor expression (transfection with increasing concentrations of receptor cDNA) causes an increased potency and maximal response to the neuropeptide Y agonist peptide YY (PYY).

Receptor density has disparate effects on the potency and maximal responses to agonists. The operational model predicts that the EC_{50} of an agonist will vary with receptor density according to the following relationship (see Section 5.9.1):

$$EC_{50} = \frac{K_A \cdot K_E}{[R_t] + K_E}, \qquad (5.1)$$

where $[R_t]$ is the receptor density, K_A is the equilibrium dissociation constant of the agonist-receptor complex, and K_E is the concentration of activated receptor that produces half-maximal response (a measure of the efficiency of the stimulus-response mechanism of the system) (see Section 5.9.1 for further details). Similarly, the agonist maximal response is given by:

$$\text{Maximal Response} = \frac{[R_t] \cdot E_{max}}{[R_t] + K_E}, \qquad (5.2)$$

where E_{max} is the maximal response capability of the system. It can be seen that increases in receptor density will cause an increase in agonist maximal response, to the limit of the system maximum (i.e., until the agonist is a full agonist). Thereafter, increases in receptor density will have no further effect on the maximal response to the agonist. In contrast, Equation 5.1 predicts that increases in receptor density will produce concomitant increases in the potency of a full agonist with no limit. These effects are shown in Figure 5.9. It can be seen from this figure that at receptor density levels where the maximal response reaches an asymptote, agonist potency increases linearly with increases in receptor density. Figure 5.9B shows the relationship between the pEC_{50} for the β_2-adrenoceptor agonist isoproterenol and β_2-adrenoceptor density in rat C_6 glioma cells. It can be seen that while no further increases in maximal response are obtained, the agonist potency increases with increasing receptor density.

Recombinant systems can also be engineered to produce receptor-mediated responses by introducing adjunct proteins. For example, it has been shown that the $G_{\alpha16}$ G-protein subunit couples universally to nearly all receptors [6]. In recombinant systems, where expression of the receptor does not produce a robust agonist response,

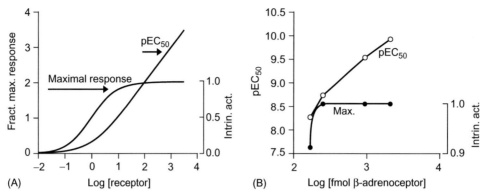

FIGURE 5.9 Effects of receptor density on functional assays. (A) Effect of increasing receptor density on potency (pEC$_{50}$) and maximal response to an agonist. Left ordinal axis is ratio of observed EC$_{50}$ and K$_A$ as $-$ log scale; right ordinal axis as fraction of system maximal response (intrinsic activity). (B) Observed pEC$_{50}$ values for isoproterenol for increases in cyclic AMP in rat glioma cells transfected with human β_2-adrenoceptors (open circles) and maximal response to isoproterenol (as a fraction of system maxima, filled circles) as a function of β_2-adrenoceptor density on a log scale (fmol/mg protein). Data redrawn from [5].

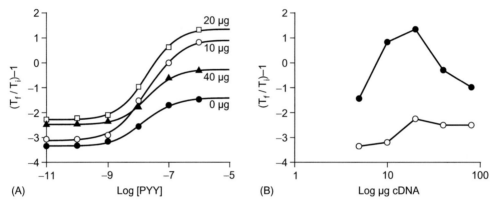

FIGURE 5.10 Effects of coexpressed G-protein (G$_{\alpha16}$) on neuropeptide NPY4 receptor responses (NPY-4). (A) Dose-response curves for NPY-4. Ordinates: *Xenopus laevis* melanophore responses (increases light transmission). Ordinates: logarithms of molar concentrations of neuropeptide Y peptide agonist PYY. Curves obtained after no cotransfection (labeled 0 µg) and cotransfection with cDNA for G$_{\alpha16}$. Numbers next to the curves indicate µg of cDNA of G$_{\alpha16}$ used for cotransfection. (B) Maximal response to neuropeptide Y (filled circles) and constitutive activity (open circles) as a function of µg cDNA of cotransfected G$_{\alpha16}$.

cotransfection of the G$_{\alpha16}$ subunit can substantially enhance observed responses. Figure 5.10 shows that both the maximal response and potency of the neuropeptide Y peptide agonist PYY is enhanced when neuropeptide Y-4 receptors are cotransfected with cDNA for receptor and G$_{\alpha16}$. Similarly, other elements may be required for a useful functional assay. For example, expression of the gluatamate transporter EAAT1 (a glutamate aspirate transporter) is required in some cell lines to control extracellular glutamate levels (which lead to receptor desensitization) [7].

While high receptor density may strengthen an agonist signal, it may also reduce its fidelity. In cases where receptors are pleiotropic with respect to the G-proteins with which they interact (receptors interact with more than one G-protein), high receptor numbers may complicate signaling by recruitment of modulating signaling pathways. For example, Figure 5.11 shows a microphysiometry response to human calcitonin produced in human embryonic kidney cells transfected with human calcitonin receptor. It can be seen that the response is sustained. In a transfected cell line with a much higher receptor density, the response is not of higher magnitude and is also transient, presumably because of complications due to the known pleiotropy of this receptor with other G-proteins. The responses in such systems are more difficult to quantify, and cumulative dose-response curves are not possible. These factors make a high receptor density system less desirable for pharmacological testing. This factor must be weighed against the possible therapeutic relevance of multiple G-protein coupling to the assay.

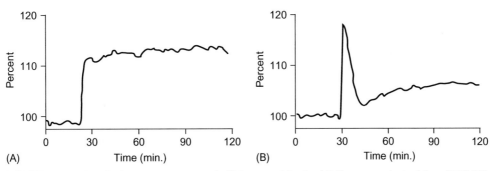

FIGURE 5.11 Microphysiometry responses to 1 nM human calcitonin. (A) Responses obtained from HEK 293 cells stably transfected with low levels of human calcitonin receptor (68 pM/mg protein). Response is sustained. (B) Response from HEK 293 cells stably transfected with high levels of receptor (30,000 pM/mg protein). Data redrawn from [8].

5.4 FUNCTIONAL EXPERIMENTS: DISSIMULATION IN TIME

A potential problem when measuring drug activity relates to the temporal ability of systems to come to equilibrium, or at least to a steady state. Specifically, if there are temporal factors that interfere with the ability of the system to return a cellular response, or if a real-time observation of response is not possible at the time of exposure to drugs, especially agonists, then the time of exposure to drugs becomes an important experimental variable. In practice, if responses are observed in real time, then steady states can be observed and the experiment designed accordingly. The rate of response production can be described as a first-order process. Thus, the effect of a drug ([E]) expressed as a fraction of the maximal effect of that drug (receptors saturated by the drug, [Em]) is:

$$\frac{[E]}{[E_m]} = 1 - e^{-k_{on}t}, \tag{5.3}$$

where k_{on} is a first-order rate constant for the approach of the response to the equilibrium value, and t is time. The process of drug binding to a receptor will have a temporal component. Figure 5.12 shows three different rates of response by an agonist, or by binding of a ligand in general. The absolute magnitude of the equilibrium binding is the same, but the time taken to achieve the effect is quite different. It can be seen from this figure that if response is measured at t = 1000 s, only drug A is at steady state. If comparisons are made at this time point, the effect of the other two drugs will be underestimated. As previously noted, if responses are observed in real time, steady states can be observed and temporal inequality ceases to be an issue. However, this can be an issue in stop-time experiments, in which real-time observation is not possible and the product of a drug response interaction is measured at a given time point. This is discussed further later in the chapter.

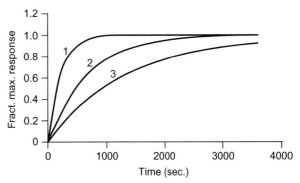

FIGURE 5.12 First-order rate of onset of response for three agonists of equal potency but differing rates of receptor onset. Ordinates: response at time t as a fraction of equilibrium response value. Abscissae: time in seconds. Curve 1: $k_1 = 3 \times 10^6$ s^{-1} mol^{-1}, $k_2 = 0.003$ s^{-1}. Curve 2: $k_1 = 10^6$ s^{-1} mol^{-1}, $k_2 = 0.001$ s^{-1}. Curve 3: $k_1 = 5 \times 10^5$ s^{-1} mol^{-1}, $k_2 = 0.0005$ s^{-1}.

Another potential complication can occur if the responsiveness of the receptor system changes temporally. This can happen if the receptor (or host system, or both) demonstrates desensitization (tachyphylaxis) to drug stimulation (see Chapter 2). There are numerous systems where constant stimulation with a drug does not lead to a constant steady state response, but rather, a "fade" in the response occurs. This can be due to depletion of a cofactor in the system producing the cellular response, or a conformational change in the receptor protein. Such phenomena protect against overactive stimulation of systems to physiological detriment. Whatever the cause, the resulting response to the drug is temporally unstable, leading to a dependence of the magnitude of the response on the time at which the response was recorded. The process of desensitization can be a first-order decay according to an exponential function, the time constant for which is independent of the magnitude of the response. Under these circumstances, the response tracings would resemble those shown in Figure 5.13A. Alternatively, the rate of

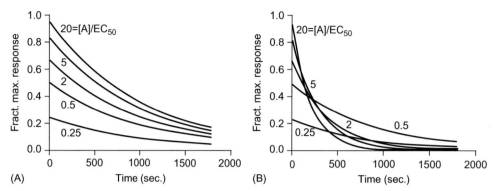

FIGURE 5.13 Fade of agonist-induced responses in systems with a uniform rate constant for desensitization (panel A) or a rate of desensitization proportional to the magnitude of the response (panel B). Abscissae: time in seconds. Ordinates: fractions of maximal response; responses ranging from 0.25 to 0.95 × maximum. (A) Temporal response multiplied by an exponential decay of rate constant 10^{-3} s^{-1}. Numbers refer to the concentration of agonist expressed as a fraction of the EC$_{50}$. (B) Rate constant for exponential decay equals the magnitude of the fractional response multiplied by a uniform rate constant 10^{-3} s^{-1}. For panel B, the rate of desensitization increases with increasing response.

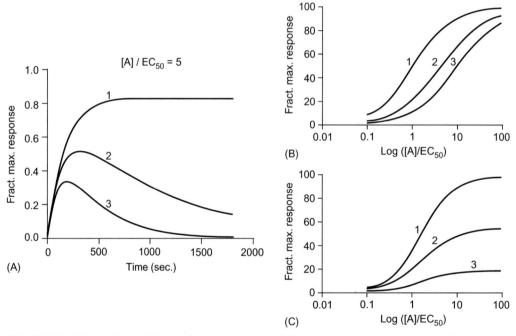

FIGURE 5.14 Temporal desensitization of agonist response. (A) Patterns of response for a concentration of agonist producing 80% maximal response. Curve 1: no desensitization. For concentration of agonist [A] = 5 × EC$_{50}$, first-order rate of onset k_1 = sec^{-1} mol^{-1}, k_2 = 10^{-3} sec^{-1}. Curve 2: constant desensitization rate = k_{desen} = 10^{-3}. Curve 3: variable desensitization rate equals ρk_{desen}, where ρ equals fractional receptor occupancy. (B) Complete dose-response curves to the agonist taken at equilibrium with no desensitization (curve 1), at peak response for constant desensitization rate (curve 2), and at variable desensitization rate (curve 3). (C) Curves as per panel B but response measured after 10 minutes equilibration with the agonist.

desensitization may be dependent on the intensity of the stimulation (i.e., the greater the response the more rapid will be the desensitization). Under these circumstances, the fade in response will resemble the pattern shown in Figure 5.13B. These temporal instabilities can lead to underestimation of the response to the agonist. If the wrong time point for measurement of response is chosen, this can lead to a shift to the right of the agonist dose-response curve (Figure 5.14A) or a diminution of the true maximal response (see Figure 5.14B). Temporal studies must be done to ensure that the response values are not dependent on the time chosen for measurement.

5.5 EXPERIMENTS IN REAL TIME VERSUS STOP-TIME

The observation of dependent variable values (in functional experiments, this is cellular response) as they happen (i.e., as the agonist or antagonist binds to the receptor and as the cell responds) is referred to as *real time*. In contrast, a response chosen at a single point in time is referred to as *stop-time experimentation*. There are certain experimental formats that must utilize stop-time measurement of responses since the preparation is irreparably altered by the process of measuring response. For example, measurement of gene activation through reporter molecules necessitates lysis of the cell. Therefore, only one measurement of response can be made. In these instances, the response is a history of the temporal process of response production from the initiation of the experiment to the time of measurement (for example, the production of the second cellular messenger cyclic AMP as a function of time). In specially constructed reporter cells, such as those containing an 8-base-pair palindrome sequence called cyclic AMP response element (CRE), receptor activation causes this element to activate a p-promoter region of cyclic-AMP-inducible genes. This, in turn, causes an increase in transcription of a protein called *luciferase*. This protein produces light when brought into contact with an appropriate substrate, making it detectable and quantifiable. Therefore, any agonist increasing cyclic AMP will lead to an increase in luciferase. This is one of a general type of functional assays (called *reporter assays*) where agonism results in the production and accumulation of a detectable product. The amount of product accumulated after agonism can be measured only once. Therefore, an appropriate time must be allowed for assumed equilibrium before reading the response. The addition of an agonist to such an assay causes the production of the second (reporter) messenger, which then goes on to produce the detectable product. The total amount of product made from the beginning of the process to the point where the reaction is terminated is given by the area under the curve that defines cyclic AMP production. This is shown in Figure 5.15. Usually the experimenter is not able to see the approach to equilibrium (real-time response shown in Figure 5.15A) and must choose a time point as the best estimate regarding when equilibrium has been attained. Figure 5.15B shows the area under the curve as a function of time. This area is the stop-time response. This function is not linear in the early stages during approach to equilibrium, but is linear when a steady state or true equilibrium has been attained. Therefore, a useful method to determine whether equilibrium has been achieved in stop-time

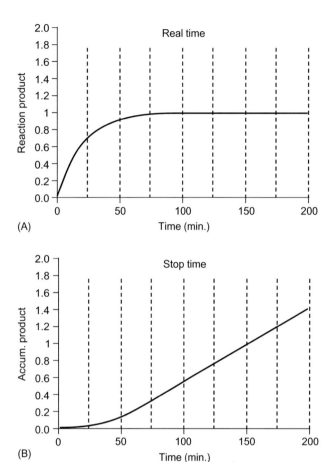

(A)

(B)

FIGURE 5.15 Different modes of response measurement. (A) Real time shows the time course of the production of response such as the agonist-stimulated formation of a second messenger in the cytosol. (B) The stop-time mode measures the area under the curve shown in panel A. The reaction is stopped at a designated time (indicated by the dotted lines joining the panels), and the amount of reaction product is measured. It can be seen that in the early stages of the reaction, before a steady state has been attained (i.e., a plateau has not yet been reached in panel A), the area under the curve is curvilinear. Once the rate of product formation has attained a steady state, the stop-time mode takes on a linear character.

experiments is to stop the reaction at more than one time point and ensure that the resulting signal (product formed) is linear with time. If the relationship between three stop-time responses obtained at three different time points is linear, then it can be assumed that the responses are being measured at equilibrium.

A potential pitfall with stop-time experiments comes with temporal instability of the responses. When a steady state sustained response is observed with time, then a linear portion of the production of reporter can be found (see Figure 5.15B). However, if there is desensitization or any other process that makes the temporal responsiveness of the system change, the area under the curve will not assume the linear character seen in sustained equilibrium reactions. For example, Figure 5.16 shows a case where the production of cyclic AMP with time is transient.

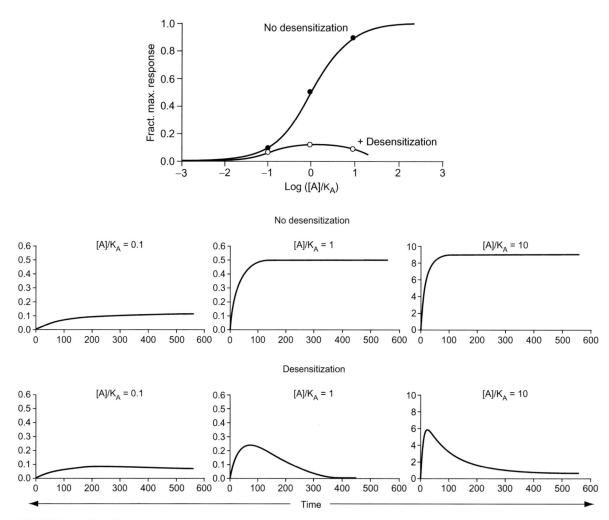

FIGURE 5.16 The effect of desensitization on stop-time mode measurements. Bottom panels show the time course of response production for a system with no desensitization, and one in which the rate of response production fades with time. The top dose-response curves indicate the area under the curve for the responses shown. It can be seen that, whereas an accurate reflection of response production is observed when there is no desensitization, the system with fading response yields an extremely truncated dose-response curve.

Under these circumstances, the area under the curve does not assume linearity. Moreover, if the desensitization is linked to the strength of signal (i.e., becomes more prominent at higher stimulations) the dose-response relationship may be lost. Figure 5.16 shows a stop-time reaction dose-response curve for a temporally stable system and a temporally unstable system where the desensitization is linked to the strength of the signal. It can be seen that the dose-response curve for the agonist is lost in the stop-time temporally unstable system.

5.6 QUANTIFYING AGONISM: THE BLACK-LEFF OPERATIONAL MODEL OF AGONISM

As discussed in Chapter 3 (Section 3.6), the operational model published by James Black and Paul Leff [9] is an excellent theoretical framework to quantify and think about agonism. For a defined agonist ([A]) in a functional system which can yield a maximal response (denoted E_m) when the target is fully activated, this model can be used to predict and quantify response. The magnitude of response is determined by the affinity of A for the receptor (expressed as the reciprocal of the equilibrium dissociation constant of the agonist-receptor complex, denoted K_A), and the term τ, which describes the intrinsic efficacy of the agonist. This term quantifies both the power of the agonist to induce response and the sensitivity of the system (containing a term quantifying the number of responding units in the system as the receptor density [R_t] and the efficiency of the coupling of each receptor to the stimulus-response mechanism of the cell). Dose-response data are fit to the Black-Leff equation [9] — see Chapter 3:

$$\text{Response} = \frac{[A]^n \tau^n E_m}{[A]^n \tau^n + ([A] + K_A)^n} \quad (5.4)$$

where n is the slope of the dose-response curve. In this model, the descriptive data of maximal response and the EC_{50} (potency described as the concentration of agonist producing 50% maximal response), which is dependent upon the specific system generating the curve, can be transformed into predictive data that are true for the drug in all systems, namely affinity (K_A^{-1}) and efficacy (τ, where the ratio of τ values for two drugs is constant and transferrable across different systems) through two equations. The first relates the maximal response to efficacy [10]:

$$\text{Maximal Response} = \frac{\tau^n E_m}{\tau^n + 1}. \qquad (5.5)$$

And the second relates potency to both affinity (K_A) and efficacy:

$$EC_{50} = \frac{K_A}{((2 + \tau^n)^{1/n} - 1)} \qquad (5.6)$$

Equation 5.4 can be used to compare agonists through an index that denotes the power of that agonist to produce activation, namely a value referred to as a transduction coefficient and defined as $\log(\tau/K_A)$ [11]. This number takes into account both the maximal response produced by the agonist and its potency (as an EC_{50} value). If the slope of the dose-response curve is not significantly different from unity, then $\log(\tau/K_A)$ is the maximal response divided by the EC_{50} (i.e., for n = 1, $\log(\tau/K_A) = \log(\text{max}/EC_{50})$): [12] — *vide infra*). Thus ratios of τ/K_A values (denoted $\Delta\log(\tau/K_A)$) are system-independent estimates of the relative ability of agonists to induce a given response. The use of $\log(\tau/K_A)$ for predicting agonist response and/or receptor selectivity is specifically discussed in Chapter 8 (see Section 8.2.1).

Unlike the analysis for full agonists, certain experimentally derived starting points for the fit are evident for partial agonists. The first step is to furnish initial parameters for computer fit to the operational model; the E_{max} for the system and K_A values for each agonist are good starting points. There are two ways in which the E_{max} can be determined in any given functional system. In some cases, the maximal response to the agonist of interest will equal the maximal response to agonists for other systems. For example, a maximal α-adrenoceptor contraction that is equal in magnitude to that produced by a complete depolarization of the tissue by potassium ion would probably indicate that both produce the tissue maximal response (E_{max}). Also, if a number of agonists for a given receptor produce the same magnitude of maximal response, then it would be likely that all saturate the stimulus-response capability of the system and thus produce the system maximal response. The EC_{50} value for a partial agonist is a good estimate of the K_A (*vide infra*). As a starting point for the K_A of even a full agonist, the $100 \times EC_{50}$ can be used for fitting (see Figure 5.17). The data then can be fitted to a general logistic function

of variable slope to estimate the Hill coefficient (Figure 5.17, top right panel). Finally, with estimates of K_A, E_{max}, and n, the complete data set can be fit with varying τ values (bottom left panel, Figure 5.17). It should be noted that unless a given agonist can be tested in a system where it produces partial agonism, the K_A value cannot be absolutely determined, since the location parameters of full agonists are controlled by a product of affinity and efficacy. For example, the relative affinity and efficacy of the full agonist in Figure 5.17 is shown as $\tau = 100$ and $K_A = 5 \mu M$, but the curve fits equally well with $\tau = 1000$ and $K_A = 50 \mu M$. In fact, there are an infinite number of combinations of τ and K_A that can fit concentration-response curves to full agonists, and it is the τ/K_A ratio that is unique for these types of molecules. Figure 5.18 shows the analysis of the full agonist isoproterenol and partial agonist prenalterol. It can be seen that once the relative efficacy values are determined in one tissue, the ratio is predictive in other tissues as well. This advantage can be extrapolated to the situation whereby the relative efficacy and affinity of agonists can be determined in a test system and the activity of the agonist then predicted in the therapeutic system — see Chapter 8.

Correct estimates of relative affinity and efficacy can furnish a powerful mechanism for predicting agonist effects in different tissues. Figure 5.19A shows the relative response of guinea pig ileum to the muscarinic agonists oxotremorine and carbachol [13]. It can be seen from this figure that oxotremorine is two -to three fold more potent than carbachol. The following question then can be posed: What will the relative potency of these agonists be in a less sensitive system? Ostensibly, a 100-fold reduction in the sensitivity of the system would cause a 100-fold shift to the right of both concentration-response curves (Figure 5.19B). What is, in fact, observed is that the carbachol curve shifts to the right by a factor of 100 and the maximum is slightly reduced, while the concentration-response curve to oxotremorine disappears completely! This effect is predicted by the operational model in this situation. An assessment of the relative efficacies and affinities of these two agonists using the operational model indicates that the affinity of carbachol is $300 \mu M$, that of oxotremorine is $0.5 \mu M$, and that carbachol has 200 times the efficacy of oxotremorine. Thus, the response to the high-affinity, low-efficacy agonist (oxotremorine) is reduced to a greater extent with diminution of tissue sensitivity than that of the low-affinity, high-efficacy agonist (carbachol), as predicted by receptor theory and, in particular, by the operational model. This effect is discussed in further detail in Section 5.6.1. These types of predictions illustrate the value of determining the relative efficacy and affinity of agonists when predicting effects in a range of systems.

Ideally, while agonist response can be quantified in terms of the parameters of efficacy (τ) and K_A for

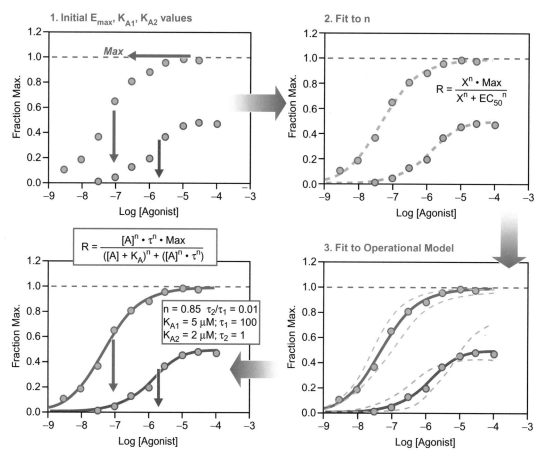

FIGURE 5.17 Fit of the operational model to experimentally determined agonist concentration-response data. The maximal response of the system either is determined experimentally (if a series of powerful agonists produce the same maximal response, this is a good indicator that the maximal response is the system maximum) or is assumed from the maximal response of the most powerful agonist. In addition, the K_A for the partial agonist is assumed to be approximated by the EC_{50}, while a first estimate of the K_A for the full agonist also may be the EC_{50} for the full agonist curve. The data are fit to the general logistic function with variable slope to determine slope n. The initial estimates for E_{max}, K_{A1}, K_{A2}, and n are used to fit the two curves simultaneously with varying τ values using Equation 11.1 until a minimum sum of squares for the difference between the predicted and experimental points is obtained.

predictionof agonism; it will be seen that there are separate methods which have been developed to quantify agonism such as equiactive agonist potency ratios that do not employ direct fitting of data to the Black/Leff operatonal model (*vide infra*). In addition to the quantification and prediction of agonism, there are other important aspects of agonist response that are relevant to the complete profile of an agonist drug; these are related to agonist selectivity, relative dependence of agonist potency on affinity vs. efficacy, secondary effects, and the actual "quality" of the efficacy these molecules express in biological systems. This latter factor is quantified under the heading of "biased signaling."

5.6.1 Affinity-Dependent versus Efficacy-Dependent Agonist Potency

In the early stages of lead optimization, agonism is usually detectable but at a relatively low level, that is, the lead

probably will be a partial agonist. Partial agonists are the optimal molecule for pharmacological characterization. This is because partial agonism allows the estimation of the system-independent properties of drugs; namely, affinity and efficacy (for partial agonists). Under these circumstances, medicinal chemists have two scales of biological activity that they can use for lead optimization. The EC_{50} of a partial agonist is a reasonable approximation of its affinity (see Section 5.9.1) therefore the observed EC_{50} for weak agonists in structure-activity relationships (SAR) studies can be used to track the effect of changing chemical structure on ligand affinity. Similarly, the relative maximal responses of partial agonists can be useful indicators of relative efficacy (see Section 5.9.4). Thus, partial agonism provides a unique opportunity for medicinal chemists to observe the effects of changes in chemical structure on either affinity or efficacy. Figure 5.20 shows the effects of increasing alkyl chain length on a series of alkylammonium muscarinic agonists

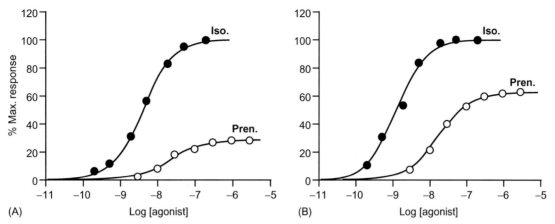

FIGURE 5.18 Concentration-response curves to the β-adrenoceptor agonists isoproterenol (filled circles) and prenalterol (open circles) obtained in (A) guinea pig left atria and (B) rat left atria. Data fit to the operational model with the following parameters: isoproterenol, $K_A = 400\,nM$ for both tissues, $\tau = 100$ for rat and 300 for guinea pig left atria; and prenalterol, $K_A = 13\,nM$ for rat atria and 20 nM for guinea pig atria, $\tau = 0.21$ for rat and 0.8 for guinea pig left atria. Notably, data for the two agonists can be fit with relatively constant ratios of τ (0.0021, 0.0027) and K_A (30, 20 nM) for both tissues illustrating the tissue independence of K_A and relative τ measurements.

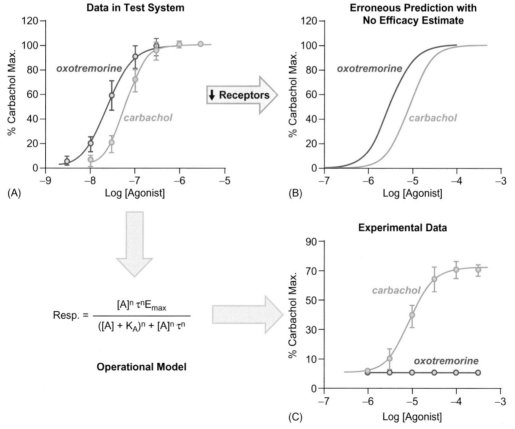

FIGURE 5.19 Concentration-response curves to the muscarinic agonists oxotremorine and carbachol in guinea pig ileum (data redrawn from [13]); oxotremorine is three fold more potent than carbachol. With no prior knowledge of the relative efficacies of these agonists and with no calculation with the operational model, it might be supposed that a 100-fold loss in system sensitivity would yield the profile shown in panel B. Calculation of predicted effects with the operational model predicts the profile shown in panel C; the curves shown are actual experimental curves obtained after alkylation of a portion of the receptor population to produce a 100-fold decrease in sensitivity.

FIGURE 5.20 The effects of chain length elongation on alkyltrimethylammonium agonists of muscarinic receptors in guinea pig ileum. Responses to C_7TMA (filled circles), C_8TMA (open circles), C_9TMA (filled triangles), and $C_{10}TMA$ (open squares). Note the selective effect on efficacy and lack of effect on affinity. Drawn from [14].

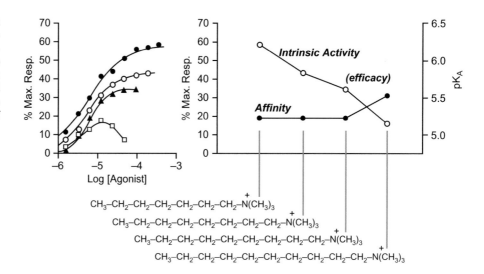

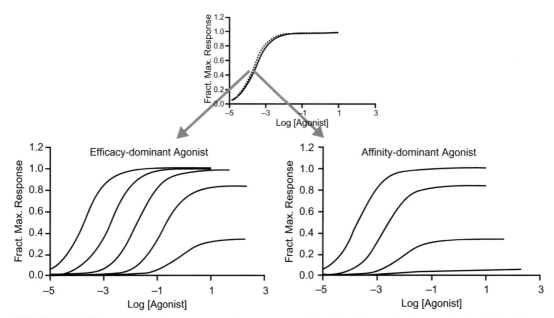

FIGURE 5.21 Effects of decreasing receptor number on two agonists. The efficacy-dominant agonist has high efficacy ($\tau = 5000$) and low affinity ($K_A = 1$), while the affinity-dominant agonist has low efficacy ($\tau = 50$) and high affinity ($K_A = 0.01$). Top curves show that both agonists are equiactive in a high receptor density system. However, as receptor density decreases in 10-fold increments, the curves for the efficacy-dominant agonist shift to the right but retain maximal response until a 100-fold shift is attained, while the curves to the affinity-dominant agonist show depressed maxima with any decrease in receptor number.

[14]. It can be seen from these data that the increased chain length selectively produces changes in efficacy while not affecting affinity to any great extent.

It is important to note that it may be very useful to determine whether an observed agonist potency is more dependent upon high efficacy or high affinity. In a given receptor system, two agonists may have identical potency and thus seem indistinguishable (see Figure 5.21A). However, the potency of one agonist may emanate from high efficacy (denoted "efficacy-dominant") while the potency of the other may emanate from

high affinity (and concomitant low efficacy; denoted "affinity-dominant"). The importance of knowing this is the fact that these agonists will deviate from such identical potency profiles in systems of different receptor number and/or receptor coupling efficiency. Specifically, the maximal response to the efficacy-dominant agonist will be more resistant to decreases in receptor number than will the lower-efficacy agonist. Therefore, the dose-response curve of the high-efficacy agonist will shift to the right with decreases in coupling efficiency, receptor number, or onset of tachyphylaxis (desensitization; see

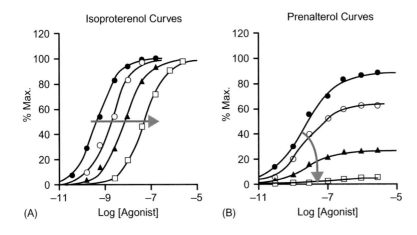

FIGURE 5.22 Dependence of agonist response on efficiency of receptor coupling and/or receptor density. Responses to the high-efficacy β-adrenoceptor agonist isoproterenol (panel A) and the low-efficacy β-adrenoceptor agonist prenalterol (panel B) in thyroxine pretreated guinea pig right atria (filled circles), rat left atria (open circles), guinea pig left atria (filled triangles), and guinea pig extensor digitorum longus muscle (filled squares). Data redrawn from [15].

TABLE 5.2 Tri-Level Testing of Agonists

Activity	Experimental Approach	Rationale
Level 1	Track extent of agonism	• Quantify pEC_{50} and Max if partial agonists • Quantify potency ratios if full agonists • Quantify agonism in a system-independent manner
Level 2	Determine if agonism is orthosteric or allosteric to endogenous agonist site	• Determine selectivity • Block effects with target orthosteric antagonist • Determine effects of partial agonist on dose–response curves to full agonist • Define agonist properties • Determine if partial agonist will block some endogenous agonism
Level 3	Measure temporal characteristics of agonism	• Measure special properties • GPCRs: Test pK inhibitors/ measure ERK activity • Proclivity for desensitization • Characterize signaling

Figure 5.21 lower left), whereas the dose-response curves to the affinity-dependent agonist will return a depressed maximal response with no shift to the right (see Figure 5.21 lower right). Thus, these agonists can be equiactive in some tissues but show completely different profiles of activity in others. In general, efficacy-dominant agonists are more resistant to tachyphylaxis (or, at least, an increase in dosage can regain response) and give a more uniform stimulation to all tissues *in vivo*. In contrast, affinity-dominant agonists are more sensitive to tachyphylaxis (and no increase in dosage can regain response, and, in fact, the agonist can then function as an antagonist of other agonists at the receptor) and demonstrate more texture with respect to organ-selective agonism *in vivo*. Figure 5.22 shows the agonist effects of two β-adrenoceptor agonists; isoproterenol is efficacy-dominant while prenalterol is affinity-dominant [15]. It can be seen that the responses to prenalterol are more sensitive to tissue type, with respect to the maximal response, than are the responses to isoproterenol. It can also be seen that the guinea pig extensor digitorum longus muscle

produces a response to isoproterenol but no agonist response to prenalterol. In this tissue, prenalterol functions as a full competitive antagonist of responses to isoproterenol.

5.6.2 Secondary and Tertiary Testing of Agonists

Table 5.2 indicates two additional levels of testing to fully characterize agonists. Once it has been determined that a series of compounds produce concentration-dependent agonism that can be measured reliably with concentration-response curves, it also is important to determine whether the test agonist binds to the endogenous orthosteric binding site of the receptor (used by the natural agonist) or a site separate from that site (see Table 5.2). In the latter case, the agonist would be allosteric. The usual method of differentiating these is to determine the sensitivity of the agonism to standard orthosteric antagonists of the target receptor. Lack of effect of such antagonists suggests an allosteric site (see Chapter 7, Figure 7.15 for an example).

FIGURE 5.23 Schematic diagram of seven transmembrane receptor signaling pathways. Activation of G-proteins results in a rapid transient intracellular response. Agonist-activated receptors also may bind β-arrestin and internalize to form an intracellular complex for kinases that produce long-term signals involved in transcription. Separate agonist assays may be required to visualize each of these activities.

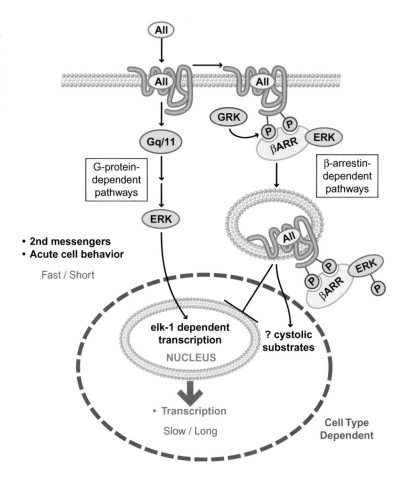

There are fundamental differences in the way orthosteric versus allosteric agonists interact with the natural system. Thus, while an orthosteric partial agonist initiates its own response, it will also block the effects of the endogenous agonist in some cases (see Chapter 6, Section 6.3.5 and Figure 6.13A). In contrast, an allosteric agonist binds to its own site to allow the natural agonist to co-bind to the receptor. The presence of the allosteric agonist may change the reactivity of the receptor toward the natural agonist, either decreasing its effect (as would an orthosteric partial agonist), not changing its effect, or increasing the effects of the natural agonist [16] (see Figure 7.15). This is discussed further in Chapter 7 under the heading of allosteric agonism.

Another possibly important aspect of agonism is the breadth of cellular pathways that an agonist stimulates and/or the temporal aspect of that stimulation. For example, as discussed in Chapter 2, 7-transmembrane receptor stimulation can result in activation of G-proteins for a rapid transient response and also a longer lasting, lower level activation of β-arrestin-mediated kinase activation that leads to transcription events in the nucleus (see Figure 5.23). While early data suggested that β-arrestin mainly causes the termination of the G-protein effects, subsequent studies have indicated a rich array of

responses emanating from the β-arrestin intracellular complex [17−20]. Presently there is a large body of evidence to implicate β-arrestin signaling in a host of diseases including diabetes [21], heart failure [22], cardiovascular disease [22−24], central nervous system diseases involving serotonin [25], diseases involving angiotensin [26,27] and adrenergic signaling [28,29], and parathyroid hormone [30]. There are data to show that different agonists favor one of these pathways over the other in some receptor systems; special agonist assays are required to detect this heterogeneity of effect, and this is becoming a part of standard characterization of response in agonist discovery programs. This leads into a major consideration in the quantification of agonism, namely the determination and quantification of biased agonism.

5.7 BIASED SIGNALING

Data have emerged in the literature that are incompatible with a scheme whereby receptors are simple switches (an active and inactive state), and now it is realized that different agonists can produce different *qualities* of agonism as well as varying quantities of agonism (for reviews see [31−34]). The source of this variance in agonist quality is

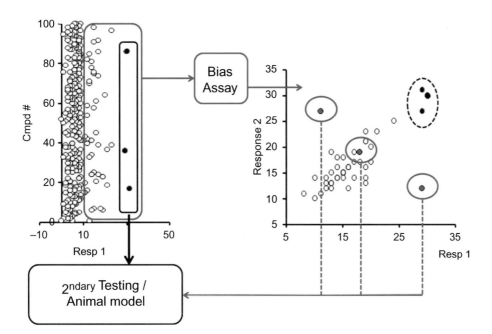

FIGURE 5.24 Screening for biased phenotypes. Panel to the left shows screening data where most active compounds are represented by open circles lying furthest to the right along the Resp1 axis. Conventional discovery schemes would progress the most active molecules (filled circles) into more sophisticated models. In light of possible biased agonism, a larger subset of the compounds outlined in the red rectangle are tested in another assay for a second signaling pathway and exemplar molecules (red filled circles) from the array progressed into further tests. These molecules would be known to be different with respect their signaling properties.

the fact that agonists can stabilize different active states of receptors. These multiple active states in turn interact differentially with signaling proteins in the cell as they produce agonism [35]; the stabilization of different receptor active states through the binding of different ligands has been observed directly by [^{19}F]-nuclear magnetic resonance [36]. When this occurs certain cellular pathways will be activated to a greater extent than others, and the ligands that produce this effect will produce biased signals. Signalling bias has the potential to produce therapeutically beneficial effects by emphasizing useful therapeutic signals and minimizing harmful secondary effects. Strategies have been employed to capitalize on biased signalling for therapeutic drugs; one is to generate data to identify where a given signal is either especially beneficial or especially harmful to a defined therapeutic treatment. Genetic knockout animals can be very helpful in this regard. For example, nicotinic acid receptor activation (GPR109) in β-arrestin null mice leads to a lowering of serum fatty acids without the accompanying flushing seen in normal mice [37]; this suggests that an agonist of GPR109 with β-arrestin activating effects could be a superior therapy. Similarly, opioid receptor agonists are known to produce analgesia with concomitant and unwanted respiratory depression. Respiratory depression to opioid agonists is greatly diminished in β-arrestin knockout mice, suggesting that a ligand that did not cause receptor association with β-arrestin would produce analgesia with less respiratory depression [38—41]. Similarly there is a possible indication for parathyroid hormone (PTH) in the treatment of osteoporosis. The fact that parathyroid hormone does not build bone or increase the number of osteoclasts in β-arrestin-2 knockout mice suggests that this signaling pathway is the therapeutically relevant

one [42,43], and that a PTH agonist with β-arrestin biased signaling would be an optimal therapy for this receptor.

Even if it is not clear whether a bias would provide a better treatment, i.e., there are no preconceived ideas as to the desirability of biased signaling, modern screening practices can be used to identify biased ligands as tools to evaluate signaling systems. Thus, selective assays for various signaling pathways are used to identify biased ligands which then are tested in more complex assays (animal models *in vivo*) to determine whether superior therapeutic phenotypes can be associated with any defined bias (see Figure 5.24).

The term "bias" suggests that receptor activation by a ligand causes one signaling pathway linked to that receptor to be activated to a greater extent than another. A useful representation of such behavior is through a "bias plot", in which the response to one process is graphed as a function of the response produced in another. For example, biased signal activation can be shown for the cardiac activity by comparing myocardial inotropy (increased isometric force of contraction) to lusitropy (increased rate of relaxation) in response to elevations in intracellular cyclic AMP. As shown in Figure 5.25, there is a curved relationship when myocardial inotropy is graphed as a function of myocardial lusitropy; i.e., the response is biased toward the production of greater lusitropy for a given increase in inotopy. Presumably this is a function of the requirements of the cell and will be referred to as "system bias"; all agonists producing elevated cyclic AMP in the myocardial cell will be subject to this signaling bias. While this conceivably might be exploited therapeutically, it is of limited application since it is a bias that cannot be manipulated pharmacologically. Bias plots also can be curvilinear due to the relative sensitivity of the assays used to

FIGURE 5.25 Effects of dibutryl cyclic AMP on myocardial relaxation (lusitropy) and force of contraction (inotropy) responses in rat atria. Panel on right shows a bias plot where the observed lusitropic effects are expressed as a function of the inotropic effects seen at the same concentration of dibutryl cyclic AMP. It can be seen that in this tissue, the lusitropic response requires less intracellular messenger to become activated than does the inotropic response. Data redrawn from [44].

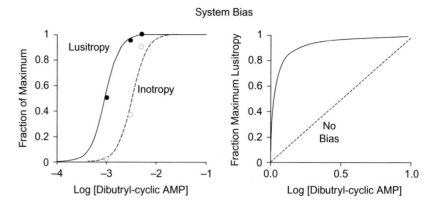

FIGURE 5.26 Effects of β-adrenoceptor agonists on G-protein activation of cyclic AMP and β-arrestin-receptor complexation in separate assays for the effects. Panel on right shows a bias plot where the observed effects on cyclic AMP are expressed as a function of the β-arrestin effects seen at the same concentration of agonist (ISO = isoproterenol, FEN = fenoterol, EPI = epinephrine). It can be seen that the cyclic AMP assay is generally more sensitive than the β-arrestin assay causing an observed bias toward the cyclic AMP response in the bias plot. However, this bias is imposed equally on all the agonists since it is simply due to the differential sensitivity of the two assays. Data drawn from [45].

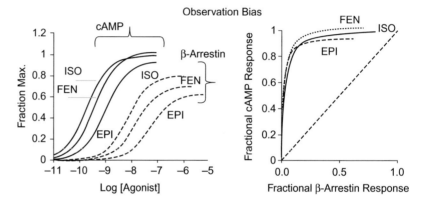

make the measurement; this is referred to as "observation bias". For example, Figure 5.26 shows how β-adrenoceptor-mediated beta-arrestin pharmacologic assays are, in this case, 30-fold less sensitive than second messenger assays [45]; a bias plot of these two responses shows a clearly skewed relationship. As with system bias, there is no distinction between agonists with this type of effect, i.e., all agonists are uniformly affected by observation bias. Observational bias will vary with types of assays and assay conditions. However, a third type of bias, termed "ligand bias" can be operable within system and observational bias which stems from the stabilization of different receptor active states by agonists [35]. This type of bias is uniquely related to the chemical structure of the agonist and thus can be manipulated using medicinal chemistry for possible therapeutic advantage. When this mechanism is operative, the bias plots of different ligands, while all subject to system and observation bias, will show a ligand-dependent heterogeneity (see Figure 5.27); it is this ligand-specific bias that can be exploited therapeutically, since it is related to the chemical structure of the molecule.

Figure 5.28A shows two ligands interacting with the same receptor; agonist A stabilizes a conformation that

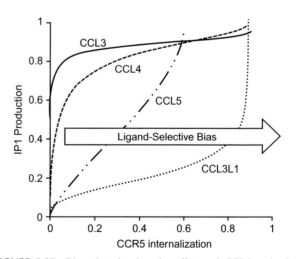

FIGURE 5.27 Bias plot showing the effects of CCR5 activation by four chemokines on inositol phosphate production (ordinate values IP1) and the internalization of CCR5 receptors (abscissae) produced by the same concentration of chemokine receptor in two separate assays. While there is a bias towards the IP1 response (which could be the result of system and/or observation bias), it is not homogeneous for all chemokines This indicates that something unique to the specific chemokines imposes an added bias to the signaling, i.e., these molecules stabilize different receptor active states. Data redrawn from [11].

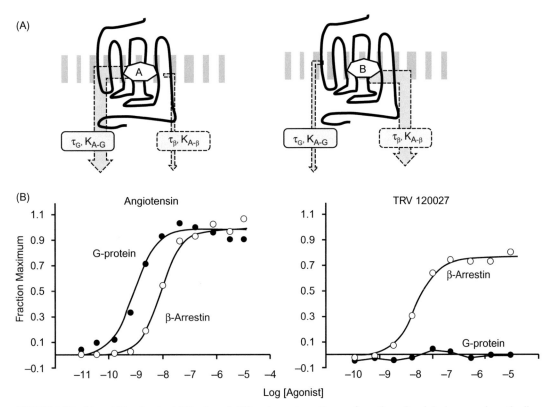

FIGURE 5.28 Ligand bias due to stabilization of different receptor active conformations. Panel A shows a schematic diagram of two receptors activated by two ligands A and B. Ligand A stabilizes a state that preferentially interacts with the G-protein signaling pathway (giving an efficacy for this pathway of τ_G with an affinity K_{AG} (but also having another efficacy for the β-arrestin pathway $\tau\beta$ and $K_A\beta$) while another agonist B has the opposite bias preferentially activating the β-arrestin pathway. Panel B shows an example of such a biased ligand. While angiotensin produces activation of G_q and β-arrestin signaling, the biased ligand TRV120027 activates only the β-arrestin pathway. Data for Panel B redrawn from [46].

favors activation of G-proteins, while agonist B stabilizes a conformation favoring the interaction of the receptor with β-arrestin. Depending on the physiological outcomes of each of these signaling pathway activations, agonists A and B could have very different activity profiles. Figure 5.28B shows the relative activation (or lack of activation) of G-protein and β-arrestin pathways produced by two ligands for angiotensin receptors. While angiotensin II produces activation of both G_q protein and causes the receptor to associate with β-arrestin (to cause another type of signaling—see Chapter 2 Section 2.5.4), the biased ligand TRV120027 does not activate G-proteins but does cause β-arrestin-based signaling [46]. In this case, the profile of TRV120027 is an improvement on standard heart failure treatments such as losartan, as the latter blocks debilitating vasoconstriction due to elevated angiotensin level while the former does so and provides beneficial β-arrestin signaling to the failing myocardial cell [47,48]. In general, biased signaling can be therapeutically useful in two settings: the emphasis of a favorable signal or the deletion of an unwanted signal. A key factor in the development of biased agonists (and antagonists) is

the system-independent quantification of the effect for use in optimization studies.

Biased agonism can be quantified with the Black/Leff operational model; the key is to assign an efficacy (τ) and affinity (K_A) to the signaling pathway and not total cell response. The index of agonism that is the theoretically most sound takes into account the potency of the agonist (i.e., the location parameter of the agonist concentration-response curve along the concentration axis; usually the pEC_{50}) and the maximal response to the agonist. To this end a transducer coefficient can be calculated for each signaling pathway in the form of log (τ/K_A) [11]. Transducer coefficients describe a molecular allosteric vector [31] comprised of the agonist (as modulator), receptor (as a conduit), and signaling protein (as a guest — see Figure 5.29). In effect, biased agonism is probe-dependent allosterism directed toward the cellular signaling apparatus; i.e., the agonist modulator modifies the affinity of the receptor toward the signaling protein and also the molecular outcome of the result (the efficacy). Biased agonism, through differing efficacies of the agonists toward signaling pathways, is intuitive but

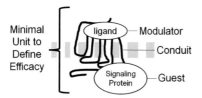

FIGURE 5.29 Biased signaling as an allosteric system comprised as the agonist functioning as an allosteric modulator of the receptor protein (the conduit) as it interacts with guest molecules (signaling proteins). All three components must be considered when quantifying efficacy.

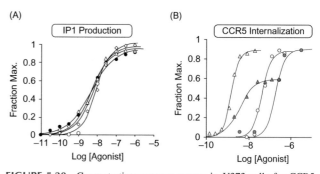

FIGURE 5.30 Concentration-response curves in U373 cells for CCR5 activation with chemokines (CCL3L1, filled circles), CCL5 (open circles), CCL3 (filled triangles), and CCL4 (open triangles). Panel A for inositol phosphate production and panel B CCR5 internalization. Data redrawn from [11].

what may not be as intuitively clear is the need to associate a unique affinity of the agonist for the receptor as it interacts with each signaling pathway as well. Thus, the same receptor can have different affinities for different signaling proteins when the agonist is bound, and since allosteric energy is reciprocal, this means also that the receptor will have different affinities for the agonist when different signaling proteins are bound. For example, there could be a K_A value for a given agonist for a receptor when it is interacting with a G-protein and another K_A for the same agonist on the same receptor when it interacts with β-arrestin; this is due to the allosteric nature of receptors [31,49,50] and is discussed in detail in Section 7.4.3).

This idea is supported by functional and binding experiments; for instance there is a 50-fold change in the affinity of [^{3}H]dimethyl-W84 with the allosteric modulator gallamine for muscarinic M_2 receptor changes in the presence of the co-binding ligand N-methylscopolamine [51]. In functional studies the affinity of the N-methyl-D-aspartate (NDMA) receptor antagonist ifenprodil changes by a factor of 10 in the presence of the co-binding ligand NMDA [52]. Changes in receptor structure also have been shown with the binding of signaling proteins to receptors; i.e., binding of $G_{\alpha 16}$ and/or $G_{\alpha i2}$ G-protein subunits to the κ-opioid receptor show changes in conformation in transmembrane domains 6 and 7 and these are concomitant with an 18-fold change in the affinity of the ligand salvanorin [53]. For this reason it is untenable to utilize a single K_A from a single source (i.e., binding) in $\log(\tau/K_A)$ estimates for different pathways. In addition, these data suggest that the binding affinity may have no relevance to the operational functional affinity in the cell.

Figure 5.30 shows chemokine-mediated effects for the CCR5 chemokine receptor for two signaling pathways; inositol phosphate production and internalization of the CCR5 receptor [11]. These concentration-response curves furnished the heterogeneous bias plots shown in Figure 5.27; $\Delta\log(\tau/K_A)$ calculations quantify this heterogeneity in bias and assign a bias number to each molecule which should be an independent measure of the ability of the molecule to induce bias for CCR5 in all cellular systems. An example of this procedure is given in Table 5.3 and can be thought of as a stepwise process:

1. Calculate $\log(\tau/K_A)$ values for each agonist for each signaling pathway and then express these for

each pathway as a $\Delta\log(\tau/K_A)$ value for each agonist when compared to a selected reference agonist. Which agonist chosen as the reference does not affect the calculations but often a natural agonist for the system is chosen as a contrast to bias of synthetic agonists. The $\Delta\log(\tau/K_A)$ values serve as a relative measure of the agonists to activate the selected signaling pathway.

2. When this is done for both pathways (with the same reference agonist used for each pathway), then cross-pathway comparisons can be made. Thus, $\Delta\Delta\log(\tau/K_A)$ values are calculated which serve to quantify the relative difference in selective pathway activation, i.e., bias. It should be noted that comparison to the reference agonist cancels both system bias and observation bias and these effects cease to be a factor in the calculations.

3. The bias of the agonist is then defined as:

$$\text{Bias} = 10^{\Delta\Delta \mathit{l}\text{Log}(\tau/K_A)} \qquad (5.7)$$

It can be seen from Figure 5.27 that CCL3L1 is uniquely the most biased towards inducing the greatest amount of CCR5 receptor internalization for a given IP1 response, when compared to CCL3, CCL4, and CCL5. This may be therapeutically relevant for this chemokine since the gene copy number for the production of CCL3L1 has been associated with favorable survival after HIV-1 infection in progression to AIDS [54]. The data suggest that CCL3L1-mediated internalization of the CCR5 receptor may yield protection from further HIV-1 infection by removing CCR5, the target protein used by the gp120 viral coat protein to infect cells. The 32.4-fold bias of CCL3L1 for CCR5 internalization shown in Table 5.3 is consistent with this idea.

It can be seen from Equations 5.5 and 5.6 that the parameters of the operational model can translate to observable indices, namely the potency of an agonist (EC_{50}) and the maximal response. Under certain

TABLE 5.3 Biased Signaling for Chemokine Activation of CCR5 Receptors

Agonist	IP₁ Production		CCR5R Internalization	
	$\text{Log}(\tau/K_A)$	$\Delta\text{log}(\tau/K_A)$[1]	$\text{Log}(\tau/K_A)$	$\Delta\text{log}(\tau/K_A)$[1]
CCL3	7.75	0	6.58	**0**
CCL4	8.01	0.26	8.2	1.62
CCL5	8.27	0.52	8.53	1.95
CCL3L1	8.48	0.73	8.82	2.24

	$\Delta\Delta\text{Log}(\tau/K_A)$[2]	BIAS[3]
CCL3	**0**	1
CCL4	1.36	23.1
CCL5	1.43	27
CCL3L1	1.51	32.4

[1]Relative to CCL3
[2]IP1 vs Internalization
[3]$10^{\Delta\Delta\text{Log}(\tau/K_A)}$

circumstances, these easily observable features of agonism can be utilized to quantify agonist bias. Specifically, an index has been proposed to characterize agonism termed the "relative activity", consisting of the maximal response divided by the EC_{50} [12,55,56]. Combining Equations 5.5 and 5.6 yields the following expression for RA in terms of the Black/Leff operational model:

$$RA = \frac{\tau^n((1+\tau^n)^{1/n} - 1)E_m}{K_A(1 + \tau^n)} \quad (5.8)$$

In the special circumstance of curves with $n = 1$, the RA then becomes $\tau E_m/K_A$ and relative RA values reduce to transduction ratios $(\Delta\text{log}(RA) = (\Delta\text{log}(\tau/K_A)))$. An additional method of determining $\Delta\text{log}(\tau/K_A)$ values is through the methods of Barlow, Scott and Stephenson [57]. This method is discussed more fully in Section 5.8.1 and yields values of $\Delta\text{log}(\tau/K_A)$ for two agonists through the slope of the linear regression (*vide infra*).

Log transducer coefficients can be used to quantify agonist-specific signaling bias and also the induction of bias into endogenous signaling through allosteric modulation (see Chapter 7). However there are factors to consider when predicting possible biased effects *in vivo* and these are discussed more fully in Chapter 8.

5.7.1 Receptor Selectivity

Since $\text{log}(\tau/K_A)$ is an index of the power that a molecule has to activate a receptor, transduction ratios $(\Delta\text{log}(\tau/K_A))$ can also be used to gage selective receptor agonism. Thus, the relative power of two agonists to activate the primary (therapeutic) receptor (quantified as Δlog

$(\tau/K_A)_{\text{therapeutic}}$ values) vs. their relative power to activate a secondary receptor (perhaps denoting a safety hazard or other unwanted activity) given as $\Delta\text{log}(\tau/K_A)_{\text{secondary}}$ values; the selectivity index would then be:

$$\Delta\Delta\text{log}(\tau/K_A)_{\text{selectivity}} = \text{log}(\tau/K_A)_{\text{therapeutic}} \\ - \Delta\text{log}(\tau/K_A)_{\text{secondary}} \quad (5.9)$$

The interpretation of $\Delta\Delta\text{log}(\tau/K_A)_{\text{selectivity}}$ values is discussed further in Chapter 8.

5.8 NULL ANALYSES OF AGONISM

Although the Black/Leff operational model is the most sound theoretical framework for agonism, and also offers the best options for characterizing and quantifying agonism, other null methods have been presented in the literature which can be used to quantify the efficacy and affinity of agonists. The most straightforward can be applied to partial agonists, since the location parameter of the partial agonist concentration-response curve (EC_{50}) is a relatively close estimate of the affinity (K_A), while changes in maximal response are good indicators of changes in efficacy (see Figure 5.31).

5.8.1 Partial Agonists

As noted in Chapter 2, the functional EC_{50} for a full agonist may not, and most often will not, correspond to the binding affinity of the agonist. This is due to the fact that the agonist possesses efficacy and the coupling of agonist binding to production of response is nonlinear. In terms

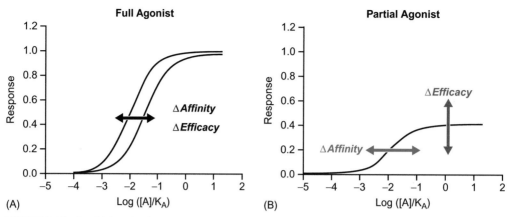

FIGURE 5.31   Sensitivity of various descriptive parameters for concentration-response curves to drug receptor parameters. (A) The location parameter (potency) of curves for full agonists depends on both affinity and efficacy. (B) For partial agonists, the location parameter (EC_{50}, potency) is solely dependent upon affinity while the maximal response is solely dependent upon efficacy.

of the Black/Leff operational model (see Section 5.10.1) the EC_{50} is related to the K_A by:

$$EC_{50} = \frac{K_A}{(1 + \tau)}, \qquad (5.10)$$

where τ is the term relating efficacy of the agonist and the efficiency of the receptor system in converting receptor activation to response (high values of τ reflect either high efficacy, highly efficient receptor coupling, or both). High values of τ are associated with full agonism. It can be seen from Equation 5.10 that full agonism produces differences between the observed EC_{50} and the affinity (K_A).

Equation 5.10 shows that as $\tau \to 0$, $EC_{50} \to K_A$. Therefore, in general the EC_{50} of a weak partial agonist can be a reasonable approximation of the K_A (see Section 5.10.1 for further details). The lower the magnitude of the maximal response (lower τ), the more closely the EC_{50} will approximate the K_A. Figure 5.32 shows the relationship between agonist-receptor occupancy for partial agonists and the response for different levels of maximal response (different values of τ). It can be seen that as the maximal response $\to 0$, the relationship between agonist-receptor occupancy and tissue response becomes linear and $EC_{50} \to K_A$.

A measure of the affinity of a partial agonist can be obtained using the method devised by Barlow, Scott, and Stephenson [57]. Using null procedures, the effects of stimulus-response mechanisms are neutralized and receptor-specific effects of agonists are isolated. This method, based on classical or operational receptor theory, depends on the concept of equiactive concentrations of drug. Under these circumstances, receptor stimuli can be equated since it is assumed that equal responses emanate from equal stimuli in any given system. An example of this procedure is given in Section 13.2.2.

Dose-response curves to a full agonist [A] and a partial agonist [P] are obtained in the same receptor preparation. From these curves, reciprocals of equiactive concentrations of the full and partial agonist are used in the following linear equation (derived for the operational model; see Section 5.10.2):

$$\frac{1}{[A]} = \frac{1}{[P]} \cdot \frac{\tau_a \cdot K_P}{\tau_p \cdot K_A} + \frac{\tau_a - \tau_p}{\tau_p \cdot K_A}, \qquad (5.11)$$

where τ_a and τ_p are efficacy terms for the full and partial agonist, respectively, and K_A and K_P their respective ligand-receptor equilibrium dissociation constants. Thus, a regression of $1/[A]$ upon $1/[P]$ yields the K_B modified by an efficacy term with the following parameters from Equation 5.11:

$$K_P = \frac{Slope}{Intercept}\left(1 - \frac{\tau_p}{\tau_a}\right). \qquad (5.12)$$

It should be noted that the logarithm of the slope from the regression described by Equation 5.11 will also furnish an estimate of the $\Delta\log(\tau/K_A)$ values for the agonists for use in calculating biased signaling. It can be seen from Equation 5.12 that a more accurate estimate of the affinity will be obtained with partial agonists of low efficacy (i.e., as $\tau_a \gg \tau_p$, $\tau_p/\tau_a \to 0$). Double reciprocal plots are known to produce overemphasis of some values, skew the distribution of data points, and be heterogeneously sensitive to error. For these reasons, it may be useful to use a metameter of Equation 5.11 as a linear plot to measure the K_P. Thus, the K_P can be estimated from a plot according to:

$$\frac{[P]}{[A]} = \frac{[P]}{K_A}((\tau_A/\tau_p) - 1) + \frac{\tau_a K_P}{\tau_p K_A}, \qquad (5.13)$$

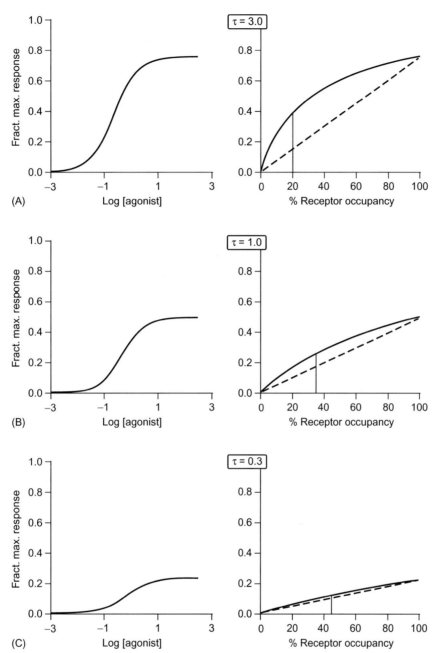

FIGURE 5.32 The relationship between the EC_{50} for partial agonists and the affinity (K_A). For higher-efficacy partial agonists ($\tau = 3$), the relationship between receptor occupancy and response is hyperbolic (note solid versus dotted line in right-hand panel, where the dotted line represents a linear and direct relationship between the occupancy of the receptor by the agonist and the production of response). This deviation lessens with lower efficacy values for the partial agonist (note panels for agonist with $\tau = 1$). With weak partial agonists, the EC_{50} and K_A values nearly coincide (see panels with $\tau = 0$).

Where:

$$K_P = \frac{Intercept}{Slope}(1 - \tau_p/\tau_a).$$ (5.14)

Another variant is:

$$\frac{[A]}{[P]} = \frac{\tau_p K_A}{\tau_a K_P} - [A]^* \frac{(1 - \tau_p/\tau_a)}{K_P},$$ (5.15)

Where:

$$K_P = \frac{(\tau_p/\tau_a - 1)}{slope}.$$ (5.16)

An example of the application of this method to the measurement of the affinity of the histamine receptor partial agonist E-2-P (with the full agonist histamine) is

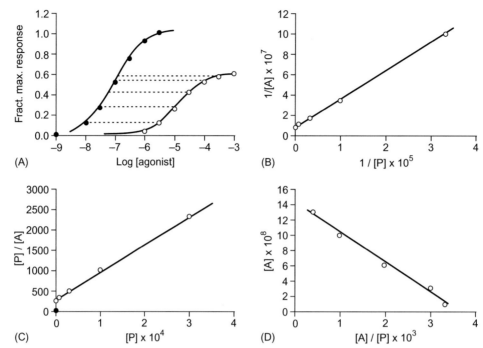

FIGURE 5.33 Method of Barlow, Scott, and Stevenson for measurement of affinity of a partial agonist. (A) Guinea pig ileal smooth muscle contraction to histamine (filled circles) and partial histamine receptor agonist E-2-P (N,N-diethyl-2-(1-pyridyl)ethylamine (open circles). Dotted lines show equiactive concentrations of each agonist used for the double reciprocal plot shown in panel B. (B) Double reciprocal plot of equiactive concentrations of histamine (ordinates) and E-2-P (abscissae). Linear plot has a slope of 55.47 and an intercept of 1.79×10^6. This yields a K_B $(1 - \tau_p/\tau_A) = 30.9$ μM. (C) Variant of double reciprocal plot according to Equation 5.8. (D) Variant of double reciprocal plot according to Equation 5.10. Data redrawn from [58].

shown in Figure 5.33. A full example of the application of this method for the measurement of partial agonists is given in Section 13.2.2.

The other system-independent measure of drug activity that can be measured for an agonist is efficacy, the power of the molecule to induce a change in the biological system. Since the maximal response to an agonist is totally dependent on efficacy and the efficiency of receptor stimulus-response coupling (receptor occupancy is maximal and thus affinity is not an issue), the relative maxima of agonists can be used to estimate the relative efficacy of agonists. In terms of operational theory, the maximal response to a given agonist (Max) is given by the following (see Section 5.10.3):

$$\text{Max} = \frac{E_{max}\tau}{1 + \tau}. \tag{5.17}$$

The relative maximal response to two agonists with τ values denoted τ and τ' is given by the following (see Section 5.9.4):

$$\frac{\text{Max}'}{\text{Max}} = \frac{\tau'(1 + \tau)}{\tau(1 + \tau')}. \tag{5.18}$$

It can be seen that the relative maxima are completely dependent on efficacy, receptor density, and the efficiency of stimulus-response coupling ($\tau = [R]/K_E$; see

Chapter 3). However, the relationship is not a direct one. At low values of receptor density the relative maximal response approximates the relative efficacy of the two agonists (as τ, $\tau' << 1$, Max'/Max $\rightarrow$ τ'/τ). Equation 5.18 indicates that if both agonists are weak partial agonists in a given receptor system, then the relative maximal response will be an approximation of the relative efficacy of the two agonists. At the least, even in cases where the maxima approach the system maximum, the rank order of the maxima of two agonists is an accurate estimate of the rank order of the efficacy of the agonists.

5.8.2 Full Agonists

As discussed previously, the location parameter of a dose-response curve (potency) of a full agonist is a complex amalgam of the affinity and efficacy of the agonist for the receptor and the ability of the system to process receptor stimulus and return tissue response. This latter complication can be circumvented by comparing the agonists in the same functional receptor system (null methods). Under these circumstances, the receptor density and efficiency of receptor coupling effects cancel each other, since they are common for all the agonists. The resulting relative potency ratios of the full agonists (providing the concentrations are taken at the same response level for

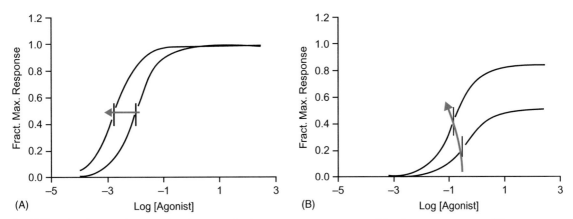

FIGURE 5.34 Comparative potencies of two agonists in two receptor systems containing the same receptor at different receptor densities. (A) Relative potency in system with high receptor density ($\tau_1 = 500$, $\tau_2 = 100$). The potency ratio = 5. (B) Dose-response curves for same two agonists in receptor system with 1/100 the receptor density. Potency ratio = 1.3.

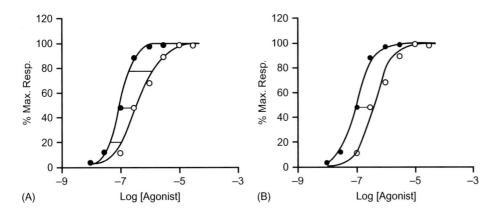

FIGURE 5.35 Full agonist potency ratios. (A) Data fit to individual three-parameter logistic functions. Potency ratios are not independent of level of response: At 20%, PR = 2.4; at 50%, PR = 4.1; and at 80%, PR = 6.9. (B) Curves refit to logistic with common maximum asymptote and slope. PR = 4.1. The fit to common slope and maximum is not statistically significant from individual fit.

each agonist) are system-independent measures of the molecular properties of the agonists; namely, their affinity and efficacy for the receptor. Such potency ratios for full agonists are sometimes referred to as EMRs (equimolar potency ratios) or EPMRs (equipotent molar potency ratios) and are a standard method of comparing full agonists across different systems.

There are three major prerequisites for the use of this tool in SAR determination. The first is that the agonists must truly all be full agonists. If one is a partial agonist, then the system independence of the potency ratio measurement is lost. This is because of the different effects that variation in receptor density, efficiency of coupling, and measurement variation have on the location parameters of dose-response curves to partial versus full agonists. For example, Figure 5.34 shows the effect of an increase in receptor number on a high-efficacy agonist ($\tau = 500$) and low-efficacy agonist ($\tau = 5$). It can be seen from this figure that the curve for the high-efficacy agonist shifts to the left directly across the concentration axis, whereas the curve for the lower-efficacy agonist rises upward along the ordinal axis with little concomitant displacement along the concentration axis: that is, the

potency of the full agonist changes, whereas the potency of the partial agonist does not. This is because potency is dependent upon efficacy and affinity to different extents for full and partial agonists. Therefore, it is inconsistent to track SAR changes for full and partial agonists with the same tool, in this case, potency ratios.

Another prerequisite for the use of potency ratios for agonist SAR is that the ratio be independent of the level of response at which it is measured. Figure 5.35 shows dose-response curves for two full agonists. It can be seen that a rigorous fit to the data points results in two curves that are not parallel. Under these circumstances, the potency ratio of these agonists varies depending on which level of response the ratio is measured (see Figure 5.35A). In this situation the measure of drug activity is system dependent and not useful for SAR. However, the nonparallelism of these curves may be the result of random variation in response measurement and not a true reflection of the agonist activity. A statistical test can be done to determine whether these curves are from a single population of curves with the same slope, that is, if the data can be described by parallel curves, with the result that the potency ratio will not be system dependent. Application of this test to the

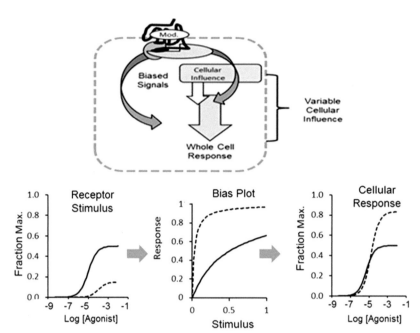

FIGURE 5.36 Non-monotonic linkage of receptor stimulus to cellular response. Top panel shows biased agonism where two receptor stimuli combine to yield a total cellular response. The cell imparts an emphasis to one of the pathways in accordance to its particular physiological requirements. As agonists produce differential production of the two stimuli, the agonist producing a greater stimulus of the cell-emphasized pathway will yield a greater cellular response than another agonist that does not. Lower panel shows two agonists activating the receptor where the stimulus from the pathway shown with the dotted line is more efficiently coupled to cellular response than other pathways. Under these circumstances, the broken line stimulus produces a greater response thus causing an aberration of the relative order of stimuli at the receptor (compare this figure to Figure 2.10).

curves shown in Figure 5.35A yields the parallel curves shown in Figure 5.35B. In this case, there is no statistical reason why the data cannot be described by parallel curves (see Chapter 12 for a detailed description of the application of this test); therefore the potency ratio can be derived from parallel curves with the result that system-independent data for SAR can be generated.

Two full agonists can be compared through EPMR values fit from curves fit to a generic sigmoidal function to yield a useful parameter dependent only upon the molecular properties of the full agonists (see Section 5.10.4):

$$\text{EPMR} = \frac{K_A(1 + \tau')}{K'_A(1 + \tau)}. \qquad (5.19)$$

For full agonists $\tau, \tau' \gg 1$, allowing the estimate $EC_{50} = K_A/\tau$. Substituting $\tau = [R_t]/K_E$, the potency ratio of two full agonists is:

$$\text{EPMR} = \frac{EC_{50}}{EC'_{50}} = \frac{K_A K_E}{K'_A K'_E}, \qquad (5.20)$$

where K_E is the Michaelis–Menten constant for the activation of the cell by the agonist-bound active receptor complex (a parameter unique to the agonist). It can be

seen from Equation 5.20 that changes in full agonist potency ratios reflect changes in either affinity or efficacy, and it cannot be discerned which of these changes with any given change in potency ratio.

The third prerequisite for accurate full agonist potency ratios is that the function connecting initial receptor stimulus given to the cellular response mechanism that yields observable response be monotonic in nature. Specifically, if the receptor stimulus is x and the tissue response is y, then there must be only one value of y for every x; this is shown in Figure 2.10. This assumption is defensible for agonists that stabilize the same receptor active conformation but may not be valid for biased agonists that do not. Therefore, if two agonists impart different degrees of stimulus to the receptor through the differential activation of two signaling pathways, then the composition of the cell may add a layer of influence into the stimulus-response function that is not constant for each agonist. In other words, if one of the signaling pathways in a given cell is more important than another, then the agonist that is biased toward that pathway will give a greater overall cellular response than a biased agonist that does not emphasize that same pathway; this is shown as an alternative version to Figure 2.10 in Figure 5.36. In practical terms, this can make full agonist potency ratios cell type

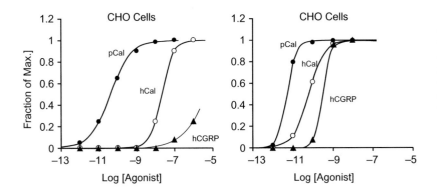

FIGURE 5.37 Cell type dependence on agonist activation of human calcitonin receptors transfected into Chinese hamster ovary (CHO) cells and CV-1 fibraoblast-like cell (COS) cells. The relative potency of the agonists is cell type dependent. Agonists are porcine (pCal), human (hCal) calcitonin and human calcitonin gene-related peptide (hCGRP). Redrawn from [59].

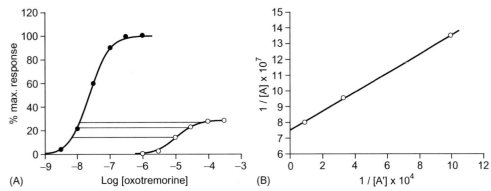

FIGURE 5.38 Measurement of the affinity of a full agonist by the method of Furchgott. (A) Concentration-response curves to oxotremorine in guinea pig ileal smooth muscle strips. Ordinates: percent maximal contraction. Abscissae: logarithms of molar concentrations of oxotremorine. Control curve (filled circles) and after partial alkylation of muscarinic receptors with phenoxybenzamine 10 μM for 12 minutes (open circles). Lines represent equiactive concentrations of oxotremorine before and after receptor alkylation. (B) Regression of reciprocals of equiactive concentrations of oxotremorine before (ordinates) and after (abscissae) receptor alkylation. The regression is linear with a slope of 609 and an intercept of 7.4×10^7. Resulting K_A estimate for oxotremorine according to Equation 5.12 is 8.2 μM. Data redrawn from [13].

dependent for biased agonists; an example is shown in Figure 5.37 for calcitonin biased agonists in two different cell types.

For full agonists, the approximation of the EC_{50} as affinity is not useful and other methods must be employed to estimate affinity. A method to measure the affinity of high-efficacy agonists has been described by Furchgott [60]. This method is based on the comparison of the responses to an agonist in a given receptor system under control conditions and again after a fraction of the receptor population has been irreversibly inactivated. For some receptors — such as α-adrenoceptors, muscarinic, serotonin, and histamine receptors — this can be accomplished through controlled chemical alkylation with site-directed alkylating agents such as β-haloalkylamines. Thus, equiactive responses obtained before and after receptor alkylation are compared in the following double reciprocal relation (see Section 5.10.4):

$$\frac{1}{[A]} = \frac{1}{[A']} * \frac{1}{q} + \frac{1}{K_A} \cdot \frac{1-q}{q}, \qquad (5.21)$$

where [A] and [A'] are equiactive agonist concentrations measured before and after receptor alkylation, respectively; q is the fraction of receptors remaining after alkylation; and K_A is the equilibrium dissociation constant of the agonist-receptor complex. Thus, a regression of 1/[A] upon 1/[A'] yields a straight line with given slope and intercept. From these, the equilibrium dissociation constant of the agonist-receptor complex can be calculated:

$$K_A = \frac{Slope - 1}{Intercept}. \qquad (5.22)$$

An example of the use of this approach is given in Figure 5.38. The method of Furchgott indicates that the affinity of the muscarinic agonist oxotremorine in guinea pig ileal smooth muscle is 8.2 μM. The EC_{50} for half-maximal contractile response to this agonist is 25 nM (a 330-fold difference). This underscores the fact that the EC_{50} for full agonists can differ considerably from the K_A. A full example of the use of this method to measure the affinity of a full agonist is given in Section 13.2.3.

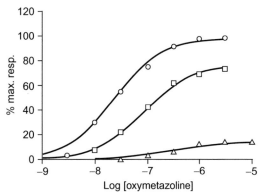

FIGURE 5.39 Measurement of affinity of a full agonist by the method of Furchgott [11] utilizing nonlinear curve fitting techniques according to the operational model. Contractions of rat anococcygeus muscle to α-adrenoceptor agonist oxymetazoline before (circles) and after irreversible receptor alkylation with phenoxybenzamine (squares: 30 nM for 10 minutes; triangles: 0.1 μM for 10 minutes). Curves fit simultaneously to Equation 5.15 with $E_{max} = 105$ and τ values for curves of ($\tau_1 = 12$), ($\tau_2 = 2.6$), and ($\tau_3 = 0.15$). The equilibrium dissociation constant for the agonist-receptor complex is 0.3 μM. Estimation by the double reciprocal plot method is $K_A = 0.32$ μM and by the Schild method (whereby oxymetazoline is utilized as a competitive antagonist of responses to the higher-efficacy agonist norepinephrine after receptor alkylation is 0.2 μM). Data redrawn from [13].

The Furchgott method can be effectively utilized by fitting the dose-response curves themselves to the operational model with fitted values of τ (before and after alkylation) and a constant K_A value. Figure 5.39 shows the use of nonlinear curve fitting to measure the affinity of the α-adrenoceptor agonist oxymetazoline in rat anococcygeus muscle after alkylation of a portion of the receptors with phenoxybenzamine. These data show how all three curves can be used for a better estimate of the affinity with nonlinear curve fitting, a technique not possible with the double reciprocal plot approach where only two dose-response curves can be used. The use of three curves increases the power of the analysis since more data are utilized for the fit and all must comply with a single estimate of K_A.

5.9 CHAPTER SUMMARY AND CONCLUSIONS

- There are practical advantages to measuring biological responses in functional experiments and numerous formats are available to do this.
- Functional responses can be measured near their cytosolic origin (immediately proximal to the activation of the biological target), further on down in the stimulus-response mechanism or as an end organ response. Amplification occurs as the progression is made from point of origin to end organ response.

- Recombinant assays have revolutionized pharmacology and now functional systems can be constructed with engineered levels of responsiveness (i.e., through difference in receptor levels or cotransfection of other proteins).
- One possible complication to consider in functional experiments is the dependence of the response on time. If fade occurs in the response, time becomes an important factor in determining the magnitude of response.
- The complications of time become much more important in stop-time measurements of response, in which a time is chosen to measure an amount of product from a biochemical reaction. Observing linearity in the production of response with respect to time allows determination that a steady state has been reached.
- The best method of quantifying agonism is through fitting agonist concentration-response curves to the Black/Leff operational model.
- The use of selective agonist assays have demonstrated that many agonists produce biased signals in cells; these biased effects can be quantified through $\log(\tau/K_A)$ values and yield therapeutic superiority over non-biased agonists.
- Biased agonists can produce cell-dependent agonist potency ratios in whole tissue experiments.

5.10 DERIVATIONS

- Relationship between the EC_{50} and affinity of agonists (Section 5.10.1).
- Method of Barlow, Scott, and Stephenson for affinity of partial agonists (Section 5.10.2).
- Maximal response of a partial agonist is dependent on efficacy (Section 5.10.3).
- Measurement of agonist affinity: method of Furchgott (Section 5.10.4).

5.10.1 Relationship Between the EC_{50} and Affinity of Agonists

In terms of the operational model, the EC_{50} of a partial agonist can also be shown to approximate the K_A. The response to an agonist [A] in terms of the operational model is given as:

$$\text{Response} = \frac{E_{max} \cdot [A] \cdot \tau}{[A](1 + \tau) + K_A}, \tag{5.23}$$

where E_{max} is the maximal response of the system, τ is a factor quantifying the ability of both the agonist (in terms of the agonist efficacy) and the system to generate response (in terms of the receptor density $[R_t]$ and the efficiency of stimulus-response coupling K_E, $\tau = [R_t]/K_E$). For a partial agonist, the maximal response $Max < E_{max}$. Therefore, from Equation 5.23:

$$Max = \frac{E_{max} \cdot \tau}{1 + \tau}. \tag{5.24}$$

For $Max < E_{max}$ (partial agonist), Equation 5.24 shows that τ is not considerably greater than unity. Under these circumstances, it can be approximated that $(\tau + 1) \to 1$. Under these circumstances, the equation for EC_{50} for a partial agonist reduces to:

$$EC_{50} = \frac{K_A}{(1 + \tau)}. \tag{5.25}$$

5.10.2 Method of Barlow, Scott, and Stephenson for Affinity of Partial Agonists

In terms of the operational model, the response to a full $[A]$ is given by:

$$Response_A = \frac{E_{max} \cdot [A] \cdot \tau_A}{[A](1 + \tau_A) + K_A}, \tag{5.26}$$

where E_{max} is the maximal response capability of the system, K_A refers to the equilibrium dissociation constant of the agonist-receptor complex, and τ_A is the term describing the ability of the agonist to produce response (efficacy, receptor density, and the stimulus-response capability of the system; see Chapter 3). Similarly, the response produced by a partial agonist $[P]$ is given by:

$$Response_p = \frac{E_{max} \cdot [P] \cdot \tau_p}{[P](1 + \tau_p) + K_P}. \tag{5.27}$$

For equiactive responses, Equation 5.26 equals Equation 5.27, and after simplification:

$$\frac{1}{[A]} = \frac{1}{[P]} \cdot \frac{\tau_a \cdot K_P}{\tau_p \cdot K_A} + \frac{\tau_a - \tau_p}{\tau_p \cdot K_A}. \tag{5.28}$$

5.10.3 Maximal Response of a Partial Agonist Is Dependent on Efficacy

In terms of the operational model, response is given by:

$$Response_A = \frac{E_{max} \cdot [A] \cdot \tau_A}{[A](1 + \tau_A) + K_A}, \tag{5.29}$$

where τ is a factor quantifying the ability of both the agonist (in terms of the agonist efficacy) and the system (in terms of the receptor density $[R_t]$ and the efficiency of

stimulus-response coupling K_E, $\tau = [Rt]/KE$). The maximal response to the agonist (i.e., as $[A] \to \infty$) is:

$$Max = \frac{E_{max} \cdot \tau}{1 + \tau}. \tag{5.30}$$

The relative maxima of two agonists is therefore:

$$\frac{Max'}{Max'} = \frac{\tau'(1 + \tau)}{\tau(1 + \tau')}. \tag{5.31}$$

It can be seen that as τ, $\tau' >> 1$ then $Max'/Max \to 1$ (i.e., both are full agonists). However, when the efficacy is low or when the stimulus-response coupling is inefficient (both conditions of low values for τ), then $\tau + 1 \to 1$ and $Max'/Max = \tau'/\tau$ (the relative maxima approximate the relative efficacy of the agonists).

5.10.4 System Independence of Full Agonist Potency Ratios

In terms of the operational model, the response to an agonist $[A]$ in terms of the operational model is given as:

$$Response = \frac{E_{max}[A]\tau}{[A](1 + \tau) + K_A}, \tag{5.32}$$

where E_{max} is the maximal response of the system, and τ is a factor quantifying the ability of both the agonist (in terms of the agonist efficacy) and the system (in terms of the receptor density $[R_t]$ and the efficiency of stimulus-response coupling K_E, $\tau = [R_t]/K_E$).

From Equation 5.31, the EC_{50} for a full agonist is:

$$EC_{50} = \frac{K_A}{1 + \tau}, \tag{5.33}$$

where K_A is the equilibrium dissociation constant of the agonist-receptor complex. For full agonists, $\tau >> 1$, therefore the $EC_{50} = K_A/\tau$. Substituting $\tau = [R_t]/K_E$, the potency ratio of two full agonists is:

$$Potency\ Ratio = \frac{EC'_{50}}{EC_{50}} = \frac{K'_A K'_E}{K_A K_E}. \tag{5.34}$$

It can be seen that the potency ratio of two full agonists, as defined by Equation 5.34, is composed of factors unique to the agonists and not the system, assuming that the stimulus-response coupling components of K_E, being common for both agonists, cancel.

5.10.5 Measurement of Agonist Affinity: Method of Furchgott

In terms of classical receptor theory, equiactive responses to an agonist are compared in the control situation $([A]$

and after irreversible inactivation of a fraction of the receptors ([A′]). Assume that after alkylation the remaining receptors equal a fraction q:

$$\frac{[A]}{[A] + K_A} = \frac{[A']}{[A'] + K_A} \cdot q, \qquad (5.35)$$

where K_A is the equilibrium dissociation constant of the agonist-receptor complex. Rearrangement of Equation 5.35 leads to

$$\frac{1}{[A]} = \frac{1}{[A']} \cdot \frac{1}{q} + \frac{1}{K_A} \cdot \frac{1-q}{q}. \qquad (5.36)$$

The equilibrium dissociation constant of the agonist-receptor complex (K_A) can be obtained by a regression of 1/[A] upon 1/[A′]. This leads to a linear regression from which:

$$K_A = \frac{\text{Slope} - 1}{\text{Intercept}}. \qquad (5.37)$$

An identical equation results from utilizing the operational model. The counterpart to Equation 5.35 is:

$$\frac{[A] \cdot \tau}{[A](1 + \tau) + K_A} = \frac{[A'] \cdot \tau'}{[A'](1 + \tau') + K_A}, \qquad (5.38)$$

where τ equals the receptor density divided by the magnitude of the transducer function, which depends on the efficiency of receptor coupling and the efficacy of the agonist: $\tau = [R_t]/K_E$. The difference between τ and τ' is that τ' represents the system with a depleted (through irreversible receptor inactivation) receptor density; that is:

$$[R_t'] < [R_t]).$$

This leads to:

$$\frac{1}{[A]} = \frac{1}{[A']} \cdot \frac{\tau}{\tau'} + \frac{(\tau/\tau') - 1}{K_A}. \qquad ([5.39])$$

Equation 5.39 can then be used to obtain the K_A from a regression of 1/[A] upon 1/[A′].

REFERENCES

[1] Chio CL, Lajiness ME, Huff RM. Activation of heterologously expressed D3 dopamine receptors: comparison with D2 dopamine receptors. Mol Pharmacol 1994;45:51–60.

[2] Roettger BF, Ghanekar D, Rao R, Toledo C, Yingling J, Pinon D, et al. Antagonist-stimulated internalization of the G protein-coupled cholecystokinin receptor. Mol Pharmacol 1997;51:357–62.

[3] Adie EJ, Kalinka S, Smith L, Francis MJ, Marenghi A, Cooper ME, et al. A pH-sensitive fluor CypHer 5, used to monitor agonist-induced G-protein coupled receptor internalization in live cells. Biotechniques 2002;33:1152–7.

[4] Chen G, Way J, Armour S, Watson C, Queen K, Jayawrickreme C, et al. Use of constitutive G protein-coupled receptor activity for drug discovery. Mol Pharmacol 1999;57:125–34.

[5] Zhong H, Guerrero SW, Esbenshade TA, Minneman KP. Inducible expression of β1-and β2-adrenergic receptors in rat C6 glioma cells: functional interactions between closely related subtypes. Mol Pharmacol 1996;50:175–84.

[6] Offermanns S, Simon MI. Gα15 and Gα16 couple a wide variety of receptors to phospholipase C. J Biol Chem 1995;270:15175–80.

[7] Johnson MP, Wisnoski DD, Leister WH, O'Brien JA, Lemaire W, Williams DL, et al. Discovery of the positive allosteric modulators of the metabotropic glutamate receptor subtype 5 from a series of N-(1,3-diphenyl-1-H-pyrazol-5-yl)benzamides that potentiate receptor function. J Med Chem 2004;47:5825–8.

[8] Kenakin TP. Differences between natural and recombinant G-protein coupled receptor systems with varying receptor/G-protein stoichiometry. Trends Pharmacol. Sci 1997;18:456–64.

[9] Black JW, Leff P. Operational models of pharmacological agonist. Proc R Soc Lond [Biol] 1983;220:141.

[10] Black JW, Leff P, Shankley NP(Appendix J. Wood). An operational model of pharmacological agonism: the effect of E/[A] curve shape on agonist dissociation constant estimation. Br J Pharmacol 1985;84:561–71.

[11] Kenakin TP, Watson C, Muniz-Medina V, Christopoulos A, Novick S. A simple method for quantifying functional selectivity and agonist bias. ACS Chem Neurosci 2012;3:193–203.

[12] Griffin T, Figueroa KW, Liller S, Ehlert FJ. Estimation of agonist affinity at G protein-coupled receptors: analysis of M2 muscarinic receptor signaling through Gi/0, Gs and G15. J Pharmacol Exp Ther 2007;321:1193–207.

[13] Kenakin TP. The pharmacologic analysis of drug receptor interaction. 3rd ed. New York: Lippincott-Raven; 19971–491.

[14] Stephenson RP. A modification of receptor theory. Br J Pharmacol 1956;11:379–93.

[15] Kenakin TP, Beek D. Is prenalterol (H 133/80) really a selective beta-1 adrenoceptor agonist? Tissue selectivity resulting from difference in stimulus-response relationships. J Pharmacol Exp Ther 1980;213:406–13.

[16] Kenakin TP. Allosteric agonist modulators. J Recept Signal Transd 2007;27:247–59.

[17] Luttrell LM, Ferguson SSG, Daaka Y, Miller WE, Maudsley S, Della Rocca GJ, et al. β-arrestin-dependent formation of β2 adrenergic-Src protein kinase complexes. Science 1999;283:655–61.

[18] DeWire SM, Ahn S, Lefkowitz RJ, Shenoy SK. Beta arrestins and cell signaling. Annu Rev Physiol 2007;69:483–510.

[19] Ibrahim IA, Kurose H. β-arrestin-mediated signaling improves the efficacy of therapeutics. J Pharmacol Sci 2012;118:408–12.

[20] Zahn X, Kaoud TS, Dalby KN, Gurevich VV. Non-visual arrestins function as simple scaffolds assembling the MKK4-JNK3 β2 signaling complex. Biochem 2011;50:10520–9.

[21] Feng X, Wang W, Liu J, Liu Y. β-arrestins: multifunctional signaling adaptors in type 2 diabetes. Mol Bio Rep 2011;38:2517–28.

[22] Noor N, Patel CB, Rockman HA. β-arrestin: a signaling molecule and potential therapeutic target for heart failure. J Mol Cell Cardiol 2011;51:534–41.

[23] Tilley DG. G protein-dependent and G protein-independent signaling pathways and their impact on cardiac function. Circ Res 2011;109:217–30.

[24] Lymperopoulos A. Beta-arrestin biased agonism/antagonism at cardiovascular seven transmembrane-spanning receptors. Curr Pharm Des 2012;18:192–8.

[25] Bohn LM, Schmid CL. Serotonin receptor signaling and regulation via β-arrestins. Crit Rev Biochem Mol Biol 2010;45:555–66.

[26] Tilley DG. Functional relevance of biased signaling at the angiotensin II type 1 recetor. Endocr Metab Immune Disord Drug Targets 2011;11:99–111.

[27] Godin CM, Ferguson SS. Biased agonism of the angiotensin II type 1 receptor. Mini Rev Med Chem 2012;12:812–6.

[28] Patel CB, Noor N, Rockman HA. Functional selectivity in adrenergic and angiotensin signaling systems. Mol Pharmacol 2010;78: 983–92.

[29] Shenoy SK. β-arrestin-biased signaling by the β-adrenergic receptors. Curr Top Membr 2011;67:51–78.

[30] Viladarga JP, Gardella TJ, Wehbi VL, Feinstein TN. Non canonical signaling of the PTH receptor. Trends Pharmacol Sci 2012;33 (423–431):1.

[31] Kenakin TP, Miller LJ. Seven transmembrane receptors as shapeshifting proteins: the impact of allosteric modulation and functional selectivity on new drug discovery. Pharmacol Rev 2010;62:265–304.

[32] Perez DM, Karnick SS. Multiple signaling states of G-protein coupled receptors. Pharmacol Rev 2005;57:147–61.

[33] Leach K, Sexton PM, Christopoulos A. Allosteric GPCR modulators: taking advantage of permissive receptor pharmacology. Trends Pharmacol Sci 2007;28:382–9.

[34] Mailman RB. GPCR functional selectivity has therapeutic impact. Trends Pharmacol Sci 2007;28:390–6.

[35] Kenakin TP. Agonist-receptor efficacy II: agonist-trafficking of receptor signals. Trends Pharmacol Sci 1995;16:232–8.

[36] Liu JJ, Horst R, Katritch V, Stevens RC, Wüthrich K. Biased signaling pathways in β2-adrenergic receptor characterized by 19F-NMR. Science 2012;335:1106–10.

[37] Walters RW, Shukla A, Kovacs JJ, Violin JD, DeWire SM, Lam CM, et al. β-arrestin 1 mediates nicotinic acid-induced flushing, but not its antilipolytic effect, in mice. J Clin Invest 2009;119: 1312–21.

[38] Raehal KM, Walker JKL, Bohn LM. Morphine side effects in β-arrestin 2 knockout mice. J Pharmacol Exp Ther 2005;314:1195–201.

[39] Bohn L, Lefkowitz RJ, Gainetdinov RR, Peppel K, Caron MG, Lin F-T. Enhanced morphine analgesia in mice lacking beta-arrestin 2. Science 1999;286:2495–8.

[40] Xu H, Partilla JS, Wang X, Rutherford JM, Tidgewell K, Prisinzano TE, et al. A comparison of non-internalizing (herkinorin) and internalizing (DAMGO) μ-opioid agonists on cellular markers related to opioid tolerance and dependence. SYNAPSE 2007;61:166–75.

[41] Groer CE, Tidgewell K, Moyer RA, Harding WW, Rothman RB, Prisinzano TE, et al. An opioid agonist that does not induce mu opioid receptor-arrestin interactions or receptor internalization. Mol PharmacolMol Pharmacol 2007;71:549–57.

[42] Gesty-Palmer D, Chen M, Reiter E, Ahn S, Nelson CD, Wang S, et al. Distinct β-arrestin- and G protein-dependent pathways for para-thyroid hormone receptor-stimulated ERK1/2 activation. J Biol Chem 2006;281:10856–64.

[43] Ferrari SL, Pierroz DD, Glatt V, Goddard DS, Bianchi EN, Lin FT, et al. Bone response to intermittent parathyroid hormone is altered in mice bull for (beta) arrestin 2. Endocrinol 2005;146:1854–62.

[44] Kenakin TP, Ambrose JR, Irving PE. The relative efficiency of β-adrenoceptor coupling to myocardial inotropy and diastolic relaxation: organ selective treatment for diastolic dysfunction. J. Pharmacol. Exp. Ther. 1991;257:1189–97.

[45] Rajagopal S, Ahn S, Rominger DH, Gowen-MacDonald W, Lam CM, DeWire SM, et al. Quantifying ligand bias at seven-transmembrane receptors. Mol Pharmacol 2011;80:367–77.

[46] Violin JD, DeWire SM, Yamashita D, Rominger DH, Nguyen L, Sciller K, et al. Selectively engaging β-arrestins at the angiotensin II type 1 receptor reduces blood pressure and increases cardiac performance. J Pharmacol, Exp Ther 2010;335:572–9.

[47] Boerrigter G, Lark MW, Whalen EJ, Soergel DG, Violin JD, Burnett JC. Cardiorenal actions of TRV120027, a novel β-arrestin-biased ligand at the angiotensin II type 1 receptor, in healthy and heart failure canines: a novel therapeutic strategy for acute heart failure. Circ Heart Fail 2011;4:770–8.

[48] Boerrigter G, Soergel DG, Violin JD, Lark MW, Burnett Jr JC. TRV120027, a novel β-arrestin biased ligand at the angiotensin II type I receptor, unloads the heart and maintains renal function when added to furosemide in experimental heart failure. Circ Heart Fail 2012;5:627–34.

[49] Christopoulos A. Allosteric binding sites on cell-surface receptors: novel targets for drug discovery. Nature Rev Drug Disc 2002;1:198–210.

[50] Christopoulos A, Kenakin TP. G-protein coupled receptor allosterism and complexing. Pharmacol Rev 2002;54:323–74.

[51] Trankle C, Weyand A, Schroter A, Mohr K. Using a radioalloster to test predictions of the cooperativity model for gallamine binding to the allosteric site of muscarinic acetylcholine (m2) receptors. Mol Pharmacol 1999;56:962–5.

[52] Kew JNC, Trube G, Kemp JA. A novel mechanism of activity-dependent NMDA receptor antagonism describes the effect of ifenprodil in rat cultured cortical neurons. J Physiol 1996;497.3: 761–72.

[53] Yan F, Mosier PD, Westkaemper RB, Roth BL. Gβ-subunits differentially alter the conformation and agonist affinity of k-opioid receptors. Biochem 2008;47:1567–78.

[54] Gonzalez E, Kulkarni H, Bolivar H, Mangano A, Sanchez R, et al. The influence of CCL3L1 gene-containing segmental duplications on HIV-1/AIDS susceptibility. Science 2005;307:1433–40.

[55] Ehlert FJ. Analysis of allosterism in functional assays. J Pharmacol Exp Ther 2005;315:740–54.

[56] Tran JA, Chang A, Matsui M, Ehlert FJ. Estimation of relative microscopic affinity constants of agonists for the active state of the receptor in functional studies on m2 and m3 muscarinic receptors. Mol Pharmacol 2009;75:381–96.

[57] Barlow RB, Scott KA, Stephenson RP. An attempt to study the effects of chemical structure on the affinity and efficacy of compounds related to acetylcholine. Br J Pharmacol 1967;21: 509–22.

[58] Kenakin TP, Cook DA. N,N-Diethyl-2-(1-pyridyl)ethylamine, a partial agonist for the histamine receptor in guinea pig ileum. Can J Physiol Pharmacol 1980;58:1307–10.

[59] Christmanson L, Westermark P, Betsholtz C. Islet amyloid polypeptide stimulates cyclic AMP accumulation via the porcine calcitonin receptor. Biochem Biophys Res Commun 1994;205:1226–35.

[60] Furchgott RF. The use of β-haloalkylamines in the differentiation of receptors and in the determination of dissociation constants of receptor-agonist complexes. In: Harper NJ, Simmonds AB, editors. Advances in drug research, Vol. 3. London, New York: Academic Press; 1966. p. 21–55.

Chapter 6

Orthosteric Drug Antagonism

One of the features of this subject which hither to has been regarded as mysterious, is that in a homologous series of drugs some members may not only fail to produce the action typical of the series but may even antagonize the action of other members.

— Alfred Joseph Clark (1885–1941)

6.1 Introduction
6.2 Kinetics of Drug-Receptor Interaction
6.3 Surmountable Competitive Antagonism
6.4 Noncompetitive Antagonism
6.5 Agonist-Antagonist Hemi-Equilibria
6.6 Resultant Analysis
6.7 Antagonist Receptor Coverage: Kinetics of Dissociation
6.8 Blockade of Indirectly Acting Agonists
6.9 Irreversible Antagonism
6.10 Chemical Antagonism
6.11 Chapter Summary and Conclusions
6.12 Derivations
References

6.1 INTRODUCTION

Drugs can actively change physiological function, either directly (agonists) or indirectly through modification of physiological stimulus. If the modification is inhibitory, this is referred to as *antagonism*. This chapter discusses the blockade of agonist-induced response through interaction with receptors. Antagonism can be classified operationally, in terms of the effects of antagonists on agonist dose-response curves, and mechanistically in terms of the molecular effects of the antagonist on the receptor protein. The interference of an agonist-induced response can take different forms in terms of its effects on agonist dose-response curves. Specifically, concentration-dependent antagonism can be saturable (coming to a maximal limit of the antagonism, irrespective of the antagonist concentration) or apparently unsaturable (concentration-dependent increases in antagonism with no limit except those imposed by the drug solubility or the induction of secondary drug effects). The antagonism can be *surmountable* (dextral displacement of the dose-response curve with no diminution of maxima) or *insurmountable* (depression of the maximal agonist response). Antagonism of receptors can produce many patterns of concentration-response curves for agonists, including concentration-dependent surmountable antagonism (Figure 6.1A), surmountable antagonism that comes to a maximal limit (Figure 6.1B), depression of dose-response curves with no dextral displacement (Figure 6.1C), and dextral displacement before depression of maximal response in systems with a receptor reserve for the agonist (Figure 6.1D). These patterns should be recognized as behaviors of antagonists in different systems, and are not necessarily characteristics of the molecular nature of the antagonism (i.e., more than one molecular mechanism can produce the same behavior of the concentration-response curve). Therefore, it is important to discover the molecular mechanism of the antagonism and not just describe the antagonistic behavior, as the latter can change with experimental conditions. For example, kinetic factors can cause some antagonists to produce surmountable antagonism in some systems and insurmountable antagonism in others.

In general, there are two basic molecular mechanisms by which receptor antagonism can take place. One is where the antagonist blocks access of the agonist to the receptor through steric hindrance (prevents the agonist binding by interfering with the agonist's binding site, referred to as *orthosteric antagonism*; see Figure 6.2A). The other is where the antagonist binds to its own site on the receptor to induce a change in the reactivity of that receptor to the agonist through a change in its conformation of the receptor (referred to as *allosteric antagonism*; see Figure 6.2B). This chapter deals with orthosteric

T. P. Kenakin: A Pharmacology Primer, Fourth edition. DOI: http://dx.doi.org/10.1016/B978-0-12-407663-1.00006-5
© 2014 Elsevier Inc. All rights reserved.

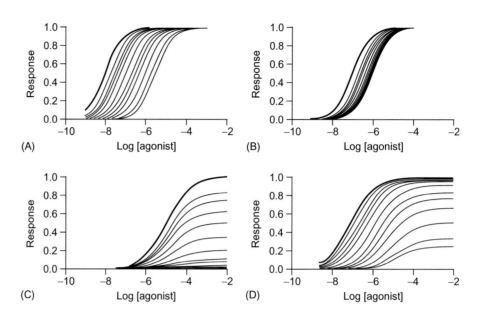

FIGURE 6.1 Effects of antagonists on agonist dose-response curves. (A) Surmountable antagonism with no diminution of maxima and no limiting antagonism (competitive antagonists). (B) Surmountable dextral displacement to a limiting value produced by an allosteric modulator. (C) Depression of dose-response curves with no dextral displacement produced by noncompetitive antagonists. (D) Dextral displacement with depression of maximum at higher concentrations produced by noncompetitive antagonists in systems with a receptor reserve for the agonist.

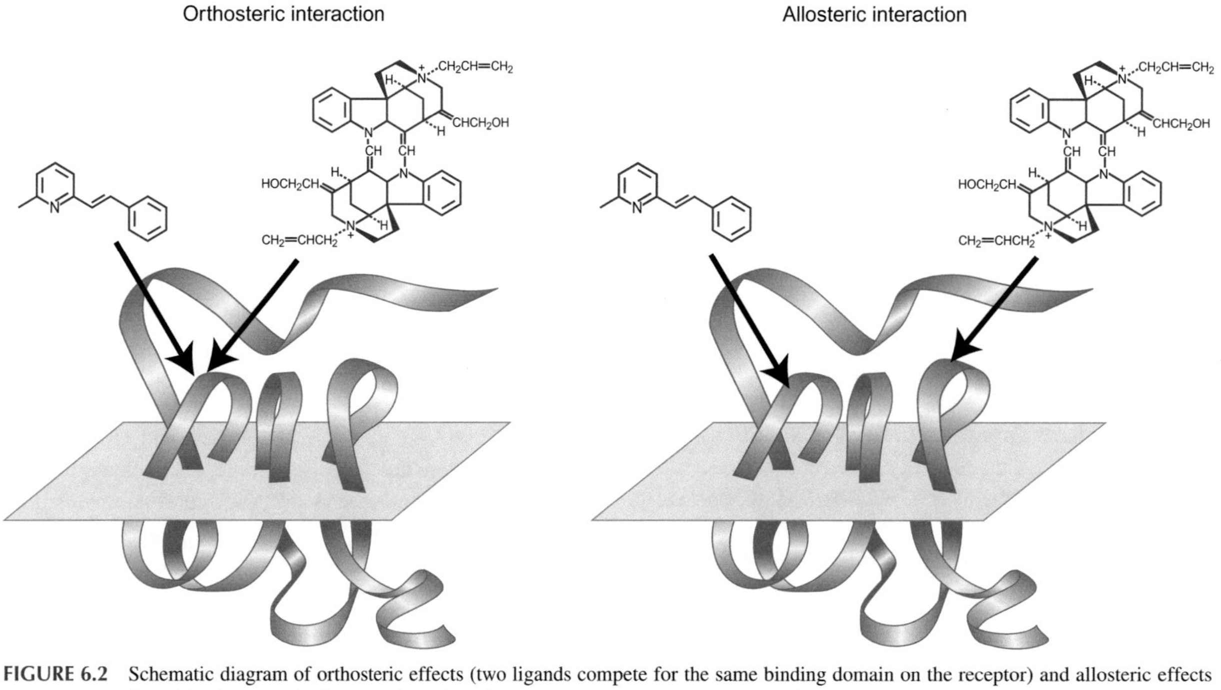

Orthosteric interaction   Allosteric interaction

FIGURE 6.2 Schematic diagram of orthosteric effects (two ligands compete for the same binding domain on the receptor) and allosteric effects (whereby each ligand has its own binding domain and the interaction takes place through a conformational change of the receptor).

antagonism, whereby the agonist and antagonist compete for the same binding site on the receptor. For orthosteric antagonism, the interaction between the agonist and antagonist is competitive and the relative affinity and concentrations of the agonist and antagonist determine which molecule occupies the common binding site. Whether this results in surmountable or insurmountable antagonism depends on the kinetics of the system. In this regard, it is worth considering kinetics as a prerequisite to a discussion of orthosteric antagonism.

6.2 KINETICS OF DRUG-RECEPTOR INTERACTION

In experimental pharmacology, the sensitivity of the preparation to the agonist is determined in a separate concentration-curve analysis, the agonist is then removed by washing, and then the preparation is equilibrated with antagonist (antagonist added to the preparation for a given period of time). This latter step is intended to cause the receptors and antagonist to come to equilibrium with

Kinetics of
equilibration

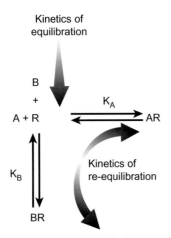

FIGURE 6.3 Antagonist potency generally is assessed by determining the sensitivity of the receptor to agonist and then equilibrating with antagonist. This first period (termed *equilibration period*) allows the antagonist and receptor to come to equilibrium in accordance with mass action (i.e., according to the concentration of the antagonist and K_B). Then, in the presence of the antagonist, agonist is added and response measured. During the period allowed for collection of response, the agonist, antagonist, and receptors must all come to a new equilibrium according to the relative concentrations of each and the K_A and K_B. This period is referred to as the *re-equilibration period*.

respect to the numbers of receptors bound by antagonist for any given concentration of antagonist in a temporally stable manner (i.e., one which will not change with time). Under these equilibrium conditions, the fraction of receptor bound by the antagonist is determined by the concentration of antagonist in the receptor compartment and the equilibrium dissociation constant of the antagonist-receptor complex (denoted K_B). Thus, the receptor occupancy by the antagonist will resemble the onset curve for binding shown in Figure 4.1. This will be referred to as the *equilibration phase* of the antagonism (see Figure 6.3). After it is thought that the receptors and antagonist have come to equilibrium according to concentration and the K_B, an agonist concentration-response curve is then obtained in the presence of the antagonist. The resulting change in the location parameter (EC_{50}) and/or maximal asymptote of the agonist concentration-response curve is then used to determine the extent of antagonism and, subsequently, to assess the potency of the antagonist. During this latter phase of the analysis, it is assumed that during the course of the determination of the agonist response the system again comes to equilibrium with the three species now present; namely, the antagonist, receptors, and the agonist. Therefore, the dissociation of the prebound antagonist from the receptor must be sufficiently rapid during the period in which the response to the agonist is obtained for the agonist to bind to the correct fraction of receptors according to the concentration of agonist and the equilibrium dissociation constant of the agonist-receptor complex. If this does not occur, a true equilibrium condition will not be attained.

This can affect how the antagonism is expressed in the system. This latter time period will be referred to as the *re-equilibration period* (see Figure 6.3). In practice, the rate of offset of antagonists generally can be much lower than the rate of offset of agonists. Under these conditions, there may be insufficient time for re-equilibration to occur, and the agonist may never occupy as many receptors as mass action dictates, especially at higher agonist concentrations where higher receptor occupancy is required.

The kinetic equation for the adjustment of receptor occupancy (ρ_t) by a pre-equilibrated concentration of an antagonist [B] with rate of offset k_2 upon addition of a fast-acting agonist [A] was derived by Paton and Rang [1] as:

$$\rho_t = \frac{[B]/K_B}{[B]/K_B + [A]/K_A + 1}$$
$$- \left(\frac{[B]/K_B}{[B]/K_B + [A]/K_A + 1} - \frac{[B]/K_B}{[B]/K_B + 1} \right) \quad (6.1)$$
$$\times e^{-k_2[([B]/K_B + [A]/K_A + 1)/([A]/K_A + 1)t]}.$$

It is worth considering the effect of varying rates of offset (k_2) and varying time periods allowed for re-equilibration of agonist, antagonist, and receptors (time t). From Equation 6.1, the equation for agonist occupancy in the presence of an antagonist for the temporal receptor occupancy for the antagonist can be rewritten as:

$$\rho_A = ([A]K_A/[A]/(K_A + 1))(1 - (\vartheta(1 - e^{-k_2\Phi_t}) + \rho_B e^{-k_2\Phi_t})),$$
$$(6.2)$$

Where:

$$\vartheta = [B]/K_B/([B]/K_B + [A]/K_A + 1) \quad (6.3)$$

$$\rho_B = [B]/K_B/([B]/K_B + 1) \quad (6.4)$$

$$\Phi = ([B]/K_B + [A]/K_A + 1)/([A]/K_A + 1) \quad (6.5)$$

Equation 6.2 can be evaluated in a number of temporal situations. Thus, if there is adequate time for re-equilibration of agonist, antagonist, and receptors, true competition between agonist and antagonist for receptors will result. Under these circumstances, the equation for agonist occupancy in the presence of antagonist can be evaluated by setting ($t \gg k_2^{-1}$) in Equation 6.2 to yield:

$$\rho_A = \frac{[A]/K_A}{[A]/K_A + [B]/K_B + 1} \quad (6.6)$$

where [A] and [B] are the agonist and antagonist concentrations, respectively, and K_A and K_B are the respective equilibrium dissociation constants of the drug-receptor complexes. These are the molar concentrations that bind to 50% of the receptor population, and, as such, quantify the affinity of the antagonist for the receptor. This is the equation used to quantify the receptor occupancy by the agonist (which is proportional to the agonist response) derived by Sir John Gaddum [2] (see Section 6.12.1).

The receptor occupancy curve can be converted to concentration-response curves by processing occupancy through the operational model for agonism (see Section 3.6). Under these circumstances, Equation 6.6 becomes:

$$\text{Response} = \frac{[A]/K_A \tau E_{max}}{[A]/K_A(1 + \tau) + [B]/K_B + 1} \quad (6.7)$$

It can be seen from Equation 6.7 that the antagonism will always be surmountable (i.e., there will be no concentration of antagonist that causes depression of the maximal response to the agonist). This is because as $[A] \to \infty$ the fractional maximal response $\to 1$ (the control maximal response in the absence of antagonism is given by $\tau/(1 + \tau)$).

The other extreme is to assume that there is no effective re-equilibration of agonist, antagonist, and receptors during the time allotted for response collection. Thus, the fractional receptor occupancy by the antagonist does not change when agonist is added. Such conditions can occur when $(t \ll k_2^{-1})$ (i.e., there is a very short period of time available for measurement of agonist response and/or there is a very slow offset of antagonist from the receptor). Under these circumstances, Equation 6.2 becomes:

$$\rho_A = \frac{[A]/K_A}{[A]/K_A(1 + [B]/K_B) + [B]/K_B + 1} \quad (6.8)$$

This is formally identical to the equation derived by Gaddum and colleagues [3] (see Section 6.12.2) for noncompetitive antagonism. In this case, it is assumed that the only available receptor population in the presence of a fractional receptor occupancy ρ_B by a noncompetitive antagonist is the fraction $1 - \rho_B$. Thus, agonist-receptor occupancy is given by:

$$\rho_A = \frac{[A]/K_A}{[A]/K_A + 1}(1 - \rho_B) \quad (6.9)$$

This equation reduces to Equation 6.8 upon simplification. In terms of agonist response, Equation 6.8 becomes:

$$\text{Response} = \frac{[A]/K_A \tau E_{max}}{[A]/K_A(1 + \tau + [B]/K_B) + [B]/K_B + 1} \quad (6.10)$$

The maximal response in the presence of antagonist is given by $(1 + \tau)/(1 + \tau + [B]/K_B)$. It can be seen that for low values of τ (low-efficacy agonist and/or low receptor density or poor receptor coupling) the maximal response to the agonist will be <1.

Thus, the two kinetic extremes yield surmountable antagonism $(t \gg k_2^{-1})$ and insurmountable antagonism $(t \ll k_2^{-1})$.

The intervening conditions can yield a mixture of dextral displacement and moderate depression of the maximal response. This is a condition described by Paton and Rang [1] as a "hemi-equilibrium" state whereby the agonist, antagonist, and receptors partially but incompletely come to equilibrium with one another. The agonist-receptor occupancy under these conditions (when $t \times k_2 = 0.01$ to 1) is given by Equation 6.2. The response is the operational metameter of that equation; specifically:

$$\text{Response} = \frac{[A]/K_A(1 - (\vartheta(1 - e^{-k_2\Phi_t}) + \rho_B e^{-k_2\Phi_t}))\tau E_{max}}{[A]/K_A((1 - (\vartheta(1 - e^{-k_2\Phi_t}) + \rho_B e^{-k_2\Phi_t}))\tau + 1) + 1} \quad (6.11)$$

It is worth considering each of these kinetic conditions in detail, as these are behaviors that are all observed experimentally and can be observed for the same antagonist under different experimental conditions. A summary of these various kinetic conditions is shown schematically in Figure 6.4.

6.3 SURMOUNTABLE COMPETITIVE ANTAGONISM

The first condition to be examined is the case where $t \gg k_2^{-1}$ (i.e., there is sufficient time for true re-equilibration among agonist, antagonist, and receptors to occur). Under these conditions, parallel dextral displacement of agonist concentration-response curves results with no diminution of maxima (Equation 6.7). This concentration-response curve pattern is subjected to analyses that utilize the magnitude of the displacement to yield an estimate of the affinity of the antagonist. Historically, the first procedure to rigorously define the quantitative relationship between such displacement and the concentration of antagonist was Schild analysis.

6.3.1 Schild Analysis

When both the agonist and antagonist compete for a common binding site, the antagonism is termed *competitive*. The equation (Equation 6.6) used to quantify the receptor occupancy by the agonist (which is proportional to the agonist response) was derived by Sir John Gaddum [2] (see Section 6.12.1 for derivation). The major pharmacological tool used to quantify the affinity of competitive antagonists is *Schild analysis*. Utilizing this method, a system-independent estimate of the affinity of a competitive antagonist can be made in a functional system. The method can also compare the pattern of antagonism to that predicted by the simple competitive model, thereby allowing definition of the mechanism of action of the antagonist. Schild analysis refers to the use of an equation derived by Arunlakshana and Schild [4] to construct linear plots designed to graphically estimate the affinity of

$$\rho_t = \frac{[B]/K_B}{[B]/K_B + [A]/K_A + 1} - \left(\frac{[B]/K_B}{[B]/K_B + [A]/K_A + 1} - \frac{[B]/K_B}{[B]/K_B + 1} \right) e^{-k_2 t} \left[\frac{[B]/K_B + [A]/K_B + 1}{[A]/K_B + 1} \right]$$

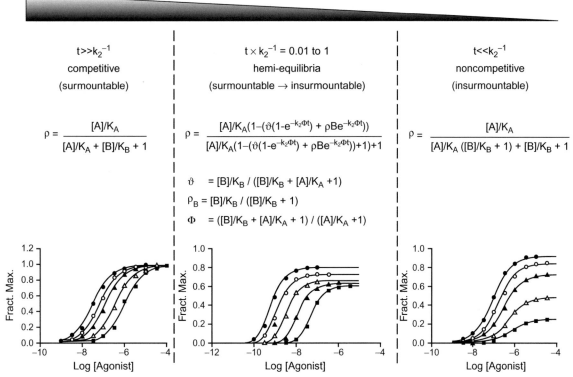

Equilibration Time x Rate of Offset

$t \gg k_2^{-1}$

competitive

(surmountable)

$$\rho = \frac{[A]/K_A}{[A]/K_A + [B]/K_B + 1}$$

$t \times k_2^{-1} = 0.01$ to 1

hemi-equilibria

(surmountable → insurmountable)

$$\rho = \frac{[A]/K_A(1-(\vartheta(1-e^{-k_2\Phi t}) + \rho_B e^{-k_2\Phi t}))}{[A]/K_A(1-(\vartheta(1-e^{-k_2\Phi t}) + \rho_B e^{-k_2\Phi t}))+1)+1}$$

$\vartheta = [B]/K_B / ([B]/K_B + [A]/K_A +1)$

$\rho_B = [B]/K_B / ([B]/K_B + 1)$

$\Phi = ([B]/K_B + [A]/K_A + 1) / ([A]/K_A +1)$

$t \ll k_2^{-1}$

noncompetitive

(insurmountable)

$$\rho = \frac{[A]/K_A}{[A]/K_A ([B]/K_B + 1) + [B]/K_B + 1}$$

FIGURE 6.4 The range of antagonist behaviors observed under different kinetic conditions. When there is sufficient time for complete re-equilibration ($t \gg k_2^{-1}$), surmountable antagonism is observed (panel furthest to the left). As the time for re-equilibration diminishes (relative to the rate of offset of the antagonist from the receptor; $t \times k_2^{-1} = 0.1$ to 0.01), the curves shift according to competitive kinetics (as in the case for surmountable antagonism) but the maxima of the curvers are truncated (middle panel). When there is insufficient time for re-equilibration, the antagonist essentially irreversibly occludes the fraction of receptors it binds to during the equilibration period ($t \ll k_2^{-1}$) and depression of the maxima occurs with dextral displacement determined by the extent of receptor reserve for the agonist (panel to the right).

simple competitive antagonists. The Schild equation was derived from the Gaddum equation (Equation 6.6, see Section 6.12.3):

$$Log(DR - 1) = Log[B] - Log K_B \qquad (6.12)$$

The method is based on the notion that both the concentration of the antagonist in the receptor compartment and its affinity determine the antagonism of agonist response. Since the antagonism can be observed and quantified, and the concentration of the antagonist is known, the affinity of the antagonist (in the form of K_B) can be calculated.

The antagonism is quantified by measuring the ratio of equiactive concentrations of agonist measured in the presence of and absence of the antagonist. These are referred to as *dose ratios* (DRs). Usually, EC_{50} concentrations of agonist (concentration producing 50% maximal

response) are used to calculate dose ratios. An example calculation of a DR is shown in Figure 6.5. Thus, for every concentration of antagonist [B] there will be a corresponding DR value. These are plotted as a regression of log (DR − 1) upon log [B]. If the antagonism is competitive, there will be a linear relationship between log (DR − 1) and log [B] according to the Schild equation. Under these circumstances it can be seen that a value of zero for the ordinate will give an intercept of the *x*-axis where log [B] = log K_B. Therefore, the concentration of antagonist that produces a log (DR − 1) = 0 value will be equal to the log K_B, the equilibrium dissociation constant of the antagonist-receptor complex. This is a system-independent and molecular quantification of the antagonist affinity that should be accurate for every cellular system containing the receptor. When the concentration of antagonist in the receptor compartment is equal to the K_B value (the concentration that binds to 50% of the receptors), then the dose ratio will be 2. Since K_B values are obtained from a logarithmic plot, they are log normally distributed and are therefore conventionally reported as pK_B values. These are the negative logarithm of the K_B, which are used much like pEC_{50} values are used to quantify agonist potency. The negative logarithm of this particular concentration is also referred to empirically as the pA_2, the concentration of antagonist which produces a twofold shift of the agonist dose-response curve. Antagonist potency can be quantified by calculating the pA_2 from a single concentration of antagonist producing a single value for the dose ratio from the equation

$$pA_2 = Log(DR - 1) - Log[B] \qquad (6.13)$$

It should be noted that this is a single measurement. Therefore, comparison to the model of competitive antagonism cannot be done. The pA_2 serves only as an empirical measure of potency. Only if a series of DR values for a series of antagonist concentrations yields a linear Schild regression with a slope of unity can the pA_2 value (obtained from the intercept of the Schild plot) be considered a molecular measure of the actual affinity of the antagonist for the receptor (pK_B). Therefore, a pK_B value is always equal to the pA_2. However, the converse (namely, that the pA_2 can always be considered an estimate of the pK_B) is not necessarily true. For this to occur, a range of antagonist concentrations must be tested and shown to comply with the requirements of Schild analysis (linear plot with slope equal to unity). A precept of Schild analysis is that the magnitude of the DR values must not be dependent on the level of response used to make the measurement. This occurs if the dose-response curves (control plus those obtained in the presence of antagonist) are parallel and all have a common maximal asymptote response (as seen in Figure 6.5).

There are statistical procedures available to determine whether the data can be fit to a model of dose-response curves that are parallel with respect to slope and all share a common maximal response (see Chapter 12). In general,

dose-response data can be fit to a three-parameter logistic equation of the form:

$$Response = \frac{E_{max}}{1 + 10^{(LogEC_{50} - Log[A])^n}} \qquad (6.14)$$

where the concentration of the agonist is $[A]$, E_{max} refers to the maximal asymptote response, EC_{50} is the location parameter of the curve along the concentration axis, and n is a fitting parameter defining the slope of the curve. A variant four-parameter logistic curve can be used if the baseline of the curves does not begin at zero response (i.e., if there is a measurable response in the absence of agonist basal):

$$Response = Basal + \frac{E_{max} - Basal}{1 + 10^{(LogEC_{50} - Log[A])^n}} \qquad (6.15)$$

In practice, a sample of data will be subject to random variation, and curve fitting with nonlinear models most likely will produce differences in slope and/or maxima for the various dose-response curves. Therefore, the question to be answered is, does the sample of data come from a population that consists of parallel dose-response curves with common maxima? Hypothesis testing can be used to determine this (see Chapter 12). Specifically, a value for the statistic F is calculated by fitting the data to a complex model (where each curve is fit to its own value of n, EC_{50}, and E_{max}) and to a more simple model (where a common E_{max} and n values are used for all the curves and the only differences between them are values of EC_{50}). (See Chapter 12 for further details.) If the F statistic indicates that a significantly better fit is not obtained with the complex model (separate parameters for each curve), then this allows fitting of the complete data set to a pattern of curves with common maxima and slope. This latter condition fulfills the theoretical requirements of Schild analysis. An example of this procedure is shown in Chapter 12, Figure 12.14.

If the data set can be fit to a family of curves of common slope and maximum asymptote, then the EC_{50}s of each curve can be used to calculate DR values. Specifically, the EC_{50} values for each curve obtained in the presence of antagonist are divided by the EC_{50} for the control curve (obtained in the absence of antagonist). This yields a set of equiactive dose ratios. If hypothesis testing indicates that individually fit curves must be used, then a set of EC_{50} values must be obtained graphically. A common level of response (i.e., 50%) is chosen and EC_{50} values are either calculated from the equation or determined from the graph. With slopes of the dose-response curves near unity, this approximation is not likely to produce substantial error in the calculation of DR values and should still be suitable for Schild analysis. However, this approach is still an approximation and fitting to curves of common slope and maxima is preferred. It should be

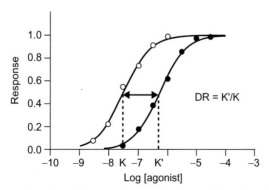

FIGURE 6.5 Calculation of equiactive dose ratios (DR values) from two dose-response curves.

noted that an inability to fit the curves to a common maximum and slope indicates a departure from the assumptions required for assigning simple competitive antagonism.

The measured dose ratios are then used to calculate log (DR − 1) ordinates for the corresponding abscissal logarithm of the antagonist concentration that produced the shift in the control curve. A linear equation of the form:

$$y = mx + b \qquad (6.16)$$

is used to fit the regression of log (DR − 1) upon log [B]. Usually a statistical software tool can furnish an estimate of the error on the slope.

The model of simple competitive antagonism predicts that the slope of the Schild regression should be unity. However, experimental data are samples from the complete population of infinite DR values for infinite concentrations of the antagonist. Therefore, random sample variation may produce a slope that is not unity. Under these circumstances, a statistical estimation of the 95% confidence limits of the slope (available in most fitting software) is used to determine whether the sample data could have come from the population describing simple competitive antagonism (i.e., having unit slope). If the 95% confidence limits of the experimentally fit slope include unity, then it can be concluded that the antagonism is of the simple competitive type and that random variation caused the deviation from unit slope. The regression is then *refit to an equation where m = 1* and the abscissal intercept taken to be the logarithm of the K_B. An example of Schild analysis for the inhibition of muscarinic-receptor-mediated responses of rat tracheae, to the agonist carbachol by the antagonist pirenzepine, is shown in Figure 6.6.

If the slope of the regression is not unity or if the regression is not linear, then the complete data set cannot be used to estimate the antagonist potency. Under these circumstances, either the antagonism is not competitive or some other factor is obscuring the competitive antagonism. An estimate of the potency of the antagonist can still be obtained by calculating a pA$_2$ according to Equation 6.13. This should be done using the *lowest positive log (DR − 1) value*. Hypothesis testing can be used to determine the lowest statistically different value for DR from the family of curves (see Figure 12.16).

A schematic diagram of some of the logic used in Schild analysis is shown in Figure 6.7. It should be pointed out that a linear Schild regression with a unit slope is the minimal requirement for Schild analysis, but that it does not necessarily prove that a given inhibition is of the simple competitive type. For example, in guinea pig tracheae, relaxant β-adrenoceptors and contractile muscarinic receptors coexist. The former cause the tissue to relax, while the latter counteract this relaxation and cause the tissue to contract. Thus, the β-adrenoceptor agonist isoproterenol, by actively producing relaxation, will physiologically antagonize contractile responses to the muscarinic agonist carbachol. Figure 6.8 shows a Schild plot constructed from the concentration-dependent relaxation of guinea pig trachea of the contractile dose-response curves to carbachol. It can be seen that the plot is linear with a slope of unity, apparently in agreement with a mechanism of simple competitive antagonism. However, these opposing responses occur at totally different cell surface receptors and the interaction is further down the stimulus-response cascade in the cytoplasm. Thus, the apparent agreement with the competitive model for these data is spurious (i.e., the plot cannot be used as evidence of simple competitive antagonism). An example of the use of this method is given in Section 13.2.4.

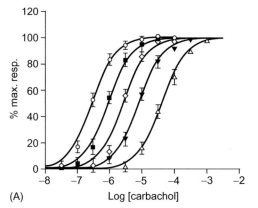

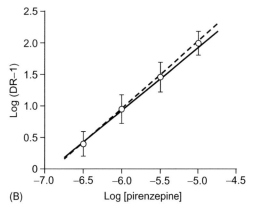

FIGURE 6.6 Schild regression for pirenzepine antagonism of rat tracheal responses to carbachol. (A) Dose-response curves to carbachol in the absence (open circles, n = 20) and presence of pirenzepine 300 nM (filled squares, n = 4), 1 μM (open diamonds, n = 4), 3 μM (filled inverted triangles, n = 6), and 10 μM (open triangles, n = 6). Data fit to functions of constant maximum and slope. (B) Schild plot for antagonism shown in panel A. Ordinates: log (DR − 1) values. Abscissae: logarithms of molar concentrations of pirenzepine. Dotted line shows best line linear plot. Slope = 1.1 + 0.2; 95% confidence limits = 0.9 to 1.15. Solid line is the best fit line with linear slope. pK$_B$ = 6.92. Redrawn from [5].

FIGURE 6.7 Schematic diagram of some of the logic used in Schild analysis.

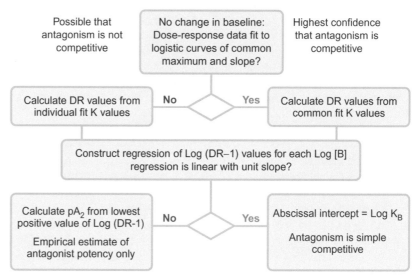

FIGURE 6.8 Apparent simple competitive antagonism of carbachol-induced contraction of guinea pig trachea through physiological antagonism of tracheal contractile mechanisms by β-adrenoceptor relaxation of the muscle. (A) Schematic diagram of the physiological interaction of the muscarinic receptor-induced contraction and β-adrenoceptor-induced relaxation of tracheal tissue. (B) Schild regression for isoproterenol (β-adrenoceptor agonist) antagonism of carbachol-induced contraction. The regression is linear with unit slope (slope = 1.02 + 0.02) apparently, but erroneously indicative of simple competitive antagonism. Redrawn from [6].

6.3.2 Patterns of Dose-Response Curves That Preclude Schild Analysis

There are patterns of dose-response curves that preclude Schild analysis. The model of simple competitive antagonism predicts parallel shifts of agonist dose-response curves with no diminution of maxima. If this is not observed it could be because the antagonism is not of the competitive type, or because some other factor is obscuring the competitive nature of the antagonism. The shapes of dose-response curves can prevent measurement of response-independent dose ratios. For example, Figure 6.9A shows antagonism in which there is a clear departure from parallelism, and in fact a distinct decrease in slope of the curve for the agonist in the presence of the antagonist is observed. This is indicative of

noncompetitive antagonism. Irrespective of the mechanism, this pattern of curves prevents estimation of response-independent DR values and thus Schild analysis would be inappropriate for this system. Figure 6.9B shows a pattern of curves with depressed maximal responses but shifts that are near parallel in nature. This is a pattern indicative of hemi-equilibrium conditions whereby the agonist and antagonist do not have sufficient time (due to the response collection window) to come to temporal equilibrium. If this could be determined, then Schild analysis can estimate antagonist potency from values of response below where depression of responses occurs (i.e., EC_{30}). The differentiation of hemi-equilibria from noncompetitive blockade is discussed in Section 6.5.

The pattern shown in Figure 6.9C is one of parallel shift of the dose-response curves up to a maximal shift.

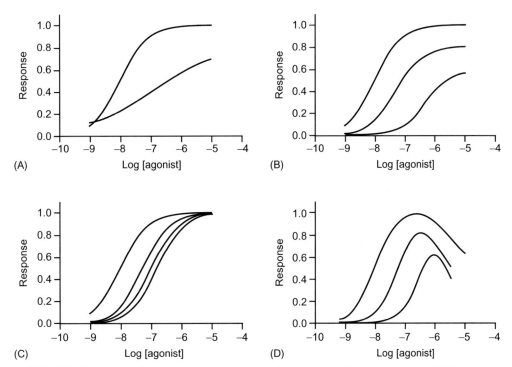

FIGURE 6.9 Patterns of dose-response curves produced by antagonists that may preclude Schild analysis. (A) Depression of maximal response with nonparallelism indicative of noncompetitive blockade. DR values are not response independent. (B) Depressed maxima with apparent parallel displacement indicative of hemi-equilibrium conditions (*vide infra*). (C) Loss of concentration dependence of antagonism as a maximal shift is attained with increasing concentrations of antagonist indicative of saturable allosteric blockade. (D) Depressed maximal responses at high concentration of agonist where the antagonist shifts the agonist response range into this region of depression (indicative of toxic or nonspecific effects of agonist at high concentrations).

Further increases in antagonist concentration do not produce further shifts of the dose-response curves beyond a limiting value. This is suggestive of an allosteric modification of the agonist's affinity by the antagonist, and other models can be used to estimate antagonist affinity under these conditions. This is discussed further in Chapter 7. Finally, if the agonist has secondary properties that affect the response characteristics of the system (i.e., toxic effects at high concentrations), then dextral displacement of the dose-response curve into these regions of agonist concentration may affect the observed antagonism. Figure 6.9D shows depression of the maximal response at high agonist concentrations. This pattern may preclude full Schild analysis but a pA_2 may be estimated.

6.3.3 Best Practice for the Use of Schild Analysis

There are two ways to make Schild analysis more effective. The first is to obtain log (DR − 1) values as near to zero as possible (i.e., use concentrations of the antagonist that produce a low level of antagonism, such as a two fold to five fold shift in the control dose-response curve).

This will ensure that the real data are in close proximity to the most important parameter sought by the analysis; namely, the abscissal intercept (pK_B or pA_2 value). If log (DR − 1) values are greater than 1.0, then the pK_B (or pA_2) will need to be extrapolated from the regression. Under these circumstances any secondary effects of the antagonist that influence the slope of the Schild regression will subsequently affect the estimate of antagonist potency. Second, at least a 30-fold (and preferably 100-fold) concentration range of antagonist (concentrations that produce an effect on the control dose-response curve) should be utilized. This will yield a statistically firm estimate of the slope of the regression. If the concentration range is below this, then the linear fit of the log (DR − 1) versus log [B] will produce large 95% confidence limits for the slope. While unity most likely will reside within this broad range, the fit will be much less useful as an indicator of whether or not unity actually is a correct slope for the antagonist. That unity is included could simply reflect the fact that the confidence range is so large.

There are Schild regressions that deviate from ideal behavior but can still be useful either to quantify antagonist potency or to indicate the mechanism of antagonism. For example, Figure 6.10A shows a linear Schild

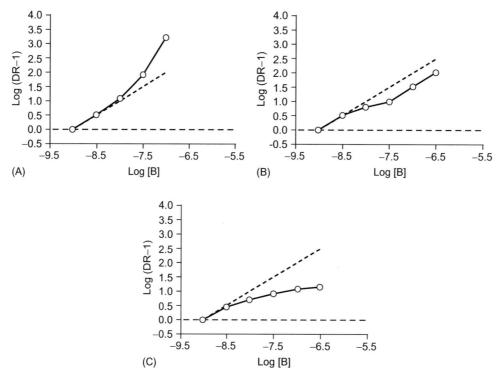

FIGURE 6.10 Some commonly encountered patterns of Schild regressions. (A) Initial linearity with increased slope at higher concentration indicative of toxic effects of either the agonist or antagonist at higher concentrations. (B) Region of decreased slope with re-establishment of linearity often observed for saturation of uptake or other adsorption effects. (C) Hyperbolic loss of antagonism indicative of saturable allosteric antagonism.

regression at low antagonist concentrations that departs from ideal behavior (increased slope) at higher antagonist concentrations. This is frequently encountered experimentally as secondary effects from higher concentrations of either the agonist or the antagonist come into play, leading to toxicity or other depressant effects on the system. The linear portion of the regressions at lower antagonist concentrations can still be used for estimation of the pK_B (if a large enough concentration range of antagonist is used) or for the pA_2 (if not).

Figure 6.10B shows a pattern of antagonism often observed in isolated tissue studies but not so often in cell-based assays. Saturation of uptake systems for the agonist or saturation of an adsorption site for the agonist can account for this effect. The linear portion of the regression can be used to estimate the pK_B or the pA_2. If there is a loss of concentration dependence of antagonism, as seen in Figure 6.10C, this indicates a possible allosteric mechanism whereby a saturation of binding to an allosteric site is operative. This is dealt with further in Chapter 7.

One of the strengths of Schild analysis is the capability of unveiling nonequilibrium conditions in experimental preparations, such as inadequate time of equilibration or removal of drugs from the receptor compartment. Figure 6.11 shows a range of possible experimentally observed but problematic linear Schild regressions that could be encountered for competitive antagonists.

6.3.4 Analyses for Inverse Agonists in Constitutively Active Receptor Systems

In constitutively active receptor systems (where the baseline is elevated due to spontaneous formation of receptor active states; see Chapter 3 for full discussion), unless the antagonist has identical affinities for the inactive receptor state, the spontaneously formed active state, and the spontaneously G-protein-coupled state (three different receptor conformations; see discussion in Chapter 1 on receptor conformation), it will alter the relative concentrations of these species; in so doing it will alter the baseline response. If the antagonist has higher affinity for the receptor active state, it will be a partial agonist in an efficiently coupled receptor system. This is discussed in the next section. If the antagonist has higher affinity for the inactive receptor, then it will demonstrate simple competitive antagonism in a quiescent system and *inverse agonism* in a constitutively active system.

The dose-response curves reflecting inverse agonism do not conform to the strict requirements of Schild analysis (i.e., parallel shift of the dose-response curves with no diminution of maxima). In the case of inverse agonists in a constitutively active receptor system, the dextral displacement of the agonist concentration-response curve is accompanied by a depression of the elevated basal response (due to constitutive activity). (See Figure 6.12A.)

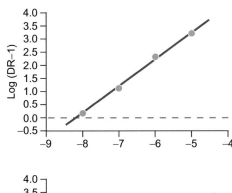

- Ideal Schild regression
- Wide concentration range
- Data near log (DR–1) = 0 value
- Linear with unit slope

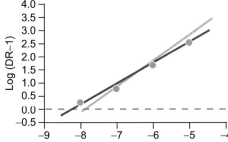

- Slope = 0.8 but not significantly different from unity
- Data near log (DR–1) = 0 value
- Wide concentration range
- Refit regression to unit slope (orange line) and calculate pK_B

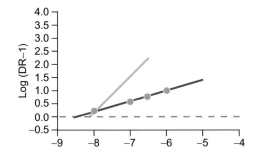

- Slope significantly less than unity–cannot fit to unit slope
- Data near log (DR–1) = 0 value
- Estimate pA_2 from single point using lowest log (DR–1) value

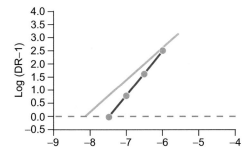

- Slope significantly greater than unity
- Probably inadequate equilibration time for antagonist
- Lowest log (DR–1) value cannot be taken for pA_2 calculation
- Repeat analysis with longer time of equilibration for antagonist

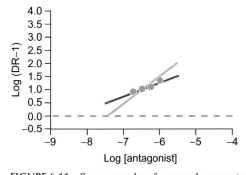

- Inadequate antagonist concentration range
- Inordinately large range on slope
- Even though slope includes unity, the ordinal intercept cannot adequately be estimated since log (DR–1) values too high
- Repeat analysis adding lower antagonist concentrations

FIGURE 6.11 Some examples of commonly encountered Schild data and some suggestions as to how antagonism should be quantified for these systems.

FIGURE 6.12 Schild analysis for constitutively active receptor systems. (A) Competitive antagonism by the inverse agonist in a constitutively active receptor system with DR values calculated at the EC_{80}. (B) Competitive antagonism by the same inverse agonist in a non-constitutively active receptor system. (C) Direct effects of an inverse agonist in systems of differing levels of constitutive activity. Open circles show midpoints of the concentration-response curves. (D) Schild regression for an inverse agonist in a non-constitutive assay where the inverse agonist produces no change in baseline (solid line) and in a constitutively active assay where depression of elevated baseline is observed (dotted line). A small shift to the left of the Schild regression is observed, leading to a slight overestimation of inverse agonist potency.

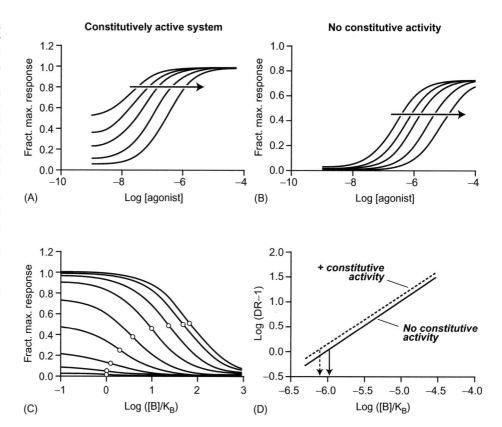

This figure shows the nonparallel nature of the curves as the constitutively elevated baseline is reduced by the inverse agonist activity. In quiescent receptor systems (nonconstitutively active), both competitive antagonists and inverse agonists produce parallel shifts to the right of the agonist dose-response curves (see Figure 6.12B).

The effects of high values of constitutive activity can be determined for functional systems where function is defined by the operational model. Thus, it can be assumed in a simplified system that the receptor exists in an active (R^*) and inactive (R) form and that agonists stabilize (and therefore enrich the prevalence of) the active form, while inverse agonists prefer the inactive form. It also is assumed that response emanates from the active form of the receptor.

Under these circumstances, the fractional response in a functional system can be derived from the expression defining the amount of active state receptor coupled to G-protein. This yields the following expression for response with a Hill coefficient of unity (see Section 6.12.4):

Response =

$$\frac{\alpha L[A]/K_A\tau + \beta L[B]/K_B\tau + L\tau}{[A]/K_A(1 + \alpha L(1+\tau)) + [B]/K_B(1 + \beta L(1+\tau)) + L(\tau + 1) + 1}$$
(6.17)

where τ is the efficacy of the full agonist, n is a fitting parameter for the slope of the agonist concentration-

response curve, K_A and K_B are the respective equilibrium dissociation constants of the full agonist and inverse agonist for the inactive state of the receptor, α and β are the relative ratios of the affinity of the full and inverse agonist for the active state of the receptor, and L is the allosteric constant for the receptor ($L = [R^*]/[R]$).

There are two ways to estimate the potency of an inverse agonist from the system described by Equation 6.17. The first is to observe the concentration of inverse agonist that reduces the level of constitutive activity by 50%, the IC_{50} of the compound as an active inverse agonist. This is done by observing the level of constitutive response in the absence of full agonist ([A] = 0) with a variant of Equation 6.17:

$$\text{Constitutive Response} = \frac{\beta L[B]/K_B\tau + L\tau}{[B]/K_B(1 + \beta L(1+\tau)) + L(\tau + 1) + 1}$$
(6.18)

Figure 6.12C shows the effect of increasing levels of constitutive activity on the midpoint of a curve to an inverse agonist. This shows that with increasing levels of inverse agonism — either through increasing intrinsic constitutive activity (increased L) or increasing levels of receptor and/or efficiency of receptor coupling (increasing τ) — the IC_{50} of the inverse agonist will increasingly be larger than the true K_B. This is important to note, since it predicts that the value of the pIC_{50} for an inverse agonist will be system dependent and can vary from cell type to cell type (just as does observed potency for positive agonists). However, in the case of inverse agonists, the effects of increasing receptor density and/or receptor coupling are opposite to those observed for positive agonists where increases cause a concomitant increase in observed potency. This trend in the observed potency of inverse agonism on system conditions (L and τ) can be seen from the midpoint of the curve defined by Equation 6.18. This is the IC_{50} for an inverse agonist inhibition of constitutive activity:

$$\text{Observed } IC_{50} = \frac{K_B(L(\tau + 1) + 1)}{(\beta L(1 + \tau) + 1)} \qquad (6.19)$$

Equation 6.19 predicts increasing IC_{50} with increases in either L or τ. In systems with low-efficacy inverse agonists, or in systems with low levels of constitutive activity, the observed location parameter is still a close estimate of the K_B (equilibrium dissociation constant of the ligand-receptor complex, a molecular quantity that transcends test system type). In general, the observed potency of inverse agonists defines only the lower *limit* of affinity.

As observed in Figure 6.12A, inverse agonists produce dextral displacement of concentration-response curves to full agonists and thus produce dose ratios that may be used in Schild analysis. It is worth considering the use of dose ratios from such curves and the error in the calculated pK_B and pA_2 produced by the negative efficacy of the inverse agonist and changes in basal response levels. It can be shown that the pA_2 value for an inverse agonist in a constitutively active receptor system is given by (see Section 6.12.5):

$$pA_2 = pK_B - \text{Log}([A](\alpha - 1)/([A](\alpha - 1) + (1 - \beta))) \qquad (6.20)$$

This expression predicts that the modifying term will always be <1 for an inverse agonist ($\beta < 1$). Therefore, the calculation of the affinity of an inverse agonist from dextral displacement data (pA_2 measurement) will always overestimate the potency of the inverse agonist. However, since $\beta < 1$ and the α value for a full agonist will be $\gg 1$, the error most likely will be very small. Figure 6.12D shows the effect of utilizing dextral displacements for an inverse agonist in a constitutively active system. The Schild regression is linear but is phase-shifted to the right in accordance with the slight overestimation of inverse agonist potency.

6.3.5 Analyses for Partial Agonists

Schematically, response is produced by the full agonist ([AR]) complex — which interacts with the stimulus-

response system with equilibrium association constant K_e — and the partial agonist (lower efficacy), which interacts with an equilibrium association constant K'_e:

B
+
A + R ⇌K_a AR
↕K_b +
BR + E ⇌K'_e BRE
↕K_e ↓
ARE ⟶ RESPONSE

Therefore, there are two efficacies for the agonism: one for the full agonist (denoted τ) and one for the partial agonist (denoted τ'). In terms of the operational model for functional response, this leads to the following expression for response to a full agonist [A] in the presence of a partial agonist [B] (see Section 6.12.6):

$$\text{Response} = \frac{[A]/K_A\tau + [B]/K_B\tau'}{[A]/K_A(1 + \tau) + [B]/K_B(1 + \tau') + 1} \qquad (6.21)$$

If the partial agonism is sufficiently low so as to allow a full agonist to produce further response, then a pattern of curves of elevated baseline (due to the partial agonism) shifted to the right of the control curve (due to the antagonist properties of the partial agonist) will be obtained. (See Figure 6.13A.) However, low-efficacy agonists can be complete antagonists in poorly coupled receptor systems and partial agonists in systems of higher receptor density and/or coupling efficiency (Figure 6.13B).

The observed EC_{50} for partial agonism can be a good estimate for the affinity (K_B). However, in systems of high receptor density and/or efficient receptor coupling where the responses approach full agonism, the observed EC_{50} will overestimate the true potency of the partial agonist. This can be seen from the location parameter of the partial agonist in Equation 6.22 in the absence of full agonist ([A] = 0):

$$\text{Observed } EC_{50} = \frac{[B]/K_B}{(1 + \tau')} \qquad (6.22)$$

Figure 6.13C shows the effect of increasing receptor density and/or efficiency of receptor coupling on the magnitude of the EC_{50} of the partial agonist. Equiactive dose ratios still can be estimated from the agonist-dependent region of the dose-response curves. For example, Figure 6.13A shows DR values obtained as ratios of the EC_{75}. The resulting Schild regression

FIGURE 6.13 Schild analysis for a partial agonist. (A) Competitive antagonism by a partial agonist. DR values calculated at EC_{75} for agonist response. (B) Schild regressions for antagonism of same receptor in a low receptor-density/coupling-efficiency receptor where no partial agonism is observed. (C) Dose-response curve for directly observed partial agonism. Under some conditions, the EC_{50} for the partial agonist closely approximates the K_B. (D) Schild regression for a partial agonist in a low receptor/coupling assay where the partial agonist produces no observed response (solid line) and in a high receptor/coupling assay where agonism is observed (dotted line). A small shift to the right of the Schild regression is observed, leading to a slight underestimation of partial agonist potency.

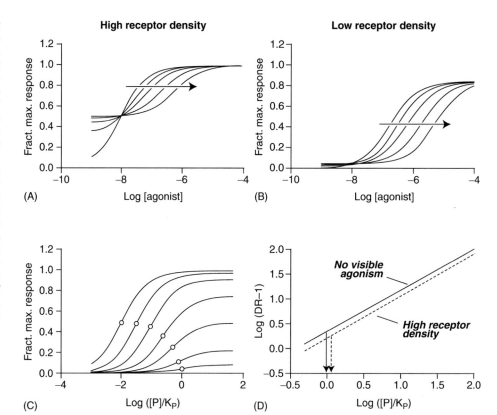

slightly underestimates the K_B (see Figure 6.13D). However, the error will be minimal. Underestimation of the true pK_B is also predicted by the operational model (Section 6.12.7):

$$pA_2 = pK_B - Log(\tau/(\tau - \tau')) \qquad (6.23)$$

It can be seen that the modifying term will always be >1, but will also have a relatively low magnitude (especially for low values of partial agonist efficacy τ'). Also, in systems where the partial agonist does not produce a response ($t' \to 0$), then $pA_2 = pK_B$ as required by simple competitive antagonism (as shown in Figure 6.13B). The use of dose ratios for partial agonists where the partial agonist produces a response will always slightly underestimate affinity by the Schild method (or calculation of the pA_2). The Schild regression for a partial agonist reflects this, in that it is still linear but slightly shifted to the right of the true regression for simple competitive antagonism (Figure 6.13D).

Another method for measuring the affinity of a partial agonist has been presented by Stephenson [7] and modified by Kaumann and Marano [8]. The method of Stephenson compares equiactive concentrations of full agonist in the absence and the presence of a concentration of partial agonist to estimate the affinity of the

partial agonist. The following equation is used (see Section 6.12.8):

$$[A] = \frac{[A']}{1 + (1 - (\tau_P/\tau_a)) \cdot ([P]/K_P)}$$
$$+ \frac{(\tau_p/\tau_a) \cdot ([P]/K_P) \cdot K_A}{1 + (1 - (\tau_P/\tau_a)) \cdot ([P]/K_P)} \qquad (6.24)$$

A regression of [A] upon [A'] yields a straight line. The K_p can be estimated by:

$$K_p = \frac{[P]slope}{1 - slope} \cdot (1 - (\tau_p/\tau_a)) \qquad (6.25)$$

A full example of the use of this method is given in Section 13.2.5.

A more rigorous version of this method has been presented by Kaumann and Marano [8]. In this method, the slopes from a range of equiactive agonist concentration plots are utilized in another regression (see Section 6.12.8):

$$Log\left(\frac{1}{slope} - 1\right) = Log[P] - Log\,K_p \qquad (6.26)$$

where m is the slope for a particular regression of equiactive concentrations of an agonist in the absence and

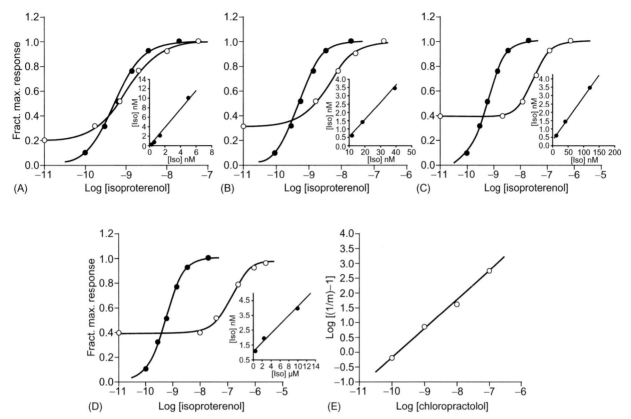

FIGURE 6.14 Method of Stephenson [7] and Kaumann and Marano [8] used to measure the affinity of the partial β-adrenoceptor agonist chlor-opractolol in rat atria. Panels A to D show responses to isoproterenol in the absence (filled circles) and presence of chloropractolol (open circles). Curves shown in the presence of 10 nM (panel A), 100 nM (panel B), 1 μM (panel C), and 10 μM (panel D) chloropractolol. Note elevated basal responses in response to the partial agonist chloropractolol. Insets to panels A through D show plots of equiactive concentrations of isoproterenol in the absence (ordinates) and presence of chloropractolol according to Equation 6.24. Slopes from these graphs used for plot shown in panel E according to the method of Kaumann and Marano [8] (see Equation 6.26). This plot is linear with a slope of 0.95, yielding a K_P estimate of 16.5 nM. Data redrawn from [9].

presence of a particular concentration of partial agonist [P]. An example of the use of this method for the measurement of the partial agonist chloropractolol is shown in Figure 6.14. The various plots of equiactive concentrations (insets to panels A to D) furnish a series of values of m for a series of concentrations of chloropractolol. These are used in a regression according to Equation 6.26 (see Figure 6.14) to yield an estimate of the K_P for chloropractolol from the intercept of the regression. Further detail on the use of this method is given in Section 13.2.5.

6.3.6 The Method of Lew and Angus: Nonlinear Regressional Analysis

One shortcoming of Schild analysis is an overemphasized use of the control dose-response curve (i.e., the accuracy of every DR value depends on the accuracy of the control EC_{50} value). An alternative method utilizes nonlinear regression of the Gaddum equation (with visualization of the data with a Clark plot [10], named for A. J. Clark). This method, unlike Schild analysis, does not emphasize

control pEC_{50}, thereby giving a more balanced estimate of antagonist affinity. This method, first described by Lew and Angus [11], is robust and theoretically more sound than Schild analysis. On the other hand, it is not as visual. Schild analysis is rapid and intuitive, and can be used to detect nonequilibrium steady states in the system which can corrupt estimates of pK_B. Also, nonlinear regression requires matrix algebra to estimate the error of the pK_B. While error estimates are given with many commercially available software packages for curve fitting, they are difficult to obtain without these (from first principles). In contrast, Schild analysis furnishes an estimate of the error for the pK_B from the linear regression using all of the data. If an estimate of the error is required and the means to calculate it are not available in the curve fitting software, manual calculation with Schild analysis is a viable alternative. In general, the method of Lew and Angus still holds definite advantages for the measurement of competitive antagonist potency. One approach to rigorously describe competitive antagonism is to use Schild analysis to visualize the data and the method of Lew and Angus to estimate the pK_B.

To apply this method, the pEC_{50} values of the control and shifted dose-response curves and the corresponding concentrations of antagonist [B] values associated with those pEC_{50}s are used to construct a Clark plot [10] according to the equation:

$$pEC_{50} = -Log([B] + 10^{-pK_B}) - Log\ c \qquad (6.27)$$

where pK_B and c are fitting constants. Note that the control pEC_{50} is used with [B] = 0. The relationship between the pEC_{50} and increments of antagonist concentration can be shown in a Clark plot of pEC_{50} versus $-\log([B] + 10^{-pK_B})$. Constructing such a plot is useful because although it is not used in any calculation of the pK_B it allows visualization of the data to ensure that the plot is linear and has a slope of unity.

Although the Clark plot can be used to visualize the slope relationship between pEC_{50} and $-\log([B] + 10^{-pK_B})$, deviation of the slope from unity is better obtained by refitting the data to a "power departure" version of Equation 6.27:

$$pEC_{50} = -Log([B]^m + 10^{-pK_B}) - Log\ c \qquad (6.28)$$

where m is allowed to vary as part of the nonlinear fit. A value of F is calculated for comparison of the fits to Equations 6.27 and 6.28, respectively. If the value of F is not significant, then there is no reason to use the power departure equation and the antagonism can be considered to be simple competitive. To test for significant deviation from linearity of the Clark plot (indicating a departure from simple competitive antagonism at some concentration used in the experiment), the data are fit to a "quadratic departure" version of Equation 6.27:

$$pEC_{50} = -Log([B](1 + n[B]10^{-pK_B}) + 10^{-pK_B}) - Log\ c \qquad (6.29)$$

where n is allowed to vary with the nonlinear fitting procedure. As with the analysis for slope, a value for F is calculated. If the quadratic departure is not statistically supported, then the regression can be considered linear.

The method of Lew and Angus uses nonlinear curve fitting procedures to estimate the pK_B. An estimate of the error calculated with Equation 6.27 is provided by the estimate of the fitting error. This is obtained from most if not all commercially available fitting programs (or can be calculated with matrix algebra). An example of this type of analysis is shown in Figure 6.15A. The pEC_{50} values for the dose-response curves and the concentrations of antagonist were fitted to the equation shown in the panel in Figure 6.15B to yield the Clark plot shown in panel B. The resulting pK_B value is 8.09 + 0.145. The data were then refit to the power departure version of the equation, to yield the Clark plot shown in panel C. The calculated F for comparison of the simple model (slope = unity) to

the more complex model (slope fit independently) yielded a value for F that is not greater than that required for 95% confidence of difference. Therefore, the slope can be considered not significantly different from unity. Finally, the data were again refit to the quadratic departure version of the equation, to yield the Clark plot shown in panel D to test for nonlinearity. The resulting F indicates that the plot is not significantly nonlinear.

6.4 NONCOMPETITIVE ANTAGONISM

From an examination of Equation 6.1, and noted in Figure 6.4, if the rate of offset of the orthosteric antagonist is slow, to the point that a correct re-equilibration cannot occur between the agonist, antagonist, and receptors during the period of response collection in the presence of antagonist, then essentially a pseudo-irreversible blockade of receptors will occur. Thus, when:

$$t \ll k_2^{-1}$$

in Equation 6.1, the agonist will not access antagonist-bound receptors and a noncompetitive antagonism will result. This is the opposite extreme of the case for simple competitive antagonism discussed in Section 6.3.

The term *competitive antagonism* connotes an obvious mechanism of action (i.e., two drugs compete for the same binding site on the receptor to achieve the effect). Similarly, the term *noncompetitive* indicates that two drugs bind to the receptor, and that these interactions are mutually exclusive (i.e., when one drug occupies the binding site then another cannot exert its influence on the receptor). However, this should not necessarily be related to binding loci on the receptor. Two drugs may interact noncompetitively but still require occupancy of the same receptor binding site. Alternatively, the sites may be separate as in allosteric effects (see next chapter).

In an operational sense, noncompetitive antagonism is defined as the case where the antagonist binds to the receptor and makes it functionally inoperative. This can occur through preclusion of agonist binding or through some other biochemical mechanism that obviates agonist effect on the receptor and thereby blocks response due to agonist. Under these circumstances, no amount of increase in the agonist concentration can reverse the effect of a noncompetitive antagonist. A distinctive feature of noncompetitive antagonists is the effect they may have on the maximal agonist response. In situations where 100% of the receptors need be occupied to achieve the maximal response to the agonist (i.e., partial agonists), any amount of noncompetitive antagonism will lead to a diminution of the maximal response. However, in systems where there is a receptor reserve there will not be a depression of the maximal response until such a point

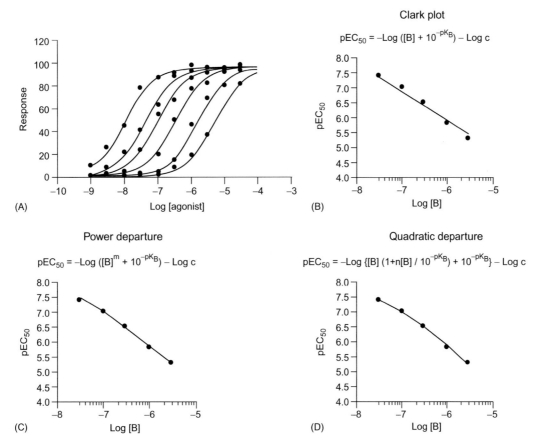

FIGURE 6.15 Example of application of method of Lew and Angus [10]. (A) Dose-response data. (B) Clark plot according to Equation 6.27 shown. (C) Data refit to "power departure" version of Equation 6.27 to detect slopes different from unity (Equation 6.28). (D) Data refit to "quadratic departure" version of Equation 6.27 to detect deviation from linearity (Equation 6.29).

where there is sufficient antagonism to block a fraction of receptor larger than that required to achieve maximal response. As discussed in Chapter 2, the magnitude of the receptor reserve is both system dependent (dependent on receptor number *and* the efficiency of stimulus-response coupling) and agonist dependent (intrinsic efficacy). Therefore, noncompetitive antagonists will have differing capabilities to depress the maximal response to the same agonist in different systems. The same will be true for different agonists in the same system.

The equation describing agonist-receptor occupancy under conditions of noncompetitive antagonism is given by Equation 6.8. The effect of antagonist on the maximal agonist-receptor occupancy (i.e., as $[A] \to \infty$) and comparison to the control maximal stimulus from Equation 6.8 is:

$$\text{Maximal agonist occupancy} = \frac{1}{1 + [B]/K_B} \quad (6.30)$$

It can be seen that at non-zero values of $[B]/K_B$ the maximal agonist-*receptor* occupancy will be depressed. However, as discussed in Chapter 2, some high-efficacy

agonists and/or some highly coupled receptor systems (high receptor density) yield maximal tissue response by activation of only a fraction of the receptor population ("spare receptors"). Thus, a noncompetitive antagonist may preclude binding of the agonist to all the receptors, but this may or may not result in a depression of the maximal response to the agonist. To discuss this further requires conversion of the agonist-receptor occupancy curve (Equation 6.8) into tissue response through the operational model:

$$A + R \underset{K_A}{\overset{}{\rightleftarrows}} AR \overset{K_E}{\longrightarrow} \text{Response}$$

(with B, + , K_B, BR shown in the scheme)

whereby the antagonist precludes agonist activation and response is produced through interaction of the [AR] complex with the tissue stimulus-response cascade

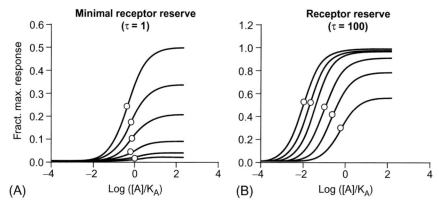

FIGURE 6.16 Effects of a slow offset orthosteric antagonist that essentially does not re-equilibrate with agonist and receptors upon addition of agonist to the system (pseudo-irreversible receptor blockade). (A) In this system a low value of τ is operative (i.e., the efficacy of the agonist is low) if there is a low receptor density and/or poor coupling of receptors. Under these circumstances, little to no dextral displacement is observed for the concentration-response curves upon antagonism (insurmountable blockade). (B) If the τ value is high (high efficacy, high receptor density, highly efficient receptor coupling, high receptor reserve), then the same antagonist may produce dextral displacement of the concentration-response curves with no depression of maximal response until relatively large portions of the receptor population are blocked.

FIGURE 6.17 Fitting of data to models. (A) Concentration-response curves obtained to an agonist in the absence (circles) and presence of an antagonist at concentrations 3 μM (triangles) and 30 μM (diamonds). (B) Data fit to model for insurmountable orthosteric antagonism (Equation 6.31) with $E_{max} = 1$, $K_A = 1$ μM, $\tau = 30$, and $K_B = 1$ μM.

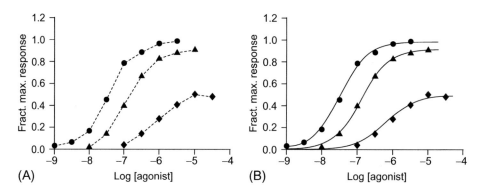

through the constant K_E according to the operational model. Under these circumstances, the response to an agonist obtained in the presence of a noncompetitive antagonist is given by:

$$\text{Response} = \frac{[A]/K_A \tau E_{max}}{[A]/K_A(1 + \tau + [B]/K_B) + [B]/K_B + 1}$$

(6.31)

Now it can be seen that the maximal response (as a fraction of the control maximal response) to the agonist (as $[A] \to \infty$) is given by:

$$\text{Maximal Response} = \frac{(1 + \tau)}{(1 + \tau + [B]/K_B)}$$

(6.32)

Here it can be seen that for very efficacious agonists, or in systems of high receptor density or very efficient receptor coupling (all leading to high values of τ), the maximal response to the agonist may not be depressed in the presence of the noncompetitive antagonist. Figure 6.16A shows

the effect of a noncompetitive antagonist on the receptor response to an agonist in a system with no receptor reserve ($\tau = 1$) is n. It can be seen that the maximal response to the agonist is depressed at all non-zero values of $[B]/K_B$. In Figure 6.16B, the same antagonist is used to block responses to a highly efficacious agonist in a system with high receptor reserve ($\tau = 100$). From these simulations it can be seen that observation of insurmountable antagonism is not necessarily a prerequisite for a noncompetitive receptor mechanism.

In terms of measuring the potency of insurmountable antagonists, the data can be fitted to an explicit model. As shown in Figure 6.17A, responses to an agonist in the absence and presence of various concentrations of an insurmountable antagonist are fitted to Equation 6.31 (Figure 6.17B) and an estimate of the K_B for the antagonist is obtained. One shortcoming of this approach is the complexity of the model itself. It will be seen in the next chapter that allosteric models of receptor antagonism can also yield patterns of agonist concentration-response curves like

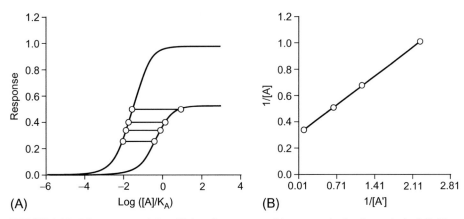

FIGURE 6.18 Measurement of the affinity of a noncompetitive antagonist by the method of Gaddum (Equation 6.33). (A) Dose-response curves for an agonist without noncompetitive antagonist present and in the presence of a concentration of antagonist of 1 μM. Dots and connecting lines show equiactive responses in the absence and presence of the noncompetitive antagonist. (B) Double reciprocal plot of equiactive concentrations of agonist in the presence (abscissae) and absence (ordinates) of noncompetitive antagonist. Plot is linear with a slope of 32.1. Method of Gaddum [3] indicates that the equilibrium dissociation constant of the antagonist-receptor complex is [B]/(Slope − 1) = 1 μM/(31.2 − 1) = 33 nM.

those shown in Figure 6.17, and that these can be fit equally well to allosteric models. Thus, model fitting can be ambiguous if the molecular mechanism of the antagonism is not known beforehand.

Historically, Gaddum and colleagues [3] devised a method to measure the affinity of insurmountable antagonists based on a double reciprocal linear transformation. With this method, equiactive concentrations of agonist in the absence ([A]) and presence ([A′]) of a noncompetitive antagonist ([B]) are compared in a double reciprocal plot describing a straight line (see Section 6.12.9):

$$1/[A] = 1/([A'][B]/K_B) + 1) + [B]/(K_B K_A) \quad (6.33)$$

According to Equation 6.33, a regression of values for 1/[A] upon 1/[A′] should give a straight line. The equilibrium dissociation constant of the antagonist-receptor complex is given by:

$$K_B = [B]/(slope - 1) \quad (6.34)$$

At the time that this method was developed, linear regression was a major advantage (in lieu of the general accessibility of nonlinear fitting). However, linearization of data is known to distort errors and weighting and to emphasize certain regions of the data set, and generally is not recommended. This is especially true of double reciprocal plots such as that defined by Equation 6.33. This shortcoming can be somewhat alleviated by a metameter such as:

$$\frac{[A']}{[A]} = [A']\frac{[B]}{K_B K_A} + \frac{[B]}{(K_B)} + 1 \quad (6.35)$$

where a regression of [A′]/[A] upon [A′] yields a straight line, with K_B being equal to:

$$K_B = [B]/(intercept - 1) \quad (6.36)$$

Figure 6.18 shows the procedure for using this method. In terms of the practical application, an important point to note is that the maximal response to the agonist must be depressed by the noncompetitive antagonist for this method to be effective. In fact, the greater the degree of maximal response inhibition, the more robust is the fit according to Equation 6.33. Moreover, data points at the concentrations of agonist yielding the higher responses (near the depressed maximal response in the presence of the antagonist) provide more robust fits with this method. An example of the use of this method is given in Section 13.2.6.

In cases where there is a substantial receptor reserve such that there is a measurable dextral displacement of the concentration-response curves, then another reliable method for determining the affinity of the noncompetitive antagonist is to measure the pA₂ (−log of the molar concentration that produces a twofold shift to the right of the agonist concentration-response curve). It can be shown that for purely noncompetitive antagonists the pA₂ is related to the pK_B with the relation (see Section 6.12.10):

$$pK_B = pA_2 - Log(1 + 2[A]/K_A) \quad (6.37)$$

Equation 6.37 predicts that the pA₂ is an accurate estimate of the pK_B at low levels of agonist-receptor occupancy ([A]/K_A → 0). For high values of agonist-receptor occupancy, the observed pA₂ will overestimate the true affinity of the antagonist. However, for low levels of response (where dose ratios for insurmountable antagonists likely will be measured) and for high-efficacy agonists, [A]/K_A ≪ EC₅₀ for response − and under these circumstances the pA₂ will be an accurate estimate of the pK_B. The use of dextral displacement to measure the affinity of noncompetitive antagonists is illustrated in Figure 6.19.

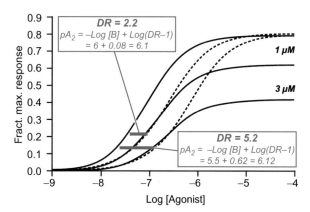

FIGURE 6.19 Use of the dextral displacement produced by an insurmountable antagonist to estimate dose ratios and subsequent pA_2 values. Response according to model for orthosteric noncompetitive blockade (Equation 6.31 with $E_{max} = 1$, $\tau = 3$, $K_A = 0.3$ µM, $K_B = 1$ µM) for 1 µM and 3 µM antagonist. Dose ratios measured at response = 0.24 for 1 µM antagonist and response = 0.15 for 3 µM antagonist. Resulting pA_2 values are close estimates of the true pK_B (6.0) as modified by the $[A]/K_A$ term (see Equation 6.37).

An example of the use of this technique is given in Section 13.2.7.

6.5 AGONIST-ANTAGONIST HEMI-EQUILIBRIA

All models of antagonism assume that sufficient time is allowed for equilibrium to be established among the receptors, the agonist, and the antagonist. For experiments carried out in real time, the approach to steady-state response for an agonist in the presence of a pre-equilibrated concentration of antagonist can be observed and the conditions of the experiment can be adjusted accordingly to make measurements at equilibrium. As discussed for binding experiments, the time required to achieve equilibrium with an agonist in the presence of an antagonist may be much longer than the time required for only the agonist if the rate of offset of the antagonist is much slower than that of the agonist. Unlike binding experiments, where the tracer ligand and displacing ligand are added together to start the reaction, functional experiments are usually done in a mode whereby the agonist dose-response curve is obtained in the presence of the antagonist in a preparation where the antagonist has been pre-equilibrated with the tissue. This pre-equilibration period is designed to be sufficient to ensure that equilibrium has been attained between the receptors and the antagonist. Under these conditions, as the agonist is added the receptors must re-equilibrate with the added agonist and the antagonist already bound to the receptor population. Given sufficient time, this occurs according to the Gaddum equation, but the time may be longer than if the agonist were equilibrating with an empty receptor

population. This is because the agonist can bind only when the antagonist dissociates from the receptor. If this is a slow process, then it may take a great deal of time, relative to an empty receptor population, for enough antagonist to dissociate for attainment of equilibrium receptor occupancy by the agonist.

As discussed in Section 6.2, the kinetic equation for the adjustment of receptor occupancy (ρ_t) by a pre-equilibrated concentration of a slow-acting antagonist [B] with rate of offset k_2 upon addition of a fast-acting agonist [A] is given by Equation 6.1 [1]. As considered in Section 6.3, if there is sufficient time for re-equilibration among agonist, antagonist, and receptors, then simple competitive surmountable antagonism results. Similarly, as further described in Section 6.4, if there is *no* re-equilibration (due to insufficient time and/or a very slow offset of the antagonist), then noncompetitive insurmountable antagonism results. Between these two kinetic extremes are conditions where the agonist, antagonist, and receptors can *partially* re-equilibrate. These conditions were described by Paton and Rang [1] as hemi-equilibria. The shortfall with respect to re-equilibration occurs at the high end of the agonist-receptor occupancy scale. Figure 6.20A shows the time course for the production of a response by a high concentration of agonist in a hemi-equilibrium system with a slow offset antagonist. It can be seen from this figure that with the parameters chosen ($k_2 = 10^{-3}$ s^{-1}, $[B]/K_B = 3$, $[A]/K_A = 100$), a true maximal response is not attained until data are collected over a period of 55 minutes. Therefore, if the period for response collection is <55 minutes, a truncated response will be measured. This will not be nearly as prevalent at lower agonist-receptor occupancies. The result of such high-level response truncation is a shifted concentration-response curve with depressed maximal responses (as shown in Figure 6.20B). It can be seen that if sufficient time is allowed the insurmountable antagonism becomes surmountable.

A characteristic of hemi-equilibria is the observation of a depressed plateau of maximal responses. Thus, while a truly insurmountable antagonist will eventually depress the concentration-response curves to basal levels, hemi-equilibrium conditions can produce partial but not complete inhibition of the agonist maximal response. This is shown in Figure 6.21.

Practical problems with hemi-equilibria can be avoided by allowing sufficient time for equilibrium to occur. However, there are some situations where this may not be possible. One is where the functional system desensitizes during the span of time required for equilibrium to be attained. Another is where the actual type of response being measured is transitory; one example is the measurement of calcium transients where a spike of effect is the only response observed in the experimental system.

Hemi-equilibria can be exacerbated in slow diffusion systems. In systems composed of cells in culture, there is

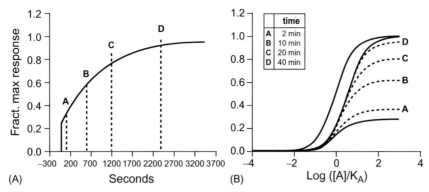

FIGURE 6.20 Increasing times for measurement of response for a slow-acting orthosteric antagonist ($k_2 = 1$ msec^{-1}) for [B]/K_B = 3. Inset shows the kinetics of response production by a concentration of the agonist producing maximal response ([A]/K_A = 100). It can be seen that a rapid initial increase in response (due to occupation of unoccupied receptors) is followed by a slower phase where the agonist and antagonist re-equilibrate with the receptor population. If only 2 minutes are allowed for measurement of response, a severely depressed concentration-response curve results. With increasing equilibration times, the maxima increase until at 40 minutes simple competition with no depression of the maximal response is observed.

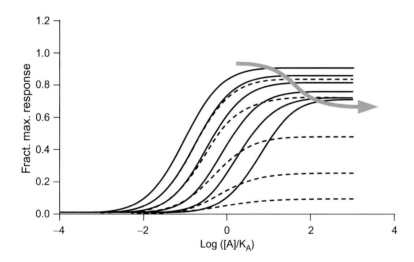

FIGURE 6.21 Hemi-equilibrium among antagonist, agonist, and receptors. Hemi-equilibrium condition according to Equation 6.11 resulting in a depressed maximal response to the agonist that reaches a plateau ($k_2 = 5 \times 10^{-5}$ s^{-1}, $\tau = 10$, t = 90 min). Antagonist concentrations of 0 = control curve farthest to the left; [B]/K_B = 1, 3, 10, 30, and 100, with dotted lines showing what would be expected from purely noncompetitive behavior of the same antagonist (no re-equilibration). Pure surmountable blockade would be observed for response times of ≥200 seconds.

little formal architecture (such as might be encountered in a whole tissue) that would hinder free diffusion. Such obstruction could intensify the effects of a removal process such as adsorption of drug to the side of the culture well. However, there is a possible effect of the thin unstirred water layer coating the surface of the cell monolayer. Free diffusion is known to be slower in unstirred, versus stirred, bodies of water. In isolated tissues where organ baths are oxygenated vigorously, the effects of unstirred layers can be minimized. However, in 96- and 384-well formats for cells in culture, such stirring is not possible. In these cases unstirred layers, for some ligands where there is an avid adsorption mechanism capable of removing the ligand from the receptor compartment, may be a factor causing an exaggeration of the apparent loss of drug potency due to adsorption. Reduced diffusion due to unstirred layers also may play a role in the observed

magnitude of agonist response in systems where hemi-equilibria could be a factor. In these cases, there could be a practical problem in classifying competitive receptor antagonism erroneously as noncompetitive antagonism (where maximal responses also are depressed).

6.6 RESULTANT ANALYSIS

Schild analysis, like all pharmacological tools, is necessarily predicated on the idea that the drugs involved have one and only one pharmacological activity. This often may not be the case and selectivity is only a function of concentration. If the concentrations used in the assay are below those that have secondary effects, then the tool will furnish the parameter of interest with no obfuscation. However, if secondary effects are operative in the

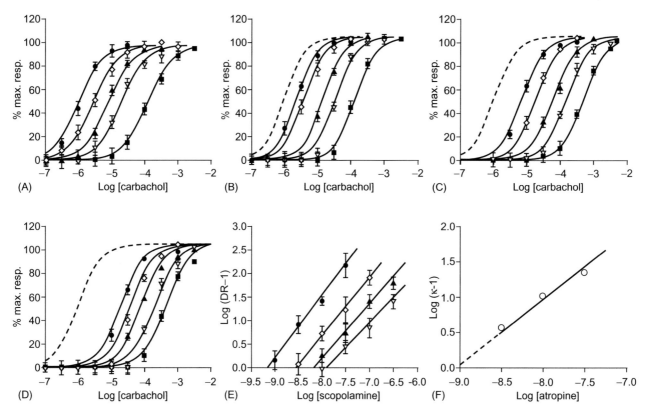

FIGURE 6.22 Pharmacological, resultant analysis of atropine. Panels A through D: dose-response curves to carbachol in the absence (filled circles) and presence of various concentrations of the reference antagonist scopolamine. (A) Scopolamine = 1 nM (open diamonds), 3 nM (filled triangles), 10 nM (open inverted triangles), and 30 nM (filled squares). (B) As for A, except experiment carried out in the presence of 3 nM atropine. Concentration of scopolamine = 3 nM, 10 nM, 30 nM, and 100 nM. Dotted line shows control curve to carbachol in the absence of atropine. (C) As for B, except atropine = 10 nM and scopolamine 10 nM, 30 nM, 100 nM, and 300 nM. (D) As for C, except atropine = 30 nM. (E) Schild regression for scopolamine in the absence (filled circles) and presence of atropine 3 nM (open circles), 10 nM (filled triangles), and 30 nM (open inverted triangles). (F) Resultant plot for atropine according to Equation 6.38. Log (φ−1) values (see text, versus log[atropine]). Data redrawn from [5].

concentration range required to measure antagonism, then the resulting parameter may be tainted by this secondary activity. One approach to nullify these effects for simple competitive antagonists is through the use of resultant analysis.

Derived by Black, Shankley, Leff, and Wood [12], this procedure essentially allows calculation of the potency of a test antagonist through measurement of the added effects this test antagonist has on another antagonist (referred to as the *reference antagonist*). The idea is that the initial response is obtained in the presence of the test antagonist and then again in the presence of both antagonists. The secondary effects of the test antagonist will be operative in both the initial and subsequent dose-response curves. Therefore, under null conditions these effects will cancel. This allows the antagonist portion of the test antagonist activity to be observed as an added component to the antagonism of a known concentration of a known reference antagonist. The principle of additive dose ratios [1] then can be used to isolate the receptor antagonism due to the test antagonist.

In practice, a series of Schild regressions is obtained for the reference antagonist in the absence and presence of a range of concentrations of the test antagonist. The dextral displacements, along the antagonist concentration axis of these regressions, are utilized as ordinates for a resultant plot in the form of ratios of log (DR − 1) values for the different Schild plots. These are designated κ. The κ values are related to the concentrations of the test antagonist by the equation (see Section 6.12.11):

$$\text{Log}(\kappa - 1) = \text{Log}[B_{test}] - \text{Log}K_{Btest} \qquad (6.38)$$

An example of the procedure is shown in Figure 6.22. Specifically, a series of Schild analyses were done for the reference antagonist scopolamine in the presence of different concentrations of the test antagonist atropine. The resultant plot according to Equation 6.38 yields an estimate of the K_B for atropine as the intercept (log $(\kappa - 1) = 0$). If atropine had secondary effects on the system, this procedure would cancel them and allow measurement of the receptor antagonism. An example of this procedure is given in Section 13.2.8.

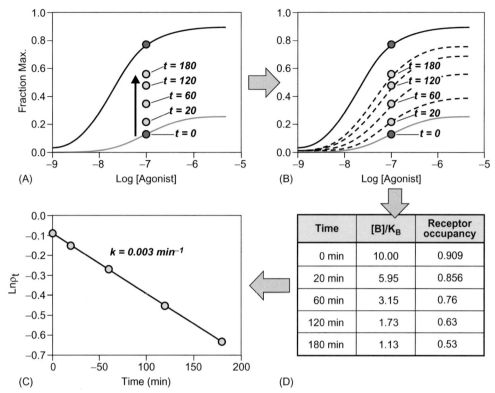

FIGURE 6.23 Measurement of offset rate for a noncompetitive antagonist. (A) Dose-response curves shown for control (no antagonist) and in the presence of a sub-maximal concentration of noncompetitive antagonist. The response to an EC_{80} concentration of agonist (blue circle) is measured at various wash times. (B) Dose-response curves fit to a model of noncompetitive blockade consistent with the potency of the antagonist (pK_B) and the position and shape of the control and blocked dose-response curves. (C) The fit dose-response curves yield virtual values of $[B]/K_B$ as the antagonist is washed off the receptor. These $[B]/K_B$ values are converted to receptor occupancies through the mass action equation. (D) A plot of ln ρ receptor occupancy versus time is used to calculate a rate of offset (slope of the straight line).

6.7 ANTAGONIST RECEPTOR COVERAGE: KINETICS OF DISSOCIATION

A key piece of data characterizing the activity of an antagonist is its persistence of binding. This is because *in vivo* systems are open systems; i.e., the concentration of antagonist is never constant, but rather increases upon absorption of drug and decreases with clearance of drug. Useful dissimulations between *in vivo* antagonist concentrations and blockade of response can be obtained if the rate of receptor dissociation of the antagonist is less than the rate of drug clearance. Since antagonist potency is the ratio of ligand dissociation (k_2) and association (k_1 — $K_{eq} = k_2/k_1$), there need not be a correlation between antagonist potency and persistence of antagonism *in vivo*. Thus, a slowly dissociating antagonist may be more valuable as a therapy than an equipotent rapidly dissociating antagonist. Because of this, it is important to quantify the dissociation rate of an antagonist from the receptor. This can be done in an *in vitro* functional assay by obtaining an equilibrium sub-maximal level of receptor blockade, fitting the obtained curve with the appropriate model, and then measuring the response to the agonist over a period of antagonist-free wash. The single values of response during the offset period are fitted to the antagonist model used to fit the equilibrium data and the virtual antagonist concentration is calculated. These virtual antagonist concentrations are then converted to receptor occupancies, and the resulting relationship of receptor occupancy with time is fitted to a first-order rate of decay to yield the rate of offset of the antagonist from the receptor. Thus, a concentration-response curve for the agonist is obtained in the absence and presence of a defined concentration of antagonist. The ideal concentration for use in this procedure is one that does not completely obliterate the response but rather produces a receptor system that still yields a concentration-response curve to the agonist. The control and antagonist-treated curves are fit to an appropriate model of antagonism (see Chapter 8); as an example, Figure 6.23 shows insurmountable antagonism fit to the model for orthosteric noncompetitive antagonism:

$$\text{Response} = \frac{[A]^n \tau^n}{[A]^n \tau_n + ([A](1+[B]/K_B) + K_A[B]/K_B + K_A)^n}$$

(6.39)

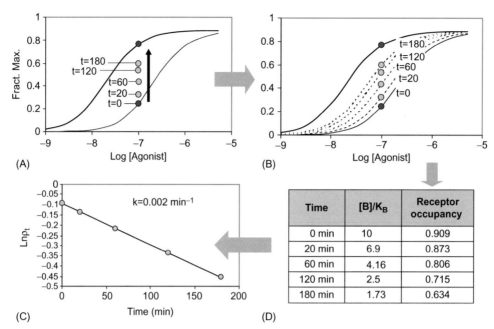

FIGURE 6.24 Measurement of offset rate for a competitive (surmountable) antagonist. (A) Dose-response curves shown for control (no antagonist) and in the presence of a sub-maximal concentration of noncompetitive antagonist. The response to an EC_{80} concentration of agonist (blue circle) is measured at various wash times. (B) Dose-response curves fit the model for simple competitive orthosteric antagonism or allosteric surmountable antagonism model; virtual values of $[B]/K_B$ used to fit the appropriate location of the shifted curves with time. (C) The fit dose-response curves yield virtual values of $[B]/K_B$ as the antagonist is washed off the receptor. These $[B]/K_B$ values are converted to receptor occupancies through the mass action equation. (D) A plot of ln ρ receptor occupancy versus time is used to calculate a rate of offset (slope of the straight line).

where [A] is the concentration of agonist; K_A and K_B are the equilibrium dissociation constants of the agonist and antagonist receptor complexes, respectively; n is a fitting coefficient; and τ is the efficacy term for the operational model. The experimental preparation is then washed free of antagonist for a period of time. During this process, the preparation is challenged with a concentration of agonist which produces approximately a 40 to 80% maximal response. In the example shown in Figure 6.23A, the assay is challenged repeatedly with 100 nM agonist periodically over a period of 180 min (while washing with antagonist-free media).The responses to the single agonist challenges are then used to fit complete concentration-response curves, according to the original model used to fit the data, with the original parameters for the curve but with different values of $[B]/K_B$ (see Figure 6.23B). The values of $[B]/K_B$ that are used to fit the agonist data then are used to calculate a receptor occupancy value according to mass action (see table in Figure 6.23C):

$$\rho_t = ([B]/K_B)/(1 + [B]/K_B) \qquad (6.40)$$

The values of ρ_t (ordinate as $\ln(\rho_t)$ values) are plotted as a function of time (abscissae) according to a first-order model of offset:

$$\rho_t = e^{-kt} \qquad (6.41)$$

As a natural logarithmic metameter:

$$Ln(\rho_t) = -kt \qquad (6.42)$$

The slope of the resulting linear regression (see Figure 6.23D) is an estimate of the negative value of the rate constant for receptor offset. For the example shown in Figure 6.23 (insurmountable blockade), $k = 0.003$ min^{-1}. This procedure can be used for any pattern of blockade. For example, surmountable (apparently competitive) blockade can be fit to the model:

$$\text{Response} = \frac{[A]^n \tau^n}{[A]^n \tau^n + ([A] + K_A(1 + [B]/K_B))^n} \qquad (6.43)$$

The same process then can be applied (see Figure 6.24).

6.7.1 Estimating Antagonist Dissociation with Hemi-Equilibria

Hemi-equilibria can be used in certain cases to estimate the rate of dissociation of antagonists. As shown in Figure 6.20, if there is an insufficient time available to measure response to an agonist in the presence of an antagonist, then the maximal response to the agonist is

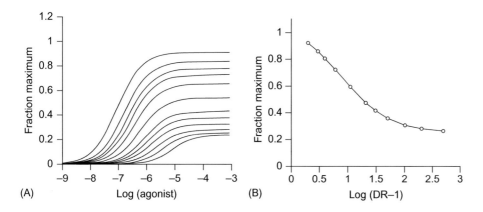

FIGURE 6.25 (A) Response to an agonist of $K_A = 1\,\mu M$, $\tau = 10$ in a system of $t = 300\,s$ for an antagonist of $K_B = 10\,nM$ and $k_2 = 10^{-4}\,s^{-1}$. (B) Maximal response to the agonist as a function of the degree of antagonism expressed as a value of dose ratio -1.

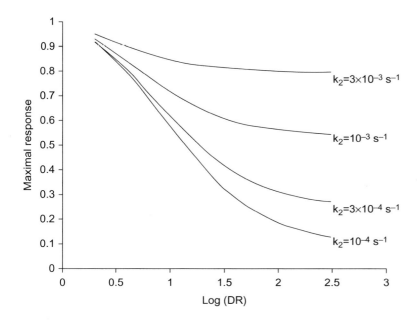

FIGURE 6.26 Relationship between magnitude of antagonism (abscissal axis as $\log(DR - 1)$ value) and maximal response in a kinetically compromised system (as shown in Figure 6.25). Response to an agonist of $K_A = 1\,\mu M$, $\tau = 10$ in a system of $t = 300\,s$ for an antagonist of $K_B = 10\,nM$ and various values of dissociation rates (from $k_2 = 3 \times 10^{-3}\,s^{-1}$ to $k_2 = 10^{-4}\,s^{-1}$).

depressed. In fact, it can be shown that the degree of depression of the maximal response is inversely proportional to the dissociation rate of the antagonist and the magnitude of the window in time available to observe response. This latter factor can be a feature of a given functional assay (i.e., calcium transient response using Fluorescence Imaging Plate Reader format) therefore the measurement in such a system can lead to a useful estimation of antagonist dissociation rate. This latter factor is a very important property of an antagonist that will be used *in vivo* since it will determine target coverage (*vide infra*). Figure 6.25A shows the effect of increasing concentrations of a slowly dissociating antagonist in a hemi-equilibrium system; it can be seen from this figure that as dextral displacements of the concentration-response curves occur, so too does the maximal response to the antagonist to a limiting value (as shown in Figure 6.21). This limiting depression of the maximal

response is dependent on the time available to measure response and the dissociation rate of the antagonist (k_2). Setting $[A]/K_A \to \infty$ in Equation 6.11 yields an expression for the maximal response to the agonist (with efficacy τ) in the presence of an antagonist with dissociation rate k_2 in a system where the time window for observation for response is t:

$$\text{Agonist Maximal Response} = \frac{(1 - e^{-k_2 t})(\tau + 1)}{(1 - e^{-k_2 t})\tau + 1} \quad (6.44)$$

The maximal response can be expressed as a function of antagonism observed (quantified as the dose ratio -1) to yield a curve that is characteristic of a given antagonist with a given dissociation rate $-$ this is shown in Figure 6.25B. Figure 6.26 shows curves for a set of antagonists with a range of dissociation rates in a given system with the same agonist (τ and t constant).

6.8 BLOCKADE OF INDIRECTLY ACTING AGONISTS

A unique pattern of antagonism can be observed if a competitive antagonist blocks the effects of an endogenously released natural agonist; the ligand doing this is referred to as an "indirect" agonist [13]. For example, tyramine is taken up by sympathetic nerve endings and this results in the release of neuronal norepinephrine, which can then act on postsynaptic β-adrenoceptors (see Figure 6.27A). The equation predicting the fractional agonist effect to the indirectly acting agonist ([A]) in these cases is given as (see Section 6.12.12 for derivation):

Fractional Effect$_{AB}$ =

$$\frac{[A]/K_A[\theta]K_E}{[A]/K_A([\theta]/K_E + [B]/K_B + 1) + [B]/K_B + 1} \quad (6.45)$$

where θ is the size of the pool of released agonist, K_E is the equilibrium dissociation constant of the released agonist-receptor complex, K_A is the equilibrium constant for the complex of the indirect agonist and site of release, [B] is the concentration of antagonist and K_B is the equilibrium

dissociation constant of the antagonist-receptor complex. Of note is the fact that the maximal response to the indirect agonist in the presence of the antagonist (as $[A]/K_A \rightarrow \infty$) is given as:

$$\text{Maximal Response}_A = \frac{\theta/K_E}{\theta/K_E + [B]/K_B} \quad (6.46)$$

It can be seen from Equation 6.46 that the size of releasable pool determines whether surmountable or insurmountable antagonism will be seen, even with fast-acting competitive antagonists. Figure 6.27B shows the effects of a competitive antagonist on an indirect agonist, and Figure 6.27C shows actual data from such a system. In this case, the β-adrenoceptor antagonist propranolol blocks the effects of endogenously released norepinephrine by the indirect agonist tyramine [13].

6.9 IRREVERSIBLE ANTAGONISM

Equilibrium between antagonists and receptors is achieved when the number of bound molecules dissociating from

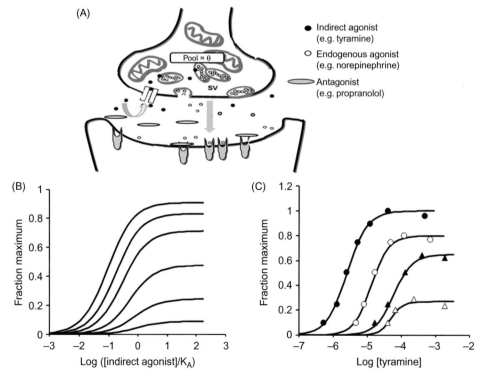

FIGURE 6.27 (A) Indirect antagonism by a competitive antagonist of responses to an indirect agonist causing the release of an endogenous agonist. A model system is shown whereby tyramine causes the release of neuronal norepinephrine acting on postsynaptic β-adrenoceptors. These postsynaptic receptors are blocked by the β-blocker propranolol. (B) The effects of an antagonist on responses to an indirectly acting agonist according to equation 6.45; for this simulation $\theta K_E = 10$. (C) Positive chronotropic responses in rat atria to tyramine blocked by propranolol. Curve shown for control (filled circles) and in the presence of propranolol 10 nM (open circles), 50 nM (filled triangles) and 200 nM (open triangles). Data for C redrawn from [13].

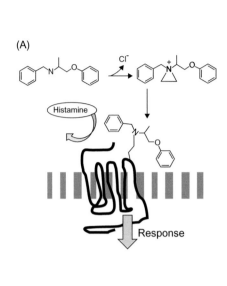

(A)

Histamine

Response

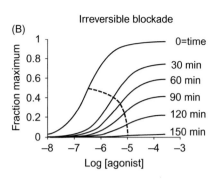

Irreversible blockade

(B)

0=time

30 min

60 min

90 min

120 min

150 min

Fraction maximum

Log [agonist]

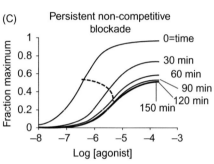

Persistent non-competitive blockade

(C)

0=time

30 min

60 min

90 min

120 min

150 min

Fraction maximum

Log [agonist]

FIGURE 6.28 Irreversible receptor antagonism. (A) Chemical alkylation of histamine receptors by phenoxybenzamine (POB). This molecule forms a chemically reactive aziridinium ion in H_2O which then can alkylate various groups on protein; the structure of POB causes it to bind to the active histamine binding site therefore this site is occluded when the POB alkylates the protein. (B) The effect of a single concentration of alkylating agent is equilibrated with the receptor preparation for increasing lengths of time. (C) For a pseudo-irreversible antagonist that has an appreciable rate of dissociation, there will be a point where an equilibrium will be reached that causes sub-maximal receptor antagonism.

receptors equals the number of molecules binding to the receptors per unit time. If there is appreciable antagonist dissociation, a sub-maximal level of antagonism can be attained, i.e., the blockade will not progress to completion at all concentrations. In cases where the rate of dissociation is extremely low (compared to the window of time available to observe effect), the rate of reversal of antagonism in the presence of drug-free medium will be correspondingly slow, a condition often referred to as "pseudo-irreversible" inhibition. However, there are cases whereby a chemical reaction between the antagonist and receptor can take place, to lead to a truly irreversible species. When this occurs, all concentrations of antagonists, when equilibrated with the receptor for a sufficient length of time, will completely block available receptors, i.e., it is a chemical reaction that goes to completion (or until the reactive chemical species reacts with other components of the system such as H_2O to dissipate). An example of this is shown in Figure 6.28A where the β-haloalkylamine, phenoxybenzamine (POB), forms a reactive aziridinium ion species which goes on to alkylate histamine, muscarinic and α-adrenergic receptors. Thus, equilibration of a receptor preparation with a β-haloalkylamine will cause increased receptor antagonism with increasing time of equilibration, until complete blockade is observed (see Figure 6.28B): this is in contrast to a pseudo-irreversible antagonist which, at some point, will reach a sub-maximal level of antagonism (see Figure 6.28C). In the case of truly irreversible blockade, washing the receptor with drug-free medium will not reverse the antagonism. Since a wide range of antagonist concentrations will produce complete blockade, it is not possible to determine an equilibrium dissociation constant for antagonism, i.e., to quantify

the potency of an irreversible antagonist, through regular means. In these cases a procedure modified from one used to quantify irreversible enzyme inactivation can be used. Figure 6.29 shows the effect of phenoxybenzamine (POB) alkylation of histamine receptors on the histamine response in guinea pig ileum; in this case, three minute exposures to increasing concentrations of POB causes irreversible dextral displacement of the concentration-response curve until the receptor reserve for the agonist is removed. This is followed by depression of the maximal response as greater receptor removal is produced. The inhibition of histamine function progresses at various rates as a function of POB concentration. The effect of alkylation on histamine receptor can be calculated by fitting the Black−Leff operational model to the data with various values for τ; as concentration-response curves shift to the right, decreasing values of τ are used to simulate the reduction in receptor number (since $\tau = [R_t]/K_E$ — see Chapter 3.6). Figure 6.29C shows the increasing antagonism with POB concentration expressed as a rate of receptor alkylation plotted as a function of POB concentration. The resulting plot can be fit with a Michaelis−Menten function according to the equation:

$$\text{Rate of Receptor Inactivation} = [POB]\upsilon / ([POB] + K_{inact})$$

(6.47)

where υ is the maximal rate of inactivation and K_{inact} the concentration of POB producing half maximal receptor inactivation. While this strategy is used to characterize time-dependent (irreversible) enzyme inhibition in pharmacokinetic studies, it is not easily applicable to irreversible antagonism of receptors. More often a given

FIGURE 6.29 Quantification of histamine receptor alkylation. (A) Concentration-response curves to histamine in guinea pig ileum in the absence (filled circles) and after 3 min exposure to POB at the concentrations shown in the key on the figure. (B) Depression of free histamine receptors at various concentrations of POB for 3 min as a rate (over the 3 min period). (C) The rates of histamine receptor alkylation obtained in panel B plotted as a function of POB concentration. This yields a plot with maximum of $\upsilon = 0.33\text{s}^{-1}$ and $K_{inact} = 0.15\mu M$.

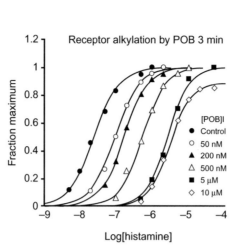

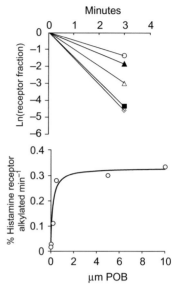

concentration and time of exposure is used to irreversibly inactivate a fraction of receptors. For example, Figure 8.5 shows responses of rat anococcygeus muscle to norepinephrine and oxymetazoline before and after irreversible alkylation of various portions of the α-adrenoceptor population; these effects were achieved by defined exposures of the preparation to specific concentrations of POB (i.e., 30 nM for 10 min and 0.1 μM for 10 min).

6.10 CHEMICAL ANTAGONISM

Antagonism of agonist responses can be produced by a chemical depletion of the agonist by a scavenging species, i.e., an antibody inactivating a peptide agonist. Agonist response can be modeled with the Black–Leff operational model (see Chapter 3, section 6);

$$\text{Response} = \frac{[A_{\text{free}}]\tau E_m}{([A_{\text{free}}](\tau + 1) + K_A)} \quad (6.48)$$

where $[A_{\text{free}}]$ is the free unbound concentration of agonist, K_A is the equilibrium dissociation constant of the agonist-receptor complex and τ the efficacy of the agonist. It is useful to consider two kinetic extremes. In the first, reversible kinetics is assumed in which the antibody, ligand, and receptor interact according to reversible mass action kinetics. A second condition assuming the binding of the chemical antagonist is essentially irreversible and thus precludes all interaction of the agonist with the receptor. It will be seen that extremely different antagonist kinetics are predicted by these two boundary conditions.

In the case of reversible kinetics it is assumed that the antibody binds reversibly to agonist and that the complex can no longer interact with the receptor (Figure 6.30A); the response is produced by free agonist $[A_{\text{free}}]$, where $[A_{\text{free}}]$ is given by (see derivations in Section 6.12.13):

$$[A_{\text{free}}] = [A_T] - 1/2([A_T] + K_B + \vartheta$$
$$- (([A_T] + K_B + \vartheta)^2 - 4[A_T]\vartheta))^{0.5} \quad (6.49)$$

$[A_T]$ is total agonist, K_B is the equilibrium dissociation constant of the agonist-Ab complex and ϑ is the concentration of Ab. This model predicts dextral displacements of the concentration-response curves to the agonist with increasing antibody concentration; these can be quantified and expressed as a pseudo-Schild regression (see Figure 6.30B). A discerning feature of this model is that there will be differences in the potency of the antibody as an antagonist with differences in the cell surface receptor density of the cell producing functional response and these are related to the magnitude of the receptor reserve to the agonist in the system. The antibody will show the highest potency in systems of high sensitivity to the agonist (largest receptor reserve for the agonist). Under these circumstances, parallel dextral displacements of the agonist concentration-response curves will be seen (see Figure 6.30C). In systems of lower sensitivity to the agonist there will be an increase in the slopes of the concentration-response curves (see Figure 6.30D) and a reduction in the potency of the antibody as an antagonist (Figure 6.30B).

Another condition was chosen whereby the antibody binds the agonist and precludes all interaction with the receptor; i.e., there is no competition between agonist, the antibody and the receptor. Under these circumstances the binding of the antibody to the receptor is given by:

$$[A_{Ab}] = \frac{[A_T])\vartheta}{[A_T])K_B} \quad (6.50)$$

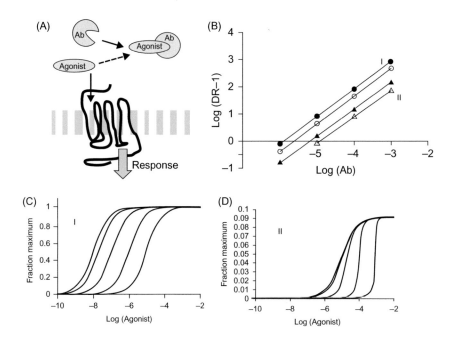

FIGURE 6.30 Reversible chemical antagonism. (A) A chemical antagonist (in this case an antibody, Ab) binds to the agonist to prevent its interaction with the receptor. (B) Apparent Schild regressions to the antibody as it blocks agonist response. Two extremes are shown: I (filled circles) is the Schild regression in a system of high agonist-receptor reserve (τ for agonist = 1000). Other systems shown are $\tau = 10$ (1% of the receptors shown in I, open circles), $\tau = 1$ (0.1% receptors, filled triangles) and system II ($\tau = 0.1$, 0.01% receptors, open triangles). (C) Effect of the antibody on concentration-response curves to the agonist in a high sensitivity system ($\tau = 1000$). (D) Effect of the antibody on concentration-response curves to the agonist in a low sensitivity system ($\tau = 0.1$). It should be noted that changes in the sensitivity to the agonist need not be solely due to differences in receptor density but rather can also be due to differences in the efficiency of receptor coupling.

Which yields another equation for $[A_{free}]$:

$$[A_{free}] = \frac{[A_T]^2 + [A_T]K_B - A\vartheta}{[A_T] + K_B} \quad (6.51)$$

Substitution of $[A_{free}]$ into Equation 6.49 yields responses to the agonist in this type of system. As shown in Figure 6.31A, the apparent Schild regressions for this type of system differ less in terms of their location parameter along the antibody concentration axis (i.e., antibody potency) but do differ in terms of increasing slope. Figure 6.31B shows the effect of the antibody on the agonist concentration-response curves in a system of high sensitivity to the agonist (high agonist-receptor reserve, $\tau = 1000$); it can be seen that the dextral displacement of the curves is accompanied by an increased slope. Figure 6.31C shows the effect of the antibody on a lower sensitivity system ($\tau = 1$). In this case, less dextral displacement is seen.

A variant on the theme of chemical antagonism is where a chemical scavenger may abstracts the concentration of competitive antagonist in a system (see Figure 6.32A). As in the previous section, the effects of the chemical antagonism (antibody binding) will be seen through changes in the effects of the receptor antagonist where two kinetic conditions are modeled. In the first, reversible kinetics are assumed between the antibody, antagonist, and receptor; it is assumed that these species interact according to reversible mass action kinetics.

Receptor antagonism is assumed to be due to interaction of the receptor with free antagonist $[B_{free}]$ which is given by (see derivations in Section 6.12.14):

$$[B_{free}] = [B_T] - [B_{Ab}] = \frac{1}{2}([B_T] + K_{B-Ab} + \vartheta \\ - (([B_T] + K_{B-Ab} + \vartheta)^2 - 4[B_T]\vartheta)^{0.5}) \quad (6.52)$$

where $[B_T]$ and $[B_{Ab}]$ refer to the total antagonist concentration and antagonist bound to the antibody respectively, ϑ refers to the concentration of antibody and K_{B-Ab} the dissociation constant for the antagonist-antibody complex. Response to the agonist [A] is then calculated from:

$$Response = \frac{([A]/K_A)\tau_A E_m}{([A]/K_A(1 + \tau_A) + ([B_{free}])/K_B) + 1} \quad (6.53)$$

where K_A and K_B refer to the equilibrium dissociation constants of the agonist and antagonist receptor complexes respectively and E_m the maximal response of the system. Figure 6.32B shows the antagonism to the antagonist in the form of a Schild regression. It can be seen that the presence of the antibody reduces the potency of the antagonist and that the slope is minimally affected; the regressions are shifted to the right with increasing concentrations of antibody.

Another possibility is that the antibody binds the antagonist irreversibly, and thus precludes all interaction with the receptor; i.e., there is no competition between the antagonist, antibody, and the receptor. Under these circumstances, the concentration of free antagonist is given by:

$$[B_{free}] = \frac{([B_T]^2 + [B_T])K_{B-Ab} - [B_T]\vartheta}{[B_T] + K_{B-Ab}} \quad (6.54)$$

The response is then calculated by substituting for $[B_{free}]$ into Equation 6.53. The antagonism is similar to that seen in the previous simulation (see Figure 6.32B), except the relationship between antagonist potency and antibody concentration differs considerably. This is reflected in the curvilinear effects on the Schild regressions to the antagonist (see Figure 6.32C).

FIGURE 6.31 Irreversible chemical antagonism. (A) Apparent Schild regressions to the antibody as it blocks agonist response. Two extremes are shown: I (filled circles) is the Schild regression in a system of high agonist receptor reserve (τ for agonist=1000). Other systems shown are $\tau=100$ (10% of the receptors shown in I, open circles), $\tau=10$ (1 % receptors, filled triangles) and system II ($\tau=1$, 0.1% receptors, open triangles). (B) Effect of the antibody on concentration-response curves to the agonist in a high sensitivity system ($\tau=1000$). (C) Effect of the antibody on concentration-response curves to the agonist in a low sensitivity system ($\tau=1$). It should be noted that changes in the sensitivity to the agonist need not be solely due to differences in receptor density but rather can also be due to differences in the efficiency of receptor coupling.

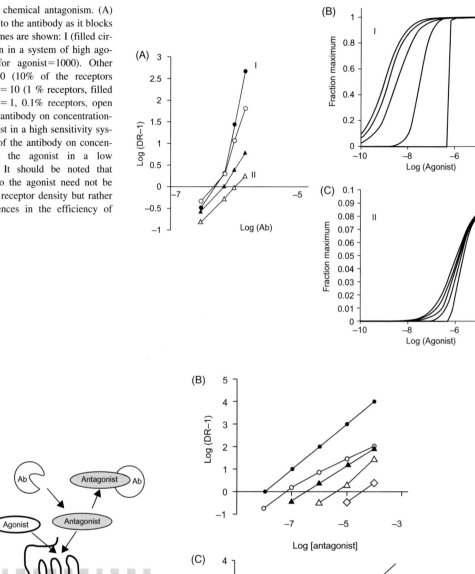

FIGURE 6.32 Chemical abstraction of an antagonist by another species (i.e. antibody). A. Response to an agonist A is blocked by a competitive antagonist B but this antagonist also may be bound to a species (i.e. in this case, antibody) that renders it unable to interact with the receptor an block agonist response. B. Reversible binding of the antagonist to the antibody. Binding of the antagonist to the antibody causes the Schild regression to the antagonist to be shifted to the right along the antagonist concentration axis. Schild regressions for the antagonist the in absence (filled circles) and presence of a range of concentrations of antibody; 1 mM (open circles), 10 mM (filled triangles), 100 mM (open triangles) and 1 mM (open diamonds). It is assumed that the equilibrium dissociation of the antagonist for the receptor (KB) is 10 nM and for the antibody complex (KB-Ab) is 1 mM. C. Irreversible binding of the antagonist to the antibody. Schild regressions for the antagonist in the absence (filled circles) and presence of various concentrations of antibody: 0.3 mM (open circles), 1 mM (filled triangles), 2 mM (open triangles) and 5 mM (open diamonds). It is assumed that the equilibrium dissociation of the antagonist for the receptor (KB) is 10 nM and for the antibody (KB-Ab) is 1 mM.

6.11 CHAPTER SUMMARY AND CONCLUSIONS

- Molecules that retard the ability of agonists to initiate biological signals are called *antagonists.*
- Two general molecular modes of antagonism are orthosteric (where the agonist and antagonist compete for the same binding site on the protein) and allosteric (where there are separate binding sites on the receptor for both the agonist and the antagonist and the effects of the antagonist are transmitted through the protein).
- These different molecular mechanisms for antagonism can produce varying effects on agonist dose-response curves ranging from shifts to the right with no diminution of the maxima (surmountable antagonism) to depression of the maximal response (insurmountable antagonism) with or without a shift of the curve.
- The kinetics of offset of the antagonist from the receptor can dictate whether surmountable or insurmountable antagonism is observed.
- The most common method used to measure the affinity of surmountable competitive antagonists is Schild analysis. This method is visual and also useful to detect non-equilibrium steady states in receptor preparations.
- The method of Lew and Angus allows the advantage of nonlinear fitting techniques to yield competitive antagonist pK_B values.
- The same principles (Schild analysis) can be applied to competitive antagonists that demonstrate either positive (partial agonists) or negative (inverse agonists) effect.
- In systems where there is insufficient time for the agonist, antagonist, and receptor to equilibrate according to mass action, slow offset antagonists can produce essentially irreversible occlusion of a portion of the receptor population. This can result in insurmountable antagonism.
- The degree of depression of the maximal response to agonists with slow offset pseudo-irreversible antagonists is inversely proportional to the efficacy of agonist and receptor density (i.e., agonists in systems with high receptor reserve are resistant to depression of maximal response by antagonists).
- In some systems with truncated response observation times and utilizing slow-acting antagonists, a depression of the maximal response can be observed that is due to the kinetics of offset of the molecules and not a molecular mechanism of antagonism (hemi-equilibrium conditions).
- A method called *resultant analysis* can be used to measure the receptor blockade produced by an antagonist with secondary properties.

6.12 DERIVATIONS

- Derivation of the Gaddum equation for competitive antagonism (6.12.1).
- Derivation of the Gaddum equation for noncompetitive antagonism (6.12.2).
- Derivation of the Schild equation (6.12.3).
- Functional effects of an inverse agonist with the operational model (6.12.4).
- pA_2 measurement for inverse agonists (6.12.5).
- Functional effects of a partial agonist with the operational model (6.12.6).
- pA_2 measurements for partial agonists (6.12.7).
- Method of Stephenson for partial agonist affinity measurement (6.12.8).
- Derivation of the method of Gaddum for noncompetitive antagonism (6.12.9).
- Relationship of pA_2 and pK_B for insurmountable orthosteric antagonism (6.12.10).
- Resultant analysis (6.12.11).
- Blockade of indirectly acting agonists (6.12.12).
- Chemical antagonism: abstraction of agonist concentration (6.12.13).
- Chemical antagonism: abstraction of antagonist concentration (6.12.14).

6.12.1 Derivation of the Gaddum Equation for Competitive Antagonism

Analogous to competitive displacement binding, agonist [A] and antagonist [B] compete for receptor (R) occupancy:

$$A \; + \; R \; \underset{K_b}{\overset{K_a}{\rightleftharpoons}} \; AR \tag{6.55}$$

where K_a and K_b are the respective ligand-receptor association constants. The following equilibrium constants are defined:

$$[R] = \frac{[AR]}{[A]K_a} \tag{6.56}$$

$$[BR] = K_b[B][R] = \frac{K_b[B][AR]}{[A]K_a} \tag{6.57}$$

Total Receptor Concentration $[R_{tot}] = [R] + [AR] + [BR]$ (6.58)

These lead to the expression for the response-producing species $[AR]/[R_{tot}]$ (denoted as ρ):

$$\rho = \frac{[A]K_a}{[A]K_a + [B]K_b + 1} \qquad (6.59)$$

Converting to equilibrium dissociation constants ($K_A = 1/K_a$) leads to the Gaddum equation [4]:

$$\rho = \frac{[A]/K_A}{[A]/K_A + [B]/K_B + 1} \qquad (6.60)$$

6.12.2 Derivation of the Gaddum Equation for Noncompetitive Antagonism

The receptor occupancy by the agonist is given by mass action:

$$\rho_A = \frac{[A]/K_A}{[A]/K_A + 1} \qquad (6.61)$$

It is also assumed that the antagonist produces an essentially irreversible blockade of receptors, such that the agonist can activate only the fraction of receptors not bound by the antagonist. If the fractional receptor occupancy by the antagonist is given by ρ_B, then the agonist-receptor occupancy in the presence of the antagonist is given by:

$$\rho_A = \frac{[A]/K_A}{[A]/K_A + 1}(1 - \rho_B) \qquad (6.62)$$

Defining ρ_B as $[B]/([B] + K_B)$, substituting this into Equation 6.60, and rearranging yields:

$$\rho_A = \frac{[A]/K_A}{[A]/K_A(1 + [B]/K_B) + [B]/K_B + 1} \qquad (6.63)$$

6.12.3 Derivation of the Schild Equation

In the presence of a competitive antagonist, the response-producing species ($[AR]/[R_{tot}] = \rho'$) is given by the Gaddum equation as:

$$\rho' = \frac{[A']/K_A}{[A']/K_A + [B]/K_B + 1} \qquad (6.64)$$

In the absence of antagonist ($[B] = 0$):

$$\rho = \frac{[A]/K_A}{[A]/K_A + 1} \qquad (6.65)$$

For equal responses ($\rho' = \rho;$):

$$\frac{[A']/K_A}{[A']/K_A + [B]/K_B + 1} = \frac{[A]/KA}{[A]/KA + 1} \qquad (6.66)$$

Defining $[A']/[A]$ as DR (the ratio of equiactive doses), and rearranging yields:

$$DR - 1 = \frac{[B]}{K_B} \qquad (6.67)$$

The logarithmic metameter of this is the Schild equation:

$$Log(DR - 1) = Log[B] - Log K_B \qquad (6.68)$$

In terms of the operational model, the equation corresponding to Equation 6.58 is:

$$\rho = \frac{[A]\tau}{[A]/K_A(1 + \tau) + 1} \qquad (6.69)$$

where τ = the receptor concentration divided by the coupling constant for tissue-agonist response production (see Chapter 3) ($\tau = [R_t]/K_E$). The counterpart to Equation 6.67 is:

$$\rho' = \frac{[A']\tau}{[A']/K_A(1 + \tau) + [B]/K_B + 1} \qquad (6.70)$$

Rearrangement of these equations leads to the Schild equation (Equation 6.66) as well.

6.12.4 Functional Effects of an Inverse Agonist with the Operational Model

$$
\begin{array}{ccccc}
BR^*E & & R^*E & & AR^*E \\
\mbig| K_e & & \big| K_e & & \big| K_e \\
BR^* & \xrightarrow{\beta K_b} & R^* & \xrightarrow{\alpha K_a} & AR^* \\
\big| \beta L & & \big| L & & \big| \alpha L \\
BR & \xrightarrow{K_b} & R & \xrightarrow{K_a} & AR
\end{array} \qquad (6.71)
$$

Equilibrium equations:

$$K_a = [AR]/[A][R] \qquad (6.72)$$

$$K_b = [BR]/[B][R] \qquad (6.73)$$

$$\alpha K_a = [AR^*]/[A][R^*] \qquad (6.74)$$

$$\beta K_b = [BR^*]/[B][R^*] \qquad (6.75)$$

$$L = [R^*]/[R] \qquad (6.76)$$

$$\alpha L = [AR^*]/[AR] \qquad (6.77)$$

$$\beta L = [BR^*]/[BR] \qquad (6.78)$$

Let $K_A = 1/K_a$, $K_B = 1/K_b$, $K_E = 1/K_e$. Thus,

$$\rho_{RESP} = \frac{[AR^*] + [BR^*] + [R^*]}{[AR^*] + [BR^*] + [R^*] + [AR] + [BR] + [R]}, \qquad (6.79)$$

$$= \frac{\alpha L[A]/K_A + \beta L[B]/K_B + L}{[A]/K_A(1 + \alpha L) + [B]/K_B(1 + \beta L) + [B]/K_B + 1}, \qquad (6.80)$$

$$\text{Response} = \frac{\rho_{RESP}[R_t]}{\rho_{RESP}[R_t] + K_E} = \frac{\rho_{RESP}\tau}{\rho_{RESP}\tau + 1}, \text{ and} \quad (6.81)$$

Response =

$$\frac{\alpha L[A]/K_A\tau + \beta L[B]/K_B\tau + L\tau}{[A]/K_A(1 + \alpha L(1 + \tau)) + [B]/K_B(1 + \beta L(1 + \tau)) + L(\tau + 1) + 1} \quad (6.82)$$

6.12.5 pA$_2$ Measurement for Inverse Agonists

The pA$_2$ calculation is derived by equating the response produced by the full agonist in the absence of the inverse agonist (Equation 6.79 with [B] = 0) to the response in the presence of a concentration of the inverse agonist that produces a dose ratio of 2 (by definition the pA$_2$). For calculation of K$_B$ from 10^{-pA_2}:

$$\frac{2\alpha L[A]/K_A\tau + \beta L[10^{-pA_2}]/K_B\tau + L\tau}{\begin{array}{c}2[A]/K_A(1 + \alpha L(1 + \tau)) + [10^{-pA_2}]/K_B(1 + \beta L(1 + \tau)) \\ + L(\tau + 1) + 1\end{array}} \quad (6.83)$$

$$= \frac{\alpha L[A]/K_A\tau + L\tau}{[A]/K_A(1 + \alpha L(1 + \tau)) + L(\tau + 1) + 1} \quad (6.84)$$

which leads to:

$$10^{-pA_2} = K_B \times \frac{([A]/K_A\tau(\alpha - 1))}{[A]/K_A(\alpha - 1) + (1 - \beta)} \quad (6.85)$$

It can be seen from Equation 6.84 that for a neutral antagonist ($\beta = 1$) the correction term reduces to unity. Therefore, as expected, $10^{-pA_2} = K_B$. The negative logarithmic metameter of Equation 6.84 yields the expression for the pA$_2$:

$$pA_2 = pK_B - \log([A](\alpha - 1)/([A](\alpha - 1) + (1 - \beta))) \quad (6.86)$$

6.12.6 Functional Effects of a Partial Agonist with the Operational Model

$$\begin{array}{c}
\text{B} \\
+ \\
\text{A} + \text{R} \xrightleftharpoons{K_a} \text{AR} \\
\big\updownarrow K_b \quad\quad + \\
\text{BR} + \text{E} \xrightleftharpoons{K'_e} \text{BRE} \\
\big\updownarrow K_e \quad\quad \big\downarrow \\
\text{ARE} \longrightarrow \text{RESPONSE}
\end{array} \quad (6.87)$$

Equilibrium equations:

$$K_a = [AR]/[A][R] \quad (6.88)$$

$$K_e = [ARE]/[AR][E] \quad (6.89)$$

$$K_b = [BR]/[B][R] \quad (6.90)$$

$$K'_e = [BRE]/[BR][E] \quad (6.91)$$

Let $K_A = 1/K_a$, $K_B = 1/K_b$, $K_E = 1/K_e$, and $K_E' = 1/K'$. Thus,

$$\rho_A = \frac{[A]/K_A}{[A]/K_A + [B]/K_B + 1} \quad (6.92)$$

$$\rho_B = \frac{[B]/K_B}{[A]/K_A + [B]/K_B + 1} \quad (6.93)$$

$$\text{Response} = \frac{[ARE] + [BRE]}{[ARE] + [BRE] + 1} = \frac{[AR]/K_E + [BR]/K'_E}{[AR]/K_E + [BR]/K'_E + 1}$$

$$= \frac{\rho_A[R_t]/K_E + \rho_B[R_t]/K'_E}{\rho_A[R_t]/K_E + \rho_B[R_t]/K'_E + 1} \quad (6.94)$$

Let $\tau = [R_t]/K_E$ and $\tau' = [R_t]/K'_E$:

$$\text{Response} = \frac{[A]/K_A\tau + [B]/K_B\tau}{[A]/K_A(1 + \tau) + [B]/K_B(1 + \tau') + 1} \quad (6.95)$$

6.12.7 pA$_2$ Measurements for Partial Agonists

As with Section 6.12.5 (inverse agonists), the pA$_2$ is derived by equating the response produced by the full agonist in the absence of the partial agonist (Equation 6.92 with [B] = 0) to the response in the presence of a concentration of the partial agonist that produces a dose ratio of 2 (by definition, the pA$_2$). For calculation of K$_B$ from 10^{-pA2}:

$$\frac{2[A]/K_A\tau + [B]/K_B\tau}{2[A]/K_A(1 + \tau) + [B]/K_B(1 + \tau') + 1} = \frac{[A]/K_A\tau}{[A]/K_A(1 + \tau)} \quad (6.96)$$

which reduces to:

$$10^{-pA_2} = \frac{K_B[A]/K_A(\tau/\tau')}{[A]/K_A(\tau/\tau' - 1)} \quad (6.97)$$

which further results in:

$$pA_2 = pK_B - \text{Log}(\tau/(\tau - \tau')) \quad (6.98)$$

6.12.8 Method of Stephenson for Partial Agonist Affinity Measurement

In terms of the operational model, the response produced by an agonist [A'] obtained in the presence of a concentration of partial agonist [P] is given by [14]

$$Response_{ap} = \frac{E_{max}[A']\tau_a}{[A'](1+\tau)+K_A(1+[P]/K_P)}$$
$$+ \frac{E_{max}[P]\tau_P}{[P](1+\tau_p)+K_P(1+[A']/K_A)} \quad (6.99)$$

where E_{max} is the maximal response of the system, K_A and K_p are the equilibrium dissociation constant of the full and partial agonist-receptor complexes, and τ_a and τ_p reflect the efficacies of the full and partial agonist. In the absence of the partial agonist, the response to the full agonist [A] is given by:

$$Response_{ap} = \frac{E_{max}[A]\tau_a}{[A](1+\tau_a)+K_A} \quad (6.100)$$

Comparing equiactive responses to the full agonist in the absence ([A]) and presence ([A']) of the partial agonist ($Response_{ap} = Response_a$) and rearranging yields:

$$[A] = \frac{[A']}{1+(1-(\tau_p/\tau_a))\cdot([P]/K_p)} + \frac{(\tau_p/\tau_a)\cdot([P]/K_p)\cdot K_A}{1+(1-(\tau_p/\tau_a))\cdot([P]/K_p)} \quad (6.101)$$

This is an equation for a straight line with slope:

$$Slope = (1+(1-(\tau_p/\tau_a))\cdot([P]/K_p))^{-1} \quad (6.102)$$

Rearranging,

$$K_p = \frac{[P]slope}{1-slope}\cdot(1-(\tau_p/\tau_a)) \quad (6.103)$$

From Equation 6.102 it can be shown that, for a range of concentrations of [P] yielding a range of slopes according to regressions of equiactive agonist concentrations, K_P can be estimated from the following regression [9]:

$$Log\left(\frac{1}{slope}-1\right) = Log[P]-LogK_p \quad (6.104)$$

6.12.9 Derivation of the Method of Gaddum for Noncompetitive Antagonism

In this model, it is assumed that the noncompetitive antagonist reduces the fraction of available receptor population. Therefore, equating stimuli in the absence and presence of noncompetitive antagonist:

$$\frac{[A]\tau}{[A](1+\tau)+K_A} = \frac{[A']\tau'}{[A'](1+\tau')+K_A} \quad (6.105)$$

The receptor population is reduced by a fraction ρ upon antagonist binding. Therefore, $[R_t'] = (1-\rho)[R_t]$, resulting in $\tau' = \tau(1-\rho)$. Rearrangement of the equation:

$$Response = \frac{[A']\tau(1-\rho)E_{max}}{[A'](1+\tau(1-\rho))+K_A} \quad (6.106)$$

Substitution for ρ in terms of the receptor occupancy by the antagonist ($\rho = [B]/K_B/([B]/K_B+1)$) results in:

$$Response = \frac{[A']/K_A\tau E_{max}}{[A]/K_A(1+\tau+[B]/K_B)+[B]/K_B+1} \quad (6.107)$$

For equiactive responses,

$$\frac{[A']/K_A\tau E_{max}}{[A']/K_A(1+\tau+[B]/K_B)+[B]/K_B+1} = \frac{[A]/K_A\tau E_{max}}{[A']/K_A(1+\tau)+1} \quad (6.108)$$

Rearrangement of the equation yields:

$$1/[A] = 1/[A']((([B]/K_B)+1)+[B]/(K_BK_A) \quad (6.109)$$

Therefore, a double reciprocal plot of equiactive agonist concentrations in the presence ($1/[A']$ as abscissae) and absence ($1/[A]$ as ordinates) of the antagonist should yield a straight line. The equilibrium dissociation constant of the antagonist is calculated from:

$$K_B = [B]/(slope-1) \quad (6.110)$$

6.12.10 Relationship of pA$_2$ and pK$_B$ for Insurmountable Orthosteric Antagonism

It is useful to describe agonist response in the presence of any antagonist as:

$$Response = \frac{\rho_A(1-\rho_B)\tau E_{max}}{\rho_A(1-\rho_B)\tau+1} \quad (6.111)$$

where ρ_A and ρ_B are the agonist and antagonist fractional receptor occupancies, respectively. For simple competitive antagonism, ρ_B is given by $[B]/K_B/([B]/K_B+[A]/K_A+1)$ to yield the well-known Gaddum equation for simple competitive antagonism for agonist-receptor occupancy in the presence of the antagonist (denoted ρ_{AB}) ($[A]/K_A/([A]/K_A+[B]/K_A+1)$). This yields:

$$Response = \frac{[A]/K_A\tau E_{max}}{[A]/K_A(1+\tau)+[B]/K_B+1}. \quad (6.112)$$

The relationship between equiactive agonist concentrations in the absence and presence of antagonist to yield a dose ratio of 2 ($[B] = 10^{-pA2}$) is then calculated by equating:

$$\frac{2[A]/K_A\tau E_{max}}{2[A]/K_A(1+\tau) + [10^{-pA_2}]/K_B + 1} = \frac{[A]/K_A\tau E_{max}}{[A]/K_A(1+\tau) + 1}$$

(6.113)

Simplifying this yields:

$$10^{-pA_2} = K_B,$$ (6.114)

as predicted by the Schild equation (i.e., $pA_2 = pK_B$) of unit slope.

An analogous procedure can equate the empirical pA_2 to pK_B for noncompetitive antagonists. Utilizing the equation for agonist response in the presence of a non-competitive antagonist (Equation 6.10), equiactive concentrations with a dose ratio of 2 in the presence and absence of antagonist are given by:

$$\frac{2[A]/K_A\tau E_{max}}{2[A]/K_A(1 + \tau + [10^{-pA_2}])/K_B + [10^{-pA_2}]/K_B + 1}$$
$$= \frac{[A]/K_A\tau E_{max}}{[A]/K_A(1+\tau) + 1}$$

(6.115)

Simplification of this relationship yields an equation relating pA_2 and K_B:

$$10^{-pA_2} = K_B/(1 + 2[A]/K_A)$$ (6.116)

$$pK_B = pA_2 - Log(1 + 2[A]/K_A)$$ (6.117)

6.12.11 Resultant Analysis

The receptor occupancy for an agonist $[A]$ in the presence of a test antagonist $[B_{test}]$ is given as:

$$\rho = \frac{[A]}{[A] + K_A(1 + [B_{test}]/K_{B\,test})}$$ (6.118)

Similarly, receptor occupancy equal to the previous occupancy (agonist concentration $[A']$) in the presence of the test antagonist and a reference antagonist $[B']$ is given as:

$$\rho' = \frac{[A']}{[A] + K_A(1 + [B']/K_B + [B_{test}]/K_{B\,test})}$$ (6.119)

If equal responses to the agonist under these two conditions (leading to equal receptor occupancies for the same agonist, $\rho = \rho'$) are compared, then equating Equations 6.117 and 6.118 and rearranging yields:

$$\frac{[A]}{[A]} = r' = 1 + \frac{[B']}{K_B} \cdot \left[1 + \frac{[B_{test}]}{K_{B\,test}}\right]$$ (6.120)

where r' is the dose ratio for the agonist. A dose ratio r for antagonism by the reference antagonist is defined in the absence of the test antagonist ($[B_{test}] = 0$):

$$r = 1[B]/K_B$$ (6.121)

Schild plots for the test antagonist alone and the test antagonist plus a range of concentrations of reference antagonist are obtained. Equieffective dose ratios are compared. Therefore, the ratio of the dose ratio produced by both the test and reference antagonist (r') is equated to the dose ratio for the reference antagonist alone (r). Equating Equation 6.119 to Equation 6.120 and simplifying yields:

$$1 + [B]/K_B = 1 + [B']/K_B(1 + [B_{test}]/K_{B\,test})$$ (6.122)

A term κ is derived, which is $[B]/[B']$; specifically, the ratio of reference antagonist concentrations giving equal log ($DR - 1$) values (the shift, along the antagonist axis, of the Schild regressions) in the presence of various concentrations of test antagonist. This yields the resultant plot:

$$Log(\kappa - 1) = Log([B_{test}]) - LogK_{B\,test}$$ (6.123)

6.12.12 Blockade of Indirectly Acting Agonists

It is assumed that a mass action process leads to the release of an endogenous agonist ψ by:

$$[\text{Endogenous Agonist}] = \frac{[A]/K_A\theta}{[A]/K_A + 1} = [\psi]$$ (6.124)

Where θ is the size of releasable pool and K_A is the dissociation constant of the indirect agonist ($[A]$) and site of release. The fractional receptor occupancy by the released endogenous agonist in the presence of a competitive antagonist ($[B]$) is given as:

$$\text{Fractional Effect}_{AB} = \frac{[\psi]K_E}{[\psi]/K_E + [B]/K_B + 1}$$ (6.125)

where K_B is the equilibrium dissocation constant of the antagonist-receptor complex. Substituting for $[\psi]$ from Equation 6.124 yields:

Fractional Effect$_{AB}$ =

$$\frac{[A]/K_A[\theta]/K_E}{[A]/K_A([\theta]K_E + [B]/K_B + 1) + [B]/K_B + 1}$$ (6.126)

6.12.13 Chemical Antagonism: Abstraction of Agonist Concentration

For reversible kinetics of an antibody binding to the agonist, it is assumed that only free agonist ($[A_{free}]$) binds to the receptor to produce the response:

$$[A_{free}] = [A_T] - [A_{Ab}] \qquad (6.127)$$

where $[A_T]$ and $[A_{Ab}]$ refer to the total concentration of agonist and concentration bound to the antibody respectively.

Considering the amount of agonist bound to the antibody as:

$$[A_{Ab}] = \frac{([A_T] - [A_{Ab}])\zeta}{([A_T] - [A_{Ab}] + K_B)} \qquad (6.128)$$

where ζ is the concentration of antibody. This leads to:

$$[A_{Ab}]2 - [A_{Ab}](\zeta + [A_T] + K_B) + [AT]\zeta = 0 \qquad (6.129)$$

One solution for which is:

$$[A_{Ab}] = \tfrac{1}{2}([A_T] + K_B + \zeta - (([A_T]+K_B+\zeta)^2 4[A_T]\zeta)^{0.5}) \qquad (6.130)$$

From 6.126:

$$[A_{free}] = [A_T] - [A_{Ab}] = \tfrac{1}{2}([A_T] + K_B + \zeta \\ - (([A_T]+K_B+\zeta)^{2-}4[A_T]\zeta)^{0.5}) \qquad (6.131)$$

Agonist response then is calculated with the Black-Leff operational model using $[A_{free}]$:

$$Response = \frac{[A_{free}]\tau E_m}{([A_{free}](\tau + 1) + K_A)} \qquad (6.132)$$

6.12.14 Chemical Antagonism: Abstraction of Antagonist Concentration

$$[B_{free}] = [B_T] - [B_{Ab}] \qquad (6.133)$$

where $[B_T]$ and $[B_{Ab}]$ refer to the total antagonist concentration and antagonist bound to the antibody respectively. The binding of the antagonist to the receptor is given by:

$$[B_{Ab}] = \frac{([B_T] - [B_{Ab}])\vartheta}{([B_T] - [B_{Ab}] + K_{B-Ab})} \qquad (6.134)$$

where ϑ refers to the concentration of antibody, and K_{B-Ab} is the dissociation constant for the antagonist-antibody complex.

This yields:

$$[B_{Ab}]^2 - [B_{Ab}](\vartheta + [B_T] + K_{B-Ab}) + [B_T]\vartheta = 0 \qquad (6.135)$$

One solution for which is:

$$[B_{Ab}] = \tfrac{1}{2}([B_T] + K_{B-Ab} + \vartheta - (([B_T]+K_{B-Ab}+\vartheta)^2 - 4[B_T]\vartheta)^{0.5}) \qquad (6.136)$$

From Equation 6.132;

$$[B_{free}] = [B_T] - [B_{Ab}] = \tfrac{1}{2}([B_T] + K_{B-Ab} + \vartheta \\ - (([B_T]+K_{B-Ab}+\vartheta)^2 - 4[B_T]\vartheta)^{0.5}) \qquad (6.137)$$

REFERENCES

[1] Paton WDM, Rang HP. The uptake of atropine and related drugs by intestinal smooth muscle of the guinea pig in relation to acetylcholine receptors. Proc R Soc Lond [Biol] 1965;163:1–44.

[2] Gaddum JH. The quantitative effects of antagonistic drugs. J Physiol Lond 1937;89:7Pe.

[3] Gaddum JH, Hameed KA, Hathway DE, Stephens FF. Quantitative studies of antagonists for 5-hydroxytryptamine. Q J Exp Physiol 1955;40:49–74.

[4] Arunlakshana O, Schild HO. Some quantitative uses of drug antagonists. Br J Pharmacol 1959;14:48–58.

[5] Kenakin TP, Boselli C. Pharmacologic discrimination between receptor heterogeneity and allosteric interaction: resultant analysis of gallamine and pirenzeipine antagonism of muscarinic responses in rat trachea. J Pharmacol Exp Ther 1989;250:944–52.

[6] Kenakin TP. The Schild regression in the process of receptor classification. Can J Physiol Pharmacol 1982;60:249–65.

[7] Stephenson RP. A modification of receptor theory. Br J Pharmacol 1956;11:379–93.

[8] Kaumann AJ, Marano M. On equilibrium dissociation constants for complexes of drug receptor subtypes: selective and nonselective interactions of partial agonists with two β-adrenoceptor subtypes mediating positive chronotropic effects of (−)isoprenaline in kitten atria. Naunyn Schmiedebeberg's Arch Pharmacol 1982;219:216–21.

[9] Kenakin TP, Black JW. The pharmacological classification of practolol and choropractolol. Mol Pharmacol 1978;14:607–23.

[10] Stone M, Angus JA. Developments of computer-based estimation of pA$_2$ values and associated analysis. J Pharmacol Exp Ther 1978;207:705–18.

[11] Lew MJ, Angus JA. Analysis of competitive agonist-antagonist interactions by nonlinear regression. Trends Pharmacol Sci 1996;16:328–37.

[12] Black JW, Gerskowich VP, Leff P. Analysis of competitive antagonism when this property occurs as part of a pharmacological resultant. Br. J. Pharmacol 1986;89:547–55.

[13] Black JW, Jenkinson DH, Kenakin TP. Antagonism of an indirectly acting agonist: block by propranolol abd sotalol of the action of tyramine on rat heart. Eur J Pharmacol 1980;65:1–10.

[14] Leff P, Dougall IG, Harper D. Estimation of partial agonist affinity by interaction with a full agonist: a direct operational model-fit approach. Br J Pharmacol 1993;110:239–44.

Chapter 7

Allosteric Modulation

When one tugs at a single thing in nature, he finds it attached to the rest of the world.

— John Muir

Whatever affects one directly, affects all indirectly… This is the interrelated structure of reality.

— Martin Luther King Jr.

7.1	Introduction	7.3	Unique Effects of Allosteric Modulators	7.5	Methods for Detecting Allosterism
7.2	The Nature of Receptor Allosterism	7.4	Functional Study of Allosteric Modulators	7.6	Chapter Summary and Conclusions
				7.7	Derivations
					References

7.1 INTRODUCTION

A major molecular mechanism of receptor interaction involves the binding of a molecule to its own site on the receptor, which is separate from the binding site of the endogenous agonist. When this occurs, the interaction between the agonist and the molecule takes place via the receptor protein. This is referred to as an *allosteric interaction* (for a schematic diagram, see Figure 6.2) and the molecules with this mode of action are referred to as allosteric modulators. Thus, an allosteric modulator produces a conformational change in the shape of the receptor, which in turn changes the affinity or efficacy of the receptor for the agonist and/or changes the receptor function.

Allosteric modulators produce saturable effects (i.e., a maximum effect is produced, after which further increases in modulator concentration have no further effect). This is because the allosteric effect is linked to occupancy of the allosteric site, and this saturates with complete occupancy of that site. Operational effects on dose-response curves do not always unambiguously indicate a molecular mechanism, in that experiments can reveal combinations of compatible operational and mechanistic classifications (i.e., an allosteric molecular mechanism can produce either surmountable or insurmountable effects on dose-response curves depending on the system). Also, since allosteric effects produce a change in shape of the receptor, it cannot be assumed *a priori* that a uniform modulatory effect on agonism will result.

In fact, it will be seen that some allosteric ligands produce antagonism of the binding of some ligands and an increase in the affinity of the receptor for other ligands (note the stimulation of the binding of [³H]-atropine by alcuronium in Figure 4.12). In addition, the effect of an allosteric ligand on a receptor probe (this can be an agonist or radioligand) is dependent on the nature of the probe (i.e., a conformational change that increases the affinity of the receptor for one agonist may decrease it for another). For example, while the allosteric ligand alcuronium produces a 10-fold change in the affinity of the muscarinic m2 receptor for acetylcholine, it produces only a 1.7-fold change in the affinity for arecoline [1]. These effects make consistent nomenclature for allosteric ligands difficult and for this reason modulation in this sense means modification, either in a positive or negative direction.

7.2 THE NATURE OF RECEPTOR ALLOSTERISM

The word *allosteric* comes from the Greek *allos*, meaning different, and *steric*, which refers to arrangement of

T. P. Kenakin: A Pharmacology Primer, Fourth edition. DOI: http://dx.doi.org/10.1016/B978-0-12-407663-1.00007-7
© 2014 Elsevier Inc. All rights reserved.

atoms in space. As a word, *allostery* literally means a change in shape. Specifically in the case of allosterism of proteins, the change in shape is detected by its interaction with a probe. Therefore, there can be no steric interference at this probe site. In fact, allosteric effects are defined by the interaction of an allosteric modulator at a so-called allosteric binding site on the protein to affect the conformation at the probe site of the protein. Since the probe and modulator molecules do not interact directly, their influence on each other must take place through a change in shape of the protein. Historically, allosteric effects have been studied and described for enzymes. Early discussions of allosteric enzyme effects centered on the geography of substrate and modulator binding. Koshland [2], a pioneer of allosteric enzyme research, classified the binding geography of enzymes in terms of "contact amino acids" and intimate parts of the active site for substrate binding, and "contributing amino acids," those important for preservation of the tertiary structure of the active site but which did not play a role in substrate binding. Finally, he defined "noncontributing amino acids" as those not essential for enzyme catalysis but perhaps serving a structural role in the enzyme. Within Koshland's hypothesis, binding to these latter two categories of amino acids constituted a mechanism of allosterism rather than pure endogenous ligand competition. Within this context, pharmacological antagonists can bind to sites distinct from those utilized by the endogenous agonist (i.e., hormone, neurotransmitter) to alter binding and subsequent tissue response (Figure 7.1). Some of these differences in binding loci can be discerned through point mutation of receptors. For example, differences in amino acids required for competitive antagonist binding and allosteric effector binding can be seen in mutant muscarinic m1 receptors where substitution of an aspartate residue at position 71, but not at positions 99 and 122, affects the affinity of the allosteric modulator gallamine but not the affinity of the competitive antagonist radiolabeled [^{3}H]-N-methylscopolamine [3].

Allosteric sites can be remote from the enzyme's active site. For example, the binding site for nevirapine, an allosteric modulator of HIV reverse transcriptase, is 10 angstroms away from the enzyme's active site [4]. Similarly, allosteric inhibition of β-lactamase occurs 16 angstroms away from the active site [5]. The binding site for CP320626 for glycogen phosphorylase b is 33 angstroms from the catalytic site and 15 angstroms from the site for cyclic AMP [6]. A visual demonstration of the relative geography of allosteric binding and receptor active sites can be seen in Figure 7.2. Here, the integrin LFA1, which binds to molecules on other cell membranes to mediate cell adhesion, has a receptor probe active site binding the intercellular adhesion molecule-1 (ICAM-1), and an allosteric binding site for the drug

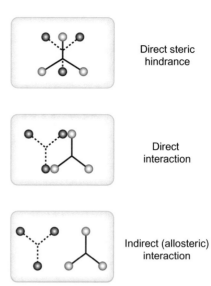

FIGURE 7.1 Enzyme ortho- and allosterism as presented by Koshland [2]. Steric hindrance whereby the competing molecules physically interfered with each other as they bound to the substrate site was differentiated from a direct interaction where only portions of the competing molecules interfered with each other. If no direct physical interaction between the molecules occurred, then the effects were solely due to effects transmitted through the protein structure (allosteric).

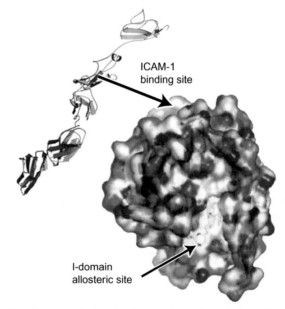

FIGURE 7.2 Model of LFA-1 showing the binding domain of ICAM-1 (the endogenous ligand for this protein) and the binding site for lovastatin, an allosteric modulator for this protein. Redrawn from [7].

lovastatin in a deep hydrophobic cleft next to the α7 helix (see Figure 7.2) [7].

While visualization of the relative binding sites for receptor probes and allosteric modulators is conceptually helpful, preoccupation with the geography of ligand binding is needlessly confining since the actual binding sites involved are secondary to the mechanism of allosterism. As shown by the preceding examples, the modulator and probe binding sites need not be near each other for allosteric effects to occur (i.e., the binding of the modulator does not necessarily need to produce a deformation near the receptor probe site). In fact, there are data to suggest that the relative geometry of binding is immaterial, except for the fact that the receptor probe and modulator must bind to exclusively different sites.

Just as the location of allosteric sites is secondary to the consequences of allosteric effect, there is evidence to suggest that the structural requirements of allosteric sites may be somewhat more permissive with respect to the chemical structures bound to them (i.e., the structure activity relationships for allosteric sites may be more relaxed due to the fact that allosteric proteins are more flexible than other proteins). For example, as shown in Figure 7.3A, structurally diverse molecules such as efavirenz, nevirapine, UC-781, and Cl-TIBO all bind to HIV reverse transcriptase [8]. Similarly, the HIV entry inhibitors Sch-C, Sch-D, UK427,857, aplaviroc, and TAK779 all demonstrate prohibitive binding (consistent with binding at the same site) for the CCR5 receptor (see Figure 7.3B [9]).

It is useful to think of allosteric binding, not in terms of deformation of the receptor active site, but rather as a lever to lock the receptor into a given conformation. As discussed in Chapter 1, receptors and other biologically relevant proteins are a dynamic system of interchanging conformations referred to as an *ensemble*. These various conformations are sampled according to the thermal energy of the system; in essence, the protein roams on a conceptual "energy landscape." While there are preferred low-energy conformations, the protein has the capacity to form a large number of conformations. An allosteric modulator may have a high affinity for some of these and thus bind to them preferentially when they are formed. Thus, by selectively binding to these conformations, the allosteric modulators stabilize them at the expense of other conformations. This creates a bias and a shift in the number of conformations toward the ligand-bound conformation (see Section 1.10 of Chapter 1, for further details).

The fact that the allosterically preferred conformation may be relatively rare in the library of conformations available to the receptor may have kinetic implications. Specifically, if the binding site for the modulator appears only when the preferred conformation is formed spontaneously, then complete conversion to allosterically modified receptors may require a relatively long period of equilibration. For example, the allosteric p38 MAP kinase inhibitor BIRB 796 binds to a conformation of MAP kinase requiring movement of a Phe residue by 10 angstroms (so-called "out" conformation). The association rate for this modulator is $8.5 \times 10^5 \, M^{-1} \, s^{-1}$, 50 times slower than that required for other inhibitors ($4.3 \times 10^7 \, M^{-1} \, s^{-1}$). The result is that while other inhibitors reach equilibrium

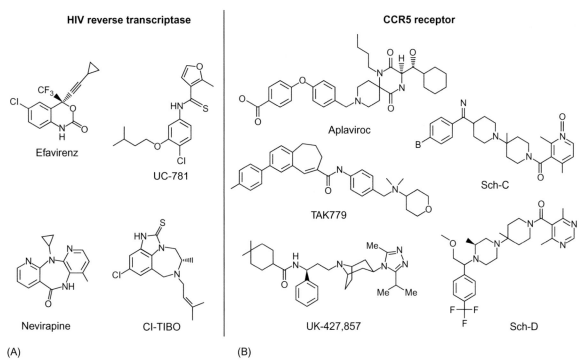

FIGURE 7.3 Diversity of structures that interact with the (A) HIV reverse transcriptase inhibitor binding site [8] and (B) the CCR5-receptor-mediating HIV-1 fusion [9].

within 30 minutes, BIRB 376 requires two full hours of equilibration time [10].

7.3 UNIQUE EFFECTS OF ALLOSTERIC MODULATORS

Orthosteric molecules (i.e., antagonists, partial agonists, inverse agonists) that preclude access of other molecules such as agonists to the receptor can be thought of as producing a preemptive type of system; i.e., there is a common maximal result for all such antagonists in the form of an inactivated (or in the case of partial agonists, a partially activated) receptor to *all* agonists. In contrast, allosteric molecules are *permissive* − allowing the interaction of the receptor protein with other molecules. The fact that allosteric effects are saturable (i.e., the effect ceases when the allosteric site is fully occupied) and that allosterism is permissive causes allosteric modulators to have a unique range of activities. These are:

a. Allosteric modulators have the potential to alter the interaction of very large proteins: The fact that global conformations of the receptor are stabilized by allosteric modulators has implications for their effects. Specifically, this opens the possibility of changes in multiple regions of the receptor instead of a single point change in conformation, and with this comes the possibility of changing multiple points of contact between the receptor and other proteins (see Figure 7.4). An example of the global nature of the conformational changes caused by allosteric interaction is evident from the interaction of CP320626 with glycogen phosphorylase b. In this case, the binding of this allosteric modulator causes the release

of 9 of 30 water molecules from a cavity capped by α-helices of the enzyme subunits [6]. Such global conformational effects means that small allosteric molecules can influence the interactions of large proteins. For example, HIV-1 entry is mediated by the interaction of the chemokine receptor CCR5 and the HIV viral coat protein gp120, both large (70 to 100 K Daltons) proteins. Analysis by point mutation indicates that all four extracellular loops of the receptor and multiple regions of gp120 associate for HIV fusion [10−13], yet small allosteric molecules such as aplaviroc and Sch-D (0.6% of their size) are able to block this interaction at nanomolar concentrations (see Figure 7.5). In general, the stabilization of receptor conformations by allosteric ligands makes possible the alteration of large protein-protein interactions, making this a potentially very powerful molecular mechanism of action.

b. Allosteric modulators have the potential to modulate but not completely activate and/or inhibit receptor function: One of the key properties of allosteric modulators is their saturability of effect. With this comes the capability to modulate but not necessarily completely block agonist-induced signals. This stems from the fact that while the allosterically modified receptor may have a diminished affinity and/or efficacy for the agonist, the agonist may still produce receptor activation in the presence of the modulator. This submaximal effect on ligand-receptor interaction is shown in Figure 4.10, where it is seen that the apparent displacement of bound ^{125}I-MIP-1α from the chemokine C receptor type 1 (CCR1) by the allosteric ligand UCB35625 is incomplete (i.e., the ^{125}I-MIP-1α still binds to the receptor but with a lower affinity). An orthosteric antagonist binding to the same

FIGURE 7.4 Schematic diagram of a GPCR in a native conformation (black) and allosterically altered conformation (red). When these are superimposed upon each other, it can be seen that more than one region of the receptor is altered upon allosteric modulation (see circled areas).

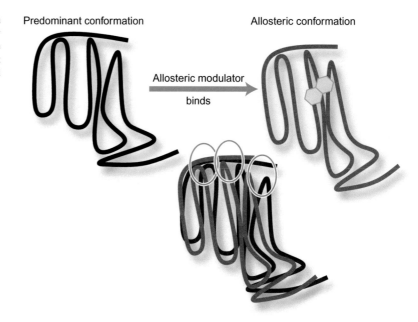

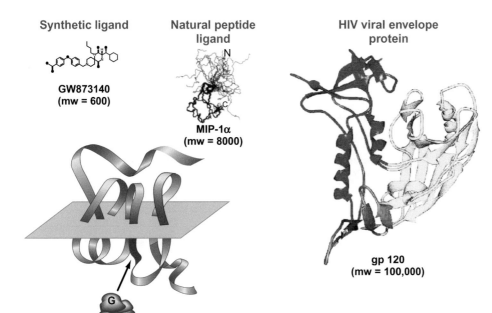

FIGURE 7.5 Cartoons showing the relative size of the CCR5 receptor, gp120 HIV viral coat protein, the natural ligand for the CCR5 receptor (the chemokine MIP-1α), and GW873140 (aplaviroc) [9], an allosteric modulator that blocks the interaction of CCR5 with both MIP-1α and gp120.

binding site as MIP-1α necessarily must completely reverse the binding of MIP-1α. In general, this leads to the possibility that allosteric modulators can modify (i.e., reduce or increase by a small amount) endogenous agonist signals without completely blocking them.

The saturability of the binding to the allosteric site also offers the potential to dissociate duration of effect from magnitude of effect. Since allosteric effects reach an asymptotic value upon saturation of the allosteric site, there is the potential to increase the duration of allosteric effect by loading the receptor compartment with large concentrations of modulator. These large concentrations will have no further effect other than to prolong the saturated allosteric response. For example, consider a system where the therapeutic goal is to produce a 10-fold shift to the right of the agonist dose-response curve. A concentration of an orthosteric simple competitive antagonist of $[B]/K_B = 10$ will achieve this, and the duration of this effect will be determined by the kinetics of washout of the antagonist from the receptor compartment and the concentration of antagonist. A longer duration of action of such a drug could be achieved by increasing the concentration, but this necessarily would increase the maximal effect as well (i.e., $[B]/K_B = 100$ would produce a 100-fold shift of the curve). In contrast, if an allosteric modulator with $\alpha = 0.1$ were to be employed, an increased concentration would increase the duration of effect but the antagonism would never be greater than 10-fold (as defined by the cooperativity factor α). Thus, the saturability of the allosteric ligand can be used to limit effect but increase the duration.

c. Allosteric modulators have the potential to preserve physiological patterns: The fact that allosteric modulators alter the signaling properties and/or sensitivity of the receptor to physiological signaling means that their effect is linked to the receptor signal. This being the case, allosteric modulators will augment or modulate function in a reflection of the existing pattern. This may be especially beneficial for complex signalling patterns such as those found in the brain. For this reason, the augmentation of the cholinergic system in Alzheimer's disease with cholinesterase inhibitors (these block the degradation of acetylcholine in the synapse and thus potentiate response in accordance with neural firing) has been one approach to treatment of this disease [14]. However, there are practical problems with this idea associated with nonspecific increase in both nicotinic and muscarinic receptor when only selective nicotinic function is required. This has opened the field for other strategies, such as selective allosteric potentiation of acetylcholine receptor function [15,16]. In general, as a theoretical approach, allosteric control of function allows preservation of patterns of innervation, blood flow, cellular receptor density, and efficiencies of receptor coupling for complex systems of physiological control in the brain and other organs.

d. Allosteric modulators may yield therapies with reduced side effects: In cases where augmentation of physiological effect is required (i.e., Alzheimer's disease), allosteric potentiation of effect would be expected to yield a lower side-effect profile. This is because modulators with this action would produce no direct effect, but rather produce actions only when the system is active through presence of the endogenous agonist.

e. Allosteric antagonists can produce texture in antagonism: Just as a given allosteric modulator can produce different effects on different receptor probes,

TABLE 7.1 The Effects of Different Allosteric Modulators on Common Agonists of Muscarinic Receptors

Receptor	Receptor Probe	Modulator	Effect[1]	Difference[2]
m3	Bethanechol	Strychnine	49 × potentiation	73 ×
		Brucine	0.67 × inhibition	
m2	P-TZTP[3]	Alcuronium	4.7 × potentiation	36 ×
		Brucine	0.13 × inhibition	
m2	Acetylcholine	Vincamine	18 × potentiation	31 ×
		Eburnamonine	0.32 × inhibition	

[1] α value for changes in potency.
[2] ratio of α values for the two modulators.
[3] 3-(3-pentylthio-1,2,5-thiadiazol-4-yl)-1,2,5,6-tetrahydro-1-methylpyridine. From [1].

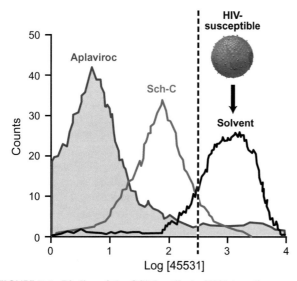

FIGURE 7.6 Binding of the CCR5 antibody 45531 to native receptor (peak labeled solvent) and in the presence of 1 µM Sch-C (blue line) and 1 µM aplaviroc (magenta peak). Different locations of the distributions show different binding sensitivities to the antibody indicative of different receptor conformations. Data courtesy of S. Sparks and J. Demarest, Dept of Clinical Virology, GlaxoSmithKline.

different modulators can produce different effects on the same modulator. For example, Table 7.1 shows the effects of different allosteric modulators on common agonists of muscarinic receptors. It can be seen from these data that different allosteric modulators have the ability to antagonize and potentiate muscarinic agonists, clearly indicative of the production of different allosteric conformational states. Similarly, the allosterically modified CCR5 receptor demonstrates heterogeneity with respect to sensitivity of antibody binding. In this case, antibodies such as 45531, binding to a specific region of the receptor, reveal different conformations stabilized by aplaviroc and Sch-C, two allosteric modulators of the receptor. This is shown by the different affinity profiles of the antibody in the presence of each modulator (see Figure 7.6). This also

has implications for the therapeutic use of such modulators. In the case of Sch-D and aplaviroc in Figure 7.6, the allosterically blocked receptors are similar in that they do not support HIV entry but quite dissimilar with respect to binding of the 45531 antibody. This latter fact indicates that the allosteric conformations produced by each modulator are not the same, and this could have physiological consequences. Specifically, it is known that HIV spontaneously mutates [17,18] and that the mutation in the viral coat protein can lead to resistance to CCR5-entry inhibitors. For example, passage of the virus in the continued presence of the CCR5 antagonist AD101 leads to an escape mutant able to gain cell entry through use of the allosterically modified receptor [19,20]. It would be postulated that production of a different conformation with another allosteric modulator would overcome viral resistance, since the modified virus would not be able to recognize the newly formed conformation of CCR5. Thus, the texture inherent in allosteric modification of receptors (different tertiary conformations of protein) offers a unique opportunity to defeat the accommodation of pathological processes to chronic drug treatment (in this case viral resistance).

f. Allosteric modulators can have separate effects on agonist affinity and efficacy: Allosteric modulators produce a new protein conformation, therefore the resulting effect on endogenous ligands need not be uniform; i.e., the changes need not be in the same direction (antagonism or potentiation). This opens the possibility that an allosteric modulator could change agonist efficacy in one direction and affinity in another. For example, the CCR5 allosteric modulator aplaviroc completely blocks CCL5-mediated agonism but only minimally affects the binding of the chemokine CCL5 to the receptor [21,22]. Thus while the steps leading to G-protein activation and subsequent cellular response are completely blocked, the high affinity binding of CCL5 is not greatly affected; i.e., aplaviroc has little effect on CCL5 affinity but a strong

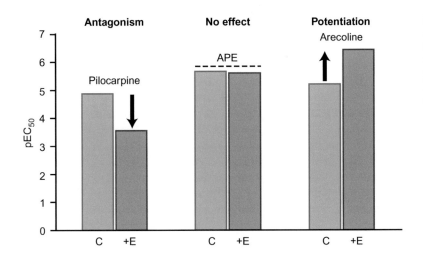

FIGURE 7.7 **Effect of the allosteric modulator eburnamonine on the affinity of muscarinic agonists on m2 receptors.** It can be seen that while no change in potency is observed for APE (arecaidine propargyl ester) pilocarpine is antagonized and arecoline is potentiated, illustrating the probe dependence of allosterism. From [1].

negative effect on CCL5 efficacy. A similar effect is seen with CPCCOEt (7-hydroxyiminocyclopropan[b]chromen-1a-carboxylic acid ethyl ester) which does not interfere with glutamate binding in CHO cells naturally expressing human GluR1b receptors, but completely blocks their responses to glutamate [23].

A useful combination of such effects is where an allosteric antagonist modulator decreases agonist efficacy but **increases** agonist affinity. The mechanism of this effect relates to the reciprocal nature of allosteric energy. Since the modulator increases the affinity of the agonist, the agonist will also increase the affinity of the modulator; this has been shown experimentally [24]. The profile of such a molecule would demonstrate increased antagonist potency with increased concentrations of agonist, i.e., the presence of higher agonist concentrations promotes higher affinity antagonist binding, and leads to more antagonism. This is observed with antagonists such as ifenprodil (for NMDA receptors [25]) and Org27569 (for cannabinoid receptors [26]).

g. Allosteric modulators may have an extraordinary selectivity for receptor types: Another discerning feature of allosterism is the potential for increased selectivity. Physiological binding sites for endogenous ligands (hormones, neurotransmitters) may be conserved between receptor subtypes, predicting that it would be difficult to attain selectivity through interaction at these sites. For example, it could be postulated that it would be difficult for orthosteric antagonists that bind to the acetylcholine recognition site of muscarinic receptors to be selective for muscarinic subtypes (i.e., teleologically these have all evolved to recognize acetylcholine). However, the same is not true for the surrounding scaffold protein of the acetylcholine receptor, and it is in these regions that the potential for selective stabilization of receptor conformations may be achieved [27–31].

h. Allosteric modulators exercise "probe dependence": Another particularly unique aspect of allosteric

mechanisms is that they can be very probe specific (i.e., a conformational change that is catastrophic for one receptor probe may be inconsequential to another). This is illustrated in Figure 7.7, where it can be seen that the allosteric modulator eburnamonine produces a 25-fold antagonism of the muscarinic agonist pilocarpine, no effect on the agonist arecaidine propargyl ester (APE), and a 15-fold *potentiation* of the agonist arecoline [1].

Allosteric probe dependence can have negative effects. For example, allosteric modification of an endogenous signaling system requires the effect to be operative on the physiologically relevant agonist. There are practical circumstances where screening for new drug entities in this mode may not be possible. For example, the screening of molecules for HIV entry theoretically should be done with live AIDS virus, but this is not possible for safety and containment reasons. In this case, a surrogate receptor probe, such as a radioactive chemokine, must be used and this can lead to dissimilation in activity (i.e., molecules may modify the effects of the chemokine but not HIV). This is discussed specifically in relation to screening in Chapter 11.

Another case is the potentiation of cholinergic signaling for the treatment of patients with Alzheimer's disease. It has been proposed that a reduction in cholinergic function results in cognitive and memory impairment in this disease [15,16]. As discussed previously, an allosteric potentiation of cholinergic function could be beneficial therapeutically, but it would have to be operative for the natural neurotransmitter — in this case, acetylcholine. This agonist is unstable and difficult to use as a screening tool and surrogate cholinergic agonists have been used in drug discovery. However, effects on such surrogates may have no therapeutic relevance if they do not translate to concomitant effects on the natural agonist. For example, the cholinergic test agonist arecoline is potentiated 15-fold by the allosteric modulator eburnamonine but no potentiation, in fact a 3-fold *antagonism*, is observed with the natural agonist acetylcholine [1]. Similarly, the allosteric potentiating ligand LY2033298 causes agonist-dependent differential potentiation of acetylcholine and oxotremorine [32]. Current data suggest that if the natural agonist (e.g., acetylcholine) cannot be used in the screening process, then the modulator must be tested early in the development process to ensure beneficial effects with the natural system. This also is relevant to targets with multiple natural agonists such as GLP-1. Specifically, it has been shown that the allosteric potentiation of GLP-1 effect by NOVO2 produces a 25-fold potentiation of the minor natural agonist for this receptor oxyntomodulin but only a 5-fold potentiation of the main natural agonist GLP-1(7−36)NH2 [33].

Allosteric probe dependence can be an issue with antagonists as well in cases where a given modulator has differential blocking effects on different interactants with the receptor. For instance, the chemokine receptor CCR5 binds HIV-1 to mediate infection and CCR5 allosteric antagonists block this effect. However, it has been shown that allosteric modulators have differing relative potency as blockers of HIV entry and CCL3L1-induced CCR5 internalization [34]. This could lead to preservation of natural CCR5 receptor internalization through chemokine binding, an effect identified as being potentially favorable in progression to AIDS after HIV-1 infection [35]. This suggests that a superior allosteric modulator would block the utilization of CCR5 by HIV-1 but otherwise allow normal chemokine function for this receptor [34]. Such effects underscore the importance of probe dependence in the action of allosteric modulators.

i. Allosteric modulators can be used for target salvage: Texture in antagonism can lead to a unique approach to the therapeutic evaluation of biological targets. For example, if a receptor is required for normal physiological function, then eliminating this target pharmacologically is prohibited. This can lead to the elimination of a therapeutic opportunity if that same target is involved in a pathological function. Such a case occurs for the chemokine X-type receptor CXCR4, since loss of normal CXCR4 receptor function may be deleterious to normal health. It specifically has been shown that deletion of the genes known to mediate expression of the CXCR4 receptor or the natural agonist for CXCR4 (stromal cell derived factor 1-α, SDF-1α) is lethal and leads to developmental defects in the cerebellum, heart, and gastrointestinal tract as well as hematopoiesis [36−38] (i.e., this receptor is involved in normal physiological function and interference with its normal function will lead to serious effects). However, this receptor also mediates entry of the X4 strain of HIV virus, leading to AIDS. Therefore, an allosteric modulator that could discern between the binding of HIV and the natural agonist for CXCR4 (SDF-1α) could be a very beneficial drug.

The probe-dependent aspect of allosteric mechanisms could still allow CXCR4 to be considered as a therapeutic target in spite of its crucial role in normal physiology. Suggestions of ligand-mediated divergence of physiological activity and mediation of HIV entry have been reported for CXCR4 in peptide agonists such as RSVM and ASLW. These peptides are not blocked by the CXCR4 antagonist AMD3100, an otherwise potent antagonist of HIV entry, suggesting a dissociation of signaling and HIV binding effects [39]. Similar dissociation between HIV and chemokine activity also is observed with other peptide fragments of SDF-1α [40]. These data open the possibility that allosteric molecules can be found that block HIV entry but do not interfere with CXCR4-mediated chemokine function.

The unique properties of allosteric modulators are summarized in Table 7.2.

7.4 FUNCTIONAL STUDY OF ALLOSTERIC MODULATORS

In essence, an allosteric ligand produces a different receptor if the tertiary conformation of the receptor is changed through binding. These different tertiary conformations can have a wide range of effects on agonist function. A different receptor conformation can change its behavior toward G-proteins (and hence the cell and stimulus-response mechanisms) or the agonist, or both. Under these circumstances, there is a range of activities that allosteric ligands can have on agonist dose-response curves.

From the point of view of agonist activation, allosteric modulation can be thought of in terms of two separate effects. These effects may not be mutually exclusive and both can be relevant. The first, and most easily depicted, is a change in affinity of the receptor toward the agonist. The most simple system consists of a receptor [R] binding to a probe [A] (a probe being a molecule that can assess receptor behavior; probes can be agonists or radioligands) and an allosteric modulator [B] [41,42]:

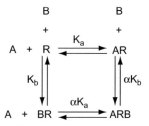

The equation for receptor occupancy for an agonist [A] in the presence of an allosteric ligand [B] is given by (see Section 7.7.1):

$$\frac{[AR]}{R_{tot}} = \frac{[A]/K_A(1 + \alpha[B]/K_B)}{[A]/K_A(1 + \alpha[B]/K_B) + [B]/K_B + 1}, \quad (7.1)$$

TABLE 7.2 Comparison of Properties of Orthosteric and Allosteric Ligands

Orthosteric Antagonists	Allosteric Modulators
Orthosteric antagonists block all agonists with equal potency.	Allosteric antagonists may block some agonists but not others (at least as well).
There is a mandatory link between the duration of effect and the intensity of effect.	Duration and intensity of effect may be dissociated (i.e., duration can be prolonged through receptor compartment loading with no target overdose).
High concentrations of antagonist block signals to basal levels.	Receptor signaling can be modulated to a reduced (but not to basal) level.
Less propensity for receptor subtype effects.	Greater potential for selectivity.
No texture in effect (i.e., patterns of signaling may not be preserved).	Effect is linked to receptor signal. Thus, complex physiological patterns may be preserved.
All antagonist-bound receptors are equal.	Texture in antagonism where allosterically modified receptors may have different conformations from each other may lead to differences in resistance profiles with chronic treatment.

where K_A and K_B are the equilibrium dissociation constants of the agonist and antagonist receptor complexes, respectively, and α is the cooperativity factor. Thus, a value for α of 0.1 means that the allosteric antagonist causes a 10-fold reduction in the affinity of the receptor for the agonist. This can be seen from the relationship describing the affinity of the probe [A] for the receptor, in the presence of varying concentrations of antagonist:

$$K_{obs} = \frac{K_A([B]/K_B + 1)}{(1 + \alpha[B]/K_B)}. \qquad (7.2)$$

It can be seen that a feature of allosteric antagonists is that their effect is saturable (i.e., a theoretically infinite concentration of [B] will cause K_{obs} to reach a maximal asymptote value of K_A/α). This is in contrast to simple competitive antagonists where the degree of antagonism is theoretically infinite for an infinite concentration of antagonist. Therefore, the maximal change in affinity that can be produced by the allosteric modulator is $K_{obs}/K_A = K_A/\alpha K_A = \alpha^{-1}$. Thus, a modulator with $\alpha = 0.1$ will reduce the affinity of the receptor for the agonist by a maximal value of 10.

As well as changing the affinity of the receptor for an agonist, an allosteric effect could just as well change the reactivity of the receptor to the agonist. This could be reflected in a complete range of receptor effects (response production, internalization, desensitization, and so on). This is depicted schematically in Figure 7.8, where the agonist-bound receptor goes on to interact with the cell in accordance with the operational model for receptor function [43]. Experimental data are fit to a mathematical model of allosteric function, the most simple version being an amalgam of the allosteric binding model [41,42] with the Black/Leff operational model for

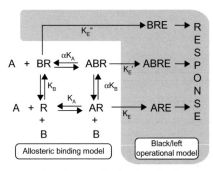

FIGURE 7.8 Parsimonious model for functional receptor allosterism [46]. A tracer ligand [A] (agonist) binds to the receptor and the resulting complex (ARE) can produce response. Similarly, the allosteric modulator B can simultaneously bind to the receptor and produce response through the complex BRE and can modify the agonist response through the species ABRE. Binding to the receptor is described by the allosteric binding model [41,42] and response is described by the Black/Leff operational model [43].

receptor function [44]. This leads to the following equation (see Section 7.7.2) [26,44,45]:

$$\text{Response} = \frac{\tau_A[A]/K_A(1 + \alpha\beta[B]/K_B) + \tau_B[B]/K_B}{\begin{array}{c}[A]/K_A(1 + \alpha[B]/K_B) + \tau_A(1 + \alpha\beta[B]/K_B)) \\ + [B]/K_B(1 + \tau_B) + 1\end{array}}$$

$$(7.3)$$

where K_A and K_B are the equilibrium dissociation constants for the agonist- and modulator-receptor complexes respectively, τ_A and τ_B the efficacies of the agonist and modulator respectively, α the allosteric effect on affinity (on both the agonist and reciprocally on the modulator), and β the modification of the efficacy of the agonist produced by the modulator. Therefore, the minimal parameters to fully characterize a modulator are K_B, τ_B, α and β — see Figure 7.9. It will be seen that affinity of modulators are conditional, and depend on the nature and concentration of the co-binding ligand and also the magnitude of α and β.

The model described by Equation 7.3 predicts virtually any effect a modulator can have on the concentration-response curve to the agonist. If the

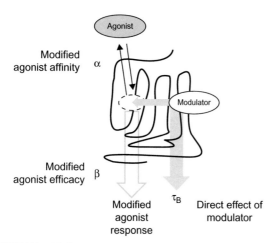

FIGURE 7.9 Minimal parameters needed to characterize and quantify receptor allosterism. Direct effects of the modulator are quantified by an efficacy term τ_B through the Black/Leff operational model while the modification of the endogenous agonist effects are described by α, the effect of the modulator on agonist affinity, and β, the effect of the modulator on agonist efficacy.

modulator has no direct action on the receptor ($\tau_B = 0$), then eight possible effects on agonism can occur; resulting from combinations of an increase, no effect, or a decrease of affinity (α) and the same possibilities with efficacy (β). These effects are shown in Figure 7.10. If the modulator has direct agonist activity ($\tau_B \neq 0$), then there are nine further possible combinations (see Figure 7.11). As can be seen from Figures 7.10 and 7.11, there are basically 17 possible patterns that can be produced by allosteric modulators [46].

As a preface to a discussion of various allosteric phenotypes, it is worth considering the general effects of allosteric modification of affinity (α) and efficacy (β). Equation 7.3 predicts that even when the modulator reduces the affinity of the receptor for the agonist ($\alpha < 1$) the effects will be surmountable with respect to the agonist (i.e., the agonist will produce the control maximal response). This can be seen from Equation 7.3 when $[A] \rightarrow \infty$ and where the maximal response therefore approaches unity. If the signaling properties of the receptor are not altered by the allosteric modulator, then the concentration-response curve to the agonist will be shifted either to the right (if $\alpha < 1$; see Figure 7.12A) or to the left ($\alpha > 1$; see Figure 7.12B). The distinctive feature of such an allosteric effect is that while the displacements are parallel with no diminution of maxima, there is a limiting value (equal to α^{-1}) to the maximal displacement.

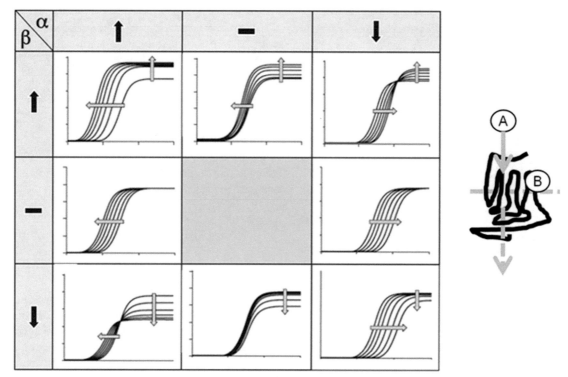

FIGURE 7.10 Effects of allosteric modulators with various properties on agonist response as predicted by Equation 7.3 ($\tau_A = 3$, $K_A = 10\,\mu M$, $K_B = 10\,nM$, $\tau_B = 0$). Panels from top row left to right ($\alpha = 30$, $\beta = 5$), ($\alpha = 1$, $\beta = 5$), ($\alpha = 0.01$, $\beta = 5$): middle row left to right ($\alpha = 30$, $\beta = 1$), middle panel no curves since $\alpha = \beta = 1$, then ($\alpha = 0.01$, $\beta = 1$), bottom row left to right ($\alpha = 30$, $\beta = 0.3$), ($\alpha = 1$, $\beta = 0.3$) and ($\alpha = 0.01$, $\beta = 0.3$).

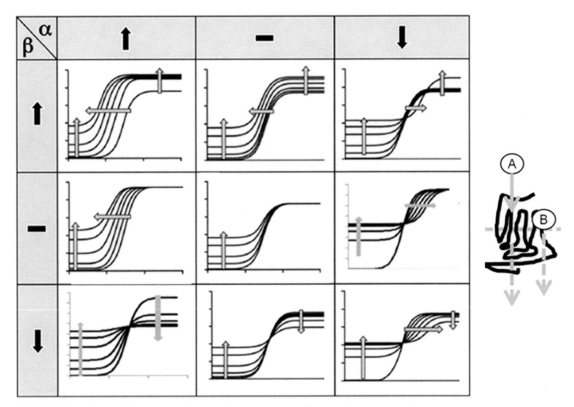

FIGURE 7.11 Effects of allosteric modulators with direct agonist efficacy and various properties on agonist response as predicted by Equation 7.3 ($\tau_A = 3$, $K_A = 10\,\mu M$, $K_B = 10\,nM$, $\tau_B = 0.25$). Panels from top row left to right ($\alpha = 30$, $\beta = 5$), ($\alpha = 1$, $\beta = 5$), ($\alpha = 0.01$, $\beta = 5$): middle row left to right ($\alpha = 30$, $\beta = 1$), middle panel no curves since $\alpha = \beta = 1$, then ($\alpha = 0.01$, $\beta = 1$), bottom row left to right ($\alpha = 30$, $\beta = 0.3$), ($\alpha = 1$, $\beta = 0.3$) and ($\alpha = 0.01$, $\beta = 0.3$).

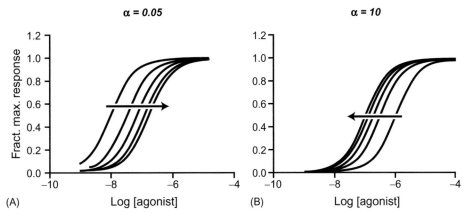

FIGURE 7.12 Functional responses in the presence of allosteric modulators as simulated with Equation 7.3 ($\tau = 30$). (A) Allosteric antagonism. Agonist $K_A = 0.3\,\mu M$, $\alpha = 0.05$, and $K_B = 1\,\mu M$. Curve farthest to the left is control in absence of modulator. From left to right, concentrations of modulator equal $3\,\mu M$, $10\,\mu M$, $30\,\mu M$, and $100\,\mu M$. Arrow indicates effect of modulator. Note the limited shift to the right. (B) Allosteric potentiation. Agonist $K_A = 30\,\mu M$, $\alpha = 10\,\mu M$, $K_B = 3\,\mu M$. Curve farthest to the right is control in absence of modulator. From right to left, concentrations of modulator equal $3\,\mu M$, $10\,\mu M$, $30\,\mu M$, and $100\,\mu M$. Arrow indicates effect of modulator. Note the limited shift to the left.

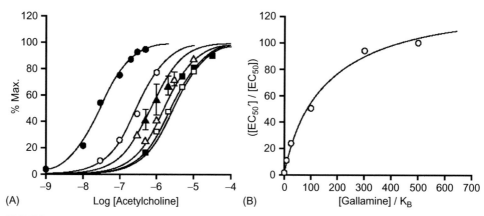

FIGURE 7.13 Operational model fit of the allosteric effects of gallamine on electrically evoked contractions of guinea pig left atrium. (A) Dose-response curves obtained in the absence (filled circles) and presence of gallamine 10 μM (open circles), 30 μM (filled triangles), 100 μM (open triangles), 300 μM (filled squares), and 500 μM (open squares). Data fit to operational model (Equation 7.4) with $K_A = 30$ nM, $E_{max} = 200$, $\tau = 1$. Data fit for gallamine $K_B = 1$ μM and $\alpha = 0.0075$. (B) Ratio of observed EC_{50} values (EC'_{50} for curve in presence of gallamine/EC_{50} control curve) as a function of concentrations of gallamine. Data fit to rectangular hyperbola of max = 134 (1/maximum = $\alpha = 0.0075$). Data redrawn from [47].

Figure 7.13A shows an experimentally observed allosteric displacement of acetylcholine effects in cardiac muscle by the allosteric modulator gallamine and the saturable maximal effect (Figure 7.13B).

7.4.1 Phenotypic Allosteric Modulation Profiles

In practical terms, there are five phenotype allosteric profiles usually seen in discovery. These phenotypes emerge because of various combinations of cooperativity with respect to affinity (α) and efficacy (β) as well as direct agonism (τ_B):

1. **Negative allosteric modulators (NAMs)**: $\alpha < 1$ and/or $\beta < 1$. These ligands reduce the affinity and/or the efficacy of agonists (panel A in Figure 7.14).
    a. **NAM-agonists**: These are NAMs that also possess intrinsic efficacy (τ_B) and thus produce response in their own right (panel C in Figure 7.14).
2. **Positive allosteric modulators (PAMs)**: $\alpha > 1$ and/or $\beta > 1$: These ligands increase the affinity and/or the efficacy of agonists (Panel B in Figure 7.14).
    a. **PAM-agonists**: These are PAMs that have intrinsic efficacy (τ_B) and thus directly produce agonist response (panel D in Figure 7.14).
    b. **PAM-antagonists**: These have $\alpha > 1$ but $\beta < 1$ and produce antagonism while

increasing the affinity of the agonist (i.e., ifenprodil [25]) — panel E in Figure 7.14.

As a preface for discussion of these allosteric phenotypes it is useful to consider a property common to many of them, namely allosteric agonism.

7.4.2 Allosteric Agonism

There is no *a priori* reason that allosteric agonism should differ from conventional agonism (i.e., the modulator stabilizes an active state of the receptor to induce response); this is underscored by setting $[A] \rightarrow 0$ in Equation 7.3 and seeing that it reduces to the standard Black/Leff equation for agonism for the modulator:

$$\text{Response} = \frac{\tau_B [B]/K_B}{[B]/K_B(1 + \tau_B) + 1} \qquad (7.4)$$

Under these circumstances, the efficacy of an allosteric agonist (τ_B) can be quantified with the Black/Leff model, as for any agonist. However, what is different from orthosteric agonism is the fact that the effect of the allosteric agonist on the endogenous agonist signaling can be complex and very different from the standard antagonism seen with orthosteric partial agonists. These effects depend on the magnitude of α and β — see Figure 7.15.

The other relevant aspect of allosteric agonism is the possibility that the allosteric agonist may produce biased agonism (see Chapter 5 Section 5.7 for further details). It is known that allosteric agonism can be associated with biased agonism [48] (see Figure 7.16), therefore this must be considered in the overall profile of the allosteric modulator.

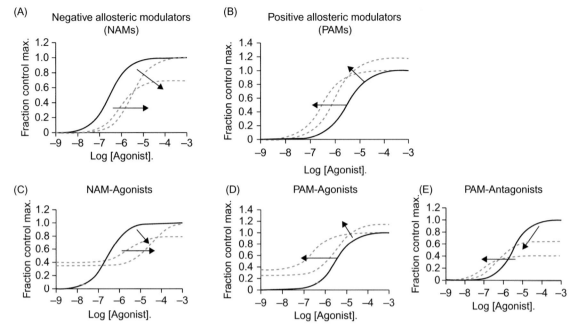

FIGURE 7.14 **Phenotypic allosteric modulators.** (A) Negative allosteric modulators (NAMs) reduce the sensitivity of the receptor to the agonist. (B) Positive allosteric modulators (PAMs) increase agonist sensitivity to agonism. (C) NAM-agonists decrease receptor sensitivity to endogenous agonism but also directly activate the receptor to produce response. (D) PAM-agonists increase receptor sensitivity to endogenous agonism and also have direct agonist action. (E) PAM-antagonists increase the binding of the agonist to the receptor but preclude this binding from producing agonist response.

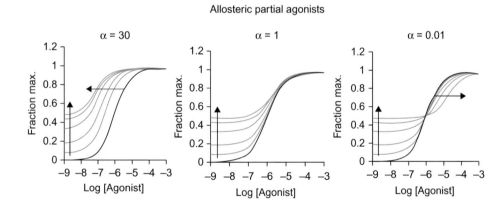

FIGURE 7.15 **Effect of allosteric partial agonists on endogenous agonist response.** For molecules with $\alpha > 1$, sensitization concomitant with direct agonism is observed (far left panel). Direct allosteric agonism with no interference with endogenous agonism also can occur ($\alpha = 1$, middle panel) as well as direct agonism and decreased sensitivity to endogenous agonism ($\alpha < 1$) — far right panel.

7.4.3 Affinity of Allosteric Modulators

A basic tenet of allosteric analysis is that the full activity of an allosteric modulator cannot be assessed in isolation; by definition, the properties of an allosteric modulator are linked to the molecule co-binding to the receptor. Because of this cooperative nature of allosteric modulators (i.e., their activity is conditional upon the co-binding ligand), it is worth examining what is meant by the observed "affinity" of an allosteric modulator. In terms of binding, radioligand binding (as denoted by ρ^*, the fraction of receptors bound to a radioligand) is given by Equation 4.10. This leads to an equation for the ratio of

the observed IC_{50} of a modulator inhibiting radioligand binding to the K_B for modulator of:

$$IC_{50} = K_B \frac{(1 + ([A^*]/K_d))}{(1 + \alpha([A^*]/K_d))} \qquad (7.5)$$

where K_d and K_B are the equilibrium dissociation constants of the radioligand-receptor complex and modulator-receptor complexes, respectively, and α is the effect of the modulator on the affinity of the radioligand. It can be seen from Equation 7.5 that the observed affinity of an allosteric modulator (IC_{50}) depends not only on the magnitude of the K_B but also on the nature (α) and

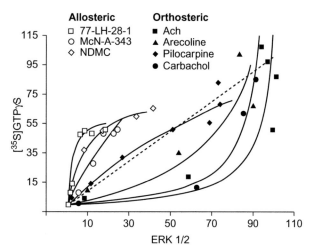

FIGURE 7.16 **Bias plot (see Section 5.7 of Chapter 5) for musca-rinic agonism on M2 receptors.** Ordinate values characterize G-protein activation through [^{35}S] GTPγS binding expressed as a function of ERK1/2 activation for the same concentration of agonist. Allosteric agonists (open symbols) show a bias toward G-protein response while muscarinic orthosteric agonists (filled symbols) have an opposite bias toward ERK1/2 signaling. Data redrawn from [48].

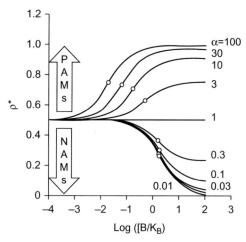

FIGURE 7.17 Radioligand binding produced by a reference concentration of radioligand [A*] = K_d. For α < 1, the affinity of the receptor is reduced causing a concomitant reduction in the radioligand binding. No effect on binding is produced with α = 1 while an enhancement of binding is seen for α > 1. Open circles show the half maximal concentrations for the various curves. It can be seen that there is little effect on IC_{50} values (concentration producing 50% inhibition of binding) for α values < 1 while dramatic effects are seen on EC_{50} values (concentrations for half maximal radioligand binding) when α > 1.

concentration [A*] of the co-binding ligand, in this case the radioligand.

Unlike orthosteric ligands, allosteric modulators have the potential to increase radioligand binding (α > 1 for PAMs) as well as decrease it (α < 1 for NAMs) − see Figure 4.12. Figure 7.17 shows the effect of various types of allosteric modulators on radioligand binding (it is assumed that [A*]/K_d = 1) where it can be seen that the IC_{50} (open circles on curves) of negative allosteric modulator antagonists is relatively stable while for PAMs the observed potency varies greatly with α.

An expression corresponding to the one for radioligand binding (Equation 7.5) for the effect of a modulator on agonist function is:

$$IC_{50}/K_B = \frac{([A]/K_A)(1 + \tau_A) + 1}{(\alpha[A]/K_A)(1 + \beta\tau_A)}. \qquad (7.6)$$

where the terms are as for Equation 7.3. As with Equation 7.5, the observed functional affinity of the modulator is subject to the magnitude of K_B as well as the concentration of [A] and the nature of the co-binding ligand as it modifies the agonist's affinity (α) and efficacy (β). Figure 7.18 shows the effect of either radioligand (for binding) or agonist concentration (for function) on the observed potency of a modulator. For this figure, standard conditions for assessing antagonist activity were used. Specifically, the level of agonist used for the IC_{50} experiment was one that gives 80% of the maximal response (R = 0.8), while the level of radioligand binding chosen was [A*]/K_d = 1 to yield 50% binding. It can be seen that the effects of ligand co-binding (either agonist for function or radioligand

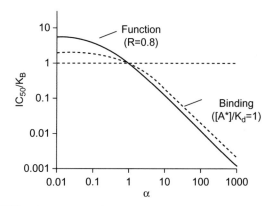

FIGURE 7.18 Potency of allosteric modulators affecting radioligand binding (where level of binding initially is equal to the K_d value) and cellular response (where the initial level of response is 80% of maximum). It can be seen that with α < 1, the IC_{50} values are greater than the K_B but the factor is < 10-fold even at very low values of α. However, for PAMs, these factors can be very high, and the observed EC_{50} value can be considerably less than the K_B, i.e., the PAM becomes much more potent in the presence of either the radioligand or agonist.

concentration for binding) is limited for allosteric antagonists but can be very substantial for positive allosteric modulators (PAMs).

7.4.4 Negative Allosteric Modulators (NAMs)

Negative allosteric modulators are antagonists with specific properties. Although their observed potency is

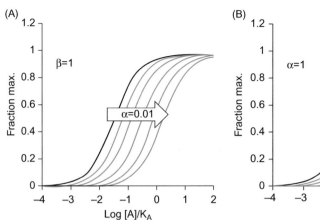

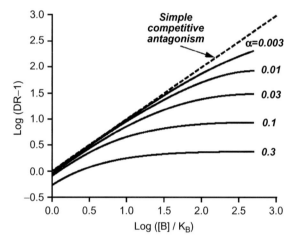

FIGURE 7.19 **Effect of varying diminutions of affinity (panel A) or efficacy (panel B) for NAMs blocking agonist response.** Changes in affinity (α values) can only change the location parameter of the agonist concentration-response curve whereas changes in efficacy (β) can change both the location parameter and the maximal response to the agonist.

FIGURE 7.20 **Schild regressions for allosteric antagonists of differing values of α.** Dotted line shows the expected Schild regression for a simple competitive antagonist. With allosteric antagonists of lower values for α, the regression reaches a plateau at higher antagonist concentrations (i.e., curvature occurs at higher antagonist concentrations).

conditional with respect to co-binding ligand, Equations 7.5 and 7.6 and Figure 7.18 (for $\alpha < 1$) indicate that these effects are relatively limited (at least when compared to PAMs). Antagonism can occur for α values < 1 and/or β values < 1 — see Figure 7.19. In cases where the maximal response is not changed ($\beta = 1$) and the antagonist produces parallel shifts to the right of the dose-response curve (due to $\alpha < 1$) with no diminution of the maximal response, the first approach used to quantify potency might be a Schild analysis (see Chapter 6 Section 6.3.1). In cases where the value of α is low (i.e., $\alpha = 0.01$), a 10-fold concentration range of the antagonist would cause shifts commensurate with those produced by a simple competitive antagonist. However, the testing of a wide range of concentrations of an allosteric antagonist would show the saturation of the allosteric binding site as revealed by an approach to a maximal value for the antagonism. The Schild equation for an allosteric antagonist is given by (see Section 7.7.3):

$$\text{Log}(DR - 1) = \text{Log}\left[\frac{[B](1 - \alpha)}{\alpha[B] + K_B}\right]. \qquad (7.7)$$

Expected Schild regressions for allosteric antagonists with a range of α values are shown in Figure 7.20. It can be seen that the magnitude of α is inversely proportional to the ability of the allosteric antagonist to appear as a simple competitive antagonist (i.e., the lower the value of α, the more the antagonist will appear to be competitive). An example of this type of analysis is given in Section 13.2.9 of Chapter 13.

The foregoing discussion has been restricted to allosteric ligands that reduce the affinity of the receptor for the agonist (i.e., allosteric antagonists or modulators). Since allosteric change is the result of a conformational change in the receptor, there is no *a priori* reason for allosterism to produce only a reduced agonist affinity, and increases in the affinity of the receptor for agonists (note the stimulation of the binding of [3H]-atropine by alcuronium in Figure 4.12) have been documented.

However, separate from ligand binding, another possible allosteric effect is to render the receptor insensitive to agonist stimulation (i.e., remove the capacity for agonist response). This may or may not be accompanied by a change in the affinity of the receptor for the agonist and is simulated in Equation 7.3 by setting $\beta < 1$.

In the special case where the modulator does not affect the affinity of the receptor or the agonist ($\alpha = 1$) and where $\beta = 0$ (the modulator prevents receptor activation by the agonist), Equation 7.3 becomes identical to the one describing orthosteric noncompetitive antagonism derived by Gaddum and colleagues [49] (see Equation 6.10). However, while the equation is identical and the pattern of concentration-response curves is the same as that for an orthosteric antagonist, it should be noted that the molecular mechanism is completely different. Whereas the system described by Gaddum et al. consists of a slow offset antagonist occluding the agonist binding

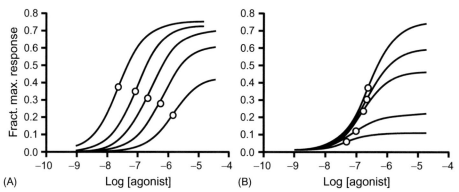

FIGURE 7.21 **Effect of insurmountable allosteric antagonists that block receptor signaling to the agonist and also affect affinity of the receptor for the agonist.** (A) Responses according to Equation 7.3 with $\tau = 3$, $K_A = 0.1\ \mu M$, $\alpha = 0.03\ \mu M$, and $K_B = 1\ \mu M$. Curves from left to right: control (no modulator present) and curves in the presence of modulator concentrations $3\ \mu M$, $10\ \mu M$, $30\ \mu M$, and $100\ \mu M$. Open circles show the EC_{50} of each concentration-response curve (and also the shift to the right of the location parameter of each curve with increasing modulator concentration). (B) Responses with $\tau = 3\ \mu M$, $K_A = 0.1\ \mu M$, $\alpha = 50\ \mu M$, $K_B = 1\ \mu M$. Curves from left to right: control (no modulator present) and curves in the presence of modulator concentrations $20\ nM$, $50\ nM$, $0.2\ \mu M$, and $0.5\ \mu M$. Open circles show the EC_{50} of each concentration-response curve. In this case, the modulator blocks signaling but *increases* the affinity of the receptor to the agonist. Note also that lower concentrations of antagonist block responses (as compared to panel A).

site, the system described by Equation 7.3 consists of the modulator binding to its own site on the receptor separate from that of the agonist. This ambiguity underscores the failure of observing patterns of concentration-response curves to determine molecular mechanism of action and how different experimental approaches to discerning allosteric versus orthosteric mechanisms are required (*vide infra*).

Equation 7.3 defines the allosteric noncompetitive antagonism of receptor function and predicts insurmountable effects on agonist maximal response (i.e., as $[A] \to \infty$); the expression for the maximal response is:

$$\text{Maximal Response} = \frac{(1 + \tau)}{(1 + \tau + \alpha[B]/K_B)}. \qquad (7.8)$$

It can be seen that, just as in the case of orthosteric noncompetitive antagonism for high-efficacy agonists or in systems of high receptor density and/or very efficient receptor coupling (high τ values, basically systems where there is a receptor reserve for the agonist), the maximal response may not be depressed until relatively high concentrations of antagonist are present. Under these circumstances, there may be dextral displacement with no diminution of maximal response until fairly considerable receptor antagonism is achieved (e.g., see Figure 6.16B). The difference between the orthosteric system described in Chapter 6, and the allosteric system described here is that there can be an independent effect on receptor affinity. No such effect is possible in an orthosteric system. Figure 7.21 shows concomitant effects on receptor affinity for the agonist in allosteric noncompetitive systems. Figure 7.21A shows the effects

of an allosteric modulator that prevents agonist-receptor activation and also decreases the affinity of the receptor for the agonist by a factor of 20 ($\alpha = 0.05$). It can be seen from this figure that the EC_{50} agonist concentrations shift to the right as the maximal response to the agonist is depressed. In contrast, Figure 7.21B shows the effects of a modulator that prevents agonist activation of the receptor but also increases the affinity of the receptor for the agonist ($\alpha = 50$). Here it can be seen that as the maximal response to the agonist is depressed by the modulator, the sensitivity of the receptor to the agonist actually increases. It should be noted that a shift of EC_{50} values to the left should not automatically be expected when an allosteric modulator increases the affinity of the receptor for the agonist. This is because if there is a large receptor reserve in the system, the EC_{50} will naturally shift to the right with noncompetitive blockade. Therefore, what is observed is an average of the effect shifting the curves to the right and the increased affinity shifting curves to the left. The example shown in Figure 7.21B was deliberately modeled in a system with little to no receptor reserve to illustrate the effect of allosterism on the EC_{50} values. Figure 7.22A shows the effect of the allosteric modulator Sch-C on the responses of the CCR5 chemokine receptor to the chemokine RANTES, and Figure 7.22B shows the effect of the allosteric modulator UK 427,857.

Since allosteric change is the result of a conformational change in the receptor, there is no reason for allosterism to produce only a reduced agonist affinity, and in fact such changes can lead to increases in the affinity of the receptor for the agonist (note the

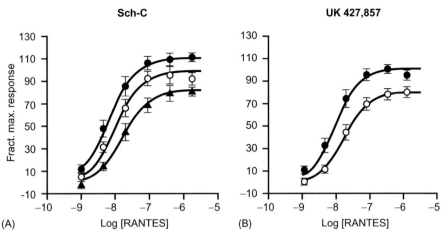

FIGURE 7.22 Insurmountable allosteric blockade of CCR5-mediated calcium transient responses produced by the chemokine agonist RANTES by (A) Sch-C: control (filled circles) and presence of Sch-C 10 nM (open circles) and 30 nM (filled triangles); n = 4. Data fit with Equation 7.3, $\tau = 16$, K_A RANTES = 120 nM, $\alpha = 0.14$, and $K_B = 12.6$ nM. (B) Blockade of RANTES response with UK 427,857 3 nM (open circles); n = 4. Data fit with Equation 7.6, $\tau = 16$, K_A RANTES = 140 nM, $\alpha = 0.2$, and $K_B = 2$ nM. Redrawn from [9].

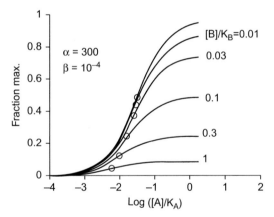

FIGURE 7.23 Increased potency of a PAM-antagonist due to the presence of the agonist. The reciprocal effect of the agonist on the affinity of the PAM causes antagonism to occur at concentrations of PAM much lower than the binding K_B. Open circles show the position of the EC_{50} values of the agonist.

stimulation of the binding of [3H]-atropine by alcuronium in Figure 4.12). Various combinations of α and β control both the location of the agonist concentration-response curve and the maximal response. A special case of NAM action is where $\beta < 1$ and $\alpha > 1$. These ligands are PAM-antagonists since they sensitize the receptor to agonism but preclude agonist function as well; this leads to the profile shown in Figure 7.23. Worthy of note for PAM-antagonists is the fact that their observed potency is considerably greater than

their binding K_B (due to the positive effect of high α values — see Equation 7.6). As noted previously, this causes the EC_{50} of the agonist to actually decrease instead of increase during the process of receptor antagonism. In practical terms this can lead to a favorable profile, in that the potency of these antagonists increases as the concentration of agonist increases; two examples of these types of ligand are ifenprodil [25] and Org27569 [26]. Another profile possible is a reverse pattern of sensitivity change to agonism, namely a reduction of affinity ($\alpha < 1$) but an increase in efficacy ($\beta > 1$): this pattern is shown in Figure 7.24A. Figure 7.24B illustrates an important feature of allosterism, namely that allosteric effects are saturable. Thus, noncompetitive blockade is produced at a range of concentrations of negative allosteric modulator up to the point where the allosteric binding sites are saturated; then antagonism reaches a limiting value.

NAM activity can be rapidly quantified by testing a range of modulator concentrations in a functional preparation pre-equilibrated with agonist (usually to an 80% response level). This leads to the standard IC_{50} type of profile yielding an inverted sigmoid concentration-response curve to the modulator — see Figure 7.25. This figure illustrates how the IC_{50} of a NAM can change with the level of agonist stimulation, and also how the maximal asymptote can be affected by the level of agonism (in keeping with the saturability of allosteric effect). Thus, at high levels of agonism with NAMs of limited α/β values (i.e., $1 < \alpha < 20$), the limited alteration of agonist affinity can be overcome by high agonist concentrations to

FIGURE 7.24 Effect of an allosteric modulator that changes both the affinity and efficacy of the agonist for the receptor. (A) Modulator increases the efficacy but decreases the affinity of the agonist for the receptor. Responses modeled with Equation 7.3 with $\alpha = 0.01$, $\beta = 5$, and $\tau = 1$. Curves shown for $[B]/K_B = 0$, 1, 3, 10, 30, and 100. (B) Modulator decreases both the efficacy and affinity of the agonist. However, the decrease in efficacy is modest and a new plateau of agonist is observed (response not blocked to basal levels). Responses modeled with Equation 7.3 with $\alpha = 0.3$, $\xi = 0.5$, and $\tau = 1$. Curves shown for $[B]/K_B = 0$, 1, 3, 10, 30, and 100.

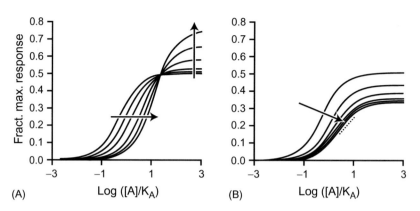

(A)   (B)

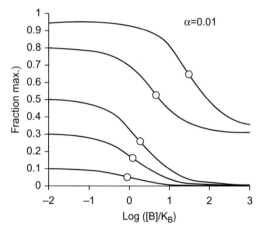

FIGURE 7.25 Effect of a NAM that reduces the affinity of the agonist by a factor of 100 on various levels of pre-equilibrated response. Open circles show the location parameter (IC_{50}) of the inhibition curves. It can be seen that with increasing levels of agonist (higher response) the curves shift to the right and also fail to reach complete inhibition.

produce IC_{50} curves that do not reach zero effect (see Figure 7.25 for agonist effect $= 0.8$ and 0.95). These types of curve are viewed as "displacement" curves for orthosteric binding (i.e., the antagonist displaces the agonist to induce antagonism), but this is not the case for allosteric modulators. Rather, these ligands re-set the affinity of the receptor for the agonist; therefore the curve does not reflect displacement but a newly adjusted binding affinity.

In general, complete NAM activity can be quantified by fitting agonist concentration-response curves in the absence and presence of a range of concentrations of modulator to Equation 7.3. It should be noted that only β effects will depress the maximal response; this is shown by a metameter of Equation 7.3 when $[A] \rightarrow \infty$:

$$\text{Maximal Response} = \tau_A(1 + \alpha\beta[B]/K_B)/(1 + \alpha[B]/K_B + \tau_A(1 + \alpha\beta[B]/K_B))$$

$$(7.9)$$

where it can be shown that if there is no effect on efficacy ($\beta = 1$), then the maximal response according to Equation 7.9 in the presence of all concentrations of modulator will be $\tau_A/(1 + \tau_A)$ which is the maximal response with no modulator present. Changes in α only affect the sensitivity along the agonist concentration axis. In general, in order to differentiate α and β effects for a NAM, it is necessary to have effects in a system where there is little to no receptor reserve for the agonist. In such a system, $\beta < 1$ will result in a depression of maximum where $\alpha < 1$ will not. The important data needed to characterize NAM activity are K_B, α and β.

As with orthosteric partial agonists, allosteric ligands can produce a direct agonist effect (quantified by τ_B) as well as affecting the affinity (α) and/or efficacy (β) of other agonists. If $\alpha < 1$ and/or $\beta < 1$, a decreased sensitivity to other agonists occurs and these will be NAM-agonists. In general, as with all allosteric ligands, these ligands can be characterized with K_B, α and β, and additionally will have a value for efficacy for direct agonism (τ_B). The effect on endogenous agonist sensitivity can be variable depending on the magnitude(s) of α and β — see Figure 7.15.

7.4.5 Positive Allosteric Modulators (PAMs)

Positive allosteric modulation of failing physiological systems can be a theoretically favorable therapy in cases where α and/or $\beta > 1$ leads to sensitization to endogenous signaling. At this point it is important to distinguish between system maximal response and target maximal response. Agonists can produce identical maximal responses in one of two ways; they could have identical efficacy values, or they both may exceed the capability of some step in the cellular stimulus-response cascade to produce saturation of that step. When this occurs for high-efficacy agonists they will have the same observed maximal response. Under these circumstances, increases in efficacy (as would be produced by $\beta > 1$) will not be registered as an increased observed

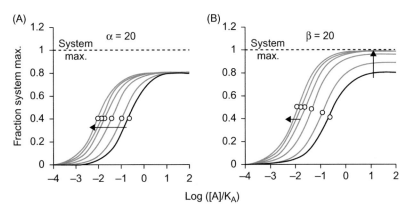

FIGURE 7.26 **Effects of PAMs on agonist concentration-response curves.** (A) Increases in the affinity of the agonist ($\alpha = 20$) can only affect the location of the concentration-response curves along the concentration axis. Shifts are concentration dependent until the allosteric site is completely occupied where a maximal asymptote for the potentiation is seen. (B) Effect of a PAM that increases the efficacy of the agonist ($\beta = 20$). If the agonist is a partial agonist, then the maximal response will increase until either the agonist saturates a step in the system stimulus-response cascade (and the system maximum is attained) or the maximal effect of the PAM on the receptor is obtained. In the example shown, the latter mechanism is not the case since a further shift to the left of the concentration-response curves is seen after the maximal response has reached a limiting value.

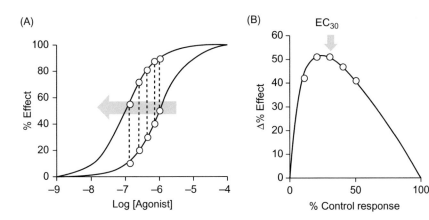

FIGURE 7.27 **Optimal levels of agonist response to view PAM effects.** It can be seen that for a PAM that produces a 20-fold sensitization to the agonist (panel A), the largest window to observe potentiation is seen at pre-existing agonist levels producing 30%; this window is not dependent upon the maximal effect of the PAM but is true for all PAM effects.

maximal response but rather as a shift to the left of the concentration-response curve with no change in maximum — see Figure 7.26. An optimal assay system has the target maximal response to be less than the system maximal response so that positive β values would be differentiated from positive α values.

Because the activity of allosteric modulators depends upon co-binding ligands, many modulator assays are conducted in the presence of a low concentration of co-binding ligand, i.e., agonist. In view of the known probe dependence of allosterism (i.e., a modulator can produce quite different effects with different co-binding ligands), it is essential that therapeutic modulators be tested with the endogenous, naturally-occurring agonist. The main assays for PAM discovery and characterization involve

the assessment of agonist sensitivity; to do this, a probe concentration of agonist must be chosen to give the optimal sensitivity to PAM activity. As shown in Figure 7.27, a concentration of agonist producing approximately 30% maximum offers the largest window to see PAM effects.

At this point it is worth considering an extremely useful PAM assay, namely the EC_{30}-sensitization assay. Here, the PAM effects are assessed by testing a range of modulator concentrations in a system with a pre-existing EC_{30} response of the agonist; increases in this activity reflect either direct modulator agonism, or PAM activity, or both — see Figure 7.28. The EC_{30}-PAM curve is very instructional as it can quantify the potency and maximal effect of a PAM. An equation for this curve can be

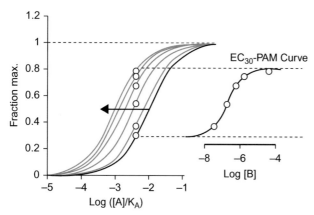

FIGURE 7.28 Potentiation of a pre-exisiting agonist response level of 30% by various concentrations of a PAM that produces a maximal sensitization of the agonist concentration-response curve to the agonist of 20-fold. The curve to the right inset is the concentration-response curve to the PAM as it produces sensitization to the agonist. This curve is a rapidly determined representation of the PAM effect with a location parameter (termed the AC_{50}) reflecting K_B, α and β (see Equation 7.11) and the maximal response reflecting aspects of α and β.

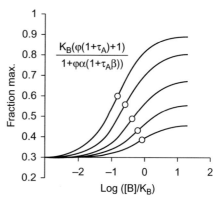

FIGURE 7.29 PAM concentration-response curves for potentiation of agonist EC_{30} effects for PAMs of varying maximal effects on agonist affinity. Shown are curves (from minimum effect to maximum) of $\alpha = 2,3,5,10$ and 20. The location parameter of the curves (AC_{50}) reflect the ability of the PAM to potentiate agonist response.

derived to illustrate this. First, the $[A]/K_A$ value for the level of basal agonism is derived where R = fraction of basal endogenous agonism. The $[A]/K_A$ value is:

$$\varphi = \frac{R}{\tau_A(1-R)-R} \quad (7.9a)$$

Substituting $[A]/K_A$ for φ, reformatting Equation 7.3 and solving for response in terms of [B] yields:

$$\text{Response} = \frac{[B]/K_B(\tau_B + \varphi\tau_A\alpha\beta)}{[B]/K_B(1+\tau_B+\varphi\alpha(1+\tau_A\beta))+\varphi(1+\tau_A)+1} \quad (7.10)$$

Equation 7.10 can be used to calculate the response to the agonist in the presence of a range of concentrations of PAMs (where $\tau_B = 0$) or PAM-agonists (where $\tau_B \neq 0$) concentrations; a sigmoidal curve is predicted — see Figure 7.29 for a PAM ($\tau_B = 0$). It can be seen from the curves shown in Figure 7.29 that the sensitivity and maximal response to PAM activity increases with the magnitude of α making the PAM-EC_{30} curve a useful index of PAM activity.

The midpoint of the EC_{30}-PAM curve (referred to as a log value of pAC_{50}) is given by:

$$pAC_{50} = \text{Log}\left[\frac{K_B(\varphi(1+\tau A)+1)}{1+\tau_B+\varphi\alpha(1+\tau_A\beta)}\right] \quad (7.11)$$

It can be seen from Equation 7.11 that the potency of a PAM producing sensitization to the agonist in an EC_{30}-PAM is dependent upon α, β and K_B and thus gives a good first estimate of PAM activity with a minimal array of concentrations. In addition, if it is known that the maximal effect of the endogenous agonist is less than the system maximum (i.e., a given target elevates cyclic AMP, and the

maximal stimulation of the target by a full agonist is below what the assay yields for forskolin), then the effects of the PAM can be tested on an EC_{100} concentration of agonist to determine the possible effects of β elevation.

In general, a logical scheme for the assessment of allosteric function can be derived which identifies the important properties of potential allosteric modulators, namely α, β, K_B and τ_B. Assuming that the initial screen for new molecules utilizes a functional system with a low level of endogenous agonism present (i.e., a one-shot EC_{30} assay), Figure 7.30 shows one example of a potentially useful approach to the quantification of all allosteric modulator activity.

7.4.6 Optimal Assays for Allosteric Function

There are some general predictions that can be made from the models and equations utilized to describe allosteric function. One is that the τ_A for the probe agonist is not necessarily relevant, i.e., the maximal effect of PAMs and NAMs will not be affected by the magnitude of the receptor reserve of the probe agonist. However, using systems where the probe agonist is a partial agonist (or at least where the E_m of the system is greater than the maximal response of the receptor target — see Figure 7.26) offers a unique capability to differentiate β from α effects. This can be useful, since the dependence of an allosteric activity on α as opposed to β can be therapeutically relevant. For the potentiation of failing physiological responses, it should be noted that potentiation of agonism through increased affinity ($\alpha > 1$) will only increase the sensitivity of the system to the existing level of endogenous agonism; if this is too low to be of physiological significance to begin with, then the modulator will not improve the situation. However, if efficacy is increased ($\beta > 1$), there is the potential to create a signal

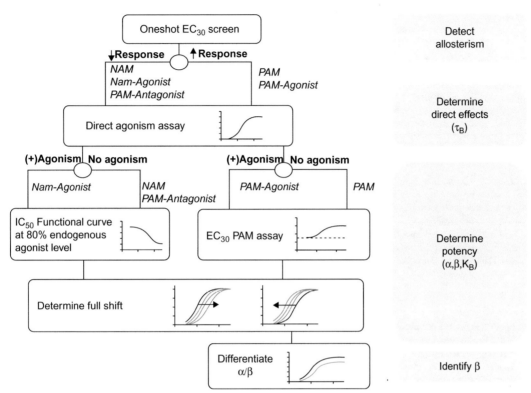

FIGURE 7.30 General scheme for quantifying allosteric effects to identify the five major allosteric phenotype molecules (see Section 7.4.1).   The major steps include determination of a direct agonist effect, identification of effect on agonist response (sensitization or antagonism) and quantification of the maximal parameters (α,β) and their relationship to the potency of the modulator (K_B). If the appropriate system is available, determination of the separate effects of the modulator on affinity and efficacy of the agonist can be done.

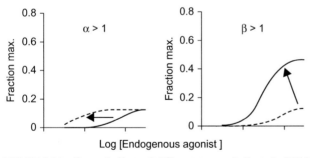

FIGURE 7.31 General effects of different types of allosteric PAM effects on agonist response. PAM effects based on increased α (affinity) will only make pre-existing agonism occur at lower levels of stimulation but will not increase maximal response; this will only be seen with changes in β.

where there was none, and thus correct pathologically low levels of endogenous signaling (see Figure 7.31).

Since allosteric molecules are permissive (i.e., there is the potential that the endogenous signal may still be physiologically present) there is always the possibility that the modulator will affect the nature of the endogenous signal. In cases where the endogenous signal involves the activation of pleiotropic cellular signaling cascades, there is the possibility, just as with the production of biased agonism (see Section 5.7 of Chapter 5)

with direct allosteric agonists, that a modulator will create bias in the endogenous agonist signal. This has been shown for PAMs (NOVO potentiation of GLP-1 [33]) and NAMs (LP1805 blockade of neurokinin A; [50] and AMD3100 blockade of SDF-1α analogs [39], Indole1 blockade of PGD2 [51]). For this reason, PAM and NAM effects must be verified for the therapeutically relevant signaling pathway.

7.5 METHODS FOR DETECTING ALLOSTERISM

Under certain conditions, allosteric modulators can behave identically to orthosteric ligands. For example, a modulator antagonist with $\alpha < 0.03$ for a number of agonists produces apparent nonspecific simple competitive antagonism within a limited concentration range. However, it can be seen from Section 7.3 that allosteric modulators possess a number of unique properties, making them different from orthosteric ligands (see also Table 7.2). For this reason it is important to differentiate allosteric from orthosteric ligands. The major approaches to doing so involve the properties of *saturability of effect* and *probe dependence* for antagonists and *loss of sensitivity to classical antagonists* for agonists.

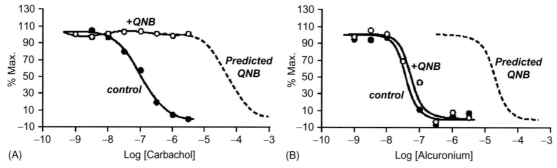

FIGURE 7.32 **Ligand-target validation.** Lack of sensitivity of putative agonist effect to classical receptor antagonists. (A) Inhibition of cyclic AMP due to activation of muscarinic m2 receptors by the classical muscarinic agonist carbachol in the absence (filled circles) and presence (open circles) of the classical muscarinic antagonist QNB present in a concentration that shifts the agonist curve to the location shown by the dotted line. This concentration of QNB completely blocks the response. (B) Inhibition of cyclic AMP through activation of muscarinic m2 receptors by the allosteric agonist alcuronium in the absence (filled circles) and presence (open circles) of the same concentration of QNB. In this case, the response is insensitive to this concentration of the antagonist. Data redrawn from [52].

FIGURE 7.33 **Schild regression for allosteric modulator of $K_B = 200$ nM that has $\alpha = 0.03$ for the agonist.** It can be seen that the regression is linear with unit slope at dose ratios < 10. However, extension of concentrations greater than 300 nM reveal saturation of the antagonism and a curvilinear portion of the Schild regression (indicative of allosteric antagonism).

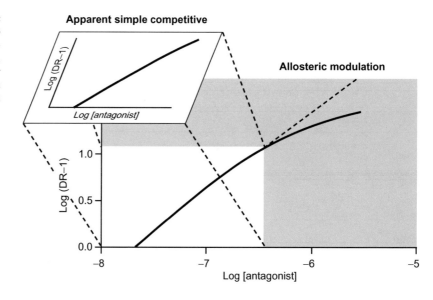

Beginning with agonists, the usual method of determining the identity of the biological target for an agonist is to block the effect with antagonists for that same target (receptor). However, if an agonist produces its effect through binding to a site separate from the one bound by the antagonist, the responses may not be sensitive to antagonism. For example, the classical muscarinic receptor agonist carbachol produces inhibition of cyclic AMP responses due to activation of muscarinic m2 receptors. The effect is blocked by the classical muscarinic receptor antagonist QNB (Figure 7.32A). However, the muscarinic m2 allosteric agonist alcuronium also activates the receptor but the effects are totally impervious to QNB (Figure 7.32B) [52]. In this circumstance, the criterion of blockade by a classical receptor antagonist is not met.

Modulators can be classified as potentiators of effect or antagonists. If potentiation is observed, it is clearly an allosteric effect, as orthosteric obfuscation of the agonist binding site cannot lead to potentiation of agonism. Antagonism can be unclear, therefore the concepts of saturability of effect and probe dependence may need to be actively pursued to tease out allosteric mechanisms. If a clear plateau of effect is observed, then allosterism is implicated (see Figure 7.24B). If an allosteric antagonism does not interfere with receptor function, then surmountable antagonism will be observed (Equation 7.3 when $\beta = 1$). A limited Schild analysis may not detect the characteristic curvilinearity of allosteric blockade (Figure 7.20). Therefore, detection of possible allosterism requires extension of normal concentration ranges for testing of blockade (see Figure 7.33).

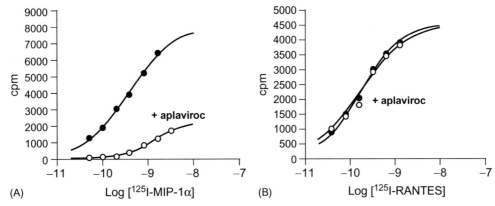

FIGURE 7.34 Effects of aplaviroc, an allosteric modulator of the CCR5 receptor, on the binding of the chemokine ^{125}I-MIP-1α (panel A) and ^{125}I-RANTES (panel B). It can be seen that aplaviroc blocks the binding of MIP-1α but has very little effect on the binding of RANTES. Such probe dependence is indicative of allosteric effect. Data from [9].

Differentiation of orthosterism and allosterism also can be made by using different receptor probes. For orthosteric antagonists, the choice of agonist is immaterial (i.e., the same pK_B will result; see Figure 12.21). However, this is not true of an allosteric effect where α and β values may be unique for every receptor probe. This is a logical consequence of the allosteric model in which it can be seen that mathematical terms exist containing the concentration of the antagonist, the α and β values for allosterism and the concentration of agonist ([A]/K_A $\tau\alpha\beta$[B]/K_B term in both the numerator and denominator of Equation 7.3). This allows the magnitude of both α and β to moderate the degree of antagonism. Since these constants are unique for every receptor probe, then the antagonism may also depend on the nature of the receptor probe (agonist). Figure 7.34 shows probe dependence on the CCR5 receptor with the allosteric modulator aplaviroc. It can be seen that the affinity of ^{125}I-MIP-1α is decreased considerably ($\alpha < 0.03$) while the affinity for ^{125}I-RANTES is unchanged (α estimated to be 0.8 [9]).

7.6 CHAPTER SUMMARY AND CONCLUSIONS

- Allosteric modulators affect the interaction of the receptor and probe molecules (i.e., agonists or radioligands) by binding to separate sites on the receptor. These effects are transmitted through changes in the receptor protein.
- Allosteric modulators possess properties different from orthosteric ligands. Specifically, allosteric effects are saturable and probe dependent (i.e., the modulator may produce different effects for different probes). Saturation occurs because allosteric effects reach an asymptote when the allosteric site is fully occupied. For this reason full shift assays are required to determine the maximal values of α and/or β.
- Allosteric effects can result in changes in affinity and/or efficacy of agonists.
- Sole effects on affinity (with no change in receptor function) result in surmountable antagonism. The dextral displacement reaches a maximal value leading to a curvilinear Schild regression.
- Allosteric modulators that block receptor function can produce insurmountable antagonism. In addition, modulators that block function also can alter (increase or decrease) affinity.
- Allosteric modulators can also potentiate agonist response (positive allosteric modulators, PAMs); this can result in a shift in the agonist concentration-response curve through increased affinity or increased agonist efficacy.
- Direct allosteric agonism can be quantified with the Black/Leff operational model and possible signaling bias should be explored.
- The observed potency of antagonists is modified by co-binding ligand activity to only a modest extent thus observed K_B values in functional or even binding assays are reasonable estimates of antagonist potency; this is not the case with PAMs.
- PAM effects through alteration of affinity (α) and efficacy (β) differ physiologically and this may be relevant to target therapeutic value.
- Both PAMs and NAMs may alter the quality of the endogenous signal by inducing bias therefore therapeutic relevance of the effect should be verified.

7.7 DERIVATIONS

- Allosteric model of receptor activity (7.7.1).
- Effects of allosteric ligands on response: changing efficacy (7.7.2).
- Schild analysis for allosteric antagonists (7.7.3).

7.7.1 Allosteric Model of Receptor Activity

Consider two ligands ([A] and [B]), each with its own binding site on the receptor with equilibrium association constants for receptor complexes of K_a and K_b, respectively. The binding of either ligand to the receptor modifies the affinity of the receptor for the other ligand by a factor α. There can be three ligand-bound receptor species; namely, [AR], [BR], and [ARB]:

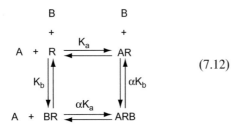

$$(7.12)$$

The resulting equilibrium equations are:

$$K_a = [AR]/[A][R], \tag{7.13}$$

$$K_b = [BR]/[B][R], \tag{7.14}$$

$$\alpha K = [ARB]/[BR][A], \text{ and} \tag{7.15}$$

$$\alpha K_b = [ARB]/[AR][B]. \tag{7.16}$$

Solving for the agonist-bound receptor species [AR] and [ARB] as a function of the total receptor species ([R_{tot}] = [R] + [AR] + [BR] + [ARB]) yields:

$$\frac{[AR] + [ARB]}{R_{tot}} = \frac{((1/\alpha[B]K_b) + 1)}{((1/\alpha[B]K_b) + (1/\alpha K_a) + (1/\alpha[A]K_aK_b) + 1)}. \tag{7.17}$$

Simplifying and changing association to dissociation constants (i.e., $K_A = 1/K_a$) yields:

$$\rho = \frac{[A]/K_A(1 + \alpha[B]/K_B)}{[A]/K_A(1 + \alpha[B]/K_B + [B]/K_B + 1)}. \tag{7.18}$$

7.7.2 Effects of Allosteric Ligands on Response: Changing Efficacy

The receptor can bind both the probe (agonist, radioligand, [A]) and allosteric modulator ([B]). The agonist-bound receptor signal through the normal operational model ([AR] complex interacting with cellular stimulus-response machinery with association constant K_e) and in a possibly different manner when the allosteric modulator is bound (complex [ABR] interacting with cell with association constant K_E'):

$$(7.19)$$

The equilibrium species are:

$$[AR] = [ABR]/\alpha[B]K_b, \tag{7.20}$$

$$[BR] = [ABR]/\alpha[A]K_\alpha, \text{ and} \tag{7.21}$$

$$[R] = [ABR]/\alpha[B]K_b[B]K_b. \tag{7.22}$$

The receptor conservation equation for total receptor [R_t] is:

$$[R_t] = [R] + [AR] + [BR] + [ABR] \tag{7.23}$$

The potential response producing species are [AR], [BR] and [ABR], therefore the fraction of receptors that may produce response is given by:

$$\rho_{A/B/AB} = \frac{[A]/K_A + [B]/K_B + \alpha[A]/K_A[B]/K_B}{[A]/K_A(1 + \alpha[B]/K_B) + [B]/K_B + 1} \tag{7.24}$$

where $K_A = 1/K_a$ and $K_B = 1/K_b$.

According to the operational model, response is given by the fractional receptor species interacting with a common pool of cellular effector (maximal effector = E_m):

$$\text{Response} = \frac{([AR]/K_E + [BR]K_E'' + [ABR]/K_E')E_m}{[AR]/K_E + [BR]K_E'' + [ABR]/K_E' + 1} \tag{7.25}$$

where K_E, K_E' and K_E'' are the operational equilibrium dissociation constants of the receptor species-cellular effector complexes.

The actual amount of receptor species (e.g., [AR]) is given by the fraction of receptor species mulitplied by the total number of receptors ($\rho_A = [AR]/[R_t]$) and defines the fractional response (ρ_{Res}) as:

$$\rho_{Res} = \frac{\rho_A[R_t]/K_E + \rho_B[R_t]/K_E'' + \rho_{AB}[R_t]/K_E'}{\rho_A[R_t]/K_E + \rho_B[R_t]/K_E'' + \rho_{AB}[R_t]/K_E' + 1} \tag{7.26}$$

Defining τ_A as [R_t]/K_E, τ_B as [R_t]/K_E'' and τ_{AB} as [R_t]/K_E' allows expression of Equation 7.26 as:

$$\rho_{Res} = \frac{\rho_A\tau_A + \rho_B\tau_B + \rho_{AB}\tau_{AB}}{\rho_A\tau_A + \rho_B\tau_B + \rho_{AB}\tau_{AB} + 1} \tag{7.27}$$

Further defining τ_{AB}/τ_A as β yields:

Response =

$$\frac{\tau_A[A]/K_A(1+\alpha\beta[B]/K_B)+\tau_B[B]/K_B}{[A]/K_A(1+\alpha[B]/K_B+\tau_A(1+\alpha\beta[B]/K_B))+[B]/K_B(1+\tau_B)+1}$$

$$(7.28)$$

7.7.3 Schild Analysis for Allosteric Antagonists

From Equation 7.3, the observed EC_{50} for the agonist, in the presence of a concentration of allosteric antagonist [B], is given by:

$$EC_{50}' = \frac{EC_{50}([B]/K_B + 1)}{(1 + \alpha[B]/K_B)}, \qquad (7.29)$$

where EC_{50} refers to the EC_{50} of the control concentration-response curve in the absence of modulator. The ratio of the EC_{50} values (concentrations of agonist producing 50% response in the presence and absence of the allosteric antagonist) is given by

$$\frac{EC_{50}'}{EC_{50}} = DR = \frac{([B]/K_B + 1)}{(1 + \alpha[B]/K_B)}. \qquad (7.30)$$

This leads to the logarithmic metameter form of the Schild equation:

$$Log(DR - 1) = Log\left[\frac{[B](1-\alpha)}{\alpha[B] + K_B}\right]. \qquad (7.31)$$

REFERENCES

[1] Jakubic J, Bacakova I, El-Fakahany EE, Tucek S. Positive cooperativity of acetylcholine and other agonists with allosteric ligands on muscarinic acetylcholine receptors. Mol Pharmacol 1997;52:172−9.

[2] Koshland DE. The active site of enzyme action. Adv Enzymol 1960;22:45−97.

[3] Lee NH, Hu J, El-Fakahany EE. Modulation by certain conserved aspartate residues of the allosteric interaction of gallamine and the ml muscarinic receptor. J Pharmacol Exp Ther 1992;262:312−6.

[4] Smerdon SJ, Jager J, Wang J, Kohlstaedt LA, Chirino AJ, Friedman JM, et al. Structure of the binding site for non-nucleoside inhibitors of the reverse transcriptase of human immunodeficiency virus type 1. Proc Natl Acad Sci U S A 1994;91:3911−5.

[5] Horn JR, Shoichet BK. Allosteric inhibition through core disruption. J Mol Biol 2004;336:1283−91.

[6] Oikonomakos NG, Skamnaki VT, Tsitsanou KE, Gavalas NG, Johnson L. A new allosteric site in glycogen phosphorylase b as a target for drug interactions. Structure 2000;8:575−84.

[7] Arkin MR, Wells JA. Small-molecule inhibitors of protein-protein interactions: progressing towards the dream. Nature Rev Drug Disc 2004;3:301−17.

[8] Teague SJ. Implications of protein flexibility for drug discovery. Nat Rev Drug Disc 2003;2:527−41.

[9] Watson C, Jenkinson S, Kazmierski W, Kenakin TP. The CCR5 receptor-based mechanism of action of 873140, a potent allosteric non-competitive HIV entry-inhibitor. Mol Pharmacol 2005;67:1268−82.

[10] Tong C, Churchill L, Cirillo PF, Gilmore T, Graham AG, Grob PM, et al. Inhibition of p38 MAP kinase by utilizing a novel allosteric binding site. Nat Struct Mol Biol 2002;9:268−72.

[11] Bieniassz PD, Fridell RA, Aramori I, Ferguson SS, Caron MG, Cullen BR. HIV-1 induced cell fusion is mediated by multiple regions within both the viral envelope and the CCR-5 co-receptor. EMBO J 1997;16:2599−609.

[12] Kwong PD, Wyatt R, Robinson J, Sweet RW, Sodroski J, Hendricks WA. Structure of an HIV gp120 envelope glycoprotein in complex with the CD4 receptor and a neutralizing human antibody. Nature 1998;393:648−59.

[13] Doranz BJ, Lu Z-H, Rucker J, Zhang T-Y, Sharron M, Cen Y-H, et al. Two distinct CCR5 domains can mediate coreceptor usage by human immunodeficiency virus type 1. J Virol 1997;71:6305−14.

[14] Flicker L. Acetylcholinesterase inhibitors for Alzheimer's disease. Br Med J 1999;318:615−6.

[15] Maelicke A, Albuquerque EX. New approach to drug therapy of Alzheimer's dementia. Drug Disc Today 1996;1:53−9.

[16] Krause RM, Buisson B, Bertrand S, Corringer P-J, Galzi J-L, Changeux J-P, et al. Ivermectin: a positive allosteric effector of the a7 neuronal nicotinic acetylcholine receptor. Mol Pharmacol 1998;53:283−94.

[17] Poignard P, Saphire EO, Parren PW, Burton DR. gp120: biologic aspects of structural features. Annu Rev Immunol 2001;19:253−74.

[18] Wyatt R, Sodroski J. The HIV-1 envelope glycoproteins: fusogens, antigens, and immunogens. Science 1998;280:1884−8.

[19] Trkola A, Kuhmann SE, Strizki JM, Maxwell E, Ketas T, Morgan T, et al. HIV-1 escape from a small molecule, CCR5-specific entry inhibitor does not involve CXCR4 use. Proc Natl Acad Sci U S A 2002;99:395−400.

[20] Korber BT, Wolinsky SM, Moore JP, Kuhmann SE, Pugach P, Kunstman KJ, et al. Genetic and phenotypic analyses of human immunodeficiency virus type 1 escape from small-molecule CCR inhibitor. J Virol 2004;78:2790−807.

[21] Maeda K, Nakata H, Koh Y, Miyakawa T, Ogata H, Takaoka Y, et al. Spirodiketopiperazine-based CCR5 inhibitor which preserves CC-chemokine/CCR5 interactions and exerts potent activity against R5 human immunodeficiency virus type 1 in vitro. J Virol 2004;78:8654−62.

[22] Watson C, Jenkinson S, Kazmierski W, Kenakin TP. The CCR5 Receptor-based mechanism of action of 873140, a potent allosteric non-competitive HIV entry-inhibitor. Mol Pharmacol 2005;67:1268−82.

[23] Litschig S, Gasparini F, Ruegg DF, Stoehr N, Flor PJ, Vranesic I, et al. CPCCOEt, a noncompetitive metabotropic glutamate receptor 1 antagonist, inhibits receptor signaling without affecting glutamate binding. Mol Pharmacol 1999;55:453−61.

[24] Trankle C, Weyand A, Schroter A, Mohr K. Using a radioalloster to test predictions of the cooperativity model for gallamine binding to the allosteric site of muscarinic acetylcholine (m2) receptors. Mol Pharmacol 1999;56:962−5.

[25] Kew JNC, Trube G, Kemp JA. A novel mechanism of activity-dependent NMDA receptor antagonism describes the effect of ifenprodil in rat cultured cortical neurons. J Physiol 1996;497(Pt 3):761−72.

[26] Price MR, Baillie GL, Thomas A, Stevenson LA, Easson M, Goodwin R, et al. Allosteric modulation of the cannabinoid CB1 receptor. Mol Pharm 2005;68:1484–95.

[27] Tucek S, Proska J. Allosteric modulation of muscarinic acetylcholine receptors. Trends Pharmacol Sci 1995;16:205–12.

[28] Ellis J, Huyler J, Brann MR. Allosteric regulation of cloned M1-M5 muscarinic receptor subtypes. Biochem Pharmacol 1991;42:1927–32.

[29] Liang JS, Carsi-Gabrenas J, Krajesewski JL, McCafferty JM, Parkerson SL, Santiago MP, et al. Anti-muscarinic toxins from dendroaspis angusticeps. Toxicon 1996;34:1257–67.

[30] Gnagey AL, Seidenberg M, Ellis J. Site-directed mutagenesis reveals two epitopes involved in the subtype selectivity of the allosteric interactions of gallamine at muscarinic acetylcholine receptors. Mol Pharmacol 1999;56:1245–53.

[31] Johnson MP, Nisenbaum ES, Large TH, Emkey R, Baez M, Kingston AE. Allosteric modulators of metabotropic glutamate receptors: lessons learnt from mGlu1, mGlu2, and mGlu5 potentiators and agonists. Biochem Soc Trans 2004;32:881–7.

[32] Suratman S, Leach K, Sexton PM, Felder CC, Loiacono RE, Christopoulos A. Impact of species variability and "probe-dependence" on the detection and *in vivo* validation of allosteric modulation at the M4 muscarinic acetylcholine receptor. Br J Pharmacol 2011;162:1659–70.

[33] Koole C, Wooten D, Simms J, Valant C, Sridhar R, Woodman OL, et al. Allosteric ligands of the glucagon-like peptide 1 receptor (GLP-1R) differentially modulate endogenous and exogenous peptide responses in a pathway-selective manner: implications for drug screening. Mol Pharmacol 2010;78:456–65.

[34] Muniz-Medina VM, Jones S, Maglich JM, Galardi C, Hollingsworth RE, Kazmierski WM, et al. The relative activity of 'function sparing' HIV-1 entry inhibitors on viral entry and CCR5 internalization: is allosteric functional selectivity a valuable therapeutic property?. Mol Pharmacol 2009;75:490–501.

[35] Gonzalez E, Kulkarni H, Bolivar H, Mangano A, Sanchez R, et al. The influence of CCL3L1 gene-containing segmental duplications on HIV-1/AIDS susceptibility. Science 2005;307:1434–40.

[36] Nagasaw T, Hirota S, Tachibana K, Takakura N, Nishikawa S, Kitamura Y, et al. Defects of B-cell lymphopoiesis and bone-marrow myelopoiesis in mice lacking the CXC chemokine PBSF/SDF-1. Nature 1996;382:635–8.

[37] Tachibana K, Hirota S, Iizasa H, Yoshida H, Kawabata K, Kataoka Y, et al. The chemokine receptor CXCR4 is essential for vascularization of the gastrointestinal tract. Nature 1998;393:591–4.

[38] Zou YR, Kottmann AH, Kuroda M, Taniuchi I, Littman DR. Function of the chemokine receptor CXCR4 in haematopoiesis and in cerebellar development. Nature 1998;393:595–9.

[39] Sachpatzidis A, Benton BK, Manfredis JP, Wang H, Hamilton A, Dohlman HG, et al. Indentification of allosteric peptide agonists of CXCR4. J Biol Chem 2003;278:896–907.

[40] Heveker N, Montes M, Germeroth L, Amara A, Trautmann A, Alizon M, et al. Dissociation of the signaling and antiviral properties of SDF-1-derived small peptides. Curr Biol 1998;8:369–76.

[41] Stockton JM, Birdsall NJM, Burgen ASV, Hulme EC. Modification of the binding properties of muscarinic receptors by gallamine. Mol Pharmacol 1983;23:551–7.

[42] Ehlert FJ. Estimation of the affinities of allosteric ligands using radioligand binding and pharmacological null methods. Mol Pharmacol 1988;33:187–94.

[43] Black JW, Leff P, Shankley NP, Wood J. An operational model of pharmacological agonism: the effect of E/[A] curve shape on agonist dissociation constant estimation. Br J Pharmacol 1985;84:561–71.

[44] Kenakin TP. New concepts in durg discovery: collateral efficacy and permissive antagonism. Nat Rev Durg Disc 2005;4:919–27.

[45] Ehlert FJ. Analysis of allosterism in functional assays. J Pharmacol Exp Ther 2005;315:740–54.

[46] Kenakin TP. Allosteric agonist modulators. J Recept Signal Transd 2007;27:247–59.

[47] Kenakin TP. Biased signaling and allosteric machines: new vistas and challenges for drug discovery. Br J Pharmacol 2012;165:1659–69.

[48] Gregory KJ, Hall NE, Tobin AB, Sexton PM, Christopoulos A. Identification of orthosteric and allosteric site mutations in M2 muscarinic acetylcholine receptors that contribute to ligand-selective signaling bias. J Biol Chem 2010;285:7459–74.

[49] Gaddum JH, Hameed KA, Hathway DE, Stephens FF. Quantitative studies of antagonists for 5-hydroxytryptamine. Q J Exp Physiol 1955;40:49–74.

[50] Maillet EL, Pellegrini N, Valant C, Bucher B, Hibert M, Bourguignon J-J, et al. A novel, conformation-specific allosteric inhibitor of the tachykinin NK2 receptor (NK2R) with functionally selective properties. FASEB J 2007;21:2124–34.

[51] Mathiesen JM, Ulven T, Martini L, Gerlach LO, Heineman A, Kostenis E. Identification of indole derivatives exclusively interfering with a G protein-independent signaling pathway of the prostaglandin D2 receptor CRTH2. Mol Pharmacol 2005;68:393–402.

[52] Jakubic J, Bacakova L, Lisá V, El-Fakahany EE, Tucek S. Activation of muscarinic acetylcholine receptors via their allosteric binding sites. Proc Natl Acad Sci U S A 1996;93:8705–9.

Chapter 8

The Optimal Design of Pharmacological Experiments

We become what we behold. We shape our tools and then our tools shape us.

— Marshall McLuhan (1911–1980)

No amount of experimentation can ever prove me right; a single experiment can prove me wrong.

— Albert Einstein (1879–1955)

...The prismatic qualities of the assay distort our view in obscure ways and degrees...

— James W. Black (1924–2010), Nobel Lectures: Physiology and Medicine

8.1   Introduction
8.2   The Optimal Design of Pharmacological Experiments
8.3   Null Experiments and Fitting Data to Models
8.4   Interpretation of Experimental Data
8.5   Predicting Therapeutic Activity in All Systems
8.6   Summary and Conclusions
8.7   Derivations
      References

8.1 INTRODUCTION

Pharmacology is unique in that it encompasses the methodology to convert descriptive data on drug effect (observed potency and activity in a given system) to predictive data (parameters that can be used to predict drug activity in all systems). This is done through a combination of the application of null experiments and the comparison of data to mathematical models. There are pharmacological tools and techniques designed to determine system-independent measures of the potency and efficacy of drugs; however, in order to apply them effectively, the molecular mechanism of the drug must be known beforehand. In new drug discovery, this is seldom the case, and in fact the observed profile of the molecules must be used to discern their molecular mechanism. In this setting, it is not always possible to apply the correct technique or model for quantification of drug activity, and the tool chosen for analysis is based on initial observation of drug activity; that is, the process is data driven.

In practical terms, a wide range of potential drug behaviors can be described by a limited number of molecular models, and it is useful to describe these and their application in the drug discovery process. In general, drugs can be divided into two initial types: those that do and those that do not initiate a directly observable pharmacological response in the tissue.

8.2 THE OPTIMAL DESIGN OF PHARMACOLOGICAL EXPERIMENTS

As discussed in Chapter 1, pharmacology is a unique discipline, in that it can interpret the behavior of molecules in different physiological systems in terms of the molecular properties of those molecules. This process can be divided into four parts:

1. **Defining the experiment:** The main objective of pharmacological experiments is to quantify the

T. P. Kenakin: A Pharmacology Primer, Fourth edition. DOI: http://dx.doi.org/10.1016/B978-0-12-407663-1.00008-9
© 2014 Elsevier Inc. All rights reserved.

molecular properties of drugs in a system-independent manner to in turn derive parameters that can be used to predict drug activity in all systems. The four minimal properties that allow characterization of all pharmacodynamic activities are [1]:

a. Drug efficacy (or efficacies) — the property of the molecule that causes the pharmacological target to change its behavior toward the cell.

b. Drug affinity: the concentrations at which the molecule binds to and stays associated with the target.

c. Whether the molecule interacts with the target in an orthosteric (same binding site as the endogenous activator of the target) or allosteric (separate site) manner.

d. Dissociation kinetics of the molecule to determine target coverage in open systems (i.e., *in vivo*).

2. **Conducting the experiment:** The application of null methods to isolate characteristic drug properties, as well as the comparison of data to pharmacological models to determine mechanism of action and system-independent parameters of drug activity.

3. **Interpretation of experimental data:** How do we gauge progress in terms of improvement of drug activity in the drug discovery and development process?

4. **Predicting drug activity in all (including the therapeutic) systems:** How do we apply the parameters quantifying drug activity to *in vivo* therapeutic systems to predict useful activity?

The first of these points to be discussed is the aim of the pharmacological experiment, namely the determination of parameters that can characterize drug activity in molecular terms.

8.2.1 Drug Efficacy

The first observable effect of a drug in a biological preparation is the initiation of some pharmacological effect (referred to as *response*). If this is seen, then it must be determined that it is specific for the biological target of interest (i.e., not a general nonspecific stimulation of the cell) and that a concentration-response relationship can be determined. Once activity for a given molecule has been confirmed by retest at a single concentration, a dose-response curve for the effect must be determined; the biological effect must be related to the concentration in a predictive manner.

A frequently asked question at this point is; does the array of responses for given concentrations represent a

true dose-response relationship, or just random noise around a given mean value? It is useful to demonstrate approaches to this question with an example. Assume that a compound is tested in dose-response mode, and 11 "responses" are obtained for 11 concentrations of compound giving a maximal ordinal response of 7.45%. On the one hand, it might not be expected that noise could present a sigmoid pattern indicative of a concentration-response curve (although such patterns might be associated with location on plates or counters). However, a maximal ordinate response of 7.45% also is extremely low. A useful rule of thumb is to set the criterion of $>3\sigma$ (where σ is the standard error of the mean) of basal noise responses as the definition of a real effect. In this case, the signal from 1325 wells (for the experiment run that same day; historical data should not be used) obtained in the presence of the lowest concentration of compound (10 μM, assumed to be equivalent to basal response) yielded a mean percent response of −0.151% with a standard deviation of 1.86%. Under these circumstances, $3\sigma = 5.58\%$. With this criterion, the response to the agonist would qualify as a signal above noise levels.

A pharmacological method for determining whether a very low level of response constitutes a real dose-response curve is to use a maximal concentration of the "very weak partial agonist" to block responses to a standard full agonist. The basis for this method is the premise that the EC_{50} of a weak partial agonist closely approximates its affinity for the receptor. For example, assume that a fit to the data points shows a partial agonist to have a maximal response value of 8% and EC_{50} of 3 μM. Under these circumstances, the dose-response curve to the standard agonist would be shifted ten fold to the right by 30 μM of the weak partial agonist. This could indicate that the 8% represents a true response to the compound. Also, it could furnish a lead antagonist series for the screening program. However, this method requires considerable follow-up work for each compound.

Another method of detecting a dose-response relationship is to fit the data to various models for dose-response curves. This method statistically determines whether or not a dose-response model (such as a logistic function) fits the data points more accurately than simply the mean of the values; this method is described fully in Chapter 12. The simplest approach would be to assume no dose-response relationship, and to calculate the mean of the ordinate data as the response for each concentration of ligand (horizontal straight line parallel to the abscissal axis). A more complex model would be to fit the data to a sigmoidal dose-response function. A sum of squares can be calculated for the simple model (response − mean of all response) and then for a fit of the data set refit to the four parameter logistic shown previously. A value for the F statistic can then be calculated, which determines whether there is a statistical basis for assuming there is a dose-response relationship. An example of this procedure is given in Chapter 12 (see Figure 12.13). The remainder of this discussion assumes that it has been determined that the drug in question produces a selective pharmacological response in a biological preparation that can be defined by a concentration-response curve, that is, it is an agonist. Once a target-related agonism has been determined, then this activity must be quantified and a structure-activity relationship for that activity determined.

A first step in this process is to compare the maximal response to the test agonist with the maximal response capability of the biological preparation. If there is no statistical difference between the maximal response of the agonist and to the maximal response of the tissue, then the drug is a full agonist. If the magnitude of the maximal response to the agonist is lower than that of the tissue, then the drug is a partial agonist. There is separate information that can be gained from either of these two categories of agonist, as discussed in Chapter 5.

It is useful to re-define what is meant by 'efficacy'. In light of the fact that receptors themselves can spontaneously form active states that impart a cellular response (see Chapter 3 Section 3.10), it is insufficient to label efficacy as the excitation of receptors to produce a response. Rather, efficacy is better defined as the property of a molecule that causes the target (receptor) to change its behavior toward the cell when the molecule is bound;

this includes negative efficacy as would be observed in an inverse agonist that reverses constitutive receptor activity. Historically, definitions of efficacy were hampered by the paucity of assay systems available to gauge the direct effect of drugs. Until as recently as 20 years ago, overt cellular response was used to assess drug effect. For example, the disappearance of response after chronic agonism was assumed to relate to the desensitization linking this process with agonism, i.e., intense activation of receptors was the impetus for internalization. However, the subsequent availability of imaging techniques measuring receptor internalization indicate that some antagonists that are devoid of direct stimulating properties can cause active internalization of receptors [2,3]. The mechanism responsible is postulated to be the stabilization of receptor conformations by these antagonists that are prone to phosphorylation and subsequent internalization.

The advent of an increasing number of assays to gauge receptor behavior has uncovered a range of different "efficacies" for drugs, and has also blurred the lines of taxonomy of drug classification [4]. In other words, the simple classes of agonist, antagonist, etc. do not fully describe drugs as they can have many efficacies that qualify for many different classifications. Figure 8.1 shows a schematic diagram of some of the known behaviors of receptors and also the phenotypic activities these behaviors can mediate. The fact that many biological targets

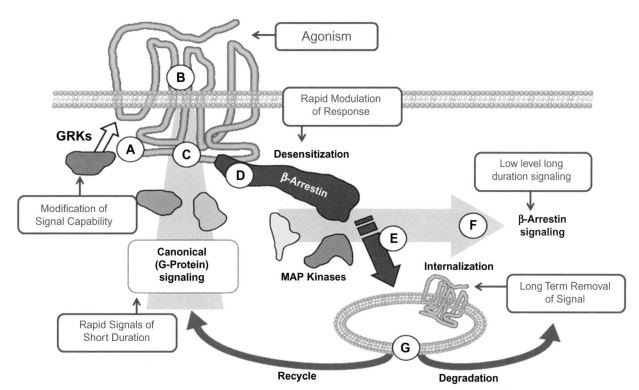

FIGURE 8.1 Various drug activities shown in red bordered rectangles caused by interference with various receptor activation and regulation mechanisms in the cell.

FIGURE 8.2 Of the 16 β-blockers that have been studied in clinical trials for treatment of congestive heart failure, three have been shown to have measurably favorable effects, with carvedilol emerging as the most efficacious. Carvedilol has a number of activities in addition to β-adrenoceptor affinity that may make it efficacious in the treatment of congestive heart failure. Data from [7].

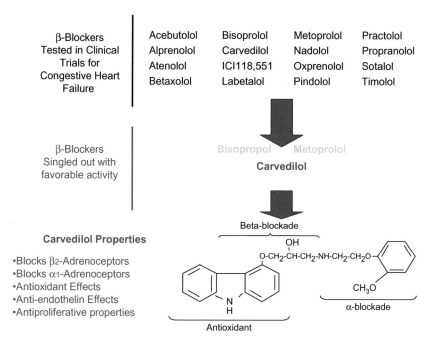

(i.e., receptors) control pleiotropic cellular signals raises the specter of multiple efficacies for a single molecule; these usually are related to the unique ensemble of receptor conformations stabilized by the molecule. Given the term "pluridimensional efficacy" [5], this property of drugs makes simple classification of efficacy difficult, i.e., a given molecule may be an agonist, antagonist, inverse agonist and/or bias agonist for a collection of pathways. For example, the cannabinoid ligand desacetyl-levonantradol is a positive agonist for CB1-mediated Gi1 and Gi2 activation but is an inverse agonist for Gi3 mediated effects [6].

The inability of simple labels to characterize drug activity is underscored by the many subclassifications of the general class of drugs known as β-blockers (antagonists of β-adrenoceptors – see Figure 2.23). In fact, one area where the secondary effects of drugs plays a prominent part is in cardiovascular drug studies for congestive heart failure [7]. There are theoretical reasons for supposing that β-blocking drugs may be of benefit in this area. Accordingly, a large number of these were tested in clinical trials and, interestingly, of 16 β-blockers tested, only three showed favorable outcome, with carvedilol emerging prominently [7] (see Figure 8.2). Interestingly, the unique combination of carvedilol activities (β- and α-blockade, antioxidant, antiendothelin, and antiproliferative effects) may be the discerning factor for utility in congestive heart failure. In accordance with the notion that disease is a complex system failure where numerous factors contribute to morbidity, the various properties of adrenoceptor-active ligands that may contribute negatively to treatment of congestive heart failure are listed in Table 8.1. In general, this underscores the fact that the

therapeutic value of a drug may be due to a constellation of efficacies, therefore these all should be explored. The increasing number of functional assays available through an increasing number of technological advances makes such efforts increasingly practical.

As discussed in Chapter 5, the Black/Leff operational model is used to quantify agonism and assigned efficacy (in the form of a parameter τ) and affinity (the term K_A) to agonists that can be used to predict agonism in other systems (*vide infra*) with the following equation [8]:

$$\text{Response} = \frac{[A]^n \tau^n E_m}{[A]^n \tau^n + ([A] + K_A)^n} \quad (8.1)$$

where n is the slope coefficient for the concentration-response curves and E_m is the maximal response capability of the system. It is essential to have independent knowledge of E_m; the n can be obtained from fitting the Hill equation to the data. The K_A is a very important parameter since it controls the value of τ given by the model; it is the equilibrium dissociation constant of the agonist-receptor complex which is roughly equal to the reciprocal of the agonist affinity. However, in terms of functional agonism and the use of this model, the K_A is specifically the concentration around where concentration-response curves collapse upon diminution of receptor density and/or reduction of signaling capability of the system (see Figure 8.3).

The K_A value (also referred to as the operational affinity) may or may not be the binding affinity measured in binding experiments so this should not be assumed. Ideally, this model should be fit to partial agonists where

TABLE 8.1 Potentially Deleterious Effects of Adrenergic Receptor Activity in Heart Failure and Cardiovascular Remodeling

Effect	β_1-Adrenoceptor Mediated	β_2-Adrenoceptor Mediated	α_1-Adrenoceptor Mediated
Positive inotropic	+ + +	+ +	+
Positive chronotropic	+ + +	+ +	0
Myocyte hypertrophy	+ + +	+	+ +
Fibroblast hyperplasia	+ + +	+	NA
Myocyte toxicity	+ + +	+	+
Myocyte apoptosis	+ +	−	−
Tachyarrhythmias	+ +	+ +	+
Vasoconstriction	0	−	+ +
Sodium retention	0	0	+ +
Renin secretion	+	0	0

+ = positive effect. − = negative effect. 0 = null effect. NA = not assessed.
From [7].

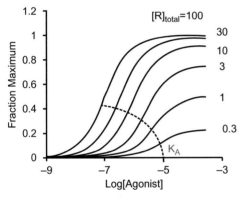

FIGURE 8.3 **The Black/Leff operational model utilizes the equilibrium dissociation constant of the agonist-receptor complex.** The model predicts that diminution of response capability (either through diminution of the receptor number or some other decrease in the translation of receptor-based stimulus into tissue response) will cause the concentration-response curves for the agonist to shift to the right until the concentrations of the agonist approach the K_A value. With further decrease in response capability the concentration-response curves will show depressed maxima with the EC_{50} values approximating the K_A value. The appropriate value for agonist affinity for any models utilizing the Black/Leff operational model for signaling must adhere to the requirement predicted for the K_A in the model shown above.

the K_A value closely approximates the EC_{50}; under these circumstances, there is no ambiguity about the K_A value. For full agonists, an infinite combination of τ and K_A values will fit a curve which is why τ/K_A ratios are used to quantify bias and receptor selectivity — see Chapter 5 Section 5.7.1. Under these circumstances, a value approximately $100\times$ the EC_{50} is routinely chosen as a starting value for the computer fit to Equation 8.1.

Efficacy has the dual properties of quantity and quality. Considering the quantity of efficacy first; this reflects the strength which a given molecule has to activate a given signaling pathway, and it is quantified as the magnitude of τ. In this regard, the receptor density of the tissue (e.g., cells) in a given functional assay can be extremely useful as a variable controlled by the experimenter. As shown in Figure 8.4, low receptor density preparations will allow facile quantification of agonist affinity (K_A) and in some cases also of τ through fitting to the operational model. Higher receptor density preparations can be used to detect efficacy and/or inverse agonism (see Figure 8.4). With regard to the magnitude of efficacy, it also is useful to determine whether the potency of the agonist is primarily due to high affinity or high efficacy, since these differences translate to how robust the agonism will be in tissues of varying sensitivity (see Chapter 5 Section 5.6.1). Figure 8.5 shows dose-response curves to two agonists for α-adrenoceptors in the rat anococcygeus muscle; oxymetazoline is an affinity-dominant agonist while norepinephrine is an efficacy-dominant agonist [9]. It can be seen that while oxymetazoline is more potent than norepinephrine in the native tissue, reduction in the sensitivity of the tissue through chemical alkylation of the receptors (reduction in receptor number) produces a disproportionate decrease in the response to the lower efficacy agonist (oxymetazoline). This would translate to a greater variability in the agonism to oxymetazoline (vs. norepinephrine) in various organ systems.

As well as the quantity of efficacy, agonists can also differ in the quality of efficacy they impart to cells if the

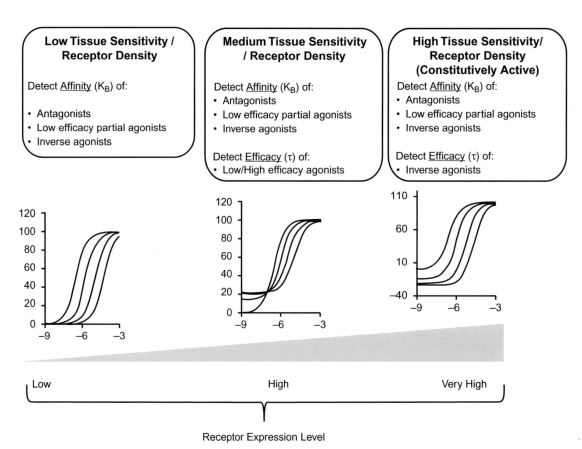

FIGURE 8.4 Effect of varying receptor density on detection capability of functional assays to characterize various types of pharmacologic ligand.

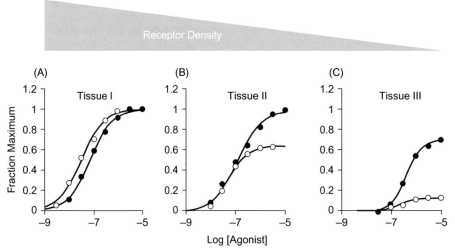

FIGURE 8.5 Rat anococcygeus muscle responses to oxymetazoline (open circles) and norepinephrine (filled circles).   Three separate tissue treatments are shown. (A) Control tissue. (B) Tissue treated with 30 nM α-adrenoceptor alkylating agent phenoxybenzamine for 10 min and then washed for 1 h with solution containing sodium thiosulfate to remove aziridinium ion and then 1 h with drug-free medium. (C) Tissue treated with a further 0.1 μM phenoxybenzamine for 10 min and then washed for 1 h with solution containing sodium thiosulfate to remove aziridinium ion and then 1 h with drug-free medium. Redrawn from [9].

receptor they activate interacts pleiotropically with multiple signaling systems. This mechanism is extensively described in the section on biased signaling (Section 5.7) and highlights the fact that it should not be assumed that new synthetic agonists will produce an identical signaling pattern to that of the natural endogenous agonist. The first requirement to quantify bias is to have the selective assays to characterize the various separate signaling pathways of

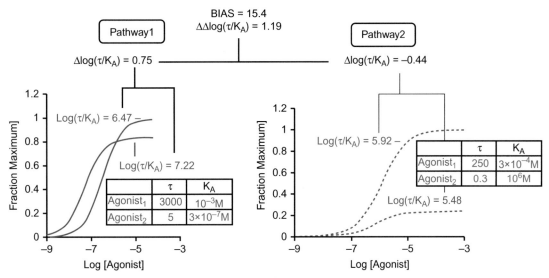

FIGURE 8.6 **The quantification of signaling bias using $\Delta\Delta\log(\tau/K_A)$ values.** Concentration-response curves for two agonists are obtained for each signaling pathway and the activity of each agonist in each pathway by fitting data with the Black/Leff operational model; a value for $\log(\tau/K_A)$ is determined for each curve in each pathway. A reference agonist is chosen and all other agonists compared to that reference through calculation of $\Delta\log(\tau/K_A)$ values for each pathway. Providing the same reference agonist is utilized for both pathways, $\Delta\Delta\log(\tau/K_A)$ values then provide an estimate of the relative activity of each pathway for activation of the various pathways, i.e., $\log(BIAS) = \Delta\Delta\log(\tau/K_A)$.

interest, eg., GTPγS for G-protein activation and BRET for β-arrestin association. Then τ and K_A values are calculated for each agonist *for each pathway* [10]; it cannot be assumed that a given agonist will have the same K_A value for activation of the two pathways [11]. The "power" of each agonist to activate each pathway is calculated as the ratio $\log(\tau/K_A)$. It is of paramount importance that all log (τ/K_A) estimates be expressed as a ratio to a reference agonist in each pathway, and that the reference must be the same for each pathway. Thus the transferrable value of relative agonism for each pathway is $\Delta\log(\tau/K_A)$ and the transferrable value for bias between pathways is $\Delta\Delta\log$ (τ/K_A); BIAS $= 10^{\Delta\Delta\log(\tau/KA)}$. This procedure cancels system and measurement bias always present due to the sensitivity of the assays and the intrinsic efficiency of each pathway in the cells. An example of this procedure is shown in Figure 8.6, where it is seen that although the agonist depicted in blue is 5.5-fold less active as an activator of pathway 1, it is 15-fold more biased for activation of pathway 1 over pathway 2. This underscores the independence of efficacy and bias; i.e., efficacy determines *if* agonism appears and bias determines *at what relative concentration* it appears when it does (between pathways).

Large scale fitting of the Black/Leff model to numerous concentration-response curves can be problematic for logistical reasons and there are circumstances where relative activity (RA) values, as defined by Ehlert [12], may suffice. The definition of RA is (maximal response/EC$_{50}$), a value that is amenable to estimation from concentration-response curve data; there are certain circumstances in which bias and receptor selectivity procedures may utilize $\Delta\log(RA)$

in the same manner as $\Delta\log(\tau/K_A)$. Thus RA values can be related to the Black/Leff operational model with the relationship [13] — see Chapter 5, Section 5.7:

$$RA = \frac{E_m(\tau^n(2+\tau^n)^{1/n} - 1)}{K_A(1 + \tau^n)} \qquad (8.2)$$

Thus, when the Hill coefficients of concentration-response curves are not significantly different from unity, it can be seen that $\Delta\log(RA) = \Delta\log(\tau/K_A)$. When $n \neq 1$, then there will be a variable error between $\log(RA)$ and the more correct $\Delta\log(\tau/K_A)$ values [10]. However, the magnitude of this error is relatively small and the use of RA values for early calculations on large data sets to identify compounds of interest may be an acceptable strategy.

A final measure of agonist value is its selectivity for the therapeutic target (over other receptors). Here transducer ratios ($\Delta\log(\tau/K_A)$ values) can be useful and offer an advantage of providing an insight that may add value to simple agonist potency ratio measurements — see Section 5.7.1. Specifically, a given agonist could have a favorable potency ratio over a secondary receptor in a sensitive tissue that may not transfer to less sensitive tissues if the therapeutic agonist selectivity depends primarily on affinity (vs. efficacy). However, since $\Delta\Delta\log(\tau/K_A)$ values take maximal response (as well as potency) into account, these may be more accurate for prediction of selectivity in a range of tissues. The procedure used for quantifying bias can also be used to quantify receptor selectivity; in this case, concentration-response curves for an agonist acting on two receptors are used instead of two pathways. As shown in Section 5.7.1, a selectivity index is obtained:

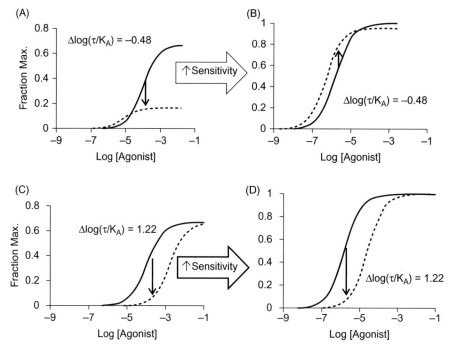

FIGURE 8.7 The use of $\Delta\log(\tau/K_A)$ values to provide predictive measures of receptor selectivity. For the agonist shown in panels A and B and another agonist shown in panels C and D, the relative capability to activate two receptor types (therapeutic receptor in solid lines, secondary receptor in dotted lines) are shown. The agonist in the top panels (A and B) is selective for the therapeutic receptor because of a low efficacy for the secondary receptor. However, this agonist does have a higher affinity for the secondary receptor and this causes the $\Delta\log(\tau/K_A)$ value to be negative. As can be seen in panel B, in tissues of higher sensitivity, the secondary receptor activity actually becomes dominant over the therapeutic receptor activity. This possibility is predicted by the $\Delta\log(\tau/K_A)$ values. In contrast, the positive $\Delta\log(\tau/K_A)$ value for the agonist shown in panels C and D suggests that this agonist is truly more selective for the therapeutic receptor in all systems, i.e., tissues of low sensitivity (panel C) and high sensitivity (panel D).

$$\Delta\Delta\log(\tau/K_A)_{selectivity} = \Delta\log(\tau/K_A)_{therapeutic}$$
$$- \Delta\log(\tau/K_A)_{secondary} \quad (8.3)$$

where $\Delta\log(\tau/K_A)_{therapeutic}$ represents the selectivity of the test agonist (over a reference agonist) for the therapeutic receptor and $\Delta\log(\tau/K_A)_{secondary}$ represents the relative activity of the test agonist (over a reference agonist) for a secondary receptor. A positive value of $\Delta\Delta\log(\tau/K_A)_{selectivity}$ indicates a positive selectivity for the therapeutic receptor even when appearances suggest otherwise; this is shown in Figure 8.7. Panel 8.7A suggests that the agonist with the solid line curve is more selective than the one with the dotted line curve, yet the $\Delta\Delta\log(\tau/K_A)$ value is negative [$\Delta\Delta\log(\tau/K_A) = -0.48$; fractional $(\tau/K_A)_{selectivity}$ values]. However, it can be seen that in a tissue of increased sensitivity, the dotted line agonist is now more potent on the secondary receptor [in keeping with the $\Delta\Delta\log(\tau/K_A)$ ratio − Panel 8.7B]. In contrast, panel 8.7C shows two agonists where the $\Delta\Delta\log(\tau/K_A)$ ratio is positive [$\Delta\Delta\log(\tau/K_A) = 1.22$]; in tissues of higher sensitivity this selectivity stays constant − panel 8.7D. This is because $\log(\tau/K_A)$ indices take into consideration whether agonists

are affinity dominant or efficacy dominant in producing their response.

In general, efficacy can be characterized in terms of the following headings:

1. What types of efficacy does the molecule possess?
2. For pleiotropic signaling, does the molecule produce a biased signal?
3. Is the agonism affinity driven or efficacy driven?
4. How selective is the agonism?

A schematic diagram illustrating the process of efficacy classification is given in Figure 8.8.

8.2.2 Affinity

The next system-independent descriptor of a drug molecule is its affinity for the target. As pointed out in Section 5.8, while the EC_{50} (concentration producing half maximal agonism) for a weak partial agonist is a close measure of the K_A (equilibrium dissociation constant of the agonist-receptor complex and also the reciprocal of the affinity), the EC_{50} cannot be used as a measure of affinity for a full agonist.

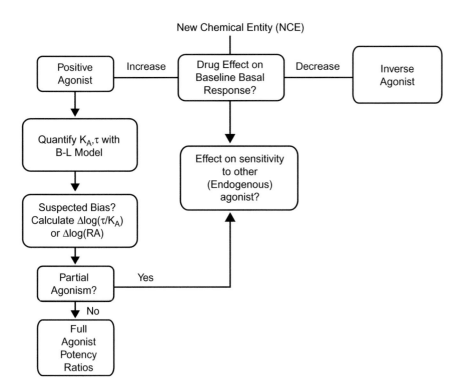

FIGURE 8.8 **Schematic diagram for logistical scheme for the evaluation of agonism.** A decrease in basal effect after addition of the agonist suggests that the system is constitutively active and that the ligand is an inverse agonist. Positive agonism is analyzed with the Black/Leff operational model to determine efficacy (τ) and affinity (K_A). This can be done in assays for different signaling systems to determine possible bias which is then quantified with $\Delta\Delta\log(\tau/K_A)$ values. Partial agonists also can be evaluated for activity in blocking responses to full agonists (see Section 6.3.5 in Chapter 6).

In general, affinity measurements are much more important descriptors of antagonists, defined as ligands that interfere with the production of pharmacological response by an agonist. Every compound made by medicinal chemists for an antagonist program must be tested for potency at the primary target, and the most expeditious means of doing this is through a pIC_{50} curve. This is where a stimulus is given to the system (i.e., an 80% maximal concentration of agonist activating the receptor) and then a range of concentrations of antagonist added to determine inhibition of that response. There are a number of reasons for this approach:

1. It is less labor intensive than analyzing full agonist concentration-response curves (see Figure 8.9).
2. It can cover a wide range of antagonist concentrations (to find where antagonism begins). This is imperative in a "data driven" system, where the activities of test molecules are unknown.
3. Unless a high concentration of agonist is used for simple competitive blockade, the pIC_{50} will be, at most, a 2−6 times underestimation of the true pK_B but not more than that. However, pIC_{50} values can still be used to track potency since a correction factor usually will be common to all molecules.
4. Effects on maximal antagonism in a pIC_{50} mode can detect partial agonists, allosteric modulation, and inverse agonism.

The determination of antagonist potency through determination of a pIC_{50} is a facile method but it does not automatically yield a system-dependent measure of potency; that is, the true aim of an antagonist program is to determine the molecular system-independent measure of affinity; namely, the pK_B ($-\log$ of the molar equilibrium dissociation constant of the antagonist-receptor complex). This latter value can be applied to all systems where the antagonist is to be tested. Therefore, it is worth considering the relationship between the readily obtainable pIC_{50} and the desired pK_B.

For competitive antagonists, the observed pIC_{50} depends upon the magnitude of the strength of stimulus given to the system. Therefore, the potency of the antagonist (as measured by the pIC_{50}) for inhibiting a 50% maximal agonism will be lower than that for driving the system at 80% maximal stimulus (see Figure 8.10A). The relationship between the pIC_{50} and pK_B under these circumstances (for pure competitive antagonism) is:

$$pK_B = pIC_{50} + \log([A]/K_A + 1), \qquad (8.4)$$

where the strength of stimulus to the system is given by $[A]/K_A$ ($[A]$ is the concentration of agonist and K_A the equilibrium dissociation constant of the agonist-receptor complex). This relation (often referred to as the *Cheng−Prusoff correction* [14]) is valid only for systems where the Hill coefficient for the concentration-response curves is unity and where the K_A is known. Most often in functional antagonist programs, the effects are against a concentration-response curve for functional activity, which is defined by a curve of observed slope and location (EC_{50}) but where the K_A is not known and $n \neq 1$. Under these circumstances it can be shown that the

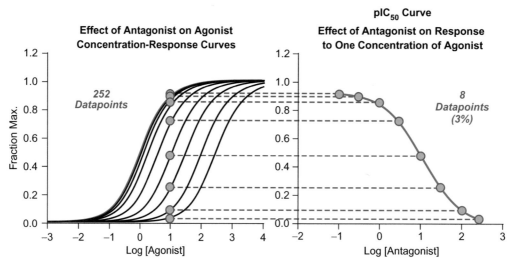

FIGURE 8.9 Panel on the left shows the effects of a simple competitive antagonist on full concentration-response curves to an agonist. An alternative method to gauge the effects of the antagonist is to add increasing concentrations of antagonist onto a preparation prestimulated with a concentration of agonist that produces 80% maximal response (red circles). The antagonist reduces the effect of the EC_{80} concentration to define the sigmoidal curve shown on the right-hand panel. This curve concisely reports the potency of the antagonist (through the pIC_{50}) with a fraction of the number of data points.

relationship between the IC_{50} and the K_B in functional experiments is given by (as defined by Leff and Dougall [15] and derived in Section 8.7.1):

$$K_B = IC_{50}/((2 + ([A]/EC_{50})^n)^{1/n} - 1), \qquad (8.5)$$

where the concentration of agonist is [A], the concentration of agonist producing 50% maximal response is EC_{50}, and n is the Hill coefficient of the agonist dose-response curve. From Equation 8.5 it can be seen that the K_B, which is a system-independent estimate of antagonist potency, can be made from an estimate of the IC_{50} that is corrected for the level of agonism. However, this is required only for a competitive antagonist and not for noncompetitive antagonists. In the latter case, the pIC_{50} corresponds directly to the pK_B (see Figure 8.10B). The reason for the difference between the pIC_{50} correspondence (or lack of it) in competitive versus noncompetitive systems is the dextral displacement of the agonist concentration-response curve produced by the antagonism. Thus, in competitive systems, the dextral displacement causes the disparity between pIC_{50} and pK_B values (Figure 8.10A). In purely noncompetitive systems, there is no dextral displacement and the pIC_{50} corresponds to the pK_B (Figure 8.10B). Between these two extremes are systems where a small dextral displacement is produced, even under conditions of noncompetitive blockade, due to a receptor reserve in the system or perhaps a hemi-equilibrium state. Under these circumstances, there will be a low-level difference between the pIC_{50} and pK_B, less than that for pure competitive antagonist systems but enough to prevent

an absolute correspondence. An example of the use of the pIC_{50} to quantify antagonism is given in Section 13.2.11.

There are two reasons why use of pIC_{50} values early in antagonist discovery programs is adequate. The first is that the absolute error, if the EC_{80} concentration for agonism is used for measurement of the IC_{50}, is small (at most a five fold error). Second, any correction will be uniform for a series of molecules with the same mechanism of action, therefore the relative changes in the pIC_{50} should reflect corresponding relative changes in the pK_B.

There are two characteristic properties of pIC_{50} curves of interest that can yield valuable information about antagonist activity. The first is the potency (pIC_{50}) discussed previously. The second is the maximal degree of antagonism. If the antagonist reduces the EC_{80} effect of the agonist to the baseline (0% response), then this is consistent with "silent" antagonism, whereby the antagonist has no efficacy, and also with a normal orthosteric mechanism of antagonism. However, if the maximal degree of antagonism does not attain baseline values, then further valuable information about the mechanism of action of the antagonism can be deduced.

There are two possible reasons for the pIC_{50} curve to fall short of the baseline (produce < 100% inhibition). One is that the antagonist demonstrates partial agonism in the system, that is, the elevated baseline is due to a direct agonism produced by the antagonist (see Figure 8.11A – see also Chapter 6, Section 6.3.5). This can be confirmed in separate experiments where the direct effects of the "antagonist" are observed. Another possibility is a limited saturable blockade of agonist effect, which does not allow complete obliteration

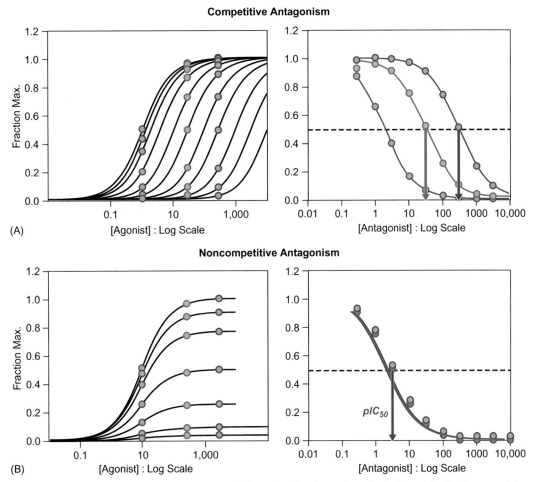

FIGURE 8.10 pIC$_{50}$ curves measured under different levels of agonist stimulation. (A) Simple competitive antagonist. In this case, the magnitude of the agonist response produces an inverse effect on the observed potency of the antagonist. The color-coded pIC$_{50}$ curves reflect full-scale inhibition (control is normalized to be 100%); it can be seen that the antagonist appears more potent in blocking the lower agonist stimulation (red curve) than the higher level of agonist stimulation (magenta). (B) The same is not true for insurmountable noncompetitive antagonism. With these types of antagonist, the level of stimulation does not affect the observed potency of the antagonist when measured in a pIC$_{50}$ mode.

of the induced agonist effect (see Figure 8.11B). This is discussed more fully in Chapter 4 (see Figures 4.8 and 4.9).

The other possibility is that the pIC$_{50}$ curve may extend below the baseline; see Figure 8.12. The most common reason for this is that what is perceived to be the baseline ("zero" response) is really a spontaneously elevated baseline due to constitutive receptor activity (see Section 3.10). If the antagonist has negative efficacy (inverse agonist activity), then this elevation will be reversed and the pIC$_{50}$ curve will extend beyond the baseline (see Figure 8.12).

Before discussing the determination of antagonist mechanism by observation of antagonist effects on full agonist concentration-response curves, it is worth considering the pA$_2$ ($-$ log molar concentration of the antagonist that causes a twofold shift to the right of the agonist concentration-response curve) as a mechanism-independent measure of antagonist potency. This estimate

of the pK$_B$ is an even better estimate than the pIC$_{50}$ since the differences between pK$_B$ and pA$_2$ values are very small. The basis for the use of the pA$_2$ stems from the fact that an antagonist will produce little to no effect on an agonist response until it occupies approximately 50% of the receptor population. In a purely competitive system, when antagonist occupancy reaches 50%, then the dose ratio for an agonist is 2 (by definition, the $-$ log of the molar concentration of antagonist is the pA$_2$). Therefore, determination of the concentration that produces a two fold shift to the right of any agonist concentration-response curve by any antagonist is a useful way to estimate antagonist potency. The major problem with this approach is the lack of parallelism in agonist concentration-response curves. However, judicious measurement of dose ratios (for example, at levels of response lower than 50%) can overcome this obstacle [16]. Figure 8.13 shows how pA$_2$ measurements can be made

FIGURE 8.11 Inhibition curves in pIC$_{50}$ mode that do not show complete inhibition. (A) A partial agonist will depress the agonist response only to the point equal to the maximal direct agonist effect of the partial agonist. (B) An allosteric modulator that produces a submaximal decrease in affinity or efficacy of the agonist can also produce an inhibition curve that does not extend to basal (zero response) levels.

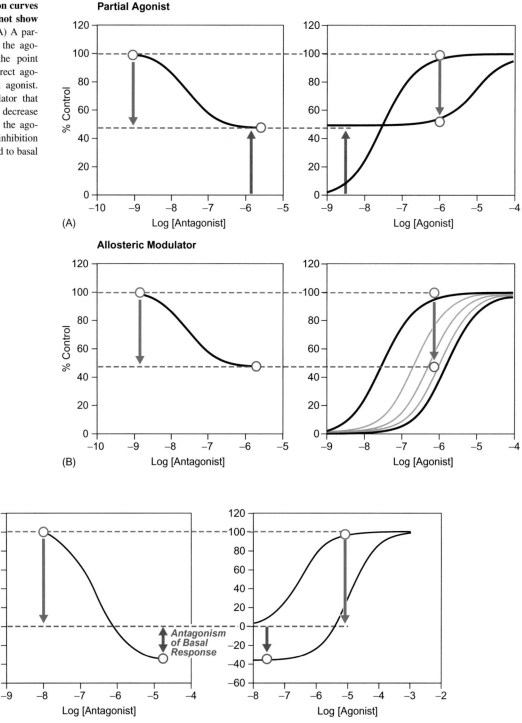

FIGURE 8.12   An inverse agonist could produce antagonism below basal levels if the basal response is due to an elevated constitutive activity.

in almost any condition of receptor antagonism. The relationships between the pA$_2$ and the pK$_B$ are derived in Section 8.7.2 for orthosteric insurmountable effects and Section 8.7.3 for allosteric insurmountable effects. An example of how pA$_2$ values are obtained is given in Section 13.2.7.

Data driven analysis of antagonism relies upon the observed pattern of agonist concentration-response curves produced in the presence of varying concentrations of the antagonist. As a prerequisite to the discussion of the various molecular mechanisms of antagonism and how they are analyzed, the effect of antagonists on the parameters

Type of Antagonism	$pA_2 =$	Correction Factor	Curve Pattern(s)
Competitive Surmountable	pK_B	None but Schild regression must be linear with unit slope	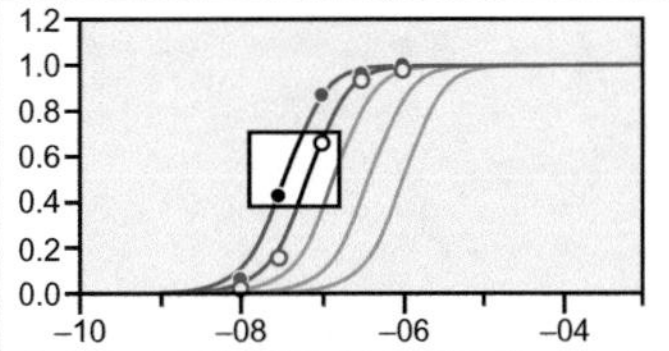
Hemi-Equilibria	$pK_B + \psi Log(1 + 2[A]/K_A)$ $\psi \ll 1$	Very slight overestimation to no correction	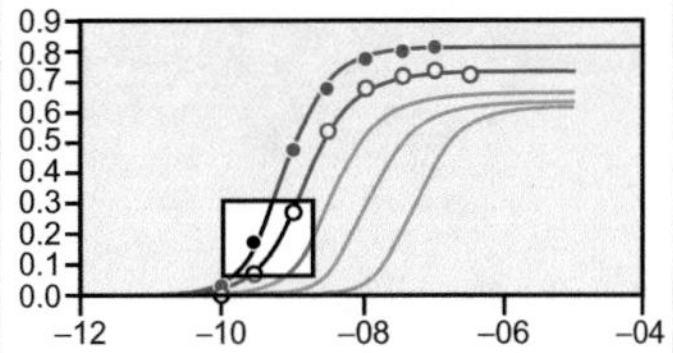
Orthosteric Insurmountable	$pK_B + Log(1 + 2[A]/K_A)$	Slight overestimation (maximal error ≈ 2)	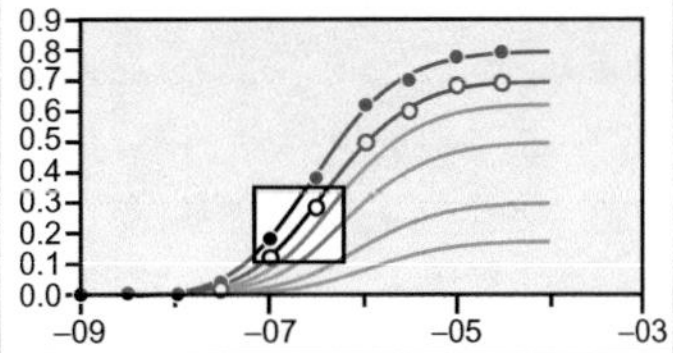
Allosteric Insurmountable	$pK_B + Log(1 + 2\alpha[A]/K_A)$	Very slight overestimation (for modulators with $\alpha < 1$)	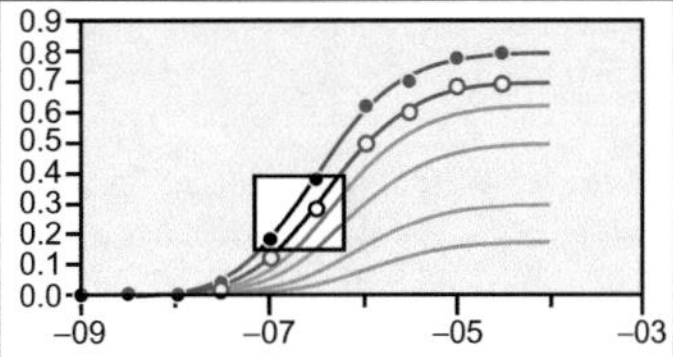

FIGURE 8.13 **Patterns of insurmountable antagonism through three different molecular mechanisms.** In each case, the concentration of antagonist that produces between a 1.8-fold to a 4-fold shift to the right of the agonist concentration-response curve can be used to calculate the pA_2, which, in turn, furnishes a reasonably accurate estimate of the pK_B. If depression of the maximal response is observed, then approximately parallel regions of the concentration-response curves should be used to calculate the dose ratios. Redrawn from [16].

of agonist concentration-response curves should be determined. This can be done statistically. In general, while antagonists can produce numerous permutations of effects on agonist concentration-response curves, there are some pharmacologically key effects that denote distinct receptor activities. Thus, an antagonist may:

1. Alter the baseline of concentration-response curves.
2. Depress the maximal response to the agonist.
3. Change the location parameter of the concentration-response curves.

A data driven process classifies curve patterns and associates them with molecular mechanism; a schematic diagram of this process for antagonists is shown in Figure 8.14. Assuming that the effects on baseline and maxima are clear (either obvious or discernible with an F-test), then certain models of interaction between receptors, agonists, and antagonists can be identified. It can be seen from Figure 8.14 that a first step would be to observe possible changes in the baseline in the presence of the antagonist. If the baseline is increased, this suggests that the antagonist is demonstrating partial agonist activity in the preparation. Under these circumstances, the data can be described by the model for partial agonism (see Chapter 6, Section 6.3.5). Alternatively, if the baseline is decreased, this could be a constitutively active

receptor system, and the antagonist could be demonstrating inverse agonism (see Chapter 6, Section 6.3.4).

The next consideration is to determine whether the antagonism is surmountable or insurmountable. In the case of surmountable antagonism, a Schild analysis is carried out (dose ratios can be used from curves generically fit to four parameter logistic equations; see Chapter 6, Section 6.3). The behavior of the relationship between log (DR−1) values and the logarithm of the molar concentrations of antagonist can be used to determine whether the antagonism best fits an orthosteric or allosteric mechanism. If the Schild regression is linear with unit slope, then a Gaddum−Schild model of orthosteric competitive antagonism is used to fit the data (see Chapter 6, Section 6.3.1). If there is curvature in the Schild regression resulting from attainment of a saturably maximal dose ratio, this would suggest that a surmountable allosteric mechanism of action is operative (see Figure 7.20). In this case, it is assumed that the allosteric modulator alters (reduces) the affinity of the agonist for the receptor but does not interfere with the agonist's ability to induce a response. The model for this type of interaction is discussed further in Chapter 7, Section 7.4.

If the antagonism is insurmountable, then there are a number of molecular mechanisms possible. The next question to ask is if the maximal response to the agonist can be completely depressed to basal levels. Alternatively,

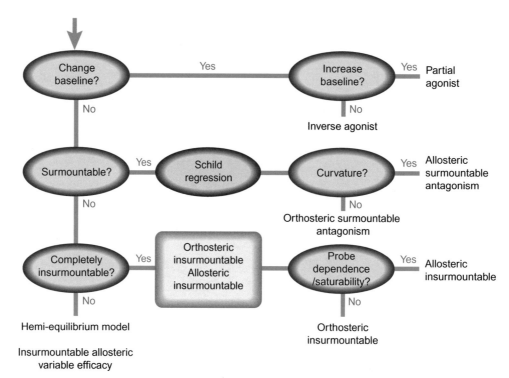

FIGURE 8.14 **Schematic diagram of steps involved in analyzing pharmacological antagonism.** Key questions to be answered are in purple, beginning with assessments of changes in baseline, followed by assessment of whether or not the antagonism is surmountable, and followed by assessment of possible probe dependence and/or saturability.

this could be due to a hemi-equilibrium condition (see Section 6.5), which produces a partial shortfall to true competitive equilibrium leading to incomplete depression of the maximal response but also antagonist-concentration-related dextral displacement of the concentration-response curve to the agonist (see Figure 6.21). Another way in which a partial depression of the maximal response could occur is through an allosteric mechanism whereby the antagonist modulator produces an alteration in the efficacy of the agonist. This can result in a different steady state, whereby the curve is partially depressed but no further dextral displacement is observed (see Figure 7.24B). The complete model for such an allosteric mechanism (with partial sparing of agonist function) is discussed in Section 7.4. While the models used to describe allosteric alteration of both affinity and efficacy of receptors are complex and require a number of parameters, the identification of such effects (namely, incomplete antagonism of agonist response) is experimentally quite clear and straightforward.

Less straightforward is the differentiation of orthosteric versus allosteric antagonism, when the antagonist produces an insurmountable and complete blockade of the agonist response. Specifically, there are two completely different mechanisms of action for receptor blockade that can present nearly identical patterns of concentration-response curves. Orthosteric insurmountable antagonism occurs when the antagonist binds to the agonist binding site and the rate of offset of the antagonist is insufficient for complete re-equilibration of agonist, antagonist, and

receptors (see Section 6.4 for further details). Allosteric antagonism, whereby the antagonist binds to its own site on the receptor and precludes receptor activation by the agonist (see Chapter 7, Section 7.4.4 for further details) can produce insurmountable blockade as well. As discussed in Chapter 7, what is required to delineate orthosteric versus allosteric mechanism is the conscious testing of predictions of each mechanism through experiment. Thus, the blockade of a range of agonists through a large range of antagonist concentrations should be carried out to detect possible saturation of effect and probe dependence (see Section 7.5 for further discussion).

As with agonism, there are a number of general statements that can be made about the study of antagonism in drug discovery programs. These are:

1. The pA_2 is a good estimate of the pK_B for any mechanism of antagonism.
2. Allosteric antagonism can masquerade as orthosteric antagonism under a variety of circumstances.
3. If a compound is an antagonist, it does not mean it also does not have efficacy (partial agonists, inverse agonists).
4. Goodness of fit is not a reliable approach to determination of mechanism of action — *vide infra*.

Empirical measures of antagonist potency can be used in discovery programs to guide medicinal chemistry to optimize activity, but the ultimate aim of pharmacodynamic studies is the measurement of the K_B, the equilibrium

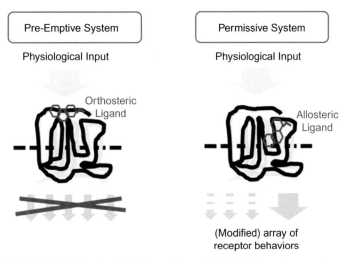

FIGURE 8.15 Panel on left shows orthosteric (steric hindrance) antagonism of signaling; this pre-empts any other activation of the target. Panel on the right shows an allosteric system where the ligand allows the signaling molecules to bind to possibly produce response (a permissive system).

dissociation constant of the antagonist-receptor complex, since this is a system-independent estimate of the activity of the antagonist. Towards this end, the mechanism of action of the molecule is required to fully understand what behaviors will be seen therapeutically. The first requirement for this process is to obtain a set of concentration-response curves for agonism in the absence and presence of a range of concentrations of the molecule (either antagonist or modulator). Inspection of these patterns often suggests the first clue as to which model should be applied for analysis; although this can be misleading, as suggested by F. Klein (Reed and Simon: Methods of modern mathematical physics): "...Everyone knows what a curve is, until he has studied enough mathematics to become confused through the countless number of possible exceptions." This initial comparison is then subjected to a rigorous quantitative analysis; the comparison of data to mathematical models will be discussed further in this chapter — see Section 8.3.

8.2.3 Orthosteric vs. Allosteric Mechanisms

As discussed previously, there are a number of important differences between molecules that interact with the biological target in an orthosteric manner (binding to the same site as the endogenous agonist or substrate) or allosterically (binding to a site removed from that site). The main differences center around the behavior of the target towards the endogenous signaling system. For orthosteric drugs, the result is pre-emptive, in that the endogenous agonist or substrate is not allowed to bind to the target and impart any effect; this leads to a defined set of behaviors of the target toward the endogenous system based on steric hindrance (see Figure 8.15). In contrast, there is a great deal more variability of the endogenous system

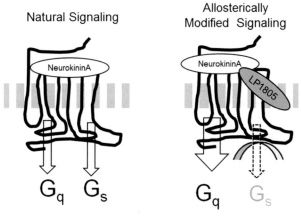

FIGURE 8.16 **Bias imposed by an allosteric ligand on a natural signaling system.** While the endogenous agonist (neurokinin A) causes the receptor to couple to and activate G_q and G_s protein, after binding of the allosteric ligand LP1805, neurokinin A only permits G_q signaling to occur. Data from [17].

behavior when an allosteric molecule is present. These effects can be permissive, in that the endogenous signaling system may still function to a certain extent, i.e., the response may be blocked, partially blocked, potentiated or otherwise altered. That is, the quality of the signal may change. For example, the allosteric modulator LP18095 (N,N-(2-methylnaphthyl-benzyl)-2-aminoacetonitrile) binds to NK-1 receptors and modifies the quality of the signal produced by the endogenous agonist neurokinin A. Specifically, while neurokinin A activates both G_s and G_q proteins, in the presence of LP1805 the G_s protein response to neurokinin A is potentiated while the G_q response is blocked [17] — see Figure 8.16.

Allosteric effects can be confirmed in separate experiments (see Chapter 7, Section 7.5). In general, allosterism, while it can appear as an orthosteric antagonism under a

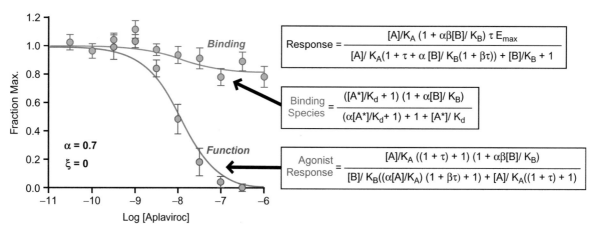

FIGURE 8.17 Inhibition curves for the allosteric modulator for CCR5 receptors, aplaviroc in blocking the binding of the chemokine RANTES (blue curve) and the CCR5-mediated calcium transient response to RANTES (red curve). It can be seen that aplaviroc produces a differentially greater inhibition of efficacy (agonist response) than affinity (binding species). Equations next to the curve illustrate that different receptor species mediate the response production in each assay. Data redrawn from [18].

variety of conditions, may be uncovered through observing the extremes of the antagonist behavior. There are three characteristic features of allosteric modulators. They are

1. Probe dependence: An allosteric effect observed with one receptor probe (i.e., agonist, radioligand) could be completely different for another probe; see Figure 7.34 and Figure 4.12.
2. Saturability of effect: That is, when the allosteric site is fully saturated, the effect stops; see Figure 4.10.
3. There can be separate effects on probe affinity and efficacy.

This latter feature can be extremely important since selective effects on efficacy can be detected only in functional, not binding, assays. Figure 8.17 shows the selective inhibition of aplaviroc on the CCR5-mediated responses to the chemokine RANTES. It can be seen that the binding of RANTES is minimally affected, while the calcium transient response to the chemokine is completely blocked [18]. This can be quantified with a functional allosteric model (Equation 7.3), where there is minimal effect on affinity ($\alpha = 0.7$) but compete inhibition of formation of the receptor state ($\xi\beta = 0$); see Figure 8.17. This separation of effect on affinity and efficacy of agonists can lead to some interesting and useful effects. For example, Figure 8.18 shows the effect of the modulator ifenprodil on responses to NMDA [19]. It can be seen that this potency of ifenprodil actually increases with increasing concentrations of NMDA, that is, the agonist increases the affinity of the antagonist. This can be observed in modulators that block function ($\xi\beta = 0$) but increase the affinity to the agonist ($\alpha > 1$). Since allosteric effects are reciprocal, the agonist will also increase the affinity of the receptor to the modulator. It can be seen that such effects may be therapeutically useful, since the activity of the antagonist increases with the activity of the system. Given that orthosteric and allosteric mechanisms produce very different

profiles of activity, it is very important to design experiments to identify these mechanisms.

8.2.4 Target Coverage *In Vivo*

It is important to note that the determination of antagonist potency is carried out in a closed system (equilibrium mass action kinetics, where the drugs and targets are equilibrated and concentrations are kept constant). However, these antagonists are then used in open systems where the concentration is variable and dependent on time (see Figure 8.19). Therefore, potency is only part of the required profile; for adequate target coverage (where the target is blocked by the antagonist for a therapeutically useful length of time), the binding of the antagonist must be persistent (i.e., of slow offset) to maximize target coverage in the face of variable pharmacokinetics [20]. For example, two hypothetical antagonists A and B are equiactive ($K_B = 10$ nM) but one has a rate of offset of 0.007 s^{-1} M and rate of onset of 7×10^5 s^{-1} ($K_B = 0.002$ s^{-1} M/7 $\times 10^5$ s$^{-1} = 10^{-9}$ M) and the other has a rate of offset of 0.002 s^{-1} M and rate of onset of 2×10^5 s^{-1} ($K_B = 0.002$ s^{-1} M/2 $\times 10^5$ s$^{-1} = 10^{-9}$ M); see Figure 8.20. At equilibrium, a concentration of 3 nM gives the same target coverage in a closed system (receptor occupancy of 75%). However, when the system is open and the concentration in the media surrounding the target goes to zero, then the target coverage is given by the amount of antagonist bound to the receptor, and this, in turn, is given by the first order rate of offset of the antagonist from the receptor, which is given by:

$$\rho_t = \rho_e e^{-kt}, \qquad (8.6)$$

where ρ_t and ρ_e are the fractional receptor occupancies at time t and equilibrium (time zero), respectively, and k is the rate of offset. A measure of target coverage can be gained from the area under the curve of the offset curves

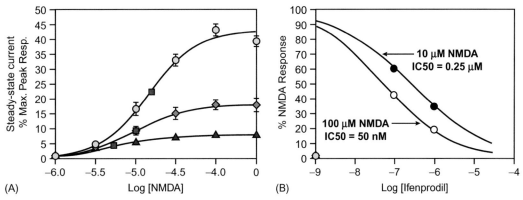

FIGURE 8.18 Noncompetitive allosteric antagonism of NMDA responses by ifenprodil. (A) Concentration-response curves to NMDA in rat cortical neurons in the absence (filled circles) and presence of ifenprodil ($0.1\,\mu M$, filled diamonds; and $1\,\mu M$, filled triangles). (B) pIC_{50} curves for ifenprodil-blocking $10\,\mu M$ and $100\,\mu M$ NMDA. Note the increase in ifenprodil potency with increasing activation by NMDA. Data redrawn from [19]. See Figure 7.21B in Chapter 7 for further details.

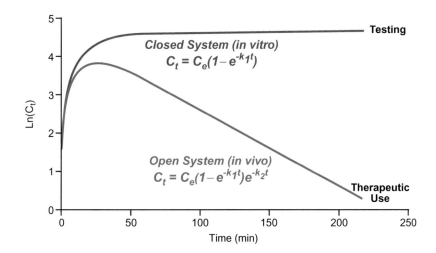

FIGURE 8.19 Concentration of an antagonist when tested in an *in vitro* test system (red curve) versus how it is used therapeutically (*in vivo* open system; blue curve). While the concentration is constant in the *in vitro* system, it is not so in an *in vivo* system. In the latter, the rate of receptor offset (k_2) becomes important in determining how well the antagonist blocks the target. The rate of receptor onset is k_1.

(as with pharmacokinetics; see Chapter 9), and this can be estimated from the integral of Equation 8.6 over a given time period. One estimate for this is the time from zero (antagonist in the bathing medium at the maximal concentration) and five times the half time for offset:

$$\int_{t=0}^{t=5\cdot t_{1/2}} \rho_e e^{-kt} = \frac{\rho_e e^{-kt}}{-k} = \frac{\rho_e (1 - e^{\frac{-k\cdot 5\cdot 0.695}{k}})}{-k} = \frac{0.97\rho e}{-k},$$

(8.7)

where $t_{1/2} = 0.693/k$. Figure 8.20 shows the target coverage for these two antagonists as calculated by Equation 8.7 for a range of concentrations. It can be seen that, for any given concentration, the coverage by the slower offset antagonist is considerably higher than for the faster offset antagonist and that this effect increases with increasing antagonist concentration. In light of this effect, it would be useful to measure the rate of offset of candidate antagonists in the final stages of a discovery program to detect differences that may be relevant therapeutically.

Examples of how these offsets are measured are given in Chapter 6, Section 6.7.

8.3 NULL EXPERIMENTS AND FITTING DATA TO MODELS

Experimental pharmacology is based on the null technique since the biochemical reactions that transform receptor activation to cellular response are largely unknown. Null methods obviate the requirement for understanding these mechanisms; i.e., it is assumed that equal receptor effects of drugs in any given system are translated in an identical fashion by the cell. Under these circumstances, equiactive ratios of drug concentration are independent of the cellular stimulus-response process. As discussed in Chapter 5, Section 5.8.2, a basic requirement of this method is that the function linking the initial membrane drug event that triggers response and the end organ response is ***monotonic***

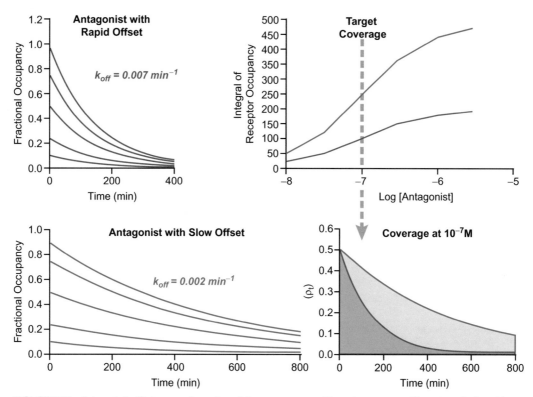

FIGURE 8.20   Integrated offset curves for antagonists as a measure of target coverage.   The antagonist in red has a rate of offset 3.5 times greater than the antagonist in blue. Red and blue lines represent receptor occupancy, with time, for six concentrations of antagonist corresponding to $[B]/K_B$ values of 0.01, 0.03, 1, 3, 10, and 30 ($K_B = 100$ nM). Integrated values of antagonist occupancy from time $t = 0$ to $5 \times t_{1/2}$ show a much higher degree of receptor occupancy for the blue antagonist (top right panel).

in nature. Failure to comply with this requirement renders null methods such as the comparison of agonist dose ratios invalid (see Section 5.8.2).

As a preface to a specific discussion of the use of data driven analyses, it is useful to consider the application of surrogate parameters. Ideally, pharmacological data should directly be fit to specific models and parameters derived from that direct fit. However, there are cases where the specific models predict surrogate parameters that can be derived without fitting data to a specific model. This can be an advantage. For example, equiactive dose ratios (DR) from parallel concentration-response curves shifted to the right by the antagonist can be used in Schild analysis; therefore, DR values can be used as surrogates for the analysis of antagonism without the need to fit to the explicit model. Under these circumstances, the data can be fit to a generic sigmoidal curve of the form:

$$\text{Response} = \text{Basal} + \frac{\text{Max} - \text{Basal}}{1 + 10^{(\text{LogEC}_{50} - \text{Log}[A])^n}} \qquad (8.8)$$

and the shift in EC_{50} values used to calculate DR estimates for Schild analysis (see Chapter 6.3.1). There are certain instances in data driven pharmacological analyses where it is useful to use such surrogate parameters.

Ultimately, drug activity must be characterized in terms of system-independent molecular parameters, and these are integral parts of mathematical models used to describe pharmacodynamics events. The usual process for determining this is to assess the veracity of various pharmacodynamic models of two molecule single target systems as descriptors of concentration-response curve data — i.e., how well does a given model fit? There are surprisingly few models required to fit a bewildering range of possible pharmacodynamic behaviors. For orthosteric surmountable effects, Figure 8.21 shows three of these, classified by their description of antagonist effects on basal tissue response; Figure 8.22 shows the model for orthosteric insurmountable effects. A wide range of allosteric effects (see Figures 7.10 and 7.11) can be described by a single equation (with a variant where $\tau_B = \text{or} \neq 0$) — see Figure 8.23. It should also be noted that "goodness of fit" is not proof of veracity of the model since a number of models often can describe the same pharmacodynamic behavior. For example, Figure 8.24 shows a pattern of dextral displacement of concentration-response curves with concomitant depression of maximal response that is consistent with three molecular modes of action. How well a given equation fits a set of data is assessed through the magnitude of the squares of the differences between

Orthosteric Surmountable Competitive Antagonism

$$\text{Response} = \frac{([A]/EC_{50})E_m}{([A]/EC_{50})+[B]/K_B+1}$$

Orthosteric Partial Agonism

$$\text{Response} = \frac{(\tau_A[A]/K_A+\tau_B[B]/K_B)E_m}{[A]/K_A(1+\tau_A)+[B]/K_B(1+\tau_B)+1}$$

Orthosteric Inverse Agonism

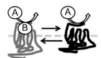

$$\text{Response} = \frac{L(\alpha\tau_A[A]/K_A+\beta\tau_B[B]/K_B+\tau_B)\,E_m}{[A]/K_A(\alpha L(1+\tau_A)+[B]/K_B(\beta L(1+\tau_B)+1)+L(1+\tau_R)+1}$$

FIGURE 8.21 **Three mechanisms of orthosteric interaction of an antagonist and agonist for a competition between the antagonist (B) and agonist (A) for a common binding site.** Top panel: the antagonist has no observable direct effect. Middle panel: the same type of antagonist but, in this case, the antagonist has sufficient positive efficacy to produce an elevated baseline. Bottom panel: an antagonist that has selective affinity for the inactive state of the receptor and where the system is such that sufficient spontaneously formed receptor active state is present to produce an elevated baseline in the absence of agonist. In this case, the ligand produces a decrease in the basal response.

Orthosteric Insurmountable (Non-Competitive) Antagonism

$$\text{Response} = \frac{(\tau[A]/K_A)\,E_m}{[A]/K_A(1+\tau+[B]/K_B)+[B]/K_B+1}$$

FIGURE 8.22 An orthosteric antagonist that produces insurmountable effects on the agonist concentration-response curves through persistent occupancy of the receptor.

the actual data and the value for the data predicted by the equation (for an explanation of sum of squares, see Chapter 12). This often can be capricious as, again, a number of equations may yield very similar values for the sum of squares. Figure 8.25 shows a hypothetical data set fit to the allosteric model in Figure 8.25A and the orthosteric model in Figure 8.25B. The circled data points were changed very slightly to cause an F-test to prefer either model for each respective model, illustrating the fallacy of relying on computer fitting of data and statistical tests to determine a molecular mechanism.

8.4 INTERPRETATION OF EXPERIMENTAL DATA

The lead optimization phase of discovery and development is the iterative process of testing molecules, assessing their activity, and synthesizing new molecules based on that

data (determining a structure-activity relationship, SAR). If there is a single index of activity, then the attainment of an improved potency (as determined by statistics) is a useful approach. One way to do this is to test the molecules repeatedly, determine a mean value with a measure of variation (standard deviation), and use those measurements to determine a confidence limit for that estimate. One proposed confidence limit that rapidly leads to comparison of multiple estimates is the 84% confidence limit of a mean [21]. For example, if four measurements yield a mean estimate pIC_{50} of 7.1 with a standard deviation (s_x) of 0.13, then the 84% confidence limits can be calculated as:

$$\text{Confidence limit} = s_x \bullet t_{0.16} \bullet (n)^{-1/2}, \qquad (8.9)$$

where the $t_{0.16}$ is the value for 84% confidence limits and the standard deviation based on a sample (s_x) is:

$$s_x = \sqrt{\frac{n\sum x^2 - (\sum x)^2}{n(n-1)}}. \qquad (8.10)$$

In this example, $t = 1.72$, therefore the 84% confidence limits for this estimate are $7.1 \pm (1.72 \times 0.13) = 7.1 \pm 0.22 = 6.9$ to 7.32. This means that 84% of the time, the true value of the pIC_{50} will lie between those values based on this estimate. The significance of the 84% confidence limits lies in the statistical evidence that it may be concluded that two samples from different populations (i.e., two pIC_{50}s) are different if their 84% confidence limits do not overlap [21]. This provides a simple method of sorting through a series of compounds

FIGURE 8.23 Models for allosteric modulation of agonist (A) response by an allosteric modulator (B) that produces no direct agonism (top panel) or produces a direct agonist response (efficacy of modulator $= \tau_B$: bottom panel). Descriptions of parameters of the main equation (Equation 7.3) described in Section 7.4 of Chapter 7.

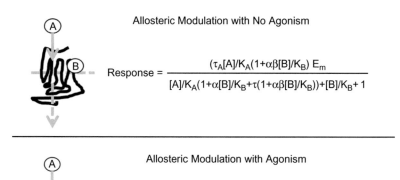

Allosteric Modulation with No Agonism

$$\text{Response} = \frac{(\tau_A[A]/K_A(1+\alpha\beta[B]/K_B)\,E_m}{[A]/K_A(1+\alpha[B]/K_B+\tau(1+\alpha\beta[B]/K_B))+[B]/K_B+1}$$

Allosteric Modulation with Agonism

$$\text{Response} = \frac{(\tau_A[A]/K_A(1+\alpha\beta[B]/K_B)+\tau_B[B]/K_B)E_m}{([A]/K_A(1+\alpha[B]/K_B+\tau_A(1+\alpha\beta[B]/K_B))+[B]/K_B(1+\tau_B)+1}$$

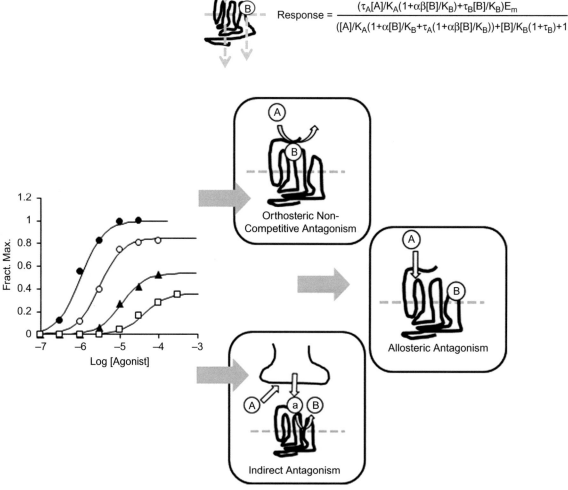

FIGURE 8.24 Three mechanisms producing dextral displacement and depression of maximal responses of agonist concentration-response curves. A slowly dissociating orthosteric antagonist (Chapter 6, Section 6.4), an allosteric antagonist that decreases agonist efficacy (Chapter 7, Section 7.4.4) or the competitive antagonism of an endogenous agonist released by the agonist (Section 6.8) all could produce the pattern of concentration-response curves seen in the left panel.

to determine which changes in chemical structure produce statistically significant improvements in activity. For example, Table 8.2 shows a series of pIC_{50} values for a range of related compounds; these data are shown graphically in Figure 8.26. It can be seen from these data that significant improvements in potency, from the base compound 1, are achieved with compounds 6, 8, 9, and 10.

The conventional level of significance chosen for true difference is 95% confidence (see Chapter 12), but there are practical reasons for using a less stringent level for structure-activity relationship analysis. Usually, a single change in chemical structure is made to assess a change in activity; this allows for a systematic analysis of the relationship between chemical structure and

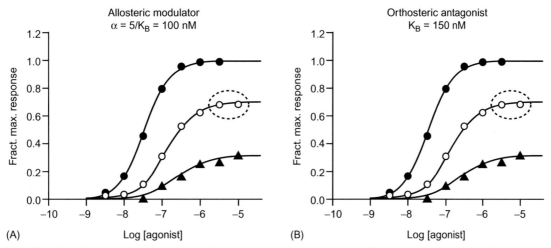

FIGURE 8.25 Simulation data set fit to an allosteric model (Equation 7.3, panel A) and to an orthosteric model (Equation 6.10, panel B). The data points circled with the dotted line were altered very slightly to cause the sum of squares for computer fit of the points to the model to favor either the allosteric or orthosteric model. It can be seen that very small differences can support either model even though they describe completely different molecular mechanisms of action.

TABLE 8.2 Primary Activity Data for a Series of Compounds

Number	Compound	pIC_{50}	STD	84% Conf. Limit
1	ACS55542	7.1	0.13	6.81 to 7.38
2	ACS55549	7.25	0.13	6.67 to 7.23
3	ACS55546	6.9	0.15	6.57 to 7.3
4	ACS55601	7.36	0.17	7 to 7.73
5	ACS55671	7.2	0.16	6.85 to 7.55
6	ACS55689	7.75	0.16	7.4 to 8.5
7	ACS55704	7.5	0.07	7.35 to 7.65
8	ACS55752	7.8	0.14	7.49 to 8.1
9	ACS55799	7.65	0.1	7.43 to 7.87
10	ACS55814	7.86	0.12	7.6 to 8.1

It is imperative to have a simple unambiguous scale of activity to guide SAR, but there can be more than one such guide required (multivariate SAR). For example, if two related targets or activities are involved and selectivity between the two is required, then the scale of absolute activity and the ratio between two activities (selectivity) are relevant [22]. Table 8.3 shows the activity of 10 compounds with activities on two receptors; the aim of the program is to optimize the activity on receptor A and minimize the concomitant activity on receptor B (optimize the potency ratio of A to B). The standard deviation for the ratio of activities on A and B is given by:

$$s_{A/B} = \sqrt{\frac{(n_A - 1)s_{xA}^2 + (n_B - 1)s_{xB}^2}{n_A + n_B - 2}}. \qquad (8.11)$$

The corresponding confidence limit on the selectivity ratio is given as:

$$\text{Confidence limit} = t \bullet s_{A/B} \sqrt{\frac{1}{n_A} + \frac{1}{n_B}}. \qquad (8.12)$$

With the assessment of the error on the ratio comes the possibility to statistically assess differences in selectivity between compounds. For example, for given compounds 1 and 2, the standard deviation of the selectivity is given as:

$$s_{\text{diff}} = \sqrt{\frac{df_1 s_{(A/B)1}^2 + df_2 s_{(A/B)2}^2}{df_1 + df_2}}, \qquad (8.13)$$

where $df_1 = N_{1-2}$ where N_1 is the sum of the values used to calculate selectivity 1 and df_2 is N_{2-1} where N_2 is the sum of the values used to calculate selectivity 2. This, in

pharmacological activity. However, it may be that a single change in structure may not produce a large improvement in activity, that is, it may take more than one change to produce a large improvement. Therefore, small improvements in activity can be utilized by choosing a less stringent criteria for compound progression — see Figure 8.27. An analogy from baseball would be to ask whether all efforts should be aimed at making a home run (>95% confidence) as opposed to a less ambitious goal of two base hits (two rounds of >84% confidence).

FIGURE 8.26 Graphical display of data shown in Table 8.2. The first compound in the series had a pIC_{50} of 7.1 (shown in red); bars represent 84% confidence limits. Compounds 2 to 5 had estimates of 84% confidence limits that cross the 84% limits of the original compound, therefore no improvement in activity was produced by these changes in structure. However, compounds 6, 8, 9, and 10 (in blue) had means and 84% confidence limits that were different from that of the original compound, therefore these represent improvements in activity.

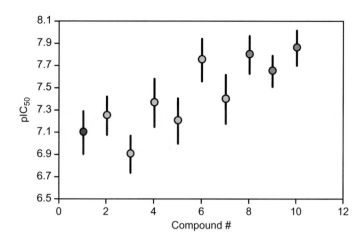

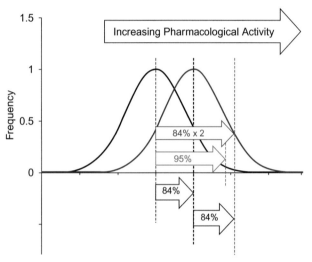

FIGURE 8.27 Compound activity depicted as a Boltzman distribution of values (with the peak representing the mean value and the width of the curve representing variation). The object is to change the mean activity to the right of the previous value (increasing activity). The compound denoted by the blue curve has a mean value that exceeds the 84% confidence band of the previous value but this is less than a value > the 95% confidence band. However, the next compound that exceeds the 84% confidence limits of the blue compound exceeds the 95% confidence limits of the original starting compound. Thus, a better compound is produced in two steps.

turn, allows the calculation of the confidence limits for the selectivity of compounds as:

$$\text{Confidence limit} = t \bullet s_{\text{diff}} \sqrt{\frac{1}{N_1} + \frac{1}{N_2}}. \quad (8.14)$$

Just as the effects of changes in chemical structure on the primary activity could be rapidly tracked through overlap of 84% confidence limits of the primary pIC_{50}s, the effects of structural changes on selectivity can be tracked through overlap of 84% confidence limits on selectivity. The data shown in Table 8.3 and Figure 8.28 illustrate a complication of multivariate SAR. Specifically, there might be separate SAR for primary activity and selectivity, making integration of both activities into one molecule

difficult. As seen in Figure 8.28A, the most potent compound is not the most selective.

The type of critical path, and whether primarily single variate or multivariate SAR is operative, sometimes depends on the type of drug the program is aimed at delivering. A therapeutically useful drug may simply be an improvement over existing therapy in the class. The primary questions to be answered are the following:

- Is the molecule active at primary target? (Potency and efficacy).
- Is the molecule promiscuous? (Selectivity).
- Is the molecule toxic? (Safety pharmacology).
- Is the molecule absorbed, distributed, and does it have sufficient $t_{1/2}$? (Adequate druglike qualities and pharmacokinetics).

A slightly more rigorous or novel approach may be required for the delivery of a drug that will be novel in the class or a completely new therapeutic entity. When the program is focused on such a chemical target, the preceding questions are still relevant, as well as a few additional questions:

- Is the molecule different from previous molecules and all other available therapy?
- Does this molecule incorporate the newest knowledge of disease and pharmacology?

Another feature of this latter type of program is the need for more critical path assays to define and differentiate unique activity.

8.5 PREDICTING THERAPEUTIC ACTIVITY IN ALL SYSTEMS

The final step in the drug discovery lead optimization process is the application of drug activity parameters to predict therapeutic utility in all systems. As pointed out in Chapter 2 (see Figure 2.1), a unique feature of

TABLE 8.3 Primary Activity Data + Selectivity Data for a Series of Compounds

	Compound	pIC_{50} Recept. A	STD_A	n_A	pIC_{50} Recept. B	STD_B	n_B	ΔpIC_{50A-B}	$STD_{A/B}$	84% c.l. of Selectivity
1	ACS66002	6.95	0.31	10	6.32	0.36	19	0.625	0.434	0.38 to 0.87
2	ACS68013	7.49	0.201	4	5.86	0.25	14	1.63	0.279	1.4 to 1.86
3	ACS62071	8.18	0.269	14	8.63	0.36	18	−0.451	0.443	−0.68 to −0.22
4	ACS64003	8.67	0.168	9	6.12	0.32	21	2.553	0.346	2.35 to 2.75
5	ACS60052	9.12	0.26	17	9.04	0.29	14	0.084	0.426	−0.14 to 0.30
6	ACS58895	9.38	0.2	10	8.32	0.33	9	1.064	0.419	0.78 to 1.35
7	ACS61004	8	0.14	8	7.9	0.32	7	0.1	0.388	−0.2 to 0.4
8	ACS64021	7.8	0.16	6	8.3	0.21	5	−0.500	0.319	−0.8 to −0.2
9	ACS67091	8.4	0.11	7	7.9	0.34	7	0.5	0.391	0.19 to 0.8
10	ACS68223	8.9	0.13	8	7.85	0.25	6	1.05	0.328	0.78 to 1.3

ΔpIC_{50A-B} = logarithm of the ratio of potencies for receptor A vs. receptor B. $STND_{A/B}$ = standard deviation of the selectivity of activity of receptor A vs. receptor B according to Equation 8.13. 84% c.l. of selectivity = the 84% confidence limits of the selectivity according to Equation 8.14.

pharmacology as a scientific discipline is that it provides the capability to use pharmacodynamic models to predict drug profiles in a host of tissues from parameters measured in just one system. The quantification of the four basic properties of drugs was discussed in Section 8.2, and these are based on the system-independent parameters of drug activity that can be used in the prediction of observed activity in the ways outlined in the following sections.

8.5.1 Predicting Agonism

The magnitude of τ for any agonist in any system is unique to that agonist in that system; it is *not transferable across different tissues*. This is because it is subject to receptor density and the efficiency of receptor coupling in the tissue as well as the intrinsic efficacy of the agonist. However, *ratios of τ values are transferable*, therefore, for any two agonists, i.e., agonist$_1$ and agonist$_2$ in a system, the desired parameter is the ratio τ_1/τ_2; this is transferable and it is this ratio that allows *prediction of relative agonism for these two agonists in any system.*

Concentration-response curves for two agonists (agonist$_1$ and agonist$_2$) are shown in Figure 8.29: the τ_1/τ_2 ratio of the agonists is 600. The relative agonist activity of agonist$_1$ and agonist$_2$ can now be calculated in any other tissue if a concentration-response curve for one of the agonists is observed in that tissue. For example, assume the τ_1/τ_2 ratio of 600 is obtained in a test system and the EC_{50} of agonist$_1$ is 330 nM. Then if agonist$_1$ is found to have an EC_{50} of 16.3 μM in a therapeutic system (a 49.4-fold diminution of potency), the τ value for agonist$_1$ in that system can be determined (Step 2, Figure 8.29). This is done

through application of one of two equations published by Black et al., [23]. These equations link the maximal response and potency (EC_{50}) to τ and K_A values through:

$$\text{Maximal Response} = \frac{\tau^n E_m}{\tau^n + 1} \quad (8.15)$$

and:

$$EC_{50} = \frac{K_A}{((2 + \tau^n)^{1/n} - 1)} \quad (8.16)$$

It is assumed that the affinity of the agonist has not changed between the test and therapeutic system (same K_A value used to fit the data). This may not be a valid assumption when this model is used to fit activation of different signaling pathways for the same agonist − *vide infra*. The efficacy of agonist$_1$ in the therapeutic system is calculated with a ratio derived from Equation 8.16:

$$\Delta\text{Potency} = \frac{EC_{50(\text{Therapeutic})}}{EC_{50(\text{Test})}} = \frac{((2 + \tau^n_{(\text{Test})})^{1/n} - 1)}{(2 + \tau^n_{(\text{Therapeutic})})^{1/n} - 1)} \quad (8.17)$$

Thus a 49.4-fold diminution of potency ($EC_{50(\text{Test})}$ = 330 nM, $EC_{50(\text{Therapeutic})}$ = 16.3 μM) and application of Equation 8.17 yields a τ value for agonist$_1$ in the therapeutic system of 60. This ratio diminution of efficacy ($\tau_{1\text{Therapeutic}}/\tau_{1\text{Test}}$ = 60/3000 = 0.02) will be imposed on all agonists in the two systems, and therefore it also applies to agonist$_2$. This means that the operational τ value for agonist$_2$ in the therapeutic system will be $\tau_{2\text{Test}} \times \tau$-ratio = 5 × 0.02 = 0.1. Application of the model thus predicts a low level of agonism for agonist$_2$ in the therapeutic system − see Step 3 in Figure 8.29).

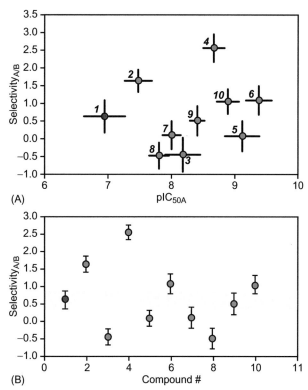

FIGURE 8.28 Multivariate structure-activity relationships. (A) Compound data summarized in Table 8.3 expressed as the pIC_{50} for the therapeutically relevant activity (activity A) as abscissae and the logarithm of the selectivity of the same compound for activity A versus B (high number is favorable) as ordinates. Bars represent standard deviations. Compound 1 (red) represents the original molecule in the active series. Note also how the most selective compound (compound 4) is not the most potent compound (compound 6). (B) Graph representing the logarithms of the selectivity of the compounds shown in panel A with bars showing 84% confidence limits. Compounds with 84% confidence limits outside of the limits of the original compound (compound 1 in red) represent compounds either less selective (compounds 3, 5, 8), of equal selectivity (compounds 6, 7, 9, 10), or greater selectivity (compounds 2, 4).

A valuable application of the above technique is in the prediction of possible observable partial agonist activity for antagonists that possess low levels of efficacy. No response (i.e., "silent" antagonism) may be observed if the test system has a low receptor level and/or low efficiency of receptor coupling. However, *in vivo*, if a low efficacy antagonist interacts with a very sensitive tissue, it may produce an agonist response, and there are cases where this may be harmful. Therefore, the determination of any possibility of agonism with antagonists should be made in very sensitive test systems (i.e., see Figure 8.4).

As noted previously, efficacy predictions using the Black/Leff operational model are valid when the agonists produce their response through the same signaling pathway, but may vary in cases of biased agonism in systems where the cell controls the relative importance of the various signaling pathways involved (see Section 5.7). For this reason, the determination of τ and K_A values should

be strictly linked with the specific signaling pathway in the form of transducer ratios $\Delta\log(\tau/K_A)$. It should also be noted that while bias estimates (in the form of $\Delta\Delta\log(\tau/K_A)$ values) determine at what relative concentration a given selective agonism will occur, they will not in themselves predict whether agonism will occur at all; this is still determined by the actual value of τ (as discussed above). This is highlighted by the array of biased ligands shown in Figure 8.30. In this case, two signaling systems (for example G-protein activation and β-arrestin signaling) controlled by the same receptor are monitored for biased agonism; the ordinate axis refers to the relative efficacy of the agonists for the two signaling pathways and the abscissal axis shows the actual bias of the agonists. Since both efficacy and affinity may vary with the signaling pathway being measured, different patterns of biased effects may be observed. Thus, a biased ligand could produce selective antagonism of an unwanted pathway or selective agonism of a preferred pathway – see Figure 8.30. This underscores the importance of linking efficacy measurements with bias measurements in the complete assessment of biased ligands.

8.5.2 Predicting Binding

The equilibrium dissociation constant of the ligand-receptor complex (K_d) can be a very predictive parameter, since it links the *in vivo* concentrations with what might be expected pharmacodynamically at the receptor (when the concentration is equal to K_d then 50% of the receptors are occupied by the ligand). The two types of drug where the K_d cannot automatically be applied to the relationship between concentration and effect are:

1. High efficacy full agonists since the efficacy of the agonist can produce large sinistral displacement of concentration-response curves for function vs. receptor occupancy.
2. Positive allosteric modulators (PAMs) where the affinity is conditional upon the co-binding ligand (usually the endogenous agonist – see Section 7.4.3 in Chapter 7).

The value of predictive parameters determined from pharmacodynamic models is illustrated by the varied effects of a PAM-agonist shown in Figure 8.31. It can be seen that a concentration of PAM-agonist equal to the K_d value can produce quite different observable profiles in tissues of varying sensitivity to the endogenous agonist (as shown by the changes in the receptor levels [R_t]). In tissues of low sensitivity, little sensitization but an increased maximal response is observed. In more sensitive tissues, increased maximal response with increased sensitivity evolving to a direct agonist effect is seen. In very sensitive tissues, no further increase in maximal response is seen but powerful agonism

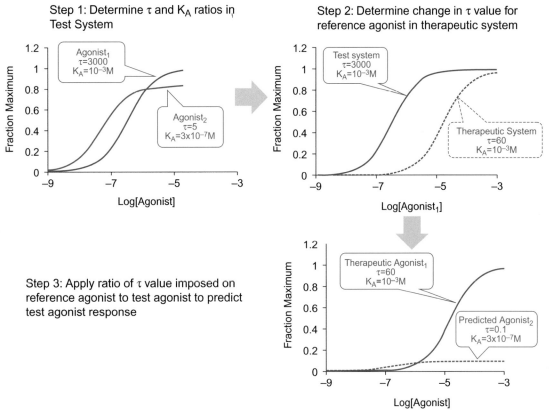

FIGURE 8.29 Prediction of agonism using the Black/Leff operational model. Top left panel: The responses to a test agonist (red) and reference agonist (blue) are quantified with the Black/Leff operational model to yield a ratio of efficacy values for the two agonists in this test system. Top right panel: The change in potency for the reference agonist in the therapeutic system is used to quantify the change in efficacy of the reference agonist through Equation 8.17. Bottom right panel: The same ratio change in efficacy (between the test and therapeutic system) is applied to the ratio of the test agonist to predict the responses of the test agonist in the therapeutic system.

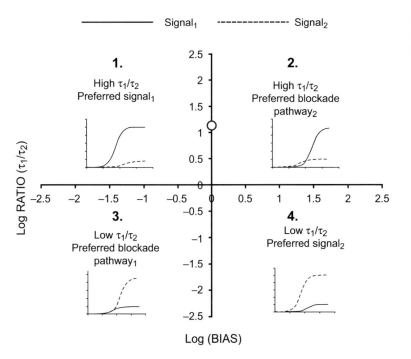

FIGURE 8.30 The interplay of relative efficacy (ordinate scale) and bias (abscissal scale). It can be seen that the antagonism of responses produced by low efficacy ligands can still be influenced by bias.

FIGURE 8.31 **Effects of a PAM-agonist in tissues of**
varying sensitivity to the endogenous agonist. Receptor
levels for the tissues written above each set of curves. For
the PAM-agonist: $\tau_B/\tau_A = 0.03$, $\alpha = 2$, $\beta = 5$.

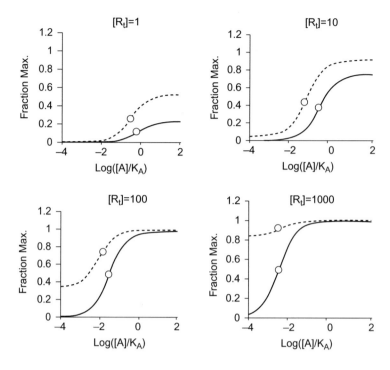

8.5.3 Kinetics of Target Coverage

The open nature of *in vivo* systems (drug concentration is
never constant) makes time an important variable in therapeutic drug activity. Thus, an antagonist is therapeutically
useful only when bound to the receptor and this, in turn,
will be dependent upon its dissociation rate from the protein surface (see Section 6.7 in Chapter 6). Under these circumstances, two antagonists could have identical affinities
but still be different in terms of their rate of dissociation
from the target and thus give very different target coverage
values — see Figure 8.20. In addition to dissociation rate
from the target, the restricted diffusion in receptor compartments *in vivo* also can lead to differences in target coverage
[20,24]. Figure 8.32A shows the plasma concentration of
the antipsychotic drug rispiradone and the dopamine D2
receptor occupancy in the brain as measured by positron
emission tomography as a function of time [25]. The dissimulation between central compartment drug concentration
and brain receptor occupancy can be seen; i.e., the plasma
concentration falls at an approximately six fold greater rate
than does receptor occupancy.

and sensitization are observed. The point of the simulation is
that these varied behaviors can **all** be predicted by a single
set of molecular parameters, in this case a low level of direct
efficacy (3.3% of the endogenous agonist) and an effect on
affinity of $\alpha = 2$ and on efficacy of $\beta = 5$ (see Section 7.4.5
in Chapter 7 for further details). This underscores the value
of determining these predictive parameters in test systems.

Persistent association of drugs with the target can be
an advantage for drugs with restricted pharmacokinetics.
Real time *in vivo* concentration of the drug is given by:

$$C_t = \frac{k_a F\,\text{Dose}}{V(k_a - K)}\left[e^{-Kt} - e^{-k_a t}\right] \qquad (8.18)$$

where k_a is the rate of absorption, K the rate of elimination,
V the volume of distribution and F the bioavailability (for
an oral drug). It can be seen from Equation 8.18 that a high
rate of clearance can lead to low *in vivo* concentrations of
drug in the receptor compartment (as discussed more fully
in Chapter 9). However, the kinetics of the actual rate of
drug dissociation from the target can be a more important
determinant of the quality of therapeutic drug action *in vivo*
since the pharmacokinetics loads the receptor compartment
and then the association (k_1) and dissociation (k_2) rates of
the molecule to and from the receptor determine reversal of
drug effect. As shown in Figure 8.32B, a persistent binding
can turn a drug with transient pharmacokinetics into one
with once-a-day dosing. For this reason it is extremely
important to measure dissociation rates of drugs, as these
can be useful predictors of effects *in vivo*.

8.5.4 Drug Combinations *In Vivo*

Drugs are often used as added treatments in ongoing therapeutic regimens and there are cases where advantages
can be gained with drug combinations. Also, there are
cases where therapy involves the modification of cellular
networks that have signaling redundancy, and action at
one single point in the system may be insufficient to

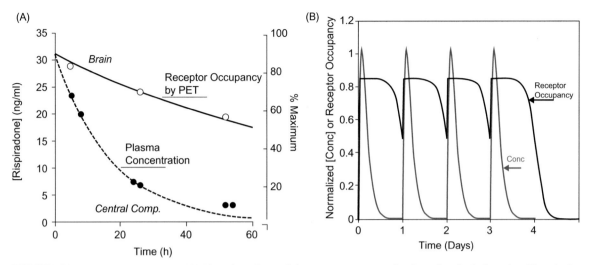

FIGURE 8.32 *In vivo* target coverage. (A) Time dependence of the receptor occupancy for the antipsychotic drug risperidone in the human brain through PET imaging (open circles, solid line) compared to the plasma levels of the drug in the central compartment (filled circles, dotted line). Redrawn from [25]. (B) An antagonist with a very slow dissociation rate from the receptor could produce complete target coverage (black line) with once-a-day dosage even if the clearance for this antagonist does not support once-a-day dosage for drug levels in the central compartment (red line).

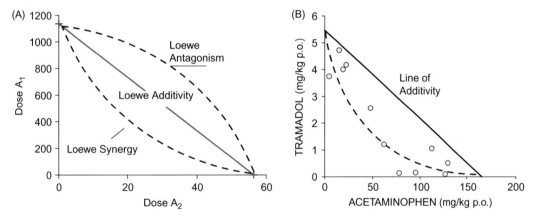

FIGURE 8.33 **Isobolograms for the ED₅₀ (effective dose of drug producing 50% maximal response) of two drugs as functions of each other.** Panel A: The prediction for additivity is a straight line. If the two drugs synergize (i.e., their combined effect is greater than additive) then there will be a downward curvature; if there is mutual antagonism, the curvature is upward. Panel B: Isobologram for the antinociceptive interaction between acetaminophen and tramadol given p.o. in mice. Redrawn from [32].

modify cellular behavior. When this occurs (i.e., diseases such as cancer, infections and AIDS), multiple drugs must be used to attack multiple control points in the network [26]. Therefore there are cases where it is important that specific drug combinations be tested for activity to detect possibly favorable synergistic effects (greater than additive) or antagonistic effects (less than additive) with defined combinations. From such studies insight may be gained into how hazardous treatment regimens (such as those required for cancer) can be optimized such that the side effects of drugs can be minimized by limiting dosage. The most common approach in these studies is the application of tools such as isobolograms [27−29], Bliss independence [30], and nonlinear blending [31].

It is useful to predict combinations of drug concentrations that produce a total effect greater than the sum of their parts, i.e., true synergy. As a starting point, additive responses must be modeled, and this can be done with sigmoidal curves for drug A_1 (Response = $[A_1]/([A_1] + K_1)$ where K_1 represents the concentration producing half maximal effect) and A_2 (Response = $[A_2]/([A_2] + K_2)$). In the simple case where both drugs produce the same maximal effect and can be described by sigmoidal curves of equal slope, the effect produced by drug A_2 can be substituted into the equation for the effect with drug A_1 to calculate the equivalent dose of A_1 producing the same effect. This calculated concentration is then virtually added to the concentrations of A_1 (A_2 is assumed to be an added

FIGURE 8.34 Surface showing the additive effects of two drugs according to Equation 8.19 and the response to a hypothetical combination dose that is above the surface (indicating a synergistic effect).

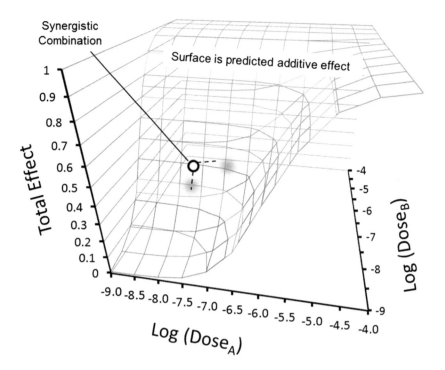

concentration of A_1) to simulate the additive response. It can then be shown that the responses to A_1, in the presence of a range of concentrations of A_2, are given by:

$$\text{Additive Effect} \frac{[A_1] + [A_2]\frac{[K_1]}{[K_2]}}{[A_1] + [A_2]\frac{[K_1]}{[K_2]} + K_1} \quad (8.19)$$

Equation 8.19 predicts a response surface showing the additive effects of A_1 and A_2; an observed response above (or below) this surface is then identified as synergy or antagonism (see Figure 8.33).

A further strategy for analyzing whether combinations of drug produce additive, supra-additive or sub-additive effects employs isobolograms [29]. These graphs consist of axes showing defined concentrations of two drugs (for example, ED_{50} values); the line (or curve) joining the two intercepts (these will be the ED_{50} of each drug) represents the pairs of doses used together giving the defined level of response that each drug gives independently. The ED_{50} values can be used in a relationship for two drugs A and B with ED_{50} values of ED_{50-A} and ED_{50-B} and maximal response values of MAX_A and MAX_B values respectively as [29]:

$$b = ED_{50-B} - \frac{ED_{50-B}}{\frac{MAX_B}{MAX_A}\left[1 + \frac{ED_{50-A}}{a}\right] - 1} \quad (8.20)$$

For two drugs with equivalent maximal responses ($MAX_A = MAX_B$) this relationship reduces to a straight line:

$$\frac{a}{ED_{50-A}} + \frac{b}{ED_{50-B}} = 1 \quad (8.21)$$

Figure 8.34A shows the additive straight line relationship for two ED_{50} values of two drugs A and B. A curved relationship for two drugs of equal maximal response indicates a supra-additive or sub-additive effect of ED_{50} values. An experimental example of this is shown in Figure 8.34B: the combination of effects of various doses of acetaminophen and tramadol for antinociception in mice indicates a curvature from additivity indicative of synergy [32].

8.6 SUMMARY AND CONCLUSIONS

- The aim of pharmacological experimentation is to define the four minimal properties of drugs: efficacy(ies), affinity, mode of binding (orthosteric vs. allosteric), and target dissociaton kinetics − with these the behavior of drugs can be predicted.
- Parameters that describe drug behavior can be determined through null experiments and the comparison of experimental data to mathematical pharmacodynamic models.
- Changes in these parameters can be evaluated statistically to confirm significant difference and then linked to molecular structure to generate structure-activity relationships.
- Predictive parameters for moelcuels (i.e., τ, K_A for agonists, K_B for orthosteric antagonists, K_B,α,β for allosteric modulators) can be used to predict drug behavior in systems of varying sensitivity. This, in turn, can be used to predict therapeutic behavior.

8.7 DERIVATIONS

8.7.1 IC$_{50}$ Correction Factors: Competitive Antagonists

The relationship between the concentration of antagonist that produces a 50% inhibition of a response to an agonist (antagonist concentration referred to as the IC$_{50}$) and the equilibrium dissociation constant of the antagonist-receptor complex (K$_B$) can be derived from the mass action equations describing the agonist-receptor response in the presence and absence of the antagonist. The response in the absence of antagonist can be fit to a logistic curve of the form:

$$Response = \frac{E_{max}[A]^n}{[A]^n + [EC_{50}]^n}, \quad (8.22)$$

where the concentration of agonist is [A], E$_{max}$ is the maximal response to the agonist, n the Hill coefficient of the dose-response curve, and [EC$_{50}$] the molar concentration of agonist producing 50% maximal response to the agonist.

In the presence of a competitive antagonist, the EC$_{50}$ of the agonist dose-response curve will be shifted to the right by a factor equal to the dose ratio; this is given by the Schild equation as [B]/K$_B$ + 1, where the concentration of the antagonist is [B] and K$_B$ is the equilibrium dissociation constant of the antagonist-receptor complex:

$$Response = \frac{E_{max}[A]^n}{[A]^n + ([EC_{50}](1 + [B]/K_B))^n}. \quad (8.23)$$

The concentration of antagonist producing a 50% diminution of the agonist response to concentration [A] is defined as the IC$_{50}$ for the antagonist. Therefore:

$$\frac{0.5E_{max}[A]^n}{[A]^n + [EC_{50}]^n} = \frac{E_{max}[A']^n}{[A']^n + ([EC_{50}](1 + [IC_{50}]/K_B))^n}. \quad (8.24)$$

After rearrangement [15]:

$$K_B = \frac{[IC_{50}]}{(2 + (([A]/[EC_{50}])^n)^{1/n}) - 1}. \quad (8.25)$$

8.7.2 Relationship of pA$_2$ and pK$_B$ for Insurmountable Orthosteric Antagonism

For simple competitive antagonism with adequate time for agonist−antagonist re-equilibration (surmountable antagonism), ρ_B is given by [B]/K$_B$/([B]/K$_B$ + [A]/K$_A$ + 1) to yield the well-known Gaddum equation for simple competitive antagonism for agonist-receptor occupancy in the presence

of the antagonist (denoted ρ_{AB}) ([A]/K$_A$/([A]/K$_A$ + [B]/K$_B$ + 1)) [33]. Under these circumstances, the equation for the response to the agonist in the presence of the simple competitive antagonist becomes:

$$Response = \frac{[A]/K_A \tau E_{max}}{[A]/K_A(1 + \tau) + [B]/K_B + 1}. \quad (8.26)$$

A relationship for equiactive agonist concentrations in the absence and presence of antagonist to yield a dose ratio of 2 ([B] = 10^{-pA2}) can be made to calculate the ratio of this empirical concentration (pA$_2$) to the true K$_B$ value:

$$\frac{2[A]/K_A \tau E_{max}}{2[A]/K_A(1 + \tau) + [10 - pA_2]/K_B + 1} = \frac{[A]/K_A \tau E_{max}}{[A]/K_A(1 + \tau) + 1}. \quad (8.27)$$

It can be seen through simplifying this relationship that:

$$10^{-pA_2} = K_B, \quad (8.28)$$

as expected from the Schild equation (i.e., pA$_2$ = pK$_B$) of unit slope.

This same procedure can be done to equate the empirical pA$_2$ to pK$_B$ for a completely noncompetitive antagonist in which the agonist and antagonist do not re-equilibrate due to kinetics. Under these circumstances, the equation for antagonist occupancy is given by mass action, and agonist-receptor occupancy in the presence of antagonist (ρ_{AB}) with no time for agonist, antagonist, or receptor re-equilibration (Equation 6.10) for noncompetitive receptor blockade is:

$$Response = \frac{[A]/K_A \tau E_{max}}{[A]/K_A(1 + \tau + [B]/K_B) + [B]/K_B + 1}. \quad (8.29)$$

The relationship between equiactive concentrations with a dose ratio of 2 in the presence and absence of antagonist is given by:

$$\frac{2[A]/K_A \tau E_{max}}{2[A]/K_A(1 + \tau + [10^{-pA_2}]/K_B) + [10^{-pA_2}]/K_B + 1}$$
$$= \frac{[A]/K_A \tau E_{max}}{[A]/K_A(1 + \tau) + 1}. \quad (8.30)$$

Simplification of this relationship yields an equation relating pA$_2$ and K$_B$:

$$10^{-pA_2} = K_B/(1 + 2[A]/K_A) \quad (8.31)$$

$$pK_B = pA_2 - Log(1 + 2[A]/K_A). \quad (8.32)$$

The magnitude of the correction term $(1 + 2[A]/K_A)$ can be scaled to the system by relating this to the EC$_{50}$ (molar concentration of agonist producing 50% maximal response to that agonist) of the control agonist concentration-response curve. The equation for response in terms of the operational model is [8]:

$$\text{Response} = \frac{[A]/K_A\tau E_{max}}{[A]/K_A(1+\tau)+1}. \qquad (8.33)$$

It can be seen from this equation that the EC_{50} concentration is given by $EC_{50} = K_A/(1+\tau)$; therefore, any value of $[A]/K_A$ can be expressed with the relation $[A]/K_A = [A]/(EC_{50} \ (1+\tau))$. Under these circumstances, Equation 8.33 becomes:

$$pK_B = pA_2 - \text{Log}(1+(2[A]/EC_{50}(1+\tau))). \qquad (8.34)$$

8.7.3 Relationship of pA_2 and pK_B for Insurmountable Allosteric Antagonism

The counterpart of Equation 8.30 for allosteric systems is:

$$\frac{2[A]/K_A\tau E_{max}}{2[A]/K_A(1+\tau+\alpha[10^{-pA_2}]/K_B)+[10^{-pA_2}]/K_B+1}$$
$$= \frac{[A]/K_A\tau E_{max}}{[A]/K_A(1+\tau)+1}.$$

$$(8.35)$$

The equation for the relationship between the pA_2 and the K_B of an allosteric modulator that produces insurmountable antagonism then becomes:

$$10^{-pA_2} = K_B/(1+2\alpha[A]/K_A) \qquad (8.36)$$

$$pK_B = pA_2 - \text{Log}(1+2\alpha[A]/K_A), \qquad (8.37)$$

in terms of functional responses expressed as multiples of the EC_{50}:

$$pK_B = pA_2 - \text{Log}(1+(2\alpha[A]/EC_{50}(1+\tau))). \qquad (8.38)$$

For allosteric modulators that decrease the affinity of the receptor for the antagonist ($\alpha < 1$), this effect actually decreases the error between the observed pA_2 and the true pK_B and thus improves the method. In contrast it can be seen that, if the allosteric modulator *increases* the affinity of the receptor for the agonist ($\alpha > 1$), then the error produced by the insurmountable nature of the blockade may become substantial.

REFERENCES

[1] Kenakin TP. Quantifying biological activity in chemical terms: a pharmacology primer to describe drug effect. ACS Chem Biol 2009;4:249–60.

[2] Gray JA, Roth BL. Paradoxical trafficking and regulation of 5-HT (2A) receptors by agonists and antagonists. Brain Res Bull 2001;56:441–51.

[3] Roettger BF, Ghanekar D, Rao R, Toledo C, Yingling J, Pinon D, et al. Antagonist-stimulated internalization of the G protein-coupled cholecystokinin receptor. Mol Pharmacol 1997;51:357–62.

[4] Kenakin TP. Pharmacological onomastics: what's in a name? Br J Pharmacol 2008;153:432–8.

[5] Galandrin S, Bouvier M. Distinct signaling profiles of β_1- and β_2 adrenergic receptor ligands toward adenylyl cyclase and mitogen-activated protein kinase reveals the pluridimensionality of efficacy. Mol Pharmacol 2006;70:1575–84.

[6] Mukhopadhyay S, Howlett AC. Chemically distinct ligands promote differential CB1 cannabinoid receptor-Gi protein interactions. Mol Pharmacol 2005;67:2016–24.

[7] Metra M, Dei Cas L, di Lenarda A, Poole-Wilson P. Beta-blockers in heart failure: are pharmacological differences clinically important? Heart Fail Rev 2004;9:123–30.

[8] Black JW, Leff P. Operational models of pharmacological agonist. Proc R Soc Lond [Biol] 1983;220:141.

[9] Kenakin TP. The relative contribution of affinity and efficacy to agonist activity: organ selectivity of noradrenaline and oxymetazoline. Br J Pharmacol 1984;81:131–41.

[10] Kenakin TP, Watson C, Muniz-Medina V, Christopoulos A, Novick S. A simple method for quantifying functional selectivity and agonist bias. ACS Chem Neurosci 2012;3:193–203.

[11] Kenakin TP, Christopoulos A. Signaling bias in new drug discovery: detection, quantification and therapeutic impact. Nat Rev Drug Disc 2013;12:1–12.

[12] Ehlert FJ. Analysis of allosterism in functional assays. J Pharmacol Exp Ther 2005;315:740–54.

[13] Griffin T, Figueroa KW, Liller S, Ehlert FJ. Estimation of agonist affinity at G protein-coupled receptors: analysis of M2 muscarinic receptor signaling through Gi/0, Gs and G15. J Pharmacol Exp Ther 2007;321:1193–207.

[14] Cheng YC, Prusoff WH. Relationship between the inhibition constant (Ki) and the concentration of inhibitor which causes 50 percent inhibition (I50) of an enzymatic reaction. Biochem Pharmacol 1973;22:3099–108.

[15] Leff P, Dougall IG. Further concerns over Cheng–Prusoff analysis. Trends Pharmacol Sci 1993;14:110–2.

[16] Kenakin TP, Jenkinson S, Watson C. Determining the potency and molecular mechanism of action of insurmountable antagonists. J Pharmacol Exp Ther 2006;319:710–23.

[17] Maillet EL, Pellegrini N, Valant C, Bucher B, Hibert M, Bourguignon J-J, et al. A novel, conformation-specific allosteric inhibitor of the tachykinin NK2 receptor (NK2R) with functionally selective properties. FASEB J 2007;21:2124–34.

[18] Kenakin TP. Collateral efficacy in drug discovery: taking advantage of the good (allosteric) nature of 7TM receptors. Trends Pharmacol Sci 2007;28:407–15.

[19] Kew JNC, Trube G, Kemp JA. A novel mechanism of activity-dependent NMDA receptor antagonism describes the effect of ifenprodil in rat cultured cortical neurons. J Physiol 1996;497:761–72.

[20] Copeland RA, Pompliano DL, Meek TD. Drug target residence time and its implications for lead optimization. Nat Rev Drug Disc 2006;5:730–9.

[21] Julious SA. Using confidence intervals around individual means to assess statistical significance between two means. Pharmaceut Stat 2004;3:217–22.

[22] Manas ES, Unwalla RJ, Xu ZB, Malamas MS, Miller CP, Harris HA, et al. Structure-based design of estrogen receptor-β-selective ligands. J Amer Chem Soc 2004;126:15106−19.

[23] Black JW, Leff P, Shankley NP. (Appendix J. Wood) An operational model of pharmacological agonism: the effect of E/[A] curve shape on agonist dissociation constant estimation. Br J Pharmacol 1985;84:561−71.

[24] Vauquelin G, Charlton SJ. Long-lasting target binding and rebinding as mechanisms to prolong *in vivo* drug action. Br J Pharmacol 2010;161:488−95.

[25] Takamo A, Suhara T, Ikoma Y, Yasuno F, Maeda J, Ichimiya T, et al. Estimation of the time-course of dopamine D2 receptor occupancy in living human brain from plasma pharmacokinetics of antipsychotics. Int J Neuropsychopharmacol 2004;7:19−26.

[26] Keith CT, Borisy AA, Stockwell BR. Multicomponent therapeutics for networked systems. Nat Drug Disc 2005;4:71−85.

[27] Loew S, Muischnek H. Uber Kombinationswirkungen. Naunyn-Schmiedeberg's Arch Exp Path Pharmacol 1926;114:313−26.

[28] Loewe S. The problem of synergism and antagonism of combined drugs. Arzneimittelforschung 1953;3:285−90.

[29] Tallarida RJ. Revisiting the isobole and related quantitative methods for assessing drug synergism. J Pharmacol Expt Ther 2012;342:2−8.

[30] Bliss CI. The toxicity of poisons combined jointly. Ann Appl Biol 1939;26:585−615.

[31] Peterson JJ, Novick SJ. Nonlinear blending: a useful general concept for the assessment of combination drug synergy. J Recept Sig Transd 2007;27:125−46.

[32] Tallarida RJ, Raffa RB. Testing for synergism over a range of fixed ratio drug combinations: replacing the isobologram. Life Sci 1995; 58:23−8.

[33] Gaddum JH. The quantitative effects of antagonistic drugs. J Physiol Lond 1937;89:7P−9P.

Chapter 9

Pharmacokinetics

Pharmacokinetics... pharmacos, a poisoner, a magician, or a sorcerer + κισισ (kinesis), movement (motion of bodies produced under the action of forces).

— Merriam-Webster's 9th Collegiate Dictionary

...never confuse motion with action...

— Benjamin Franklin (1706−1790)

Everything is in motion. Everything flows. Everything is vibrating.

— William Hazlitt (1778−1830)

9.1 Introduction
9.2 Biopharmaceutics
9.3 The Chemistry of "Druglike" Character
9.4 Pharmacokinetics
9.5 Nonlinear Pharmacokinetics
9.6 Multiple Dosing
9.7 Practical Pharmacokinetics
9.8 Placement of Pharmacokinetic Assays in Discovery and Development
9.9 Summary and Conclusions
References

9.1 INTRODUCTION

In the general scheme of pharmacology-based therapeutics, a drug must be made into a stable form amenable to introduction into the body, pass into the body, reach its biological target of action, remain there for a sufficient length of time to achieve its therapeutic end, not induce harm while in the body, and then exit the body after its task is done (Figure 9.1). This chapter discusses the various processes involved in this complex journey.

9.2 BIOPHARMACEUTICS

Biopharmaceutics is the process of determining the best form to use in the study of a molecule in toxicological and clinical studies, and also the most stable preparation for dispensability as a drug product. The pharmaceutical development of drug candidates is an important step that must go on in partnership with the study of pharmacokinetics. Ideally, the oral absorption of the molecular substance in capsule form should be equal to or greater than its absorption when administered as a soluble aqueous solution. Absorption via the oral route (preferably in a capsule) should be adequate to allow $30 \times -100 \times$ dosing for toxicological studies. The substance should also be stable in a crystalline form, as this can affect drug absorption. For example, chloramphenicol exists in two stable crystal polymorphs, A and B, with the B form being $2.5 \times$ better absorbed than the A form [1]. If stable crystals are not evident, nanomilled solid suspensions or spray-dried preparations can be made. Alternatively, polyethylene glycol surfactant enhanced solutions can be used to model soft gel caps. In general, while these techniques can assist in the presentation of molecules for *in vivo* study, pharmaceutical preparation is limited in terms of making a molecule suitable as a drug substance.

The first step to drug absorption is dissolution of the solid drug into aqueous media. A concise relationship defining this process is the Noyes−Whitney equation:

$$\frac{dW}{dt} = \frac{DA\,(C_s - C)}{L}, \tag{9.1}$$

T. P. Kenakin: A Pharmacology Primer, Fourth edition. DOI: http://dx.doi.org/10.1016/B978-0-12-407663-1.00009-0
© 2014 Elsevier Inc. All rights reserved.

FIGURE 9.1 Schematic diagram illustrating the interdependence of biopharmaceutics, pharmacokinetics, and pharmacodynamics in therapeutic drug action.

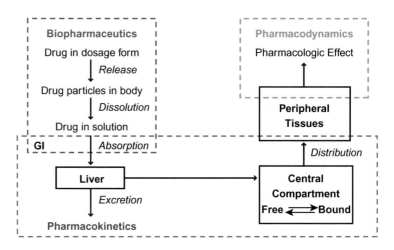

where A is the surface area of the solid; C and C_s are the concentrations of the solid in the bulk media and in the diffusion layer surrounding the solid, respectively; D is the diffusion coefficient of the media; and L is the diffusion layer thickness around the solid. It can be seen that factors such as stirring (reducing the diffusion layer L) or milling the particles to a smaller diameter (increasing A, the surface area for absorption) will increase the rate of dissolution, whereas decreasing the diffusion coefficient (i.e., dissolving in oil versus water) will reduce the dissolution. Similarly, coating tablets (reducing $C - C_s$) will hinder dissolution, so causing sustained release. In general, tablet ingredients include materials to break up the tablet such as a granulating agent, filler (should be water soluble and not interact with the drug), a wetting agent (to help the penetration of water into the tablet), and a disintegration agent (to help break the tablet apart). Formulation of a drug can be very important, and the Food and Drug Administration (FDA) requires bioavailability studies for any change in formulation of a drug therapy. This is in response to results from clinical studies which indicate that different drug products produce different therapeutic results, and also data from bioavailability studies indicating that different products are not bioequivalent. Especially vulnerable to nuances in formulation are drugs that have a narrow therapeutic range, drugs with low solubility, drugs that might require large doses, and drugs demonstrating incomplete absorption.

Formulation is a common method of developing sustained release preparations such as erosion tablets, drugs in a waxy matrix (matrix erodes or drug leaches from matrix), coated pellets (different pellets have different release properties), and coated ion-exchange preparations. There are special considerations for sustained release systems, since complicated formulations may be more erratically absorbed; the sustained release product may contain a larger dose (and failure of the controlled release mechanism may result in release of a large toxic dose) and is a more expensive technology.

Pharmaceutics is a complete discipline within itself, the full discussion of which is beyond the scope of this present book. Therefore, from this point in this chapter, it will be assumed that the drug has been formulated to a point where a predictable concentration can be introduced into the body and is available to be absorbed into the body.

9.3 THE CHEMISTRY OF "DRUGLIKE" CHARACTER

The absorption, distribution, metabolism, and excretion of a molecule defines its pharmacokinetics, and many of these processes, in turn, are controlled by the physicochemical properties of the molecule. In pharmacokinetics terms, this is often referred to as the molecule's *druglike* properties. It is worth considering the effects of various chemical structural groups on druglike properties, as these, at least to some extent, are factors that can be controlled by the medicinal chemist in the lead optimization phase of drug development. The effects of chemical functional groups on acid-base properties, water solubility, the partition coefficient (octanol-water), molecular weight, and stereochemistry are all relevant to the druglike properties of molecules.

Chemical groups in molecules have intrinsic proclivities to donate protons (acids such as phenols, sulfonamides, alkylcarboxylic acids) or accept protons (bases such as amides, nitriles, diarylamines) to the aqueous environment (intrinsic acid-base properties); these control the proportion of the molecule that exists as a charged ionic species in water at any pH. The relative amounts of charged and uncharged species of any given molecule are defined by the molecule's pK_a and the pH of the medium, according to the Henderson−Hasselbach equation (see Figure 9.2):

$$pK_a = pH + \log - \frac{[\text{acid form}]}{[\text{base form}]}. \qquad (9.2)$$

It can be seen that, when $pK_a = pH$, the ratio of the acid to the base form will be unity. These forms of the

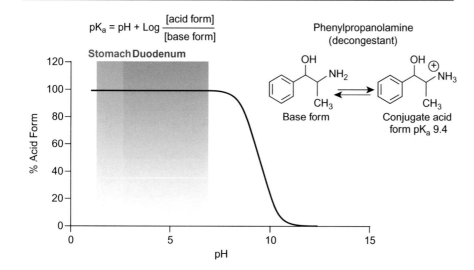

$$pK_a = pH + Log \frac{[acid\ form]}{[base\ form]}$$

FIGURE 9.2 The formations of conjugate base from acidic compounds and conjugate acid from basic compounds. The Henderson–Hassalbach equation equates the pK_a of a molecule to the pH and yields logarithm of the ratio of acid to base form of the molecule. The graph shows the ratio of acid to base form of phenylpropanolamine ($pK_a = 9.4$) at various pH values. In the stomach pH (1.5 to 2) nearly 100% of the molecule is in the acid form, and this ratio persists throughout the physiological pH range in the duodenum. For a substantial amount of basic form to be formed, the pH would need to be >8 to 9.

molecule have relevance to its absorption through biological membranes, since charged species do not readily cross lipid barriers spontaneously and may need specialized carrier processes to enter cells (*vide infra*). Organic molecules can have a very wide range of pK_a values; from as low as 2.5 (penicillins) to as high as 12 (guanethidine), and these interact with the limited pH range in the body (1.5 in the stomach to 7.5 in the blood). Figure 9.2 shows the calculated acid (charged) and base (uncharged) form of phenylpropanolamine and the predicted ratio of charged to uncharged species for this molecule at various pH values. It can be seen that, in the stomach and human gut (where the pH is acidic), this molecule is essentially uncharged and thus would penetrate lipid membranes readily. Table 9.1 shows the amounts of various drugs absorbed at different pH values.

The aqueous solubility of a drug depends on its acid-base properties and the pH, the ionization of functional groups, and the ability of chemical groups to form hydrogen bonds with water. The formation of drug salts can be a powerful method of increasing aqueous solubility, and the type of salt can be critical. For example, physostigmine salicylate has a solubility of 1 g/75 mL, while the solubility of physostigmine sulfate is 0.25 g/mL. Similarly, hydroxyzine pamoate has an aqueous solubility of 1 g/liter, while hydroxyzine hydrochloride is 1000 times more soluble (1 g/mL). Penicillin solubility (and subsequent absorption) changes with the type of salt, with K^+ salt > Ca^{2+} salt > free acid > benzathine salt.

TABLE 9.1 Differential Absorption at Varying pH

		% Absorption at			
	pK_a	pH = 4	pH = 5	pH = 7	pH = 8
Acid					
S-nitrosalicylic acid	2.3	40%	27%	0%	0%
Salicylic	3	64%	35%	30%	10%
Acetylsalicylic	3.5	41%	27%	–	–
Benzoic	4.2	62%	36%	35%	5%
Bases					
Aniline	4.6	40%	48%	58%	61%
Aminopyrene	5	21%	35%	48%	52%
Quinine	8.4	9%	11%	41%	54%

From [2].

One method to gauge the lipophylic versus hydrophilic character of chemicals is to determine their relative solubility in a lipid-like medium (i.e., octanol) and water. Thus, the log P (if experimentally determined, it is referred to as the *Mlog P*; if calculated, it is the *Clog P*) is the logarithm of the relative concentration of a molecule dissolved in octanol versus water (logarithmically related to free energy). For example, a log P value of 0.5

indicates that in a separatory funnel containing a total of 1 mole of a substance, the ratio of concentrations in octanol versus water is 2 (the concentration in the octanol layer is twice that in the water layer). As discussed previously the pK_a of the molecule and the pH of the medium determine the extent of ionization of the molecule. Since the ionic species is water soluble, the ionic character then also determines the water solubility of the compound. When the water solubility of the non-ionized and ionized form of the molecule are considered, the ratio of solubilities in water and organic medium is referred to as the log D and must be reported with the pH of the aqueous medium in which the determination was made. The relationship between the water solubility of a compound and the pH of the medium is given by:

$$\text{Acid:} \quad S = S_0(1 + 10^{(pH-pKa)})$$
$$\text{Base:} \quad S = S_0(1 + 10^{(pKa-pH)})$$
(9.3)

where S_0 is the "intrinsic solubility" of the compound; i.e., the solubility of the compound when $pH = pK_a$. For example, the water solubility of amobarbital is increased by a factor of 13.6 at $pH = 9$ ($S_0 = 1.2$ mg mL^{-1}, at $pH = 9.9$ S $= 16.3$ mg mL^{-1}). Insofar as molecules must be dissolved in aqueous media for absorption to occur, the dependence of solubility on pH can lead to substantial effects in the oral absorption of drugs. The hydrogen ion concentration in the human gastrointestinal tract varies by a factor of 6 million (pH of the stomach $= 1.2$, that of the lower colon is up to 8.0) leading to differences in drug solubility. For example, the solubility of the anti-inflammatory drug naproxen ($pK_a = 4.9$) varies by nearly a factor of 5 as it travels through the gastrointestinal tract.

Clog P values can be calculated by summing π values for log P (Clog P $= \Sigma p_{fragments}$) that have been calculated for chemical groups [3,4] (see Figure 9.3A). The example shown in Figure 9.3A shows the values for each group

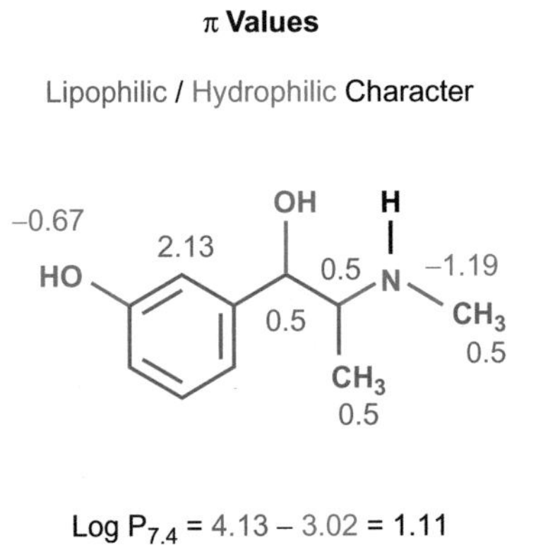

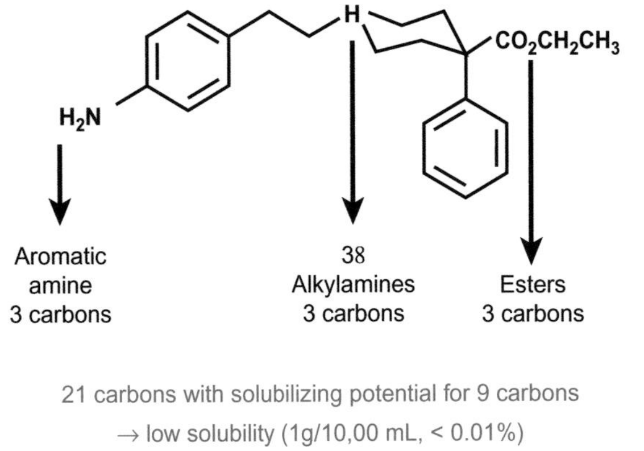

FIGURE 9.3 Calculated values to predict aqueous solubility. (A) The octanol-water partition ratio (log P) can be estimated through calculation; each chemical group has a theoretical score contributing to the total log P (if calculated, this is Clog P) [5]. For epinephrine, the scores for the lipophilic groups (red) total 4.13, while those for the hydrophilic groups (blue) total −3.02, for a total Clog P = 1.11. (B) Various chemical groups have theoretical indices denoting their "power" to solubilize carbon atoms into water. For the molecule shown, the score indicates a power to solubilize 9 carbon atoms; this is below the number of carbon atoms in the molecule, therefore aqueous solubility would be predicted to be low (experimentally determined to be <0.01%). Formation of a salt of this compound adds solubilizing power for 20−30 carbon atoms, making this molecule very water soluble. Data for part B from [6].

and the sum, which in this case is 1.11. A Clog P value of <0.5 generally ensures water solubility. Another method of estimating water solubility is through an empirical approach devised by Lemke [6], whereby the solubilizing power of various chemical groups to solubilize carbon atoms (see table in Figure 9.3B) is summed for any given molecule to yield a score. If the score of the solubilizing groups provides a number greater than the number of carbons in the molecule, then it is predicted that the molecule will be soluble in water. Figure 9.3B shows an example in which the chemical groups yield the power to solubilize 9 carbon atoms; but since the molecule has 21 carbon atoms, this would predict a low water solubility for this molecule, and this is borne out in experiments where the solubility was found to be <0.01%. However, a large measure of solubilizing power can be gained by making an ionic salt of the molecule (20–30 carbon atoms), and under these circumstances, the resulting score for the molecule would be in a range of 29–39 carbon atoms. This is larger than the number of carbons in the molecule and would predict good water solubility, which is seen in experimental studies (20%).

A useful parameter in pharmacokinetics is the MAD (maximal absorbable dose). This is a product calculated as:

$$MAD = S \times K_{ar} \times SIWV \times SITT \qquad (9.4)$$

where S = aqueous solubility in mg mL^{-1} usually at pH = 6.5, K_{ar} = transintestinal absorption rate constant, SIWV is the small intestine water volume (250 mL in humans), and SITT is the small intestine transit time (approximately 4.5 hours in humans). The MAD can yield useful guidelines for choosing compounds for progression, as it gives the maximal amount of compound that could reasonably be expected to be absorbed from a single oral dose. For example, if a required therapeutic concentration after a single dose is 0.5 mg kg^{-1}, then the dosage must yield an absorbed dosage of 35 mg. For a compound with K_{ar} of 0.3 min^{-1} and a solubility of 0.001 mg mL^{-1}, the MAD is only 2 mg, far short of the therapeutic requirement. The MAD underscores the importance of aqueous solubility to drug absorption. As will be seen, the absorption of compounds through cell monolayers is an important determinant of drug pharmacokinetics, and this factor can be altered by chemical synthetic alteration by a factor of approximately 50 in the drug development process. In contrast, aqueous solubility can be altered by far larger factors (up to a million-fold) by chemical alteration, therefore, according to the MAD calculation, aqueous solubility offers a more flexible alternative for increasing oral absorbability than does intestinal permeation. However, as will be seen when cellular permeation is discussed, a delicate balance of aqueous and lipid solubility is required for the cellular penetration needed for adequate drug absorption. The interplay between solubility and permeation is underscored by the Biopharmaceutics Classification System (BCS) for drug intestinal absorption. This classifies molecules in terms of their aqueous solubility and membrane permeation. Thus, BCS Class 1 compounds are highly soluble, have good lipid permeation and are excellent oral drugs (i.e., nortriptylene, diltiazem, labetolol, enalapril, propranolol). BCS Class 2 compounds are lipophilic but have limited aqueous solubility and require unique formulation for oral activity (i.e., phenytoin, naproxen, diclonefac). BSC Class 3 compounds have high aqueous solubility but poor lipid solubility and thus may require prodrug strategies for oral activity (vide infra) — i.e., nadolol, ranitidine, famotidine. BCS Class 4 compounds can pose problems for oral activity due to limited aqueous solubility and lipid permeability (i.e., furosemide, ketoprofen, hydrochlorthiazide).

There are two methods used to measure aqueous solubility. Kinetic solubility measurements determine the amount of compound dissolved in water when added from a stock solution in dimethylsulfoxide. These measurements are rapid, are not made at equilibrium, and are useful for detecting absorption and bioassay liabilities. Another measurement, thermodynamic solubility, is made by equilibrating the solid with water for 24–72 hours, and is used to guide formulation and in vivo studies. In light of the limited time window available for the intestinal absorption of oral drugs (approximately 4.5 hours), kinetic solubility measurements made within these time scales may be the most relevant measurement for drug development. Further discussion of the aqueous solubility of drugs can be found in Chapter 2, Section 2.9.1.

In general, water solubility is needed to carry the drug into the aqueous environment of the body and the cells within it. However, lipid solubility is also required in order to cross the bilipid membrane of the cell, so the ideal drug would have enough hydrophobicity to pass though the lipid bilayer, but not so much as to cause the molecule to be unable to partition out again. Drug hydrophobicity can affect the way that the drug distributes and is metabolized and excreted in the body. Specifically, hydrophobic drugs are generally more toxic and widely distributed, have less selective binding, are more extensively metabolized to reactive metabolites, and are retained for longer periods in the body.

Another somewhat controllable property of a drug is its molecular weight. In general, most drugs have a molecular weight of between 300 and 400 g M^{-1} (see Figure 9.4), although there are exceptions such as those seen with HIV protease inhibitors and rennin inhibitors (see Figure 9.4). There are data to show that excessively high molecular weight compounds are poorly absorbed, therefore it is advantageous to keep this parameter between 250 and 350 g M^{-1}. This may be difficult, since enhancement of biological activity from the original hit

FIGURE 9.4 **Histogram showing relative numbers of known drugs of various molecular weights.** A general Boltzman distribution indicates that most known drugs have a molecular weight between 300 and 400 g mole^{-1}. Various classes of drugs are also shown; β-adrenoceptor-blocking drugs and benzodiazepines have mean molecular weight values consistent with most known drugs. However, some drug classes have much higher molecular weights, such as HIV protease and rennin inhibitors. Data redrawn from [5].

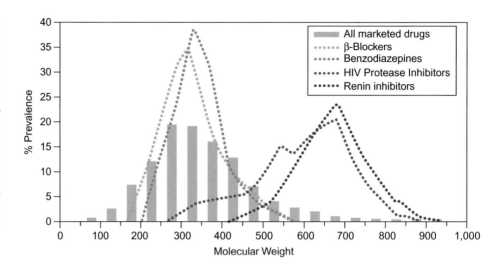

found in a screening program usually entails adding chemical groups to the molecule, not removing them.

Another chemical property relevant to druglike behavior is stereochemistry. There are molecules which contain a *chiral center* (a carbon with four different attachments), and those molecules with different chiral centers (to which the groups are attached in different orientations) are nonsuperimposable. These molecules present different three-dimensional arrays to proteins, and it is presumed that this controls their biological potency and efficacy. For instance, the Easson–Stedman hypothesis proposes that a biologically active enantiomer interacts with at least three points on a receptor to produce biological activity. Since three points define a distinct geometry in three-dimensional space, any rearrangement of those three points on the molecule, as would be produced by a different optimal isomer, would destroy the correspondence on the protein. Enantiomers are mirror-image isomers that have identical physicochemical properties (i.e., solubility, melting points) but refract polarized light in opposite directions (+ and −). An equal mixture of enantiomers is called a *racemic mixture*. Diastereoisomers have multiple chiral centers and are non-mirror-image isomers with different physicochemical properties. In general, many biomolecules are *chiral* (60% of all drugs are optically active), and in most cases one of the enantiomers produces the desired biological effect while the other may have no effect, a toxic effect, a desirable effect, or an adverse effect on absorption, distribution, metabolism, and protein binding (i.e., ketoprofen levels are much higher when both enantiomers are present than when a single enantiomer is present). The ratio between the primary active form and "inactive" form is referred to as the *eudismic index*. Optical activity can be a powerful biological discriminator. For example d-carvone is the taste of caraway, while l-carvone is the flavor of spearmint. Similarly, S-(+)ketamine produces anesthesia, while R-(−)-ketamine causes postemergent distress and spontaneous motor activity.

In general, the physicochemical properties of molecules that are known to be "druglike" furnish guidelines for medicinal chemists as they iteratively produce analogs of lead molecules in discovery and development programs. The druglike character of molecules has also been analyzed in terms of chemical structure *in silico* and some useful ideas have emerged. Thus, a set of rules, referred to as a "Rule of 5", has been derived from an analysis of 2,245 known druglike molecules. The analysis showed that 89% of the molecules have a molecular weight <550, only 10% have Clog P values >5.0, only 8% have a sum of OH and NH groups (hydrogen bond donors) >5, and only 12% have a sum of N and O atoms (hydrogen bond acceptors) >10 [7,8]. From these findings, the following rules (also referred to as "Lipinski Rules") were derived, which are now used as guidelines when looking for druglike activity. Thus, if a compound violates more than one of the following rules, it is likely that it will have suboptimal solubility and permeability characteristics:

1. More than five hydrogen bond donors.
2. More than 10 hydrogen bond acceptors.
3. A molecular weight >500.
4. A Clog P value >5.

9.4 PHARMACOKINETICS

The essence of pharmacology is the relationship between the dose of a drug given to a patient and the resulting change in physiological state (the response to the drug). Qualitatively, the type of response is important, but since, as put by the German pharmacologist Walter Straub in 1937, "... there is only a quantitative difference between a drug and a poison," the quantitative relationship between the dose and the response is paramount. Thus, the concentration (or dose) of drug is the *independent variable* (that set by the experimenter), and the pharmacological effect returned by the therapeutic system is the *dependent variable*. The value of the dependent variable has meaning only if the value of the independent variable is correct (i.e., if the experimenter truly knows the magnitude of this variable). Pharmacokinetics furnishes the tools for the clinician to determine the true value of the independent variable.

Drugs can be effective only if enough is present at the target site, and they can be harmful if enough is present to produce toxic side effects. Any attempt to draw conclusions about the clinical efficacy of a drug in a clinical trial without knowledge of the concentration at the target site is premature. The science of pharmacokinetics basically seeks to answer the following questions:

- How much of the drug that is given to the patient actually reaches the target organ?
- Where in the body does the drug go?
- How long does the drug stay in the body?

Therefore, as a prerequisite to pharmacodynamics (study of drug-receptor interactions), pharmacokinetics examines the journey of drugs into the body toward their intended therapeutic target organ. For example, a drug taken by the oral route is absorbed from the gastrointestinal tract into the systemic circulation and carried by the bloodstream throughout the body. Thus, an antiarrhythmic drug intended to prevent fatal arrhythmia of the heart must travel through the systemic circulation, through the coronary arteries, and be absorbed through the wall of capillaries and into the heart muscle. As it diffuses through layers of cells, it finally encounters the sinus node and interacts with specific sites on the cell membrane to mediate the electrical activity of the cell. Each barrier to this distribution can affect the concentration of

the drug reaching the target site. A useful acronym to describe pharmacokinetics is ADME. This generally describes the process of drug *absorption* into the body, *distribution* throughout the body, *metabolism* by degradative and metabolizing enzymes in the body, and finally *elimination* from the body. It is useful to consider each of these steps, as together they summarize pharmacokinetics.

9.4.1 Drug Absorption

While there is interstitial space between cells, drugs generally must go through (i.e., penetrate membranes), not around, cells and gain access to internal organs. Under these circumstances, the ability of molecules to pass through cell membranes is a very important determinant of absorption. The two main mechanisms available for drugs to pass through lipid membranes are simple bulk diffusion and active transport (or a variant, facilitated diffusion). For simple diffusion, the concentration gradient drives entry. The lipophilicity of the molecule is important, that is, a nonlipophilic molecule will not pass through a lipid bilayer easily, and the state of ionization is relevant (ionized charged molecules do not pass easily). The rate of diffusion also is inversely related to the size of the molecule (a general target maximal size for most orally available drugs is $MW < 600$) and also to the extent of protein binding (protein-bound drugs do not diffuse well into membranes: *vide infra*). The rate of passage through lipid membranes via bulk diffusion is linearly dependent on concentration (see Figure 9.5):

$$dC/dt = K(C_1 - C_2), \qquad (9.5)$$

where C_1 and C_2 are the concentration at the outside and inside of the permeable membrane, respectively. At time zero, $C_2 = 0$, therefore rate is linear ($dC/dt = KC_1$). As $C_2 \to C_1$, the gradient diminishes to zero, the diffusion process through the membrane proceeds in both

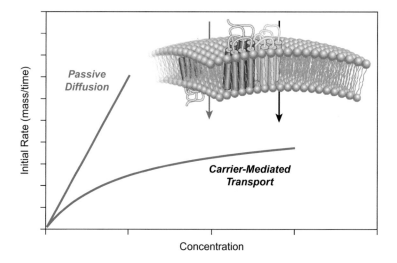

Passive Diffusion

Carrier-Mediated Transport

Initial Rate (mass/time)

Concentration

FIGURE 9.5 Graph showing initial velocity of transport processes across lipid membranes. Passive diffusion (compound dissolves directly into lipid membrane) is driven by a concentration gradient and is not saturable. In contrast, carrier-mediated transport is saturable, reaching a maximal rate when the carrier molecules are saturated with substrate. Transport proteins mediate these processes.

directions, and net bulk flow of drug through the membrane to the cytoplasm stops.

While lipophilicity is important for entry into a lipid membrane, too high a value of log P can also be detrimental to the ability of a molecule to pass through a membrane. This is because, at log P values >3 to 4, some molecules (such as dihydropyridines) actually dissolve into the cell membrane and remain there without emerging into the cytoplasm and beyond. As shown in Figure 9.6A, the ideal range for lipid penetration and passage is log P 1–3; values below this denote molecules that are too soluble in water to enter the lipid, while values >3 denote molecules that may not pass through the lipid membrane. Thus, a bell-shaped relationship between log P and passage through a lipid membrane through bulk diffusion is defined, as shown in Figure 9.6B. This figure also shows exemplar molecules defining the relationship [8].

For some molecules, active processes of transport into the cell are operative, and in these cases, general lipophilicity and size issues may be less important. A characteristic feature of active transport is that it is saturable (when the transporter is fully loaded, increases in concentration will produce no further permeation). Transport can be described by a Michaelis–Menten-like relationship between concentration and rate of diffusion (see Figure 9.5):

$$\frac{dC}{dt} = \frac{[C] \bullet V_{max}}{[C] + K_m}, \tag{9.6}$$

where V_{max} is the maximal rate of transport and K_m is the concentration of drug that causes the transport process to run at half speed. It can be seen that when $[C] \gg K_m$, then dC/dt will be constant (equal to V_{max}), and further increases in concentration will not change the rate of transport. Other features of active transport are that it requires energy and can proceed against a concentration gradient; such processes are important in the liver, kidney, gut epithelium, and across the blood-brain barrier.

These processes generally accumulate compounds essential for growth, remove waste products, and protect against toxins. A related process, in that a protein carrier is involved, is facilitated diffusion. This process depends on an oscillating carrier protein, is driven by a concentration gradient, and does not require energy. These processes are more important for the transport of sugars and amino acids and not as important for drugs. Examples of these are the insulin-sensitive glucose transporter protein GLUT4, Na^+/K^+ ATPase, Na^+/Ca^{2+} exchange protein, and the Na^+-dependent glucose transporters SGLT1 and SGLT2.

Not all transport processes facilitate drug absorption; some are designed to prevent absorption of foreign chemicals into the body. For example, P-glycoprotein (P-gp, encoded by MDR1, the multidrug resistance gene) is an ATP-dependent glycoprotein efflux pump with broad substrate specificity that has evolved as a defense mechanism against harmful substances. It is extensively expressed especially in the cells of the intestine, liver, renal proximal tubule, and the capillary endothelial cells of the blood-brain barrier. P-gp can confer variable resistance to drugs by operating as a reverse transporter out of cells back into the lumen. It is considered to be one of the most important transporters, but it is not the only one; there are over 2,000 genes in the human genome that code for transporters.

The fact that transporters are saturable can be important for drug development, since the concentration of drug presented to the transporter can be an important variable in therapeutics. For example, if a molecule is a substrate for P-gp, this will hamper entry through cell layers at low concentrations but may not at higher concentrations where this process is saturated; this is seen with the phosphodiesterase V inhibitor UK-343,664 which is a substrate for P-gp in LLc-PK1 cells transfected with the gene for the efflux transporter. At a concentration of 2 μM, P-gp produces a 5.5-fold barrier to cell entry, but this reduces to non-existent levels at concentrations of

FIGURE 9.6 Dependence of passage through lipid membranes on Log P. (A) For molecules with Log P values <1, the extreme water solubility can prevent significant entry into a lipid membrane (Pathway A). For molecules with a log P of 1–3, the balance of water and lipid solubility is ideal for entry and passage through lipid membranes (Pathway B). For molecules with Log P > 3, the extreme lipid solubility may cause them to enter the lipid membrane and remain there (Pathway C). (B) The log P behavior depicted in panel A leads to a bell-shaped relationship between log P and passage through lipid membrane. Data from [8].

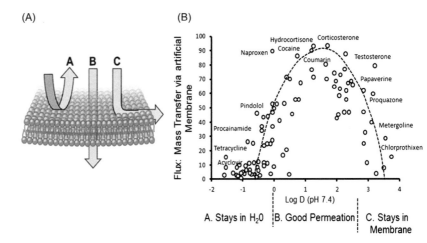

50 μM [9]. At these higher concentrations, the molecule passes through the membrane via bulk diffusion at levels much greater than can be extruded by P-gp. This defines concentration regions where active transport (either into or out of the cell) are important and where bulk diffusion dominates (see Figure 9.7). It will be seen that for oral absorption (where concentrations of compound usually are high), transport processes may be of less importance than for entry into specialized areas (i.e., the brain) from the bloodstream where concentrations are much lower.

There are a number of useful *in vitro* measures of permeability that can be used to assess how well a given molecule will be absorbed. One of the simplest is the permeation of molecules through artificial (hexadecane) membranes (referred to as *PAMPA studies*). These measure transcellular permeation by bulk diffusion in systems that avoid the complexity of active transport. With these types of assays, compounds can be ranked on the basis of lipid permeation alone; this can be a useful gauge of their ability to penetrate the gut intestinal wall. Table 9.2 shows some permeation values (in cm s^{-1}) of sample drugs; a value of log $P_{app} < -5.0$ indicates poor diffusion (less than 10^{-5} cm s^{-1}) through the membrane, and a value of log $P_{app} > -5.0$ describes good permeation. Other more sophisticated but more complicated systems utilize a monolayer of cells. In these systems, the compound is added to a chamber separated from a drug-free chamber by a permeable membrane covered by a monolayer of cells. The rate at which the drug diffuses through to the drug-free chamber is then used as a measure of permeation. These systems have the advantage of estimating the effect of active transport, efflux, and facilitated diffusion on the drug (see Figure 9.8). One of the most

common cell types used in this type of assay is Caco-2 cells. These are derived from human colonic adenocarcinomas but are morphologically and functionally very similar to intestinal (absorptive) enterocytes. They allow the

TABLE 9.2 Rates of Permeation through an Artificial Hexadecane Membrane (PAMPA)

Drug	Log P_{app}
Testosterone	−3.69
Desipramine	−3.75
Verapamil	−3.8
Lansoprazole	−4.45
Quinidine	−4.55
Antipyrene	−4.9
Naproxen	−5.04
Guanabenz	−5.32
Acyclovir	−5.79
Ceftriaxone	−5.89
Digoxin	−6.6
Sulfasalazine	−6.7
Amiloride	−7.04
Chloramphenicol	−7.13
Ranitidine	−7.16
Fluvastatin	−7.24

P_{app} in cm s^{-1}/log $P_{app} > -5.0$ is high; log $P_{app} < -5.0$ is low.

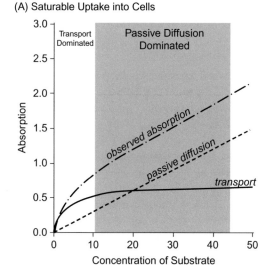
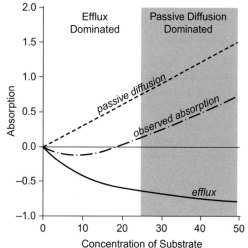

FIGURE 9.7 Overall entry into cells containing an active saturable uptake mechanism (panel A) and an active saturable efflux mechanism (panel B). It can be seen that in both cases, when concentrations of substrate reach saturating levels, bulk diffusion dominates and the mass transfer becomes linear with concentration. Thus, in both cases, the effects of saturable processes are minimal at high saturating concentrations.

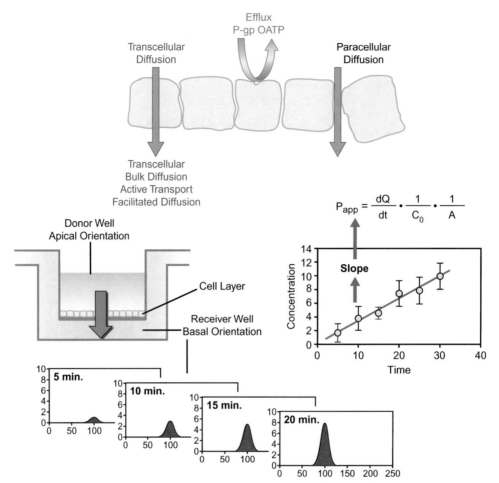

FIGURE 9.8 *In vitro* **measurement of permeation of molecules through lipid and cellular membranes.** Schematic diagram shows a common method of permeation through cellular layers (transcellular diffusion) and between cells (paracellular diffusion). In addition, efflux uptake (i.e., P-gp) excludes molecules from cells and forms an active barrier to absorption. Dual-chamber systems (separated by a permeable membrane coated with cells or lipid bilayer) constitutes an apparatus for measuring permeation. A drug can be introduced into one chamber (i.e., donor well apical cell orientation) and the rate of drug appearing in the basal receiving chamber (parameter dQ/dt) is then used to measure permeation according to the equation shown. The rate of basal to apical transfer can also be measured, and the difference used to estimate the importance of active efflux (unidirectional basal to apical) for any compound.

study of passive transcellular mechanisms, passive paracellular mechanisms, and carrier-mediated influx. In addition, Caco-2 cells contain many intestinal transporters and metabolic enzymes (aminopeptidases, P450 superfamily enzymes, esterases, phenol sulfotransferase, glucuronyltransferases). Figure 9.9A shows the permeation of some common drugs through a Caco-2 cell monolayer. The effect of drug efflux also can be assessed in Caco-2 cell systems, since permeation can be measured in two directions (apical to basolateral versus basolateral to apical); this can yield a measure of the importance of active transport (mainly P-glycoprotein: P-gp) as characterized by an asymmetry index $(B-A)/(A-B)$. An asymmetry index >1 suggests active efflux and, if observed, this can be confirmed through use of an active efflux inhibitor such as verapamil (for P-gp). Figure 9.9B shows the ratios of

basal-to-apical versus apical-to-basal permeation for a range of drugs; it can be seen that this ratio ranges from <1 to >1. Ratios of >1 indicate drugs that may undergo efflux; ratios <1 may indicate drugs that are actively transported across the Caco-2 cell monolayer. A useful method for identifying transporter processes is through the addition of specific inhibitors of these various processes and observing changes in permeation; Table 9.3 shows some common inhibitors of transporter systems. The permeation of compounds in cell monolayers can be used to generally classify absorption patterns for some drugs; see Figure 9.10 [10].

While the Caco-2 cell line is widely used, there are limitations with this system. For example, some pharmacologically important transporters are underexpressed and/or variably expressed in Caco-2 cells. Thus, β-lactam

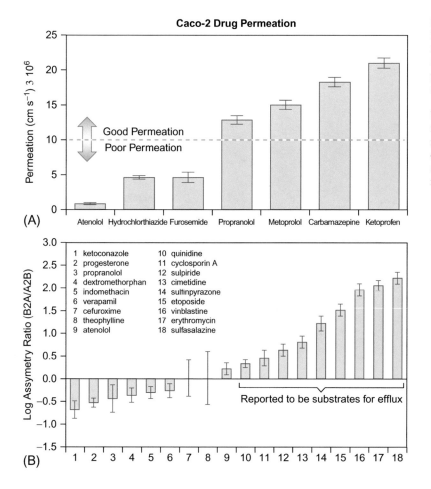

Caco-2 Drug Permeation

(A)

(B)

1 ketoconazole
2 progesterone
3 propranolol
4 dextromethorphan
5 indomethacin
6 verapamil
7 cefuroxime
8 theophylline
9 atenolol
10 quinidine
11 cyclosporin A
12 sulpiride
13 cimetidine
14 sulfinpyrazone
15 etoposide
16 vinblastine
17 erythromycin
18 sulfasalazine

FIGURE 9.9 *In vitro* **permeation data.** (A) Permeation of drugs through a Caco-2 cell monolayer. Good permeation is log $P_{app} > -5$ ($>10^{-5}$ cm s^{-1}). (B) Log of asymmetry ratios of permeation from basal to apical divided by permeation from apical to basal in MDCK cells. Ratios >1 indicate that the permeation from apical to basal is somewhat selectively hindered; one reason for this could be an outwardly oriented efflux mechanism such as P-gp. This can be confirmed by elimination of the ratio >1 by an efflux inhibitor such as verapamil. Compounds 10 to 18 have been noted to be substrates for efflux.

TABLE 9.3 Some Inhibitors of Active Transport/Efflux Mechanisms

Transporter	Inhibitor
P-gp[1]	Verapamil
BCRP[2]	Fumitremorgin
OATPB1[3]	Estrone 3-sulfate
OATPB3[3]	Estradiol-17β-D-glucuronide
OCT2[4]	Cimetidine
OAT1[3]	Diclofenac
OAT3[3]	Probenecid

[1]*P-glycoprotein.*
[2]*Breast cancer resistant protein.*
[3]*Organic anion transporter.*
[4]*Organic cation transporter.*

antibiotics (cephalexin, amoxicillin) and angiotensin converting enzyme (ACE) inhibitors are good substrates for peptide transporters. While they are completely absorbed in humans, they are very poorly permeable to Caco-2 cells. There also are poor correlations with compounds that enter through a paracellular route (i.e., mannitol). In addition, Caco-2 cells do not naturally express CYP3A4 (the principle enzyme in human gut epithelial cells), have a sensitivity to cosolvents (e.g., DMSO), and can demonstrate significant levels of nonspecific drug binding, sometimes referred to as *cacophilicity*. For these reasons, other cell lines have been explored for *in vitro* testing of permeability; a list of these is given in Table 9.4 [11]. Among the most prominent of alternative cell lines are Madin–Darby canine kidney (MDCK) cells. A special feature of these cells is that they are ideal for transfection of various transporters or enzymes. For example, MDCK cells transfected with human MDR1 gene encoding for P-glycoprotein (P-gp) transporter allows the control of levels of P-gp as opposed to using cells with heterogeneous transporters; these types of systems have been found to have some correlation with brain penetration.

A consideration in the use of permeation assays such as Caco-2 cells is the need to account for the total mass of compound. As noted previously, a ratio of (B2A)/(A2B) >1 indicates the possible presence of an efflux mechanism causing a reduction in the permeation rate from the apical side of the cell monolayer; this is seen as

FIGURE 9.10   Graph correlating data from PAMPA (parallel artificial membrane permeability assay) studies (lipid bilayer permeation) with cellular permeation studies (i.e., Caco-2 monolayer). A direct correlation would indicate that the compound passes through membranes mainly via passive diffusion (no special mechanisms are operative for permeation through cells). Compounds in the upper-left quadrant permeate more easily through cell monolayers, indicating that an active transport mechanism may be operative. Compounds in the lower-right quadrant have been selectively hindered through cell monolayers, indicating they are substrates for efflux mechanisms such as P-gp. Graph drawn after [10].

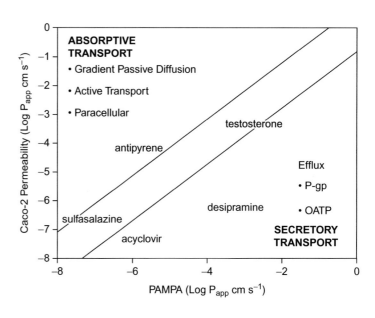

TABLE 9.4 *In Vitro* Cell Systems for Permeability Measurements

Cell Line	Species or Origin	Special Characteristics
Caco-2	Human colon adenocarcinoma	Most well-established cell model / Differentiates and expresses some relevant efflux transporters / Expression of influx transporters variable
MDCK	Canine kidney epithelial cells	Polarized cells with low intrinsic expression of transporters / Ideal for transfections
LLC-PK1	Pig kidney epithelial cells	Polarized cells with low intrinsic transporter expression / Ideal for transfections
2/4/A1	Rat fetal intestinal epithelial cells	Temperature sensitive / Ideal for paracellular absorbed compounds (leaky layers)
TC-7	Caco-2 subclone	Similar to Caco-2
HT-29	Human colon	Contains mucus-producing goblet cells
IEC-18	Rat small intestine	Provides size-selective barrier for paracellularly transported molecules

From [11].

a reduction in slope of the concentration-time relationship shown in Figure 9.8. However, any process that retards the appearance of the compound in the basolateral side of the monolayer will give the appearance of an efflux mechanism, and one of these types of effect is an irreversible binding or metabolic destruction of the compound within the cell. Such a process would yield a lower permeation value for apical to basolateral transfer, but

ascription of the effect to an efflux mechanism would be erroneous. Therefore, it is important to collect the amount of compound from the basolateral compartment to ensure that everything is accounted for and that the compound is not being selectively sequestered in the cell or otherwise destroyed. For example, the anticancer compound 2'-hydroxycinnamaldehyde (HCA) is metabolized in Caco-2 cells by aldehyde oxidase to o-coumaric acid to yield a reduced recovery of HCA in the basolateral compartment which, if not detected, would be seen erroneously as the presence of an efflux mechanism [12].

There are special regions where absorption is unique. For example, blood capillaries contain fenestrations to allow rapid interchange between blood and interstitial fluid. Similarly, glomerular capillaries (in the kidney) are extremely porous, allowing passage of all plasma constituents except macromolecules MW > 30,000. At the other end of the scale, there are certain regions where drug entry is extremely restricted. One such area is the brain where the brain and spinal cord are isolated from the periphery by the blood-brain barrier (BBB). This vascular bed forms a permeability barrier to the passive diffusion of substances from the bloodstream, and contains specialized transport systems to allow the entry of certain molecules. It is permeable to unionized and lipophilic drugs or drugs that can utilize these carrier processes (capillaries of the BBB have no pores). In addition to bulk diffusion, substances gain entry into the brain via various mechanisms across the BBB, including carrier-mediated influx transport (i.e., transporters for monocarboxylates, valproic acid, amines, amino acids, hexose, nucleosides, glutathione, small peptides), receptor-mediated transcytosis (i.e., transferrin, insulin), and adsorptive-mediated transcytosis (histone, avidin, cationized albumin, ebiratide, cationic peptides). The brain is protected by extensive efflux mechanisms as well (i.e., ABC transporters [P-gp, MRP] and transporters for organic anions [CRH, anionic cyclic peptides]). In general, the BBB can pose a significant barrier to the absorption of many drugs. For example, "non-sedating" antihistamines such as *loratadine* are simply standard histamine H1 receptor blockers that are poorly lipid soluble. Therefore, they do not cross the blood-brain barrier to gain access to brain histamine receptors (cause of sedation).

There are some general principles that assist in the understanding of drug absorption. While ionization and lipid solubility are very important, surface area is paramount. For example, salicylate is weakly acidic and unionized in stomach, and exists as an ionized species in the intestine (pH $\approx$ 6). In spite of these ionic conditions, salicylate is mainly absorbed from the intestine. This is because the surface area of intestine is orders of magnitude greater than the surface area of stomach (i.e., while the stomach presents a surface area of 3.5 m^2, the jejunum has 194 m^2 and the ileum 276 m^2, roughly the area of a tennis court). Table 9.5 summarizes some general effects that modify drug absorption.

9.4.2 Route of Drug Administration

There are numerous routes of administration of drugs into the body. The choice of which route to use in a given therapeutic situation is determined by convenience, maximization of compliance (for example, a drug taken once a day by the oral route is much easier to sustain on a chronic basis than one that needs to be injected twice a day), and attainment of concentration bias to gain advantage therapeutically. For example, topical (where there is a local effect and the drug is applied directly where needed) is used for asthma (inhalation), skin treatment (epicutaneous), antibiotics (eye drops, ear drops), decongestants (intranasal) and estrogen (vaginal). Enteral application (systemic [nonlocal] via the digestive tract) is used for the majority of drugs where possible, and parenteral (systemic route other than digestive tract) is used for vaccines, antibiotics, psychoactive drugs (intravenous), insulin (subcutaneous), and anesthesia and chemotherapy (intrathecal). The various advantages of routes of

administration are given in Table 9.6. The route of administration can completely determine what effects a given drug might have. For instance, intravenous naloxone (opiate antagonist) treats opiate overdose when given intravenously, yet by the oral route it acts exclusively on the bowels to treat constipation during pain therapy without affecting the central pain-reducing effect of opiates. Sublingual administration provides rapid absorption for lipid-soluble drugs, for example, nitrates. This route avoids the first pass effect (shunts straight into superior vena cava); if nitrates are given orally, none escape the liver. Administration by aerosol leads to very rapid absorption that also avoids first pass degradation in liver. In this case, the absorptive surface area is very large (also tennis court sized) and provides a very good area for local application. Thus β-adrenoceptor agonists such as salbutamol are very useful for rapid relaxation of constricted bronchioles in asthma. These drugs also can produce some tachycardia and notably a debilitating digital

TABLE 9.5 Factors that Modify Absorption

- Drug solubility
- Dissolution of drug into medium
- Nature of the vehicle dispersing the drug
- Concentration of drug
- pH (for ionizable drugs)
- Circulation to the site of absorption
- Absorbing surface
- Route of administration

TABLE 9.6 Features of Various Routes of Drug Administration

	Advantages	Disadvantages
Parenteral		
Intravenous	rapid attainment of concentration/precise delivery of dosage/easy to titrate dose	high initial concentration/toxicity invasive risk of infection/requires skill
Subcutaneous	prompt absorption from aqueous medium/ little training needed/ avoid harsh GI environment/can be used for suspensions	cannot be used for large volumes/ potential pain/tissue damage/variable absorption
Enteral		
Oral	convenient (storage/ portability)/ economical/non invasive/safe requires no training	delivery can be erratic/ incomplete/depends on patient compliance/drugs degrade in GI environment/first pass effect
Sublingual	rapid onset/avoids first pass	few drugs adequately absorbed/patients must avoid swallowing/ difficult compliance
Pulmonary	easy to titrate dose/ rapid onset local effect/ minimize toxic effects	requires coordination/ lung disease limits variable delivery
Topical	minimize side effects/ avoids first pass effect	cosmetically unappealing/erratic absorption

tremor. However, if taken by aerosol, salbutamol reaches the target organ first (bronchioles) for maximal effect and then diffuses throughout the bloodstream in a reduced concentration for minimal effect on the heart and skeletal muscles. Thus, side effects are minimized. Similarly, ocular drugs for glaucoma can be introduced as eye drops directly into the eye for maximal concentration effect and minimal cardiovascular side effects. The antidepressant monoamine oxidase inhibitor selegiline avoids the common monoamine oxidase inhibitor (MAOI) side effect of possible hypertensive crisis (when large amounts of cheese containing tyramine are ingested) through transdermal absorption with a patch over 24 hr periods. It is interesting to note that, while oral administration appears to be the patient-preferred method of drug administration, it constitutes only 32% of the market share of drug delivery technologies for known drugs, with pulmonary administration forming 27%, nasal 11%, injection and implants 9%, transdermal delivery 8%, and other devices 13%.

One method of enhancing absorption is by synthesizing prodrugs. These are analogs of the active molecule that are more readily absorbed than the parent drug, and are metabolized in the body to generate the parent active drug. In general, prodrugs offer a way of maximizing concentration at the required site of action, increasing the selectivity of drugs (i.e., tumors are often hypoxic, producing large quantities of reductase enzyme; this idea can be used for prodrugs that are activated by reductase), and reducing adverse effects.

This conversion of drugs to prodrugs is called *latentiation* and consists of the conversion of hydrophilic drugs into lipid-soluble drugs, usually by masking hydroxyl, carboxyl, and primary amino groups. A concentrating effect can be achieved once the prodrug enters a compartment and the active moiety is released, and trapped, by enzymatic hydrolysis. This can be a useful strategy for drug therapy in the central nervous system, which is protected by the blood-brain barrier, an obstacle relatively impervious to polar molecules. For example, a lipid-soluble diacetyl derivative of morphine crosses the blood-brain barrier at a rate 100 times faster than morphine. Once in the brain, precapillary pseudocholinesterase deacylates the molecule to form morphine (Figure 9.11A). Similarly, the delivery of gamma-aminobutyric acid (GABA) into the central nervous system (CNS) for treatment of depression, anxiety, Alzheimer's disease, parkinsonism, and schizophrenia is difficult due to the presence of the blood-brain barrier. However, the Schiff-base progamide crosses into the CNS to release gabamide and then GABA (Figure 9.11B). A particularly effective prodrug strategy is the use of the dual ester dipivalylepinephrine for the treatment of glaucoma. Epinephrine reduces intraocular pressure and is an effective treatment for the disease; however, it does not readily penetrate the cornea (it is unstable and short acting). Dipivalylepinephrine easily penetrates the cornea, and active epinephrine is released in the eye through enzymatic hydrolysis, making the prodrug 17 times more potent than the parent by the ocular route (see

FIGURE 9.11 Latentiation of morphine and gamma-aminobutyric acid (GABA) allows entry through the blood-brain barrier and subsequent trapping by enzymatic hydrolysis. Diacetylmorphine is converted to morphine by pseudocholinesterase, while progamide is converted to gabamide and subsequently to the active drug GABA.

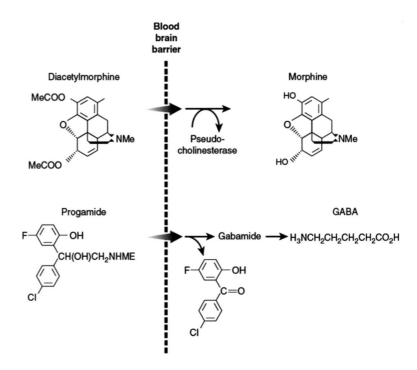

Figure 9.12). Since epinephrine itself is metabolically unstable, it degrades before reaching the general circulation, thereby eliminating side effects. The use of the prodrug optimally produces a maximally effective concentration of the active drug in the eye, the target organ. Other examples of well-known prodrugs are enalapril, which is activated by esterase to produce enalaprilat (treatment of hypertension); valaciclovir, also activated by an esterase to acyclovir (treatment of herpes); and levodopa (activated by L-3,4-dihydroxyphenylalanine (L-DOPA) decarboxylase) to yield dopamine for treatment of Parkinson's disease. Prodrug strategies also can be used to prolong drug action, as in the use of the phenothiazene antipsychotic prodrugs fluphenazine enanthate or decanoate (1−2 and 2−3 week durations of action, respectively), which yield fluphenazine upon hydrolysis by esterases.

Another type of special control of drug absorption is found with antedrugs. These are molecules that are stable and active at the point of application but then are degraded as they are absorbed into the body; this can avoid toxic systemic effects (see Figure 9.13). For example, glucocorticoids are useful as treatments for inflammation but can lead to harmful effects on the adrenal glands if absorbed systemically. Thus, topical application of specifically designed glucocorticoids that degrade to inactive metabolites can be used to treat dermal inflammation − see Figure 9.13 for an example of a steroid antedrug.

9.4.3 General Pharmacokinetics

If the entry of a molecule into the body were simply a temporally restricted absorption process, then a steady

FIGURE 9.12 The prodrug dipivalylepinephrine enters the cornea of the eye to allow esterase to produce epinephrine in the eye to alleviate high pressure in glaucoma.

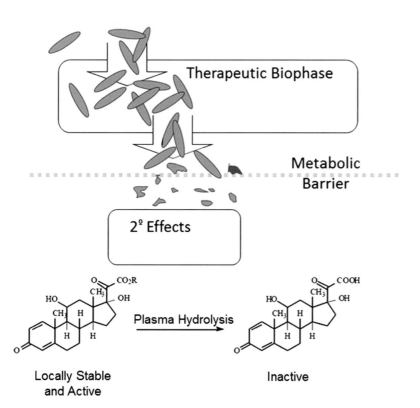

FIGURE 9.13 Antedrugs are delivered to their primary site of action and then are degraded as they enter the rest of the body. Shown is a steroid-21-oic acid that is topically active as an anti-inflammatory compound and is degraded by plasma esterases as it is absorbed into the body. Data for example from [13].

state concentration would be achieved, given enough time for complete absorption. However, what in fact is observed in drug pharmacokinetics is a complex curve reflecting absorption of the drug into the body and the diminution of the concentration that is absorbed back down to negligible levels. The reason for this complex pattern of rise and fall in drug concentration *in vivo* is due to the number of processes that impinge on the drug concentration as it passes into and out of the body; these are summarized in Figure 9.14. First, the drug must pass into the systemic circulation via the chosen route of administration. Once it is in the circulation, it is subject to a number of processes that reduce the concentration of freely accessible drug. One of these is binding to proteins in the blood, usually albumin for acidic drugs and alpha1-acid glycoprotein for basic drugs. The complex between proteins and drug can cause a sequestration of free drug into a pool not readily accessible for therapeutic purposes; that is, only free drug can cross plasma membranes. Human plasma contains more than 60 proteins, and most drugs are bound by three types, namely albumin (60% total plasma, mostly of a homogeneous type in humans), which binds anionic drugs (i.e., salicylates, sulfonamides, barbiturates, phenylbutazone, penicillins, tetracyclines, probenecid), α1-acid glycoprotein (AAG; can exist in polyforms in humans), and lipoproteins (both of these bind cationic drugs such as adenosine, quinacrine, quinine, streptomycin, digitoxin, ouabain, coumarin), and transcortin, thyroxine-binding globulin (found to bind some select drugs). In general, high lipophilicity in drugs promotes high protein binding, and the extent of protein binding for some drugs can be quite high (i.e., caffeine is 90%, theophylline 85% protein bound).

Drug protein binding is usually nonlinear and unsaturable. The effects of protein binding on free drug concentration have been described in Chapters 2 (see Section 2.9.2) and 4 (see Section 4.4.1). Drug protein binding can be relevant to therapy in a number of contexts. For instance, it can cause a drug to be unavailable for metabolism, affect drug distribution throughout the body, and restrict pharmacological action and glomerular filtration in the kidney. This last effect can delay drug onset and prolong drug action. Furthermore, free drug concentration can change in response to changes in protein binding brought on by disease (i.e., renal failure, septicemia, AIDS, inflammation, depression, trauma, myocardial infarction, cancer) and displacement by other protein-binding drugs. For example valproic acid can displace protein-bound carbamazepine, naproxen, and diazepam, while salicylic acid can displace phenytoin, imipramine, methotrexate, and valproic acid. Some of these effects can be serious, as in the displacement of warfarin by nalidixic acid to cause hemorrhage. The clearance of drugs such as propranolol, verapamil, diazepam, and warfarin is restricted by protein binding.

One of the most obvious effects of high protein binding is that it decreases the volume of distribution of a drug by keeping it in the central compartment (*vide infra*). This can decrease the elimination of a drug (in cases where drugs are filtered by the glomerulus in the kidney, since the protein-bound drug is unavailable for filtration). Interestingly, protein binding also can increase drug elimination (since the decrease in the volume of distribution keeps the drug in the central compartment and thus keeps it available for elimination either through renal tubular secretion or biliary excretion). In general, protein binding is not a significant problem with drug levels, as the system readjusts to levels of free drug (although there are exceptions to this rule). However, on a practical level, most drug measurements of plasma concentration measure total drug and do not distinguish between free and bound drug, thus extensive protein binding can lead to misinterpretation of drug levels in the clinic.

The liver (and other organs) removes active drugs through two general processes. One is through the conversion of biologically active to inactive molecules. The other is to the conversion into polar metabolites that are readily excreted (to a greater extent than the parent drug); these will be discussed in more detail in the next section.

Pharmacokinetics is the science of drug disposition in the body, and the field of clinical pharmacokinetics is concerned with the practical presentation of drugs to the target organ(s) for the therapy of disease. There are two main parameters that are of paramount importance in the study of clinical pharmacokinetics. The first is the *clearance*; this yields a measure of the body's efficiency in eliminating the drug. Clearance is measured as the volume of fluid per unit time from which the drug would

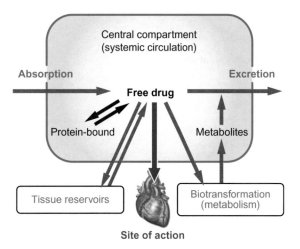

FIGURE 9.14 Schematic representation of the pharmacokinetic processes involved in drug absorption, distribution, and elimination.

have to be completely removed to account for its elimination from the body. The efficiency of clearance is dependent upon the ability of the organ to remove the drug, and also on the rate of blood flow through the organ. The second parameter is the *volume of distribution* of the drug, which is the apparent volume of fluid containing the drug in the body. From these two parameters, the *half life,* the measure of the length of time the drug stays in the body, can be calculated. Specifically, this is the length of time it takes for the concentration of the drug to be reduced to half its initial value. Another very important parameter is the *bioavailability* of the drug; this is a measure of the efficiency of absorption and presentation to the systemic circulation via the enteral route of administration. For example, a drug taken by the oral route may have a bioavailability of only 20%; that is, only 20% of the orally ingested amount reaches the general systemic circulation after ingestion.

Referring to the observed temporal relationship between the concentration of an ingested drug in a central compartment (such as the systemic circulation) and concentration in the biological compartment, there are various parameters that can be used to describe the drug's pharmacokinetic performance; these are summarized in Figure 9.15. There is a required level of drug needed for therapeutic effect (minimal effective concentration for desired response), and usually a toxic level of drug as well (minimum effective concentration for adverse effects). Thus, the therapeutic aim is to exceed the first limit but stay below the second. The time at which the level of drug achieves the minimal therapeutic level describes the time to onset of effect. The difference between the minimal effective concentration for response and highest concentration (peak effect) is referred to as the *intensity of effect*. The length of time that the concentration exceeds the minimal effective therapeutic concentration is called the *duration of action*.

A measure of the actual amount of drug in the body can be obtained from the area under the curve of the temporal concentration curve (calculated by integration). However, the temporal behavior of a drug can be extremely important in therapeutics. For example, consider three preparations of a drug that present identical values for area under the curve (i.e., amount of drug absorbed) but have different kinetics of absorption (Figure 9.16). As shown, preparation B produces a useful profile whereby the concentration exceeds the minimal effective concentration but stays below the toxic level. In contrast, preparation A exceeds this level (to produce toxic effects), and preparation C never achieves the minimal effective concentration — although very similar amounts of the drug are absorbed. In general, unfavorable pharmacokinetics can completely preclude the therapeutic effect of an active molecule.

9.4.4 Metabolism

While there are a number of organ systems that can metabolize drugs (lungs, intestinal and nasal mucosa, kidney), the main tissue for this is the liver. The actual metabolic processes that go on in the liver can be biochemically classified into two types of reaction, so-called phase I and phase II metabolism. Phase I (nonsynthetic) reactions usually (but not always) precede phase II reactions and place a functional group on parent molecules to render them biologically inactive (in some rare instances, retention or even enhancement of activity can result). The main enzymes responsible for these reactions are cytochrome P450 enzymes (the most important enzyme class in phase I metabolism, coded by 63 human genes for this enzyme in 18 families). CYP450 enzymes are found in the mitochondria and smooth endoplasmic reticulum and can metabolize multiple substrates. Of

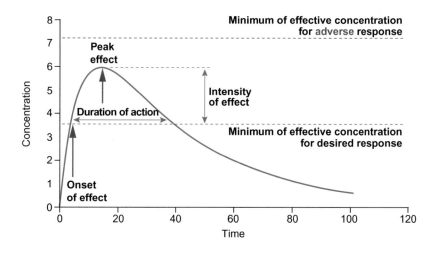

FIGURE 9.15 Kinetics of drug absorption and elimination as viewed by the plasma concentration of an orally administered drug with time.

FIGURE 9.16 Kinetic profiles of the plasma concentrations of three different drugs taken by the oral route. If absorption is rapid, toxic effects may ensue (red line); if too slow, a therapeutically effective level may not be attained (blue line).

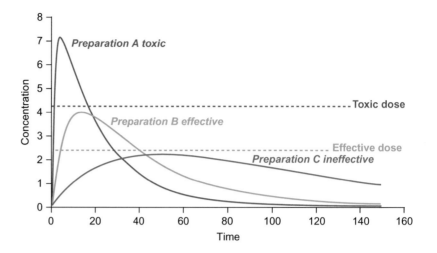

FIGURE 9.17 **Metabolism of the anticonvulsant phenytoin.** The Phase 1 hydroxylation yields an inactive molecule with reduced lipophilicity and greater water solubility. The molecule then undergoes Phase 2 metabolism to form an extremely water soluble glucuronide through conjugation with uridine diphosphate glucuronide.

the cytochrome P450 enzymes, CYP3A4, CYP2C9, CYP2C19, and CYP2D6 have the highest impact on metabolism (50% of *all* drugs metabolized by P450 enzymes are substrates for CYP3A4). Flavin monooxygenase is another prominent Phase I metabolic enzyme. The most important Phase I reaction is oxidation (mediated by cytochrome P450 monoxygenase, flavin-containing monoxygenase, alcohol dehydrogenase, monoamine oxidase, and peroxide co-oxidation); this reaction requires O_2 and NADPH. Other Phase I reactions include reduction (through NADPH-cytochrome P50 reductase and ferrous cytochrome P450) and hydrolysis (through esterases, amidases, and epoxide hydrolase). Phase II reactions (conjugation reactions such as glucuronidation, sulfation, methylation, acetylation, mercapture formation) covalently link a functional group onto the molecule to create highly polar metabolites that are rapidly excreted in urine. Figure 9.17 shows the metabolism of the anticonvulsant phenytoin and the coordination of Phase 1 and Phase 2 enzymes. The product of the Phase 1 reaction is pharmacologically inactive, less lipid soluble and more water soluble. The glucuronide product of the Phase 2 reaction is much more water soluble and is excreted by the renal system.

There are external factors such as age, gender, hormonal state, and disease that can cause variations in drug metabolism. Genetic factors also can be important. For example, the genes for CYP2A6, CYP2C9, CYP2C19, and CYP2D6 are functionally polymorphic. CYP2C19 polymorphism affects 20% of Asians and 3% of Caucasians, leading to susceptibility to ethanol intoxication. As seen in Figure 9.18, the CYP2D6 mediated metabolism of debrisoquin (as measured by the urinary ratio of debrisoquin and the metabolite 4-hydroxydebrisoquin) in 1,011 Swedish subjects shows a clear delineation in rate of metabolism. The bars in red represent subjects with genetically no or very low levels of CYP2D6 [14]. Phenotypic and genetic differences in CYPs are considered to be a major, if not *the* major, reason for PK variability. Metabolic enzyme-inducing agents such as co-administered drugs, charbroiled meats, cigarette smoke, and ethanol can also be important sources of variation. Some food interactions also are relevant, as in the CYP3A4 interaction of a number of drugs (e.g., nisoldipine, nitrendipine, saquinivir, atorvastatin, sildenafil, lovastatin, diazepam, ciclosporin, methadone) with grapefruit; this effect was discovered when grapefruit juice was used to mask the taste of ethanol in felodipine clinical trials. While metabolism is primarily regarded as a mechanism for deactivation, there are instances where enzymes produce active metabolites and the original

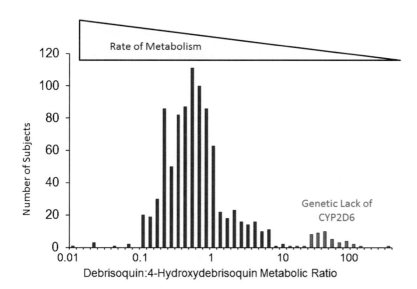

FIGURE 9.18 Genetic variation in CYP2D6 levels in 1,011 Swedish subjects lead to differences in hydroxylation of debrisoquin. Blue bars represent subjects with normal levels of CYP2D6 while red bars represent subjects with little or no CYP2D6. Data redrawn from [14].

drug takes on the role of a prodrug (e.g., amitriptyline → nortriptyline, codeine → morphine, primidone → phenobarbital). In other cases, metabolism may activate molecules to become toxic and/or carcinogenic, as with CYP1A1 (for benzolpyrene and other polycyclic aromatic hydrocarbons), CYP1A2 (4-aminobiphenyl, 2-naphthylamine, 2-aminofluorene, 2-acetylaminofluorene, 2-aminoanthracene, heteropolycyclic amines), CYP2E1 (benzene, styrene, acylnitrile, vinylbromide, trichloroethylene, carbon tetrachloride, chloroform, methylene chloride, N-nitrosodimethylamine, 1,2-dichloropropane, ethyl carbamate), and CYP3A4 (aflatoxin B1, aflatoxin G1, estradiol, 6-aminochrysine, polycyclic hydrocarbon dihydrodiols). In other cases, first pass liver metabolism (*vide infra*) is critical in preventing overdose, as in the case of terfenadine, astemizole, cisapride, and pimozide, where CYP3A4 metabolism prevents the appearance of bolus concentrations that can lead to life-threatening *torsades de pointes* (often fatal cardiac arrhythmia). This effect can be used to advantage in other cases, with inhibition of CYP3A4 with ritanavir to increase absorption of heavily metabolized drugs such as ciclosporin and saquinavir. Variations in drug levels with alterations in metabolism are most readily seen with drugs that have low bioavailability and high first pass metabolism.

As with *in vitro* estimation of drug absorption, a number of hepatic metabolic issues can be addressed early on in drug discovery and development. These are [15]:

- Identification of metabolites.
- Prediction of *in vivo* pharmacokinetic parameters from *in vitro* data.
- Identification of the P450 enzymes involved in drug metabolism.

- Interspecies comparison of metabolic profile to select species for preclinical studies (safety pharmacology).
- Drug-drug interactions due to enzyme induction-inhibition — see Chapter 10.
- Drug toxicity associated with drug metabolism — see Chapter 10.

These studies can be done with liver microsomes, hepatocytes, and recombinant preparations of CYP enzymes. Microsomes are membrane fragments prepared from homogenized liver, while hepatocytes are liver cells that have been collected from collagenase-perfused liver. These are then co-cultured with collagen and fibroblasts to yield a long-term culture of hepatocytes. Cryopreservation preserves partial function, but long-term culture may produce a shift in relative P450 content. Hepatocytes are generally considered to be preferable for determining intrinsic clearance through liver metabolism since they contain both phase I and II enzymes + cofactors. In addition, literature reports generally cite higher *in vitro−in vivo* correlation with hepatocytes than with microsomes. A technical limitation of hepatocyte usage has been the difficulty in cryopreservation, but important advances have been made to the point where this is no longer a serious drawback. Uptake transporter protein activity (i.e., OATP uptake [organic anion transporting polypeptides], NTCP uptake [sodium taurocholate cotransporting polypeptide]) also can be preserved in hepatocytes. Microsomes are mainly useful when only CYP450-mediated reactions dominate the metabolism of the drug. Table 9.7 contrasts and compares the study of metabolism with liver microsomes and hepatocytes. In addition to microsomes and hepatocytes, a centrifugation fraction of liver cell cytosol called S9 can also be used

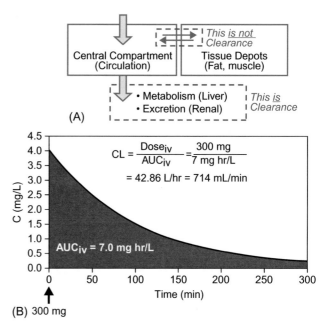

TABLE 9.7 Assays to Measure Hepatic Metabolism of Drugs

A. Hepatocytes

Advantages

Most physiologically relevant

Contain full complement of enzymes drug will encounter in first pass

Contain cofactors as well

Exposure to relevant transporters

Commercial sources increasing

Higher published correlations with *in vivo* clearance data

Cryostorage still a problem but improving

Natural orientation for linked enzymes

Limitations

Can give incorrect data when Phase II conjugation or active uptake predominates

New preparation needed for each experiment – low throughput

B. Microsomes

Advantages

Good or oxidative biotransformations

Ease of preparation

Availability

Long-term storage

Suitable when only CYP450-mediated reactions dominate

Good for oxidation and glucuronide conjunction

Limitations

Requires cofactors, for example, NADPH, O_2

Hydrolysis, reduction, and other conjugation reactions catalyzed by nonmicrosomal enzymes

Lack Phase II cytosolic enzymes (glutathione S-transferase, sulfotransferases, alcohol dehydrogenase, xanthine oxidase, etc.)

From [15,16].

FIGURE 9.19 (A) Schematic diagram emphasizing the fact that transfer of drug between compartments in the body does not constitute clearance even though it might remove drug from a primary target compartment (i.e., the brain is a rapidly equilibrated compartment that might lose drug with time to other parts of the body). Only true removal of the drug from the body constitutes clearance. (B) Oral dose yielding an absorbed amount of drug that is cleared with time. Area under the curve is a measure of total drug absorption; when this value is divided into the dose given, a measure of clearance results (volume of water cleared of the drug per unit time).

the measure of the re-equilibration of the drug within various body compartments, but rather the actual removal of drug from the body with time (usually by hepatic metabolism and/or renal excretion); see Figure 9.19A. It is worth considering drug clearance in some detail, as, along with volume of distribution, this parameter can be used to determine nearly every other pharmacokinetic parameter for any drug, and also, to answer three pragmatic questions about the drug and how it is to be used in the clinic:

- What will be the therapeutic dosage of drug?
- By what route will this dosage be administered?
- What will be the dosage interval (τ)?

It is important to consider these questions early on in the drug discovery and development program, since the drug properties that constitute the answers to these questions may reside in different chemical scaffolds, requiring structure-activity relationship data for optimization.

Clearance is measured in units of volume per unit time, as an expression of the rate at which the blood volume is cleansed of the drug. Thus, a low clearance value in humans for a drug is <500 mL min^{-1}, a medium clearance would be $500-1000$ mL min^{-1} and a high clearance value would be $1000-1500$ mL min^{-1}. One way to measure clearance is to measure the

9.4.5 Clearance

The driving force in pharmacokinetics is the speed with which a drug is cleared from the body. Clearance is not

for metabolic studies. Thus, while microsomes can primarily be used only for the study of Phase I enzymes, S9 contains Phase I and some phase II enzyme activity.

pharmacokinetics of an intravenous dose of drug with the following relationship:

$$\text{Clearance} = \text{CL} = \text{DOSE}_{iv}/\text{AUC}_{iv}, \quad (9.7)$$

where DOSE_{iv} is the dosage given by the intravenous route and AUC_{iv} is the area under the curve of the plasma concentration with time (see Figure 9.19B). One reason why it is important to determine clearance is that it enables the maintenance dose rate for infusions. Specifically, knowing the clearance enables the ready calculation of a plasma steady state concentration for any given dosage rate via intravenous drip:

$$\text{Steady-State [Conc]} = C_{ss} = \frac{\text{Dose Rate(mg hr}^{-1})}{\text{Clearance(L hr}^{-1})}. \quad (9.8)$$

Clearance also enables the determination of dosing schedules (how often a drug must be administered) — *vide infra*.

Clearance is additive, as drugs see all clearance sites in parallel (with the exception of the lungs, where elimination is in series with the rest of the body). Thus:

$$\text{CL}_{plasma} = \text{CL}_H + \text{CL}_R + \text{CL}_{other}, \quad (9.9)$$

where CL_H is hepatic clearance through the liver, CL_R is renal clearance, and CL_{other} is clearance via any other means, e.g. perspiration. Organs (processes) have an intrinsic ability to remove a drug, and this is characterized by an extraction ratio:

$$\text{Extraction Ratio} = E_H = 1 - \frac{\text{Concentration out}}{\text{Concentration in}}. \quad (9.10)$$

For example, an E_H (hepatic extraction ratio) for the liver of 0.8 means that only 20% of the drug emerges out of the liver as it enters the portal vein circulation. Measurement of clearance and knowledge of organ blood flow enables calculation of extraction ratios:

$$\text{CL}_H = Q_H \bullet E_H, \quad (9.11)$$

where Q_H is the rate of hepatic blood flow. For example, if a drug that is known to be cleared completely by the liver (Q_H; liver blood flow is 90 L h^{-1}) has a CL of 60 L h^{-1}, then the extraction ratio is 60 L h^{-1}/90 L h^{-1} = E_H = 0.66. Drugs such as diltiazem, imipramine, lidocaine, morphine, and propranolol are restricted in their clearance, not by hepatic metabolism but rather by hepatic blood flow. For these drugs, all the drug that reaches the liver is removed. In some cases the plasma clearance of some drugs exceeds organ blood flow; this can occur if the drug partitions into red blood cells. This leads to a condition whereby the delivery of drug to the organ is higher than suspected from its measured free form in plasma.

It is useful to calculate the intrinsic clearance of an organ like the liver by considering the whole organ as a virtual enzyme. The intrinsic clearance (CL_{int}) (ability of

liver to remove drug with no restriction) of a substrate drug [S] is given by:

$$\text{CL}_{int} = V_H/[S], \quad (9.12)$$

where V_H is the rate of hepatic metabolism estimated by a Michaelis−Menten equation:

$$V_H = \frac{[S] \bullet V_{max}}{[S] + K_m} \quad (9.13)$$

and where the maximal rate of metabolism is denoted V_{max}, and K_m is the concentration of drug at which metabolism proceeds at half-maximal speed. In cases where the metabolizing capability of the liver for a given drug is high, the concentration of drug is much lower than the capacity of the liver and $[S] << K_m$. This reduces Equation 9.13 to $V_H = [S] V_{max}/K_m$ and, from Equation 9.12, $\text{CL}_{int} = V_{max}/K_m$ (the rate of intrinsic clearance is constant). The intrinsic clearance can be used to calculate the extraction ratio (which, through Equation 9.11, can be used to calculate hepatic clearance). Another equation for calculating extraction ratio E_H is:

$$E_H = \frac{f_u \bullet \text{CL}_{int}}{Q_H + f_u \bullet \text{CL}_{int}}, \quad (9.14)$$

where f_u is the fraction of drug unbound by protein. It can be seen from Equation 9.14 that, if the extent of drug protein binding is very high (small f_u), then the extraction by the liver will be small. It can also be seen from Equation 9.14 that hepatic extraction is controlled by liver blood flow (Q_H), f_u (drug protein binding), and CL_{int} (intrinsic rate of clearance) to varying extents. For example, under conditions of high hepatic extraction, Q_H dominates (constant/[constant + Q_H]). Thus, compromise of cardiovascular function (changes in Q_H) has more effect on the metabolism of highly metabolized drugs than compromise of liver function, but only in the case of i.v. administration. This can be seen from an examination of Equation 9.11 as well. For highly metabolized drugs, $\text{CL}_{int} >> Q_H$, causing $E_H \rightarrow$ unity and therefore $\text{CL}_H \rightarrow Q_H$. The metabolism of such drugs is referred to as *flow limited* (one example of this is glyceryl trinitrate). In contrast, for drugs of low hepatic metabolism, CL_{int} and f_u (liver function and protein binding) dominate hepatic clearance. For these drugs, liver function is the most important determinant of metabolism and clearance. For poorly metabolized drugs, $Q_H >> f_u \text{CL}_{int}$, causing $\text{CL}_H \rightarrow f_u \text{CL}_{int}$; see Equation 9.14. The metabolism of these drugs is referred to as *capacity limited* (one example of this is diazepam). It should be noted that the route of administration is extremely important in terms of clearance. If a drug is administered via the oral route, then the first organ through which it must pass is the liver (the "first pass" effect, *vide infra*). Under these circumstances, even drugs exhibiting "flow capacity" metabolism are highly dependent on the rate of liver metabolism. This is not true of flow capacity drugs given by the intravenous route. Therefore, the only case where blood flow controls hepatic clearance is intravenous administration of a drug that is highly metabolized by the liver. Table 9.8 shows hepatic clearances for a range of common drugs.

9.4.6 Volume of Distribution and Half Life

It is worth considering the actual mechanics of clinical pharmacokinetics, to get an idea of what data actually drive the conclusions around determining ADME proper-

TABLE 9.8 Hepatic Clearances for a Range of Common Drugs

Drugs with >30% Hepatic Clearance

Low Extraction $E_R < 0.3$	Med. Extraction $E_R = 0.3$ to 0.7	High Extraction $E_R > 0.7$
Diazepam	Codeine	Propranolol
Digitoxin	Nortriptylene	Pentazocine
Indomethacin	Aspirin	Meperidine
Theophylline	Quinidine	Isoproterenol
Warfarin	Alprenolol	
Valproic Acid	Desipramine	
Procainamide	Lidocaine	
Salicylic Acid	Propoxyphene	
Phenobarbital	Nitroglycerin	
Tolbutamide	Morphine	
Doxepin		

ties of drugs. A basic and important process is the measurement of the concentration of drug in the bloodstream at various times after administration. The elimination of a drug from the body can be approximated by the exit of a substance from a single compartment via a first order elimination process. With this process, the second fundamental parameter of pharmacokinetics can be estimated; namely, the volume of distribution of the drug. From the temporal relationship of concentration also comes the half life of the drug. The volume of distribution is the quotient of the total amount of drug in the body divided by the central compartment (plasma) concentration. For example, if 10 mg of drug is given and yields a drug concentration of $1.2 \, \text{mg} \, \text{L}^{-1}$, then the volume of distribution is 10 L. This is determined by estimating the concentration of an intravenously administered dose of drug at time zero after injection. Figure 9.20A shows the waning concentration of a 10 mg dose of drug given intravenously with time; in this case, the relationship follows a first order decline in concentration given by:

$$C_t/C_0 = e^{-kt}, \qquad (9.15)$$

where C_t and C_0 refer to the concentration of drug at time t and time zero, respectively, and k is the first order rate constant for elimination of the drug. One useful feature of exponential relationships is the fact that they are linear when plotted on a semilogarithmic scale. Thus, $\ln C_t$ as a function of time yields a straight line, the slope of which can readily be measured for an estimate of the elimination rate constant (Figure 9.20B). This is the fraction of drug eliminated from the body per unit time. The linear plot of $\ln C_t$ against time can be used to estimate the volume of distribution. Specifically, the linear relationship is extrapolated to time zero to yield the concentration of drug at time zero (C_0). The volume of distribution is then calculated by:

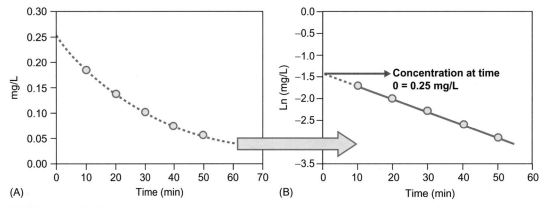

FIGURE 9.20 (A) First order clearance of a drug from a single compartment (central compartment). Concentration wanes, with time, in accordance with Equation 9.15. (B) When the data shown in panel A are expressed as a semilogarithmic plot (ordinate values ln C_t), a straight line results. Extrapolation of the line to time zero indicates a measure of the concentration at time zero. This can, in turn, be divided into the known amount of drug given to yield the theoretical volume that the drug is dissolved in at time zero to yield that concentration (the volume of distribution).

TABLE 9.9 Volumes of Distribution of Various Compartments in the Body

Compartment	Volume L/kg	Liters in 70 kg Male	% Total Body Weight
Plasma water	0.045	3	4.5
Extracellular water	0.2	14	20
Plasma + erythrocytes	0.07 to 0.08	5 to 6	7 to 9
Intracellular water	0.42	28	41
Total body water	0.6	42	60
Extensively bound to tissues	>0.64	>45	>66

$$V = (\text{Dose of Drug}) \text{ mg}/C_0 \text{ mg L}^{-1}. \qquad (9.16)$$

For the example shown in Figure 9.20B, a 3 mg dose gives a calculated concentration at time zero of 0.25 mg L^{-1}, which yields a volume of distribution of 12 liters. The volume of distribution can then be used to determine the apparent size of the compartments containing the drug. From this, the relative distribution of the drug can be determined. Table 9.9 shows some body compartment volumes as measured by tracer molecules known to have confined distribution in various compartments (i.e., inulin, Na^{23}, Br^-, I^- for extracellular fluid, Evans blue, ^{131}I-albumin, dextran for plasma, antipyrene, $D_2 0$, ethanol for total body water). The 12 L volume in the example shown in Figure 9.20B indicates that the drug is confined to the extracellular space (see Table 9.9). There are certain compartments that have restricted distribution, such as cerebrospinal, endolymph, fetal, ocular, synovial, and pleural fluids, that drugs do not enter readily.

The physicochemical properties of drugs can cause them to have a wide range of volumes of distribution. For example, 500 μg of digoxin given to a 70 kg patient yields a concentration at time zero of 0.75 ng mL^{-1}. This yields a calculated volume of distribution of 665 L, 16 times the volume of a normal 70 kg male. In this case, it indicates that digoxin is extensively bound to muscle and adipose tissue. This removes the drug from the free plasma compartment, causing a very low concentration to be measurable in the central (plasma) compartment; the low concentration is divided into the known amount of drug placed in the body (but not accessible to the measurement) to yield an abnormally large volume. Therefore, volumes of distribution >45 L (see Table 9.9) indicate sequestration of drug in depots not accessible to the sampling compartment (greater circulation). Such uneven tissue distribution can be extraordinary. For example, levels of quinacrine can be several thousand-fold higher in the liver than in the blood. Similarly, 70% of the lipid-soluble barbiturate thiopental is present in body fat 3 hours after administration. There are a number of reasons for such heterogeneous distributions of drugs in the body, such as binding to plasma proteins, cellular tissue binding, concentration in body fat, mammary transfer of drugs, and restricted diffusion due to barriers such as the blood-brain barrier and placenta. By measuring the volume of distribution, the distribution pattern of the drug in the body can be determined. Table 9.10 shows the volumes of distribution of some common drugs.

What the analysis of distribution makes evident is that the body is a heterogeneous collection of compartments. This is reflected by the fact that the elimination of a drug, as described in Figure 9.20 as a simple first order process, often does not, in fact, follow such simple kinetics. The first order process shown in Figure 9.20 assumes that the drug enters and leaves a single compartment. However, if the drug enters and leaves a more complex system (such as a system of two or three compartments in series or parallel), then a more complex kinetic relationship for drug concentration will be observed. Under these circumstances, the concentration of drug over time may follow a model

TABLE 9.10 Volumes of Distribution of Some Common Drugs

Warfarin	8 L
Tolbutamide	8 L
Theophylline	35 L
Quinidine	150 L
Lidocaine	120 L
Digoxin	420 L
Imipramine	2100 L
Nortryptilene	1500 L
Chloroquine	6600−17500 L

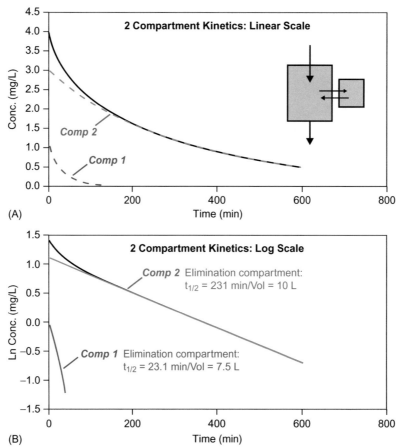

FIGURE 9.21 Multicompartment clearance. (A) The relationship between time and concentration in a two-compartment system. There is an initial rapid clearance followed by a slower phase. (B) The two phases are more clearly shown on a semilogarithmic plot (a single compartment would yield a straight line as seen in Figure 9.20B). This particular example is composed of rapid transfer from a compartment of 7.5 L (with $t_{1/2}$ of 23.1 min) and clearance from the body from the central compartment for this drug (10 L with $t_{1/2}$ of 231 min).

whereby efflux from multiple compartments are additive. For example, for a two-compartment system:

$$C_t = C_1 e^{-k_1 t} + C_2 e^{-k_2 t}, \qquad (9.17)$$

where C_1 and C_2 refer to the initial (at time zero) concentrations in each compartment, and k_1 and k_2 refer to the respective rate constants for elimination out of each of the two compartments. Figure 9.21 shows the elimination of a drug from a two-compartment system; it can be seen that a two-phase elimination is observed, and this is made more evident in the semilogarithmic plot with time. A common reason for apparent two-compartment kinetics is the fact that, upon initial entry, the drug may distribute rapidly to highly perfused regions of the body (liver, kidney, brain, lung; on a timescale of minutes); with time, the drug will then re-equilibrate with other regions of the body (i.e., viscera, muscle, skin, fat, on a timescale of hours). Thus, the initial kinetic phase is referred to as the *distribution phase* (see Figure 9.21B), while the later phase is the *elimination phase*.

In addition to detecting drug sequestration in the body, the volume of distribution can be used to determine loading dosage of drugs and the determination of dosage adjustments. For example, in the process of intravenous dosing it takes time to achieve a steady state in concentration because of varying rates of drug entry and clearance. If time is important therapeutically, this may be eliminated if the system is "loaded" with drug upon first i.v. infusion. The loading dose needed to do this is given by the target plasma concentration multiplied by the volume of distribution. For example, for a drug with a volume of distribution of 12 L, a loading dose of 120 mg will allow the rapid attainment of a concentration of 10 mg L^{-1}.

Dosage adjustment through determination of the volume of distribution can be very useful for special therapeutic compartments for some drugs. For example, if the therapeutic organ has rapid and preferred distribution (i.e., the brain), then the drug may have to be administered more often than the elimination of the drug suggests. Figure 9.22A shows the distribution out of the

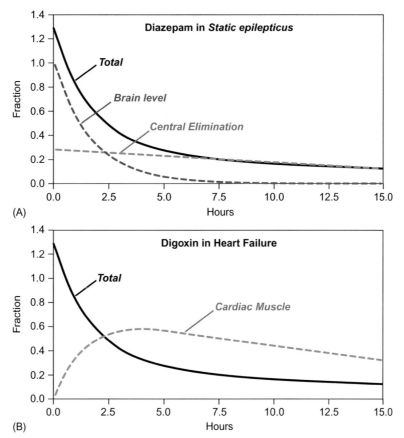

FIGURE 9.22 Two therapeutically relevant special compartments. (A) Diazepam is required to perfuse the brain in treatment of *static epilepticus*. Upon i.v. administration, diazepam rapidly equilibrates with the brain but then redistributes into the central compartment. The levels in the brain diminish much more rapidly than in the rest of the body. (B) The therapeutically relevant compartment for digoxin is cardiac muscle, but this compartment equilibrates much more slowly than the central compartment. In this case, concentrations in the muscle lag behind those in the central compartment.

brain for diazepam in *static epilepticus*. Figure 9.22B shows a different scenario; namely, a therapeutic organ with slow and restricted distribution (i.e., cardiac muscle for digoxin). In this case it can be seen that digoxin slowly redistributes into poorly accessible tissue, causing the pharmacodynamic effect to increase as the plasma levels decrease. This indicates that the loading should be done (in this case) 6 hours apart and that there is no advantage to i.v. dosing (oral is preferred).

Regarding the diffusion of drugs into restricted diffusion compartments (i.e., Figure 9.22B), it is useful to note the importance of clearance. The temporal kinetics of the concentration in the central compartment will drive the concentration going into the restricted compartment, thus it is not surprising that the amount of drug entering the restricted compartment will increase with an increased maximal peak concentration in the central compartment. However, this relationship can be harmful if the concentration in the central compartment becomes high enough to cause harmful side effects. However, if the elevated

concentrations in the central compartment are prolonged, as would be seen with a drug of lower clearance value, then the increase in the amount of time over which the concentration in the central compartment is elevated will greatly increase the amount of drug entering the restricted compartment. This is presumably because the rate of entry into the restricted compartment is low, and the longer time will allow a greater mass of drug to enter the compartment; Figure 9.23 shows this effect. The drug drawn in blue has a higher rate of clearance from the central compartment than the drug in red (left panel). The dosages of the two drugs have been adjusted to give the same peak concentration values (lower clearance drug dosage is 0.11 × concentration of higher clearance drug). In the right panel of Figure 9.23 it can be seen that, even though the dosage of the drug in red is nearly 1/10 that of the higher clearance blue drug, the amount of red drug entering the restricted diffusion compartment is nearly three times greater. This shows the remarkable influence of clearance on driving concentrations into restricted diffusion compartments.

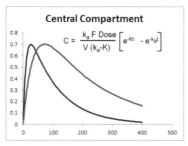
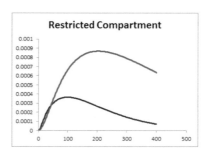

Central Compartment					Restricted Compartment		
Reference Values		Value	Ratio	New value	Ref	Ratio	Value
Rate of Absorption	k_a	1.00E-02	3	0.03	Rate in	1.00E-03	1.00E-05
Rate of Elimination	K	1.00E-01	1	0.005	Rate out	1.00E-03	1.00E-04
Vol of Distribution	V	1	1	1	Vol	1	1.00E+00
Bioavailability	F	1	1	1			
Dose	Dose	9	1	1			

FIGURE 9.23 **Hypothetical *in vivo* system showing two drugs with different values of clearance from the central compartment driving entry of drug into a restricted diffusion compartment.** Panel on left shows the central compartment concentrations of a high clearance drug (blue line) and lower clearance drug (red line); the dosages of the drugs have been adjusted to give equal C_{max} values (red drug dosage = 0.11 × blue drug dosage). Right panel shows entry of the drugs into a compartment with 0.1 × the rate of entry of the central compartment and 0.01 × the rate of efflux of the central compartment. It can be seen that the C_{max} of the lower clearance drug (red) in the restricted compartment is nearly 3 × that of the higher clearance drug despite the fact that it was given at 0.11 × the dosage.

The relationship between concentration and time (Figure 9.20B) given by Equation 9.15 can be used to determine k, the elimination rate constant, and this in turn can be used to calculate the half life ($t_{1/2}$) of the drug. This is the time it takes for the concentration to be reduced to half of its initial value. It is calculated by dividing -0.693 (ln 0.5) by k, according to a linear logarithmic metameter of Equation 9.15:

$$Ln \, (C_t/C_0) = -kt. \quad (9.18)$$

The elimination rate constant k is inversely proportional to the rate of elimination; that is, a drug with a $t_{1/2}$ of 4 hours is present in the body for approximately twice as long as one with a half time of $t_{1/2}$ of 2 hours. Relating the temporal concentration of a drug in the body during the elimination phase with k values is not intuitive. Therefore, it is frequently expressed in terms of $t_{1/2}$. Thus, a period of one $t_{1/2}$ is the time required for the drug concentration to fall to 50% of its original value, and 96.9% of the drug is eliminated after five periods of $t_{1/2}$.

As discussed previously, clearance and volume of distribution are the primary fundamental parameters required to describe pharmacokinetics. They are related to the elimination rate constant by:

$$k = \frac{CL}{V}. \quad (9.19)$$

And since $t_{1/2} = 0.693/k$, then:

$$t_{1/2} = \frac{0.693 \bullet V}{CL}. \quad (9.20)$$

These relationships assist in describing how these various parameters affect each other. For example, it can be seen that a reduction in clearance leads to a slower elimination and therefore a longer half life. Similarly, an increase in volume of distribution (increased tissue binding and sequestration of drugs away from the central compartment) leads to a reduction of accessibility to elimination and a subsequent increase in half life. Figure 9.24 shows the interplay between volume of distribution and clearance in terms of $t_{1/2}$.

The half life of a given drug can be a useful parameter for a number of reasons. First, it can determine the duration of action after a single dose. As a general rule, doubling the dose increases duration by one half life. Second, the $t_{1/2}$ can determine the time to reach steady state for chronic dosing, since this is the mirror image of disappearance. Thus, by five half lives the plasma concentration will be 96.9% of steady state (Figure 9.25A). This relationship can have practical therapeutic consequences. Thus, while a drug like morphine ($t_{1/2} = 3$ hrs) may need 12 hours to achieve a steady state drug level, drugs like digoxin ($t_{1/2} = 40$ hrs) and chloroquine ($t_{1/2} = 200$ hrs) may take 1 and 5 weeks, respectively, to reach a steady state. In the latter case, chloroquine prophylaxis requires some weeks before a patient enters a malaria-risk area. Finally, the $t_{1/2}$ can relate a single repeated dosage to steady state plasma level. Specifically, if a drug is given every $t_{1/2}$, the plateau will approach twice the peak concentration after a single dose (see Figure 9.25B).

For a one-compartment elimination, the visualization and quantification of elimination is straightforward. However, for a multi-compartment system consisting of

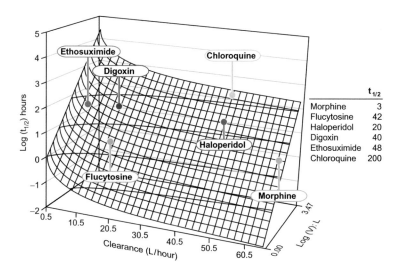

FIGURE 9.24 **Inter-relationship between clearance, volume of distribution, and $t_{1/2}$.** It can be seen that as volume of distribution increases, so too does $t_{1/2}$. In contrast, as clearance increases, $t_{1/2}$ decreases. Points on this surface reflect actual clearance, volume of distribution, and $t_{1/2}$ values for the sample of drugs shown in the table to the right of the figure.

	$t_{1/2}$
Morphine	3
Flucytosine	42
Haloperidol	20
Digoxin	40
Ethosuximide	48
Chloroquine	200

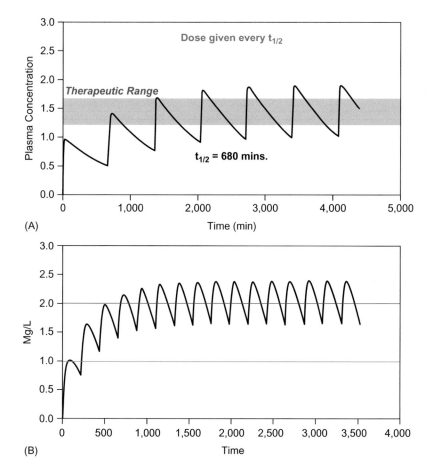

FIGURE 9.25 **Multiple dosing regimens.** (A) Intravenous effect of a drug with $t_{1/2}$ of 680 min administered every half life. A steady state (therapeutic range) is attained after five half lives have elapsed. (B) A drug given every $t_{1/2}$. It can be seen that the steady state concentration attained after approximately five half lives is twice the peak concentration of the first dose.

distribution followed by elimination, two (or more) half lives can be calculated. Usually, the first and most rapid $t_{1/2}$ relates to drug distribution, while the second (slower) $t_{1/2}$ relates to elimination (and therefore is of more clinical relevance; see Figure 9.26). However, as was seen in Figure 9.22A, if the distribution relates to a therapeutically relevant compartment, such as the brain in the diazepam treatment of epilepsy, then the first $t_{1/2}$ may also be therapeutically relevant.

Complex pharmacokinetics also can be observed when a drug metabolite has biological activity. In fact, for pro-drugs, the metabolite is the active species (kinetics of metabolite determines effect). There also are numerous cases of an active drug forming a biologically active metabolite (i.e., the acetylation of procainamide to N-acetylprocainamide). In cases where the elimination of metabolite >> disposition of parent, then the disposition of metabolites is dependent on their formation, and the pharmacokinetics follow that of the parent drug; see Figure 9.27A. However, in cases where the elimination of metabolite

<< disposition of parent, then the decay of effect is dependent on elimination of metabolite. If dosing is based on the pharmacokinetics of the parent, then accumulation of metabolite may result; with concomitant toxicity. In addition, the time to achieve a steady state of metabolite will be greater than that required for the parent. Under these circumstances the drug may not have to be administered as frequently as parent pharmacokinetics indicate (see Figure 9.27B). Figure 9.28 shows the pharmacokinetics of a 1 g dose of acetohexamide [10]. It can be seen that, while the concentration of the parent drug acetohexamide wanes after 5 hrs, the active metabolite hydroxyhexamide takes considerably longer to be eliminated.

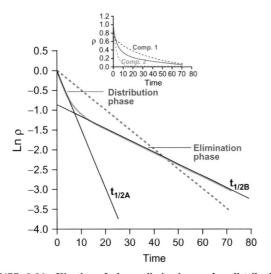

FIGURE 9.26 Kinetics of drug elimination and redistribution.
(A) First order elimination from a single compartment. Inset shows fractional concentration with time; larger graph shows the same with natural logarithmic ordinates. (B) Plasma concentration in a two-compartment system. The initially rapid elimination from the plasma in all probability represents redistribution of the drug out of the plasma into portions of the body. The slower phase represents elimination from the single body compartment. Inset shows elimination from each compartment as dotted lines with the observed combined effects shown in the solid blue line. This results in a curvilinear semilogarithmic plot.

9.4.7 Renal Clearance

A major route of drug elimination is through the kidney. The kidney has a filtration rate of 110 to 130 mL min^{-1} and receives 173 liters a day, of which 171 to 172 liters a day is recirculated to deliver a volume of urine of 1 to 2 liters a day. The various processes that the plasma is subjected to as it passes through the kidney are shown schematically in Figure 9.29. The first process is glomerular filtration, where all but large proteins pass through the glomerulus to enter the renal tubule. Specifically, blood passes through the glomerulus at 1200 mL min^{-1} and 10% is filtered through as plasma water (125 mL min^{-1}); the fraction of unbound (by protein) drug goes with it. Glomerular filtration rate (125 mL min^{-1}) is measured by creatinine or inulin clearance (these are not secreted or reabsorbed). From there, the drug passes through the proximal tubule, where the process of secretion takes place. There are two main processes of secretion: one for

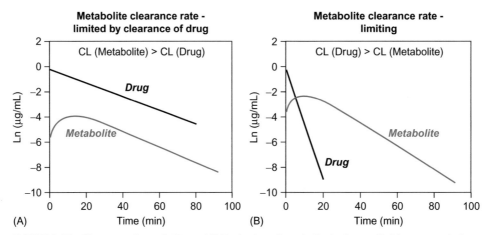

FIGURE 9.27 Clearance of metabolites. (A) Production of metabolite is the rate-limiting step, and clearance of the metabolite is faster than that of the parent drug. Under these circumstances, clearance of the metabolite is approximated by clearance of the parent drug. (B) Clearance of the metabolite is slower than clearance of the parent drug. Under these circumstances, metabolite clearance is the rate-limiting step, and clearance of the parent drug cannot be used as an indicator of elimination of effect if the metabolite is the active drug species.

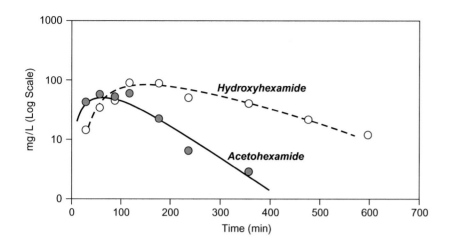

FIGURE 9.28 **Oral absorption and elimination of acetohexamide and its active metabolite hydroxyhexamide.** It can be seen that effect will follow elimination of the active metabolite, which lags behind clearance of the parent drug. Data redrawn from [17].

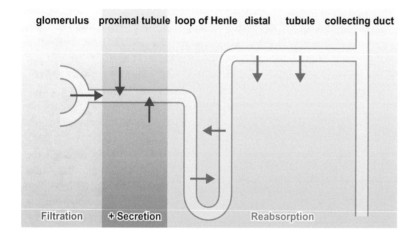

FIGURE 9.29 **Schematic diagram of path of filtered fluid through kidney tubules.** Blood is filtered through the glomerulus to pass through the proximal tubule. In this region, the process of active secretion can take place. Fluid then passes through the loop of Henle and into the distal tubule, where active reabsorption takes place. Any fluid that is not reabsorbed passes to the collecting duct and into the urine.

negatively charged (weak acids) and one for positively charged (weak bases) species. This process generally works on unbound drug, although some powerful secretion processes can strip a protein of drug. Drugs can compete for these processes and they are saturable. P-gp and multidrug resistance-associated protein 2 (MRP2) secrete amphipathic anions and conjugated metabolites, for example, glucuronides, sulfates, and glutathione adducts, while ATP-binding cassette (ABC) transporters secrete organic bases. Further on in the loop of Henle and distal tubule, the process of reabsorption takes place. In this region, all but 1–2 mL of 125 mL of filtered water is reabsorbed, and membrane-soluble drugs are reabsorbed according to a concentration gradient. Reabsorption is controlled by urine volume (high volume = low gradient = low reabsorption). Since only unionized drugs are reabsorbed, pH is a factor in drug reabsorption.

Total renal clearance (CL_R) is given by an expression that incorporates consideration of all these processes:

$$CL_R = f_u \bullet (GFR + CL_s) \bullet (1 - FR), \quad (9.21)$$

where f_u is the fraction of unbound (by protein) drug, GFR is the glomerular filtration rate (125 mL min^{-1}),

CL_S refers to active secretion of drug, and FR is the fraction reabsorbed. For a drug that is rapidly cleared by the kidney, the unbound drug clearance will essentially be the GFR = 125 mL min^{-1}. However, for instance, if the drug is 99% protein bound, then the renal clearance will be GFR/100 = 1.25 mL min^{-1}. Some drugs are cleared by kidneys so rapidly that they clear in one pass (e.g., p-aminhippuric acid, PAH); under these circumstances, clearance is equal to entire renal blood flow = 660 mL min^{-1}. Renal clearance is related to urine flow by the expression:

$$CL_R = \frac{Conc_U \ (mg \ mL^{-1}) \bullet U \ (mL \ min^{-1})}{Conc_{plasma} \ (mg \ mL^{-1})}, \quad (9.22)$$

where $Conc_U$ and $Conc_{plasma}$ are the concentrations of the drug in the urine and plasma, respectively, and U is the rate of urine flow.

A useful question to answer is how can it be known if a drug is secreted or reabsorbed by a renal process? All drugs are subject to basal renal clearance (f_u GFR), so if the renal clearance is greater than this value, then the drug is secreted (may be reabsorbed but secretion > reabsorption). If the renal clearance is less than the filtration

TABLE 9.11 Relationships of Renal Clearance Processes

Observation	Renal Effect
>GFR	Subject to renal secretion
Equal to GFR	Freely filtered/no net secretion or reabsorption
<GFR	Reabsorption or protein binding

clearance, then the drug is reabsorbed (may be secreted but reabsorption > secretion). Some useful diagnostic checks for these processes involve the use of secretion competitors (probenicid for acid, cimetidine for base) and the observation of dependence on varying urine flow rate and/or pH (i.e., if flow rate changes clearance, the drug is reabsorbed). The relationships among these various renal clearance processes are summarized in Table 9.11.

It also is useful to summarize some drug properties that may determine whether or not a given drug is subject to renal clearance. Thus, highly ionized drugs will be filtered or secreted without being reabsorbed (they will appear rapidly in the urine), while nonpolar drugs (or drugs in their nonpolar form) will be subject to reabsorption. Under these circumstances, the pH of the urine and the pK_a of the drug are very important for the process of reabsorption. The degree of renal clearance can be measured by determining the fraction of drug excreted that is unchanged (f_e):

$$f_e = \frac{\text{Renal Clearance}}{\text{Total Clearance}}. \qquad (9.23)$$

Similarly, f_m (the fraction of drug metabolized) is given by:

$$f_m = \frac{\text{Total Clearance} - \text{Renal Clearance}}{\text{Total Clearance}}. \qquad (9.24)$$

For example, for drugs that are essentially completely metabolized and not excreted unchanged (such as propranolol, morphine, tolbutamine, theophylline), $f_e = 0$. In contrast, for drugs that are not metabolized, all of the drug is excreted unchanged ($f_e = 1$, e.g., penicillin, amoxycillin, gentamicin, digoxin).

9.4.8 Bioavailability

An important concept in clinical pharmacokinetics is the bioavailability of a drug. This is the actual fraction of drug that enters the central systemic circulation upon administration via the chosen therapeutic route. For example, drugs taken by the oral route must be absorbed either through the stomach or, most likely, the small intestine, into the bloodstream. The blood preferentially flows through the liver from the GI tract; thus, the drug is subjected to metabolism before it enters the general circulation. This first barrier of metabolism is referred to as the *first pass effect*. Bioavailability is calculated as the ratio of area under the curves when the drug is given intravenously (assume 100% bioavailability) versus the chosen route of administration; see Figure 9.30.

Drugs given by the oral route must pass through the liver before they emerge in the circulation. This "first pass effect" can be devastating for highly metabolized drugs, such as for organic nitrates (i.e., glycerol trinitrate F = 1%); for this reason these are given sublingually, because they can be so completely cleared by first pass metabolism that they are ineffective by the oral route. Drugs subject to high first pass extraction are more dependent on liver function, causing drug levels to be much more variable (i.e., verapamil). High first pass drugs are more subject to enzyme induction and/or inhibition and liver disease. Intravenous and oral doses of drugs with high bioavailability are comparable. In contrast, a drug with 10% bioavailability will require 10 times more

FIGURE 9.30 Estimation of oral bioavailability is made by measuring the area under the curve for a dose of drug given intravenously and by the oral route. The bioavailability (as a fraction F) is obtained by dividing the AUC oral by the intravenous AUC.

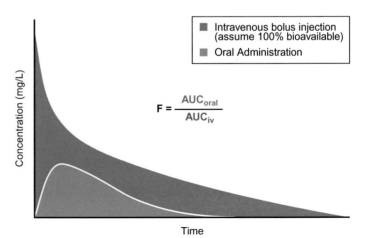

TABLE 9.12 Some Factors Affecting Oral Bioavailability

	Increased	Decreased
Stomach Emptying	i.e., hunger, exercise, metoclopramide **Increased absorption**	hot meals, pain, narcotics, antidepressants **Decreased absorption**
Intestinal Motility	gastroenteritis / decreased transit time **Decreased absorption**	narcotics, anticholinergics, tricyclics **Increased absorption**
Chemical Interaction	chelation of tetracyclines with metal ions **Decreased absorption**	

drug orally than when given i.v. The maximal total bioavailability (F) of a drug can be predicted from the expression:

$$F = f_g \bullet f_H, \qquad (9.25)$$

where f_g is the fraction of drug absorbed by the gut, and f_H is the fraction escaping the liver ($f_g = 1 - E_H$, where E_H is the hepatic extraction ratio). If it is assumed that the drug is completely absorbed from the gut ($fg = 1$), then the maximal bioavailability (F_{max}) is given by:

$$F_{max} = 1 - \frac{CL_{int}}{Q_H}, \qquad (9.26)$$

where CL_{int} is the intrinsic hepatic clearance and Q_H liver blood flow. In general, a value of $F > 0.2$ is preferred, but there are exceptions to this rule. For example, the bisphosphonate used for stabilizing bone matrix in osteoporosis is given by the oral route, yet for this drug $F = 0.03$.

Low metabolic clearance is a good predictor of good oral bioavailability and long half life, while high clearance leads to high rate of elimination and lack of oral bioavailability. There are many other factors involved in oral bioavailability. These involve drug dissolution (chemical properties of drug, crystal form[s], dosage form [sustained release, coated tablets], pH of stomach and intestine), the gastric emptying rate (stability of drug at stomach pH, solution-solid form [liquids empty more quickly], effects of food, antacids, drugs [opiates], disease), intestinal motility (mainly affects slowly soluble drugs [i.e., sustained release], degradation and/or metabolism in gut microflora), drug interactions in gut lumen (complexation [i.e., tetracyclines + divalent metal ions], adsorption [i.e., anion exchange resins], food interactions [i.e., antibiotics]) and passage through the gut wall (chemical properties [i.e., quarternary ammonium compounds], and metabolism by enzymes in intestinal epithelium [i.e., CYP3A4 in the GI tract leading to poor oral bioavailability]). Some other factors which affect oral bioavailability are given in Table 9.12.

Finally, some drug absorption is affected by the enterohepatic cycle, specifically the secretion of some drugs into the bile for subsequent reabsorption in the GI tract. Many drugs (i.e., high molecular weight drugs [approx. 500], large polar molecules, glucuronide conjugates, i.e., chloramphenicol) are secreted into the bile unchanged, and these are available for reabsorption via the GI tract. Some other drugs that are reabsorbed via the enterohepatic cycle are reabsorbed as glucuronides and other conjugates, e.g., estradiol, valproic acid, digitoxin, spironolactone, and imipramine. There can be practical consequences to enterohepatic recirculation. For example, the $t_{1/2}$ of digoxin changes from 6 days to 4.5 days upon blockade of enterohepatic recirculation by cholestyramine, while the $t_{1/2}$ for dapsone changes from 20.5 hours to 10.8 hours in the presence of charcoal, a biliary excretion inhibitor.

9.5 NONLINEAR PHARMACOKINETICS

Under normal circumstances, the velocity of elimination is first order; that is, the rate of the process is linearly related to the concentration. However, drug elimination may not be first order at high doses due to saturation of the capacity of the elimination processes at high doses of drug. In this region, the process is zero order. This means that a constant amount, not a constant fraction, of drug is eliminated until the process is no longer saturated. Zero order elimination produces a reduction in the slope of the elimination curve, since elimination is governed by the V_{max}. However, once the concentration falls below saturation levels, first order kinetics prevail.

To discuss nonlinear pharmacokinetics, it is first useful to consider linear pharmacokinetics, Thus, for a drug that does not exceed the metabolic capability of the removal process ($[S] << K_m$), the clearance is given by V_{max}/K_m. For a given steady state plasma concentration (C_{ss}), the dosage rate (DR) required is given by:

$$DR = CL \bullet C_{ss} = \frac{V_{max}}{K_m} \bullet C_{ss}. \qquad (9.27)$$

It can be seen from Equation 9.27 that there is a linear relationship between the plasma concentration and dosage of drug required to maintain it (linear pharmacokinetics).

FIGURE 9.31 Nonlinear pharmacokinetics. Phenytoin demonstrates linear pharmacokinetics within a dose range (150 to 300 mg/day) until doses are attained that saturate its metabolism. At this point, the C_{ss} obtained by increases in dosage becomes nonlinear. From the previous linear relationship, a dosage of 450 mg/day would have been expected to produce a C_{ss} of 22.5 mg/L. However, saturation of phenytoin metabolism caused a massive increase in C_{ss} to 150 mg/L.

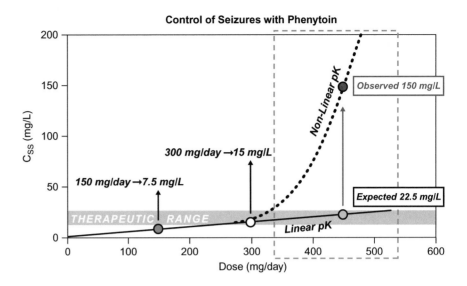

For example, for a drug with a clearance of $10\,L\,h^{-1}$, a dosage rate of $30\,\mu g\,h^{-1}$ is required for a C_{ss} of $3\,\mu g\,L^{-1}$. If an increase in the steady state concentration to $6\,\mu g\,L^{-1}$ is required, a concentration of $60\,\mu g\,h^{-1}$ would have to be administered. In the case of nonlinear pharmacokinetics, [S] is not $<< K_m$ and the relationship between DR and C_{ss} is given by:

$$DR = CL \bullet C_{ss} = \frac{V_{max}}{C_{ss} + K_m} \bullet C_{ss}. \quad (9.28)$$

An example of the way this can lead to practical problems is shown in Figure 9.31. In the control of seizures, phenytoin concentrations must be monitored and kept within a range. As shown in Figure 9.31, a linear pharmacokinetic relationship should allow control of C_{ss} in the range 7.5 to 22.5 mg L^{-1}. However, once the nonlinear range is reached (dosage >300 mg/day), increased dosage leads to an unpredictable C_{ss} considerably higher than the desired value (a goal of 22.5 mg L^{-1} is exceeded by a factor of 6.7 to 150 mg L^{-1}). There are several possible reasons for the appearance of such nonlinear pharmacokinetics:

- **Decrease in absorption**: For example, amoxicillin absorption decreases with dose.
- **Saturation of plasma protein binding**: For example, disopyramide shows increase in volume of distribution with increased dose.
- **Saturated renal excretion**: For example, dicloxacillin demonstrates saturable active renal secretion showing decreased renal clearance with increased dose.
- **Saturation of metabolism (capacity-limited metabolism)**: Phenytoin and ethanol saturate hepatic metabolism, showing decreased hepatic clearance with increased dose.

Another factor contributing to or causing nonlinear pharmacokinetics is auto-induction of metabolizing enzymes.

This is where the drug itself induces its own metabolism (increased CYP450 levels), which is the case for carbamazepine. Two other possible causes are co-substrate depletion, when the co-substrate for conjugation is depleted leading to reduced elimination (i.e., theophylline), and product (metabolite) inhibition, for example, phenylbutazone. Other factors may include low f_g (fraction absorbed in the gut) such as that seen with riboflavin (saturable gut wall transport), salicylamide (saturable gut wall metabolism), and griseofulvin (poor solubility). Yet other causes of nonlinear pharmacokinetics involve the kidney, such as that seen for penicillin G (active tubular secretion), ascorbic acid (active tubular reabsorption), salicylic acid (alteration in urine pH), theophylline (alterations in urine flow), and gentamycin (nephrotoxicity).

Some consequences of nonlinear pharmacokinetics are

- Compromised clearance; $t_{1/2}$ may become very large; that is, phenytoin $t_{1/2}$ may change from 12 hours to 1 week (since $t_{1/2}$ affects time to steady state, it may take 1 to 3 weeks to attain steady state with these long $t_{1/2}$ values).
- Drug levels may be somewhat unresponsive to cessation of treatment until clearance increases.

One useful method to detect nonlinear kinetics is to note when the ratio of AUC/dose does not remain constant; this ratio is constant over a large range if linear pharmacokinetics are operative.

9.6 MULTIPLE DOSING

The half life of a drug characterizes the kinetic aspect of pharmacokinetics, and this, in turn, is important for multiple dosing; this is the mainstay of drug therapy. For example, consider three multiple dosing treatment schedules where the aim is a steady state concentration of drug, indicated by the regimen described by the blue curve in Figure 9.32. Under these circumstances, the rate of absorption and rate of clearance combine with the dosage interval to produce a useful therapeutic effect. If elimination is too slow for the frequency of dosing, then an accumulation to possibly toxic levels will result (curve in red; Figure 9.32). If elimination is too rapid, then the therapeutic level of dosage may never be achieved (curve in green; Figure 9.32). The aim of multiple dosing is to attain a steady state of drug concentration (C_{ss}) that is therapeutically adequate but not toxic. As noted in Section 9.4.6 and Figure 9.25A, a steady state is attained after a drug has been administered every half time for five half lives. However, there may be conditions where waiting for five half lives may not be practical or advised (i.e., if the drug has a very long half life or where immediate responses are needed). Under these circumstances, a loading dose can be administered to quickly reach the steady state C_{ss}. This dose is calculated by multiplying the required C_{ss} by the volume of distribution; Figure 9.33 shows the attainment of C_{ss} after five intravenous doses of a drug given every half life and the effects of administering a loading dose along with the first dose.

An important parameter in drug therapy is the frequency of dosing (referred to as the *dosing interval,* denoted τ). There are four main determinants of τ:

- Target dosing schedule for compliance (i.e., once a day?).
- Drug half life ($t_{1/2}$).
- Dosage in tablet.
- Formulation (control of absorption).

It is worth considering τ as a therapeutic parameter. The half life for elimination from a given compartment may pose special problems, as in the case of the diazepam brain perfusion problem shown in Figure 9.22A. If the drug were to be given often enough to keep an adequate C_{ss} in the brain (a rapidly eliminated compartment), it can be seen from Figure 9.34A that toxic concentrations would soon be reached, due to the much slower elimination from the central compartment. Figure 9.34B defines the relationship between τ and $t_{1/2}$, and shows that if a drug is given too often, it will accumulate to levels far in excess of the predicted C_{ss} attained by normal dosing after a period of five half lives.

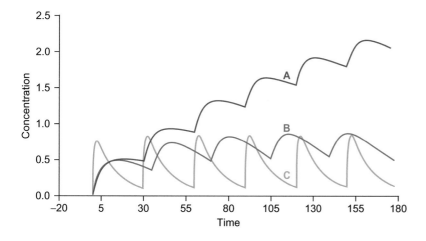

FIGURE 9.32 Repeated oral administration of drugs leads to steady state plasma concentrations. If elimination is rapid and administration too infrequent, then an elevated and therapeutically effective steady state concentration may not be achieved (green lines). In contrast, if elimination is very slow (or administration too frequent), then an accumulation of the drug may be observed with no constant steady state (red line). Blue line shows a correct balance between frequency of administration and elimination.

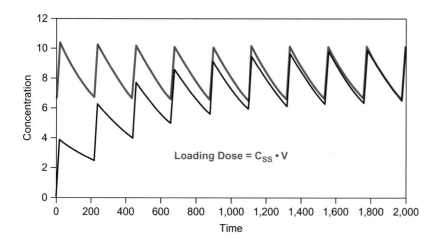

FIGURE 9.33 Use of a loading dose to eliminate the time required to achieve steady state concentrations with intravenous dosing. With no loading dose, the black line indicates the rise in C_{ss}; after approximately five half times, a steady state is achieved. The red line shows the effect of administering the first dose plus adding a loading dose (calculated by multiplying the desired C_{ss} by the volume of distribution).

FIGURE 9.34 **Variation between C_{max} and C_{min} and dosage interval.** (A) Example for diazepam (given in Figure 9.16A) where the drug is given in accordance with the $t_{1/2}$ for the rapid clearance from the brain in an attempt to sustain a therapeutically relevant C_{ss} in the brain. It can be seen that when the drug is administered this often, the much slower elimination from the central compartment precludes adequate clearance and very high concentrations accumulate in the central compartment. (B) Increased levels of C_{ss} as a multiple of the peak first dose. It can be seen that when drugs with long $t_{1/2}$ are given often (short τ), then drug levels accumulate to give levels considerably higher than those obtained with the first dose (ordinate). To avoid this accumulation, the τ must be prolonged.

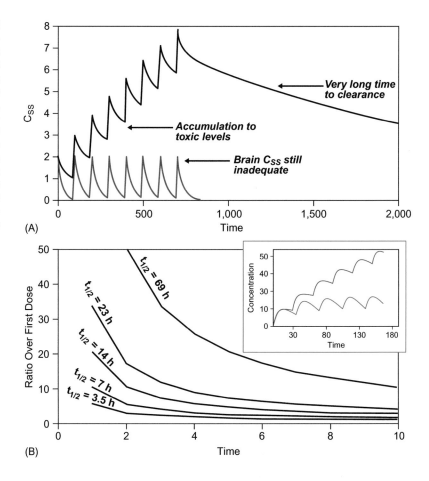

Previous discussions have been confined to administering the drug every $t_{1/2}$; this is instructive to relate certain temporal characteristics of drug behavior. However, τ also relates to patient compliance; it would be difficult for patients to take a pill every hour if the $t_{1/2}$ were 1 hour — a preferred guideline is to strive for a once-a-day dosing for maximal patient compliance. Figure 9.35A shows multiple dosing for a drug with a $t_{1/2}$ of 90 min that is given every 2 hours. The object of treatment is to obtain a C_{ss} of 2.8 to 3 $\mu g\,L^{-1}$. A better compliance would be achieved if the patient could take the drug every 6 hours, but as shown in Figure 9.35B, at the dose shown in Figure 9.29A, this would attain the required C_{ss} for only a small fraction of the time needed. One approach to achieving the C_{ss} needed is to increase the dose for drugs with little dose-related toxicity such as penicillins (amoxicillin is given in very large doses to allow once-a-day compliance for children with ear infections). This is an option for drugs that are as nontoxic as amoxicillin, but in other cases increasing the dose can be problematic from two points of view. As shown in Figure 9.35C, the peak concentrations required are extremely high (giving the possibility of toxic effects), and also, the extremes in concentration are large, leading to an

extremely variable C_{ss}. The magnitude of the ratio of C_{max} to C_{min} can be calculated by:

$$\frac{C_{max}}{C_{min}} = \frac{1}{e^{-\frac{0.693}{t_{1/2}}\tau}}. \qquad (9.29)$$

It can be seen from Equation 9.29 that large $t_{1/2}$ or small τ values will lead to large differences between C_{max} and C_{min} (as those shown in Figure 9.35C). These can be avoided by matching τ to $t_{1/2}$ (in this case, giving the drug more often), but this may pose a problem with compliance. In general, mismatched τ and $t_{1/2}$ values for a drug can lead to practical therapeutic concerns. Compliance and dose regimens are easiest to control when the therapeutic end point is clearly measurable, e.g., blood pressure, heart rate, or if there are clearly measurable biomarkers available. This can be a difficult problem for prophylaxis or for drugs with therapeutic end points that are not easily measured and there is a risk of administering subtherapeutic-to-toxic levels of drug. For some drugs, this margin is very small, for example, digoxin, theophylline, lidocaine, aminoglycosides, ciclosporin, warfarin, and anticonvulsants. One approach that is useful in some cases is to administer the drug in a sustained

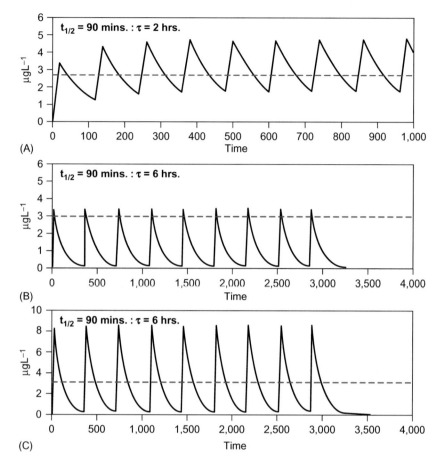

(A)

(B)

(C)

FIGURE 9.35 **Relationship between sustained therapeutic steady state level of drug dosage and frequency of administration.** (A) A drug with $t_{1/2}$ of 90 min given every $t_{1/2}$ attains a therapeutically relevant C_{ss} of 2.8 μg L^{-1}. (B) If the dosage interval is increased to allow better compliance ($\tau = 6$ hours), it can be seen that the therapeutic level of 2.8 μg L^{-1} is rarely attained. (C) Some level of coverage with 2.8 μg L^{-1} is obtained if the dosage is greatly increased and compliance is satisfied ($\tau = 6$ hours). However, the ratio of C_{max} to C_{min} is very large, raising the possibility of toxic effects at peak concentrations.

release formulation that will not cause the sharp rises in C_{max}. This allows the use of larger doses without the risk of high C_{max} values.

9.7 PRACTICAL PHARMACOKINETICS

A great deal of information can be obtained from a single dose pharmacokinetic experiment and a single dose experiment with oral administration (for an oral drug). As shown in Figure 9.36, plasma concentrations can be measured over time after a single intravenous dose; this yields the temporal relationship for concentration due to elimination. The area under the curve then can be used to calculate clearance. It should be noted that the area under the curve must be calculated from time zero to the point where drug levels diminish to zero ($t \rightarrow \infty$). The waning of concentration with time, converted to a logarithmic scale, yields a straight line, the slope of which is the elimination rate constant (see Figure 9.36). This, in turn, yields the $t_{1/2}$, and from that, the volume of distribution. The clearance can be confirmed by observing the effects of an oral dose. Also, the bioavailability of the drug can be determined by the ratio of AUC via the oral route divided by the AUC via the intravenous route.

Multiple dose studies can add information as well. As shown in Figure 9.37A, multiple i.v. doses show an accumulation when the drug is given every $t_{1/2}$ due to a time-dependent increase in $t_{1/2}$. This is characterized by the rising C_{ss} and inability to attain a constant steady state drug level. Such behavior is characteristic of nonlinear pharmacokinetics. In contrast, a decrease in $t_{1/2}$ (as shown in Figure 9.37B) suggests autoinduction of metabolism.

9.7.1 Allometric Scaling

The studies involved in candidate selection in drug discovery and development programs are done in animals and *in vitro* systems; the process of predicting the dose of the candidate that will be tested in humans for efficacy and safety is obtained by using allometric scaling. Specifically, this is the discipline of predicting human pharmacokinetics based on preclinical data, and the studies are designed to answer the following questions:

- Will the compound support once-daily dosing?
- Will the compound be well absorbed?
- What will the efficacious dose be?
- What dose will be toxic?

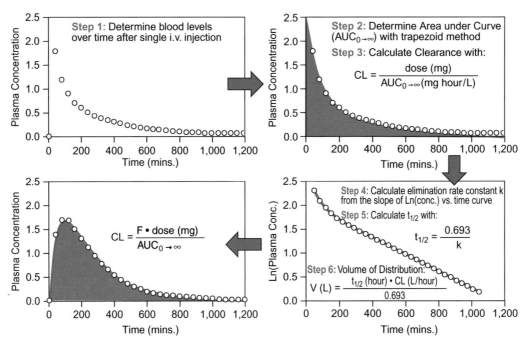

FIGURE 9.36 Single dose pharmacokinetics. A drug is administered intravenously and the plasma concentration measured at various intervals until it disappears from the bloodstream. The area under the curve is calculated and used to calculate clearance. The disappearance of drug with time from the intravenous dose also can be used to calculate $t_{1/2}$. A semilogarithmic plot of the graph shown in the top left quadrant yields a curve with a linear portion that can be used to estimate the k for elimination (and subsequent $t_{1/2}$); this then can be used to calculate the volume of distribution. The same dose of the drug given via the oral route can be used to estimate bioavailability (F) by the ratio of AUC_{oral} and AUC_{iv}.

FIGURE 9.37 Multiple dose pharmacokinetics. (A) Nonlinear pharmacokinetics are operative if the $t_{1/2}$ for elimination increases with increasing dose. If τ is chosen to be $t_{1/2}$ and $t_{1/2}$ remains constant, then a steady state will be obtained after five half life periods. However, if no steady state is achieved (and plasma concentrations keep increasing, as shown in the graph), then elimination is being reduced with time (nonlinear pharmacokinetics). (B) Metabolic enzyme induction is operative if no steady state is obtained after five half lives and the plasma concentrations decrease. This indicates that the $t_{1/2}$ is reducing with repeated dosage, and this is indicative of metabolic enzyme auto-induction.

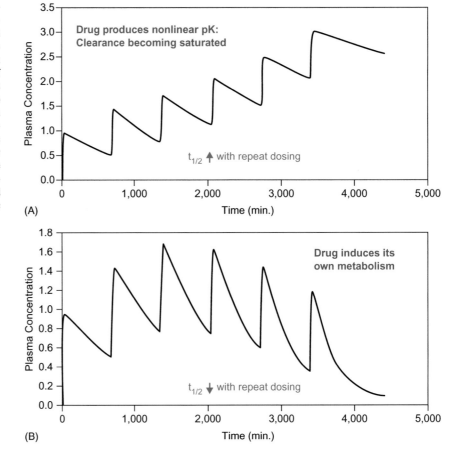

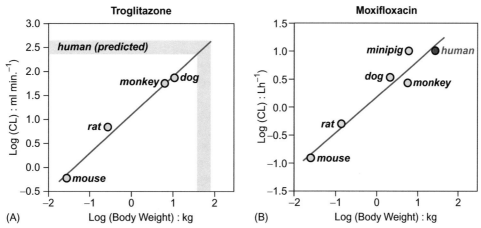

FIGURE 9.38 Allometric scaling for prediction of clearance in humans. (A) Troglitazone log clearance in mouse, rat, monkey, and dog defines a linear relationship with logarithm of body weight. These data predict a clearance of 316 mL min^{-1} for humans. Data drawn from [18]. (B) Moxifloxacin clearance in mouse, rat, monkey, dog, minipig, and human. In this case, the human experimental data agree well with the allosteric scaling prediction. Data drawn from [19].

Allometric scaling is based on body size, according to the general equation:

$$Y_{human} = Y_{animal} (W_h/W_a)^b, \qquad (9.30)$$

where W_h and W_a refer to the body weight of humans and animals, respectively, and b is a scaling power factor that changes with the nature of the index being predicted ($t_{1/2}$, b = 0.25; volume of distribution, b = 1; biological rates [hepatic flow], b = 0.75). Equation 9.30 can be used as a logarithmic metameter to yield a straight line of the form $Y = aW^b$. The logarithmic metameter is:

$$Log\ Y = Log\ (a) + b\ Log\ (W). \qquad (9.31)$$

Therefore, a plot of animal values (Y) on a log scale versus log body weight yields a straight line of slope b; this can then be used to predict the human value. Figure 9.38A shows the allometric scaling for predicting the clearance of the antidiabetic troglitazone. The data from studies in mouse, rat, monkey, and dog predict that the clearance in humans should be approximately 316 mL min^{-1} [18]. Figure 9.38B shows a similar type of study for the antibacterial moxifloxacin. In this case, clearance data from studies in mouse, rat, dog, monkey, and minipig predict a human clearance of 11.8 L h^{-1}. This is a reasonable prediction of the experimentally derived value of 9.6 L h^{-1} (see Figure 9.38B) [19].

9.8 PLACEMENT OF PHARMACOKINETIC ASSAYS IN DISCOVERY AND DEVELOPMENT

A drug candidate must be adequately absorbed, reside in the body for a time sufficient to reach its target organ(s),

and be excreted or degraded completely. There are general guidelines that can be used to determine early in the process whether or not a given molecule will fulfill these criteria. For example, a molecule with a clearance of >25% of liver blood flow by the intravenous route or <10% oral availability (assuming it is designed to be a drug taken by the oral route) would not augur well for further development. In contrast, a molecule with <25% liver blood flow clearance and >30% oral bioavailability would be a good candidate. In addition to pharmacokinetics, the chemical form of the candidate also is important; this issue can be addressed by pharmaceutical studies [20].

It is useful to consider the types of studies that can be done at various stages in the drug discovery and development process. A good starting point is to consider the end product and what clinical characteristics are required. These can be summarized by three basic properties (assuming efficacy is given):

- Route of administration,
- Magnitude of the dose of drug,
- Dosage interval (τ),

These properties summarize how the drug will be used and therefore define, early in the discovery and development process, what type of molecule will be successful. The route of administration is determined by the need for compliance and also by therapeutic bias. This latter factor incorporates the balance between how important the therapy is to health and patient preference. For example, while it may be acceptable for patients to inject insulin for life-threatening diabetes, it may not be so for an injectable weight loss drug. If a once-a-day oral drug is the aim of the program, then this raises early criteria for clearance (i.e., high first pass metabolism would be a negative) and $t_{1/2}$ (a short half life would make it difficult to formulate a once-a-day regimen). The dosage relates to drug potency, which, in turn, is related to basic pharmacological properties (affinity, efficacy), the safety margin (concentrations required for therapeutic effect versus those that cause untoward side effects), how well the drug is absorbed (for oral drugs), and f_u, the degree of protein binding. The dosage interval (τ) relates to the pharmacokinetic parameters $t_{1/2}$, volume of distribution (f_u), clearance kinetics, and dose. Many of these parameters can be estimated in rapid *in vitro* tests early on in the discovery and development process.

One of the earliest sets of parameters that can be addressed at the drug synthesis stage concerns the physicochemical properties of a molecule. As discussed in Section 9.3, the process of lead optimization usually involves the addition of chemical groups to the basic molecular scaffold. Assuming that this lead optimization process will increase both the lipophilicity and molecular weight of a lead, a molecular end point for a screening hit would be molecular weight <350, ClogP < 3, with a primary affinity for the biological target of approximately <0.1 μM. Some guidelines for medicinal chemists are contained in a set of rules known as the "rule of 5" derived by Lipinski (see Section 9.3); in general, any molecule that violates any two of these rules would be predicted to yield poor absorption *in vivo*. Figure 9.39 shows how these factors can influence the chemical properties required for a successful drug; Table 9.13 shows

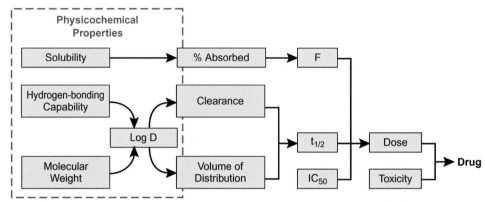

FIGURE 9.39 Schematic diagram showing how physicochemical properties of molecules affect various parameters of pharmacokinetics. The log D (log P) defines lipophilicity, which, in turn, contributes to protein and tissue binding. This can affect volume of distribution and clearance. Solubility affects presentation to the gastrointestinal tract, which, in turn, affects absorption. The absorption and clearance define bioavailability (F), while the clearance and volume of distribution define half life. The dosage, $t_{1/2}$, and F define how much drug is given and how often. If a margin of safety is operative, then the molecule will be a useful drug. Drawn from [19].

TABLE 9.13 *In Vitro* Assays for Estimating Physicochemical Properties

Solution Properties	Assay	Potential Benefits
Lipophilicity	cLogP (cLogD) or mLopgP (mLogD)	• Measure a compound potential for crossing lipid membranes • Also may indicate potential for tissue sequestration (high volume of distribution), CYP metabolism and general toxicity
Lipophilicity	Chromatographic hydrophobicity	• As above
Chemical stability	Measure stability of compounds in solution through non-enzyme degradation	• Estimate compound stability
Protein binding	Measure plasma protein binding through dialysis	• Gauge potential for sequestration from renal and hepatic clearance • Measure possible effects on volume of distribution • Estimate possible depot/sink effect
Plasma stability	Measure disappearance of compound when incubated in plasma	• Gauge how stable the compound will be in the central plasma compartment (clearance)

some *in vitro* assays available to determine the physico-chemical properties of potential drugs. Table 9.14 shows *in vitro* assays that can be used to estimate membrane permeability, and the metabolic stability of compounds can be assessed with the *in vitro* assays listed in Table 9.15.

In terms of pharmacokinetics and the probability that a molecule will evolve as a therapeutic entity active by the oral route, drug clearance is paramount. While poor absorption is detrimental, there are cases where changes in formulation or simple increases in dosage can overcome this drawback. However, if a molecule is rapidly cleared by the body, then it is unlikely ever to have the half life and system exposure required for useful therapeutic application. Figure 9.40 shows some strategies available for exploring poor system exposure in any chemical scaffold. An example of developability being a key factor in the emergence of a drug from an active molecule can be found in the histamine H2 receptor antagonist molecules. The first active histamine H2 antagonist burimamide, while active by the parenteral route, did not have the oral absorption properties required for an oral drug (Figure 9.41). The second in the series, metiamide, was active by the oral route but had fatal bone marrow toxicity which precluded clinical utility.

TABLE 9.14 *In Vitro* Assays for Estimating Permeability

In Vitro Permeability	Assay	Potential Benefits
Absorption	PAMPA permeability	• Gauge potential to cross gut wall • Estimates ability to cross lipid membranes through passive diffusion without active transport or efflux
Absorption / gut transport	Caco-2 (MDCK) permeability	• Gauges ability to cross gut wall • Also can estimate active efflux / transport properties (i.e., P-gp)
Blood brain barrier	Application of Caco-2 assay	• Measure logPS (permeability × surface area) to estimate ability of compounds to cross blood-brain barrier

TABLE 9.15 *In Vitro* Assays for Estimating Metabolism

In Vitro Metabolism	Assay	Potential Benefits
Metabolic stability	Human hepatocytes	• Contain both Phase I and II enzymes to gauge overall metabolic stability • More accurate due to inclusion of some transport processes and enzyme orientation effects
Metabolic stability	Human microsomes	• Gauge general stability and potential for liver degradation • Also can gauge general stability and non-NADPH-mediated degradation
Metabolic stability	S9 fraction human liver enzymes	• Unlike microsomes, contain both Phase I and II (i.e., glucuronidation, sulfation) enzymes thus can be used to deduce the importance of Phase II metabolism
CYP450 inhibition	Microsome stability (when CYP450 activity predominates)	• Estimate inhibition potential for major CYPs (i.e., CYP1A, CYP2C9, CYP2C19, CYP2D6, CYP3A4) • Gauge possible drug interactions
CYP450 isozyme inhibition	Recombinant system, bactosomes	• Identify which CYP important to associate with possible problems with polymorphisms
CYP450 induction	Human hepatocytes	• Gauge potential to cause CYP450 induction • Identify isozyme induced to associate with polymorphism
Metabolite identification	Human liver microsomes and/or hepatocytes + LC-MS identification	• Identify major metabolites

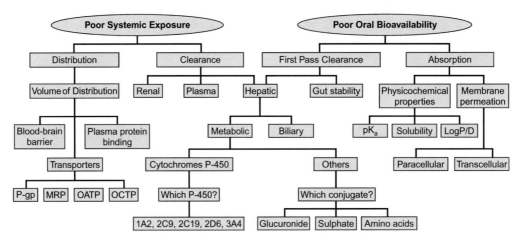

FIGURE 9.40 Troubleshooting poor pharmacokinetics. If a compound has poor system exposure, this may be due to either restricted distribution (tissue sequestration, high protein binding), where the compound cannot access the therapeutic target, or high clearance, whereby the compound cannot reside long enough in the central compartment to elicit therapeutic effect. If a compound has poor bioavailability, then it may not be absorbed or it may be highly metabolized by first pass metabolism. From [21].

FIGURE 9.41 Drugs as subsets of clinical profiles. While burimamide, cimetidine, and metiamide are all active histamine H2 antagonists with ulcer healing activity, burimamide lacks a suitable toxicity and pharmacokinetic profile, while cimetidine is adequately absorbed but still toxic. Only metiamide fulfills the requirements of a clinically useful drug.

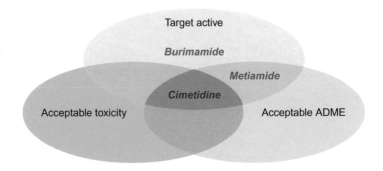

The third in the series fulfilled the requirements of target activity, acceptable absorption and toxicity profile and thus became a prototype blockbuster drug in the new series (Figure 9.41).

9.9 SUMMARY AND CONCLUSIONS

- Pharmacokinetics is concerned with the accurate determination of the magnitude of the independent variable in pharmacology and therapeutics; namely, the concentration of drug in the body at the biological target of interest.
- "Druglike" character for a molecule entails a molecular weight of 350−400, if possible, and sufficient water solubility to be dispersed in aqueous media with concomitant lipophilic property to dissolve into and diffuse through lipid bilayer membranes.
- *In vitro* assays can be used to measure the ability of a molecule to diffuse through lipid membranes (PAMPA) and biological layers of cells (i.e., Caco-2, MDCK).

- Assistance in absorption and or selectivity can be achieved by judicious choice of drug route of entry.
- The two main independent parameters in pharmacokinetics are drug clearance and volume of distribution; from these, the third important parameter of half life can be determined.
- Clearance is mainly hepatic or renal; hepatic clearance is quantified by treating the liver as a virtual enzyme. Renal clearance is determined by glomerular filtration, active secretion, and reabsorption.
- The volume of distribution of a drug can be used to determine where it is sequestered in the body.
- Drug half life can be used to determine dosing schedule and the time to attain a steady state equilibrium concentration.
- Bioavailability involves the interplay of absorption and the first pass effect, whereby an orally absorbed drug must first pass through the liver before it enters the central compartment.
- Nonlinear pharmacokinetics occur when elimination processes are saturated or the normally linear relationship between dosing and plasma concentration is exceeded either in capacity or sensitivity.

- Clearance, volume of distribution, and $t_{1/2}$ can be determined from a single i.v. dose experiment; addition of an oral dosing yields F.
- Multiple dosing experiments can quickly detect nonlinear pharmacokinetics and enzyme induction.

REFERENCES

[1] Aguiar AJ, Krc Jr. J, Kinkel AW, Samyn AC. Effect of polymorphism on the absorption of chloramphenicol from chloramphenicol palmitate. J Pharm Sci 1967;56(7):847−53.

[2] Schanker LS, Tocco DT, Brodie BB, Hogben CAM. Absorption of drugs from the rat small intestine. J Pharmacol Exp Ther 1958;123:81−8.

[3] Lemke TL. Review of organic functional groups: Introduction to medicinal organic chemistry. 3rd ed. Philadelphia: Lea and Febiger; 1992.

[4] Cates IA. Calculation of drug solubilities by pharmacy students. Amer J Pharm Ed 1981;45:11−3.

[5] Navia MA, Chaturvedi PR. Design principles for orally bioavailable drugs. Drug Disc Today 1996;1:179−99.

[6] Williams DA, Lemke TL. Foye's principle of medicinal chemistry, 5. New York: Lippincott, Williams, Wilkins; 2002.

[7] Lipinski CA. Drug-like properties and the causes of poor solubility and poor permeability. J Pharm Tox Meth 2000;44:235−49.

[8] Sugano K, Kansy M, Artursson P, Avdeef A, Bendels S, Di L, et al. Coexistence of passive and carrier-mediated processes in drug transport. Nature Rev Drug Disc 2010;9:597−614.

[9] Abels S, Beaumont KC, Crespi CL, Eva MD, Fox L, Hyland R, et al. Potential role for P-glycoprotein in the nonproportional pharmacokinetics of UK-343,664 in man. Xenobiotica 2001;31:665−86.

[10] Kerns EH, Di L, Petusky S, Farris M, Ley R, Jupp P. Combined application of parallel artificial membrane permeability assay and Caco-2 permeability assays in drug discovery. J Pharm Sci 2004;93:1440−53.

[11] Balimane PV, Chong S. Cell culture-based models of intestinal permeability: A critique. Drug Disc Today 2005;10:335−43.

[12] Lee K, Park P-K, Kwon B-M, Kim K, Yu HE, Ryu J, et al. Transport and metabolism of the anti-tumour drug candidate 2'-benzoyloxycinnamaldehyde in Caco-2 cells. Xenobiotica 2009;39:881−8.

[13] Lee HJ, Soliman MR. Anti-inflammatory steroids without pituitary-adrenal suppression. Science 1982;215:989−91.

[14] Bertilsson L, Lou YQ, Du YL, et al. Pronounced differences between native Chinese and Swedish populations in the polymorphic hydroxylations of bebrisoquin and S-mephenytoin. Clin Pharmacol Ther 1992;51:388−97.

[15] Gomez-Lechon M, Castell JV, Donato MT. Hepatocytes − the choice to investigate drug metabolism and toxicity in man: *In vitro* variability as a reflection of *in vivo*. *Chemico Biol.* Interactions 2007;168:30−50.

[16] Soars MG, McGinnity DF, Grime K, Riley RJ. The pivotal role of hepatocytes in drug discovery. *Chemico-Biol.* Interactions 2007;168:2−15.

[17] Galloway JA, McMahon RE, Culp HW, Marshall F, Young EC. Metabolism, blood levels and rate of excretion of acetohexamide in human subjects. Diabetes 1965;16:118−27.

[18] Izumi T, Enomoto S, Hosiyama K, Sasahara K, Shibukawa A, Nakagawa T, et al. Prediction of the human pharmacokinetics of troglitazone, a new and extensively metabolized antidiabetic agent, after oral administration, with an animal scale-up approach. J Pharmacol Exp Ther 1996;277:1630−41.

[19] Siefert HM, Domdey-Bette A, Henninger K, Hucke F, Kohlsdorfer C, Stass HH. Pharmacokinetics of 8-methoxyquinoloe, moxifloxacin: a comparison in humans and other mammalian species. J Antimicrob Chemother 1999;43(Suppl. B):69−76.

[20] Lipinski CA, Lombardo F, Dominy BW, Feeney PJ. Experimental and computational approaches to estimate solubility and permeability in drug discovery and development settings. Adv Drug Deliv Rev 1997;23:3−25.

[21] van de Waterbeemd H, Gifford E. ADMET *in silico* modeling: Towards prediction paradise?. Nature Rev Drug Disc 2003;2:192−204.

Chapter 10

Safety Pharmacology

Belladonna — in Italian a beautiful lady; in English a deadly poison. A striking example of the essential identity of the two tongues.

Ambrose Bierce (1842−1913)

Poison is in everything, and no thing is without poison. The dosage makes it either a poison or a remedy.

Paracelsus (1493−1541)

I would in particular draw the attention to physiologists to this type of physiological analysis of organic systems which can be done with the aid of toxic agents...

Claude Bernard (1813−1878)

The worst thing about medicine is that one kind makes another necessary.

Elbert Hubbard (1856−1915)

10.1 Safety Pharmacology
10.2 Hepatotoxicity
10.3 Cytotoxicity
10.4 Mutagenicity
10.5 hERG Activity and *Torsades De Pointes*
10.6 Autonomic Receptor Profiling
10.7 General Pharmacology
10.8 Clinical Testing
10.9 Summary and Conclusions
References

10.1 SAFETY PHARMACOLOGY

There are numerous reasons why a molecule with good primary activity may still fail as a drug, and it is becoming increasingly clear that the factors that lead to this failure need to be addressed as early as possible in lead optimization. Figure 10.1 shows the outcome of a risk analysis for the probability of a new compound emerging as a drug; it can be seen that attrition is extremely high. An active molecule must be absorbed into the body, reach the biological target, be present for a time period sufficient for therapeutic activity, and not produce untoward side effects. It will be seen that an important part of the lead optimization process is to incorporate these properties into the primary lead molecule early on in the process [1]. One reason why this is important is that the concepts involved are, in some cases, diametrically opposed. For example, while low molecular weight is a known positive property of drugs, the lead optimization process generally results in increased molecular weight as pharmacophores are added to increase potency. For this reason, the concept of "lead likeness" [2] can be used to determine the suitability of lead molecules for beginning the lead optimization process (*vide infra*). The problems involved in introducing lead likeness into screening hits is exacerbated by the fact that, as analogs become more potent, there is less tolerance for chemical analoging to improve physicochemical properties. In fact, it is a general observation that there often are relatively minor differences between leads and launched drug candidates (see Figure 10.2) [9]. On the other hand, there is abundant evidence to show that apparently very minor changes in chemical structure can impose large effects on biological activity (see Figure 10.3).

New drugs must be efficacious, reach the site of action, and do no harm; this latter condition is the subject of drug

T. P. Kenakin: A Pharmacology Primer, Fourth edition. DOI: http://dx.doi.org/10.1016/B978-0-12-407663-1.00010-7
© 2014 Elsevier Inc. All rights reserved.

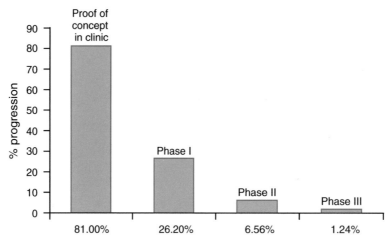

FIGURE 10.1 Attrition of molecules as they are taken through the clinical testing procedure. It can be seen that very few become drugs (1.34%). Redrawn from [1].

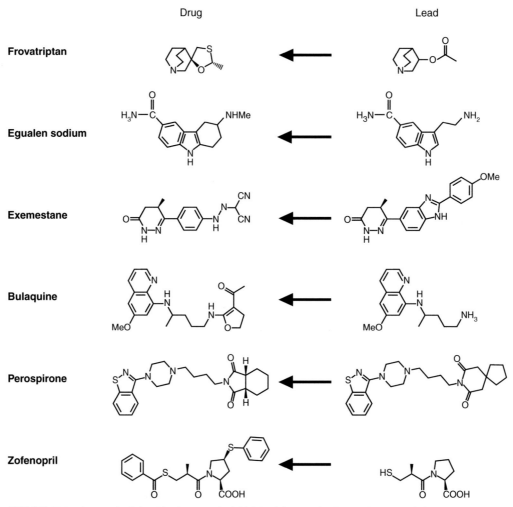

FIGURE 10.2 Structural relationships between the initial lead for a molecule and the eventual drug. It can be seen that changes in structure are, in some cases, not extensive. Data shown for frovatriptan [3], egualen sodium [4], exemestane [5], bulaquine [6], perospirone [7], and zofenopril [8]. Drawn from [9].

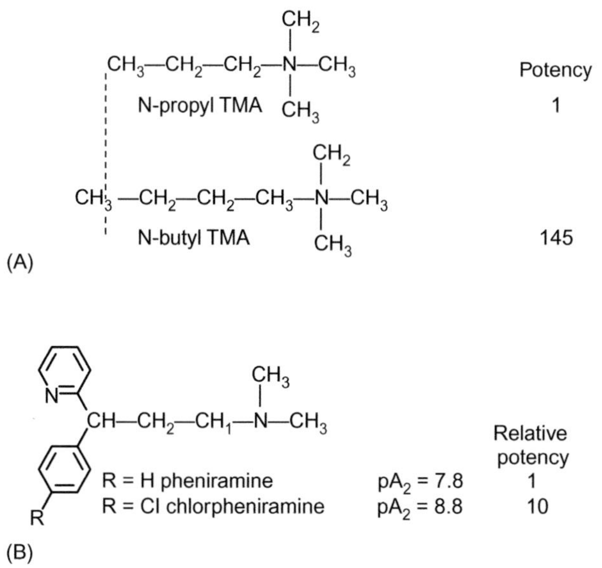

(A)

(B)

FIGURE 10.3 Small changes in the chemical structure of N-propyl tetramethylammonium and pheniramine produce 145- and 10-fold increases in potency respectively.

liability studies. In the decade 1991−2000, new drug registration was a mere 11% of compounds submitted for first human studies, with toxicity and safety issues accounting for approximately 30% of the failures. There are clear "zero tolerance" toxicities and those that are tolerable with tolerance depending on the indication, patient population (i.e., age and gender), length of treatment, and seriousness of illness. Table 10.1 shows a number of common side effects of drugs when tested in clinical trials. Toxicity is assessed in a number of ways; a commonly used index is the therapeutic index, which is the ratio of the concentration of drug required to produce 50% maximal therapeutic effect (or therapeutically active in 50% of the population) and the concentration producing 50% toxic effect (toxic in 50% of the population); see Figure 10.4A. Another, and more stringent, scale is the "margin of safety," which is the ratio of drug that is 99% effective over the concentration that produces 1% incidence of toxic effect (Figure 10.4A). The margin of safety of some commonly used drugs can be strikingly low; for example, Figure 10.4B shows the incidence of side effects with theophylline; with a less than twofold margin between effect and incidence of mild side effects to a 3.5-fold margin between effect and serious side effects [10]. Side effects commonly arise from exaggerated effects at the primary target (mechanism-based toxicity), or problems with dosing, prolonged use, or cytotoxicity (i.e., hepatoxicity and bone marrow toxicity). Table 10.2 shows some classifications of toxicity. Type A toxicity is usually dose dependent and has a 75% rate of detection in safety pharmacology testing. In contrast, Type B toxicity may not be detected until postmarketing surveillance and is not predictable. In fact, in the worst case scenario, some drugs have been seen to have such rare but serious toxicity in this phase that they had to be withdrawn from the market (i.e., practolol for

oculomucocutaneous reactions; troglitazone for liver damage, Vioxx for cardiovascular toxicity, and terfenadine for *Torsades de Pointes*). Type C toxicity involves long term adaptive changes and may be detected only with chronic dosing. Type D are delayed effects such as carcinogenicity or teratogenicity and, finally, Type E toxicity which may only be encountered upon cessation of therapy.

It should be noted that the structure-activity relationships controlling safety issues need not be in any way related to the structure-activity relationship for primary activity (or the pharmacokinetic properties − see Figure 10.5 and also Figure 9.41 for an example). This independence of effect is illustrated in Figure 10.6, where it can be seen that the liability issue of cytochrome P450 inhibition for a series of IGF-receptor antagonists can be decreased by a factor of nearly 1000, while leaving the primary IGF-receptor activity nearly unchanged [11].

Twenty-five years ago there was more of a presumption that potential drugs should not be put forward for approval if they possessed any untoward activity whatsoever; experience has tempered this unrealistic view with the realization that all foreign molecules, when introduced into the human body in sufficient quantity, will eventually produce an unwanted side effect (note the quotation by Paracelsus at the beginning of this chapter). Thus a more constructive approach to drug development strives to define the constraints within which a new molecule may be used for therapeutic benefit; i.e., define the hazards associated with the molecule and then assess the risk that those hazards will be realized with therapy. This process views some general questions [12]:

1. **What is the safety margin?** An acceptable safety margin depends upon the nature of the dose-limiting adverse event, the therapeutic indication, the intended patient population, the competitive environment, and the present standard of care.
2. **Is the toxicity reversible?** Irreversible toxicity is usually unacceptable.
3. **Is there a biomarker?** Toxicity that cannot be monitored could develop into irreversible toxicity.
4. **What is the mechanism?** Some mechanisms of toxicity are species dependent and thus not relevant to humans.

Attempts to answer these questions for a drug candidate involve testing in model systems designed to detect pharmacological hazard. These tests can be classified in terms of where they occur in the drug development process and their specific format:

1. *In vitro* testing in hepatic cellular assays to detect effects on enzymes designed to protect the body from foreign chemicals and also to determine possibly harmful interactions between these molecules and other drug therapies taken concomitantly (drug-drug interactions). These assays also can determine possible long-term effects on the

TABLE 10.1 Major Adverse Side Effects Associated with Clinical Use of Drugs

Cardiovascular	Hematology	Renal
arrhythmias	agranulocytosis	nephritis
hypotension	hemolytic anemia	nephrosis
hypertension	pancytopenia	tubular necrosis
congestive heart failure	thrombocytopenia	renal dysfunction
angina, chest pain	megaloblastic anemia	bladder dysfunction
pericarditis	clotting, bleeding	nephrolithiasis
cardiomyopathy	eosinophilia	
Dermatology	**Musculoskeletal**	**Respiratory**
erythemas	myalgia, myopathy	airway obstruction
hyperpigmentation	rhabdomyolysis	pulmonary infiltrates
photodermatitis	osteoporosis	pulmonary edema
eczema	respiratory depression	
urticaria	nasal congestion	
acne		
alopecia		
Endocrine	**Metabolic**	**Ophthalmic**
thyroid dysfunction	hyperglycemia	disturbed color vision
sexual dysfunction	hypoglycemia	cataract
gynecomastia	hyperkalemia	optic neuritis
Addison syndrome	hypokalemia	retinopathy
galactorrhea	metabolic acidosis	glaucoma
hyperuricemia	corneal opacity	
hyponatremia		
Gastrointestinal	**Neurological**	**Otological**
hepatitis, hepatocellular damage	seizures	deafness
constipation	tremor	vestibular disorders
diarrhea	sleep disorders	
nausea, vomiting	peripheral neuropathy	
ulceration	headache	
pancreatitis	extrapyramidal effects	
dry mouth		
Psychiatric		
delirium, confusion		
depression		
hallucination		
drowsiness		
schizophrenia, paranoia		
sleep disturbances		

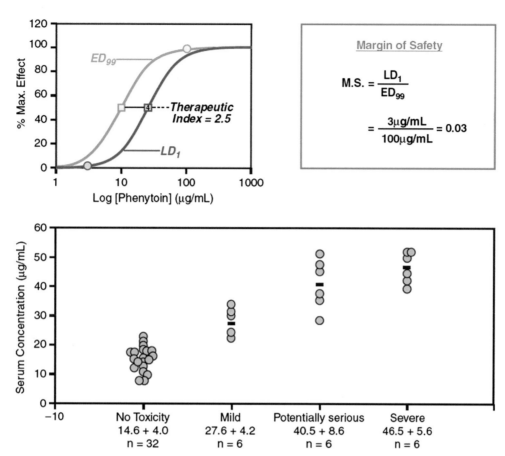

FIGURE 10.4 **Expressions of relative safety of drugs.** (A) Dose-response curves for phenytoin therapeutic activity (green) and toxicity (red). Shown also are the ED_{50} values used to calculate therapeutic index and ED_{99} values used to calculate margin of safety. (B) Toxic effects of theophylline illustrating the narrow margin between the no toxic effect dose (14.6 µg/mL), mild toxic effects (1.9-fold>), potentially serious side effects (2.8-fold>), and severe side effects (3.2-fold>). Data redrawn from [10].

TABLE 10.2 **Classifications of Toxic Effects**

Type of Toxicity	Example
Undesired expected effects	Digital tremor with β-agonist bronchodilators due to β_2-adrenoceptor stimulation
Desired excessive effects	Insulin-induced hypoglycemic reaction
Undesired, unexpected	Hypertensive crisis for treatment of depression with monoamine oxidase (MAO) inhibitor: consumption of cheddar cheese and beer (tyramine)
Poorly predictable	Drug allergies, idiosyncratic, mutagenesis, carcinogenesis, drug dependency

hepatic system (i.e., mechanism-based enzyme inhibition, hepatic enzyme induction).

2. Simple *in vitro* cellular or biochemical assays designed to detect cytotoxic activity employed in the early stages of the development process to detect possible liability in chemical scaffolds to enable elimination of these properties through synthesis or pursuit of another chemical scaffold.

3. *In vivo* studies on complete systems to determine possible harmful effects on bodily functions.

Before discussion of these various strategies, it is worth considering the function of a pharmacological safety test. In general, these assays need to be sensitive, specific, and predictive. One scheme through which these properties can be assessed is by a comparison of the outcome of pharmacological safety test with that of a subsequent clinical test. Thus, a defined side effect could be detected in the safety test and confirmed in the clinical test; this would be a "true positive" outcome; or it could be predicted in the safety test and not confirmed in the clinical test ("false positive"). Similarly, the event could not be confirmed in the safety test but found in the clinical test ("false negative") or found in the safety test and confirmed to be absent in the clinical test ("true negative") [13]. Within this scenario, the sensitivity of the test can be calculated from the formula:

$$\text{Sensitivity} = (\text{True Positives})/((\text{True Positives}) + (\text{False Negatives})) \quad (10.1)$$

Under these circumstances, the sensitivity reflects the incidence of effects correctly identified by the model, i.e., a measure of the true positive outcomes as a ratio of true positives and true positives plus false negatives (a high sensitivity reflects a low rate of false negatives). Similarly, the specificity is defined as:

$$\text{Specificity} = (\text{True Negative})/((\text{True Negative}) + (\text{False Positive})) \quad (10.2)$$

This is a measure of the drug activity in humans without any negative effect that is correctly identified by the safety pharmacology assay (a measure of the true negatives). Finally, the predictive power of the assay is given as:

$$\text{Prediction} = ((\text{True Positives}) + (\text{True Negatives}))/ \text{Total} \quad (10.3)$$

Where Total = TN + TP + FN + FP. This is the ratio of true positives and true negatives divided by the total number of drugs evaluated. A high predictive value represents the confidence in the safety pharmacology assay to predict a negative side effect. These various calculations are shown in Figure 10.7 along with an example calculated for a number of compounds in three predictive tests of cardiac arrhythmia (hERG assay, *in vivo* QTc interval, Langendorf heart – *vide infra*). In general, a predictive capacity of 65−74% is considered adequate, 75−84% good, and >85% excellent [14].

Clearly it is advantageous to detect possible safety issues with candidate molecules as early in the selection process as possible so as to not waste time and resource on the development of drugs that will fail in the clinic. In fact, a drug project has expended 90% of its cost by the time the molecule reaches Phase 3 clinical testing. As with pharmacokinetic *in vitro* testing (*vide infra*), there are a number of simple *in vitro* tests that can be done to detect future safety issues. Even before the initiation of such activity, *in silico* methods can be used to optimize the prevention of progressing toxic compounds. For example, a rapid potential method of detecting safety issues is pharmacophore modeling of "antitargets" [15]; these can be used to "virtually screen" for potential problematic drug activity. Figure 10.8 shows some known "toxicophores" associated with mutagenicity (and hence, a risk for the production of cancer). Such data can assist medicinal chemists as they produce analogs for candidate

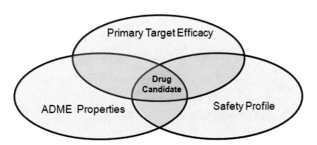

FIGURE 10.5 Venn diagram showing the three essential but independent structure-activity realtionships required for a successful drug candidate. Thus, all drugs must have primary therapeutic activity, be able to enter the body, distribute to the required therapeutic organ(s) and remain there for a period sufficient to produce useful activity (all referred to as ADME properties) and finally cause no harm (have an acceptable safety profile). An example of three drugs defining this process is shown in Figure 9.41.

FIGURE 10.6 pK$_i$ values (negative logarithms of equilibrium dissociation constants) for 3-(1 H-benzoyl[d]imidazole-2-yl)pyridine-2-(1 H)-one inhibitors of insulin-like growth factor receptor-1 (IGF-1 R) as a function of varying R groups. It can be seen that the primary activity of these molecules (pKi for ICG-1 R) varies little while the liability activity of CYP1A2 and CYP2A4 inhibition (*vide infra*) changes by a factor of 200−300. Data redrawn from [11].

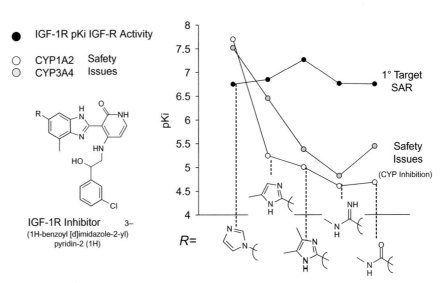

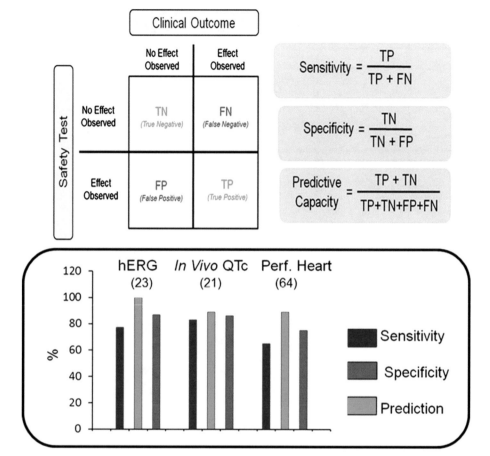

FIGURE 10.7 **Prediction of cardiac arrhythmias with safety pharmacological testing.** Top panel shows the various possibilities for observing untoward side effects clinically (abscissal axis) and in safety testing (ordinates). Bottom panel shows data for compounds tested in various assays to predict cardiac arrhythmia. Estimates of sensitivity (blue bar), specificity (red bar) and predictive power (green bar) shown for hERG channel assays, *in vivo* QTc interval studies, and Langendorf perfused heart assays. Data redrawn from [13].

selection. As seen in Figure 10.8B, while such modeling can potentially predict mutagenicity [16], these predictions are not absolute (i.e., compounds A and C are mutagenic but compound B, although predicted to also be mutagenic, is not). Physicochemical properties can be predictive of toxic effects; i.e., hydrophobic drugs have been shown to have affinity for calcium channels and, notably, potassium channels. This latter activity is a clear liability, since blockade of the hERG potassium channel can lead to cardiac QTc prolongation and a condition called *Torsades de Pointes*, a potentially fatal cardiac arrhythmia (*vide infra*). In terms of rapid *in vitro* tests done in early development programs, early testing involves hepatic cells and essentially is an extension of the metabolism studies done to determine hepatic stability, as discussed in Chapter 9.

10.2 HEPATOTOXICITY

The first line of defense for the human body against foreign chemicals (certainly for orally ingested substances but, in general, chemicals absorbed through any route) is the liver. Foreign substances can be metabolized in many other organs as well (i.e., gastrointestinal tract, brain, lungs, etc) but the enzymes involved are very often the same as those found in the hepatic system, namely the cytochrome P450 enzymes and those involved in Phase 2 analog formation (see Chapter 9). Foreign chemicals also attain their highest concentrations at the liver, thus it is not surprising that it is a prime candidate for the detection of toxic effects (i.e., one of the top five causes of death in the United States, resulting in over 100,000 deaths a year, is attributed to hepatic drug-drug interactions). The first possible untoward outcomes to be considered are drug-drug interactions from interference with hepatic enzyme function.

10.2.1 Drug-Drug Interactions

Especially in an aging population, it is unlikely that a given patient will be on a regimen of single drug therapy (i.e., the drug candidate) but, rather, the new drug candidate will be taken by patients who already are titrated on regimens of other drug therapies. This should be considered a steady-state condition, i.e., dosages may be individually optimized and steady-state drug levels are the result of a given dosage being absorbed and cleared at specific rates in the patient. If some part of this steady

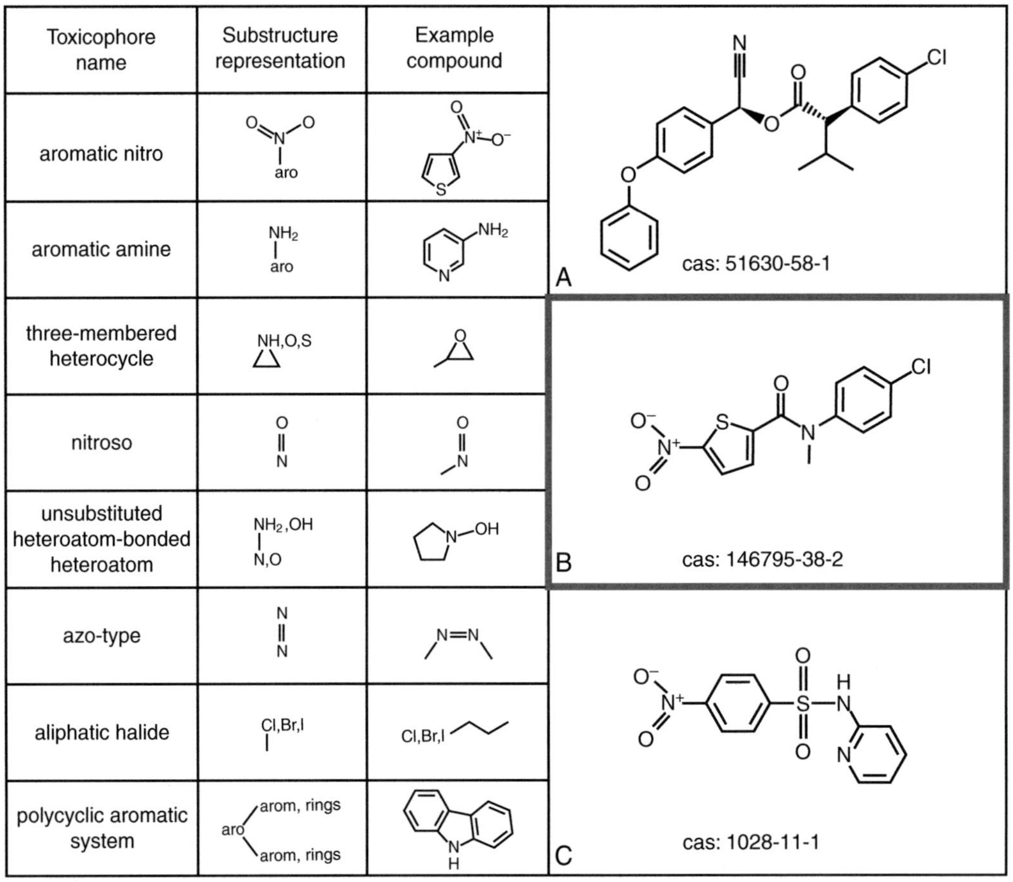

Toxicophore name	Substructure representation	Example compound
aromatic nitro	O₌N₊–O (aro)	
aromatic amine	NH₂ (aro)	
three-membered heterocycle	NH,O,S (triangle)	
nitroso	O₌N	
unsubstituted heteroatom-bonded heteroatom	NH₂,OH / N,O	
azo-type	N₌N	
aliphatic halide	Cl,Br,I	Cl,Br,I
polycyclic aromatic system	aro(arom, rings / arom, rings)	

A cas: 51630-58-1

B cas: 146795-38-2

C cas: 1028-11-1

FIGURE 10.8 **Chemical functional groups that have been associated with toxicity in drugs.** These pharmacophores can be used to predict potential mutagenic activity that can, in turn, lead to cancer. These data predict mutagenicity for compounds A, B, and C; mutagenic activity was verified only for compounds A and C, not B, illustrating how there can be exceptions to these predictions. Data drawn from [16].

state involves hepatic enzyme metabolism, then addition of another chemical that utilizes the same hepatic enzyme system has the potential to disrupt the initial steady state. When this occurs, it is called a drug-drug interaction. Drug-drug interactions can occur at any interface involving a saturable process; Table 10.3 shows a list of drug-drug interactions occurring at the level of saturation of transport processes. Cytochrome P450 enzymes are particularly susceptible to drug activity due to their broad substrate specificity. Four of these enzymes, CYP3A4, CYP2C9, CYP2C19, and CYP2D6 account for 80% of known oxidative drug metabolism [18] and blockade of these enzymes can lead to detrimental interactions with other drugs. For example, the antihistamine terfenadine has a high affinity for the hERG channel (leading to serious liability). This drug is rapidly metabolized and the metabolite fexofenadine is weakly active at the hERG channel. However, in the presence of other drugs that interfere with terfenadine metabolism (cytochrome enzymes), this antihistamine poses a serious risk of life-threatening arrhythmia. In fact, drug-drug interactions due

to interactions at the cytochrome P450 level have led to a number of drug withdrawals due to emergence of *Torsades de Pointes* (as with terfenadine) with the antihypertensive mibradil, the anti-allergic drug astemizole, the gastrointestinal (GI) heartburn treatment cisapride, and the antidepressant nefazodone [18]. Well known substances such as caffeine, which is almost exclusively metabolized by CYP1A2, cause drug-drug interactions with a number of commonly used therapies including the antidepressants Prozac, Paxil and Luvox, and other drugs such as aspirin, acetaminophen and the anti-schizophrenic clozapine; the alteration of the levels of these medications occurs because of co-usage of CYP1A2 in metabolism. When two molecules utilize the same hepatic enzyme then, in effect, one becomes a competitive antagonist of the enzyme for the metabolism of the other. It is worth considering the various mechanisms of enzyme antagonism, as these relate to drug-drug interactions at the hepatic enzyme level; this has relevance to the relative concentrations of drugs as they may or may not produce interactions at the enzyme level.

TABLE 10.3 Drug-Drug Interactions Caused by Interference with Saturable Transport Systems

Victim(s)	Perpetrator(s)	Mechanism	Outcome
Talindolol	Verapamil	Saturation of P-gp Efflux	Variable plasma concentrations, decreased intestinal secretion
Fexofenadine	Ketoconazole Erythromycin	Saturation of P-gp, OATP ETransport	Variable plasma concentrations, decreased intestinal secretion
Digoxin	Quinidine, Verapamil, Itraconazole	Saturation of P-gp, OATP Transport	Increased plasma concentrations / decreased renal clearance
Loperamide	Quinidine	Saturation of P-gp Efflux	Increased CNS effects
Dofetilide, Procainamide, Levofloxacin	Cimetidine	Saturation of P-gp, OCT, OAT, OATP	Increased AUC, decreased renal clearance
Penicillins, ACE inhibitors, Antiviral drugs	Probenecid	Saturation of OAT Transport	Decreased renal clearance, increased $t_{1/2}$

Data from [17].

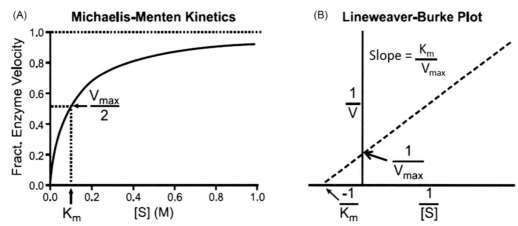

FIGURE 10.9 Enzyme reactions according to the Michaelis–Menten equation (Equation 10.4). (A) Graphical representation of the rate of the enzyme reaction as a function of the substrate concentration. (B) Linear transformation of the equation to a format referred to as the Lineweaver-Burke plot.

A useful representation of an enzyme reaction is to express the rate of production of an enzymatic product as a function of the substrate concentration; the standard equation to describe enzyme velocity as a function of substrate concentration is the Michaelis–Menten equation:

$$V = \frac{[S]V_{max}}{[S] + K_m} \qquad (10.4)$$

where V_{max} is the maximum velocity of the metabolic enzyme reaction and K_m is the Michaelis–Menten constant for the reaction denoting the sensitivity of the enzyme to the substrate (i.e., when the substrate concentration is equal to K_m then the enzyme reaction proceeds at 50% maximum). The K_m also defines at which concentrations the enzyme is saturated, since at $[S] \gg K_m$, $V \rightarrow V_{max}$, and the enzyme reaction rate is no longer sensitive to increases in substrate concentration.

Figure 10.9A shows an enzyme velocity curve according to Equation 10.4 which illustrates the increase in enzyme velocity with increasing substrate concentration until the enzyme is saturated (and the velocity attains an asymptotic value at V_{max}). A convenient manipulation of this relationship, (developed before computer programs for fitting non-linear curves were widely available) is the Lineweaver–Burke transform of Equation 10.4. This utilizes a metameter of Equation 10.4 to yield a linear relationship:

$$1/V = (1/[S])\ (K_m/V_{max}) - 1/V_{max} \qquad (10.5)$$

Thus, as shown in Figure 10.9B, a double reciprocal plot of $1/V$ as a function of $1/[S]$ yields a straight line with a slope of (K_m/V_{max}) and an x intercept of $(-K_m)^{-1}$.

There are a number of ways in which a molecule can antagonize enzyme function, but there is a simple

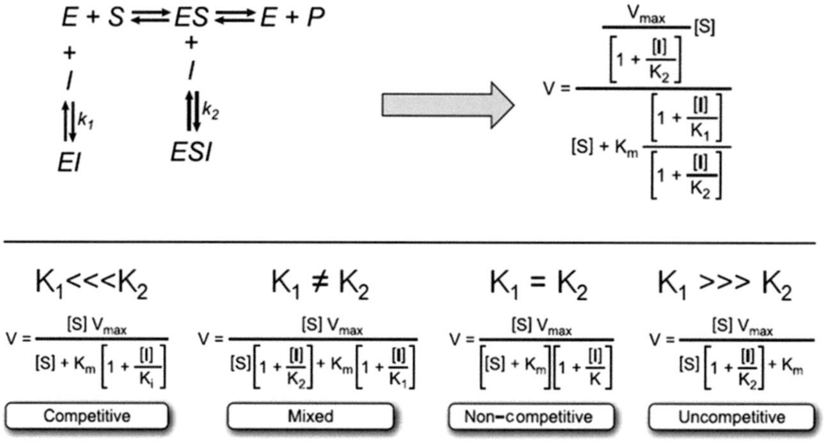

FIGURE 10.10 **Mechanisms of enzyme inhibition.** The substrate S is converted to a product P through interaction with the enzyme E. The enzyme-substrate complex is denoted ES. The enzyme inhibitor I can interact with E with equilibrium dissociation constant k_1 or ES with constant k_2. To the right of the arrow is a general equation relating enzyme velocity to substrate and inhibitor concentration. Lower panel shows various kinetic extremes leading to characteristic patterns of enzyme inhibition as discussed in the text.

$$E + S \rightleftharpoons ES \rightleftharpoons E + P$$

$$V = \frac{\frac{V_{max}}{\left[1 + \frac{[I]}{K_2}\right]}[S]}{[S] + K_m \frac{\left[1 + \frac{[I]}{K_1}\right]}{\left[1 + \frac{[I]}{K_2}\right]}}$$

$K_1 <<< K_2$

$$V = \frac{[S]\,V_{max}}{[S] + K_m\left[1 + \frac{[I]}{K_i}\right]}$$

Competitive

$K_1 \neq K_2$

$$V = \frac{[S]\,V_{max}}{[S]\left[1 + \frac{[I]}{K_2}\right] + K_m\left[1 + \frac{[I]}{K_1}\right]}$$

Mixed

$K_1 = K_2$

$$V = \frac{[S]\,V_{max}}{\left[[S] + K_m\right]\left[1 + \frac{[I]}{K}\right]}$$

Non-competitive

$K_1 >>> K_2$

$$V = \frac{[S]\,V_{max}}{[S]\left[1 + \frac{[I]}{K_2}\right] + K_m}$$

Uncompetitive

molecular scheme that organizes these effects; a molecule can block enzyme function either through interaction with the enzyme itself (with no substrate present), or the enzyme-substrate complex, or both. The relative affinity of the molecule for the bare enzyme vs. the enzyme-substrate complex determines the pattern of inhibition and also the relationship between the concentration of inhibitor and the sensitivity of the enzyme reaction for that inhibition. As shown in Figure 10.10, there are basically four schemes for enzyme inhibition. A general form for the inhibition of an enzyme by these mechanisms is [19]:

$$V = \frac{\left[\frac{[S]V_{max}}{1+[I]/K_2}\right]}{[S] + K_m\left[\frac{1+[I]/K_1}{1+[I]/K_2}\right]} \qquad (10.6)$$

where [I] is the concentration of enzyme inhibitor, [S] the concentration of substrate, and K_1 and K_2 are the equilibrium constants referring to the equilibrium dissociation constant of the inhibitor and the bare enzyme and enzyme-substrate complex respectively. Using Equation 10.6, various classifications of enzyme inhibition can be isolated through manipulation of the relative magnitudes of K_1 and K_2.

If the molecule binds to the enzyme but not the enzyme-substrate complex ($K_1 <<< K_2$; as would be seen if the inhibitor binds to the substrate binding site), then a pattern of competitive inhibition is observed. The effects on the enzyme function curve and Lineweaver–Burke plot are shown in Figure 10.11. In competitive inhibition, very high concentrations of substrate can overcome the competitive inhition, therefore the V_{max} is not affected (much like simple competitive antagonism for receptors; see Figure 6.6). In fact, this idea is utilized in hospital emergency rooms where potentially fatal methanol poisoning (the substrate methanol is converted to the fatal molecule formaldehyde by alcohol dehydrogenase) is treated with administration of ethanol to compete for the methanol substrate, so producing a non-toxic product instead. The

constancy of V_{max} is shown by the common y-axis intercept of the Lineweaver–Burke plot (no change in the intercept which is V_{max}^{-1}). Such competitive effects could lead to drug-drug interactions for drugs sharing the same cytochrome P450 enzymes for metabolism; i.e., an unduly high concentration of one of the drugs could lead to a decrease in the hepatic clearance of the other drug. For instance, the antifungal itraconazole and antidiabetic metformin share CYP 3A1/2 as their main metabolizing enzymes. Therefore, when orally co-administered to rats, each affects the total area under the curve (AUC) for oral dosing (reflecting central compartment concentration and clearance) of the other; a dose of itraconazole yielding a normal AUC of 1370 µg min^{-1}mL^{-1} increases to 2320 µg min^{-1}mL^{-1} when metformin is co-administered. Similarly, the same dose of metformin, which normally yields an AUC of 2930 µg min^{-1}mL^{-1} increases to 5340 µg min^{-1}mL^{-1} when co-administered with itraconazole [20]. Not considering drug-drug interactions with CYP3A4 can be dissimulating, as in the historical cases where double-blind placebo drug trials were conducted using grapefruit juice to mask the taste of new investigational compounds. In these cases it was subsequently found that grapefruit juice contains psoralens, which are potent inhibitors of CYP3A4, and that this had produced artificially elevated drug levels.

Another mechanism of enzyme inhibition involves binding of the inhibitor to both the bare enzyme and enzyme-substrate complex. If the affinity of the inhibitor for both protein species is the same ($K_1 = K_2$), then the inhibition is labeled noncompetitive; the patterns on the enzyme curve and Lineweaver–Burke plot are shown in Figure 10.12. It can be seen that while V_{max} is diminished, the location parameters of the substrate-activation curves do not change; this is similar to noncompetitive antagonism of receptors as shown in Figure 6.16A. Figure 10.12B shows the distinctive pattern of the

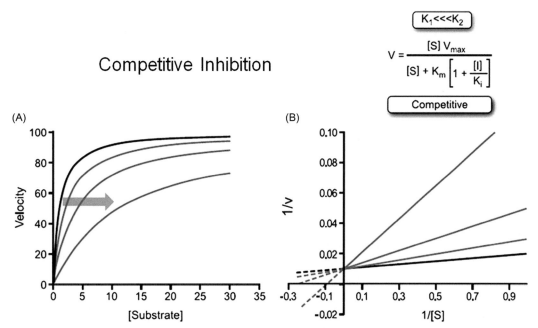

$$K_1 <<< K_2$$

$$V = \frac{[S] \, V_{max}}{[S] + K_m \left[1 + \frac{[I]}{K_i} \right]}$$

Competitive

FIGURE 10.11 **Competitive enzyme inhibition.** Competitive inhibition is characterized by a constant V_{max} and an increase in K_m. The Lineweaver–Burke plots increase in slope with inhibition but the y-axis intercept remains constant. The inhibitor has a very low affinity for ES since the substrate occupies the binding site.

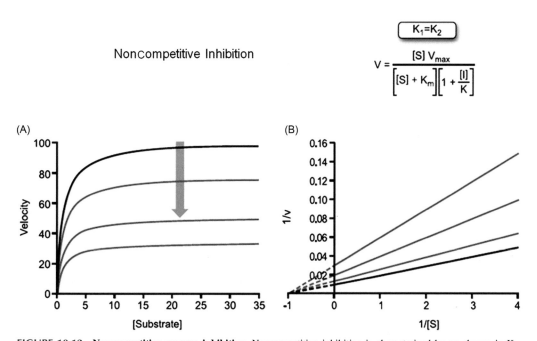

$$K_1 = K_2$$

$$V = \frac{[S] \, V_{max}}{\left[[S] + K_m \right] \left[1 + \frac{[I]}{K} \right]}$$

FIGURE 10.12 **Noncompetitive enzyme inhibition.** Noncompetitive inhibition is characterized by no change in K_m and a decreasing V_{max}. In this case the enzyme inhibitor has equal affinity for E and ES.

Lineweaver–Burke plots, namely a common x-axis intercept and varying intercepts of the y-axis. If the inhibitor interacts with both the enzyme and enzyme-substrate complex to varying degrees ($K_1 \neq K_2$), then a mixed type of inhibition involving a mixture of depression of V_{max} and dextral displacement of the curves (increasing K_m) is observed (see Figure 10.13). This pattern is similar to the

non-competitive antagonism of receptors in a system with a receptor reserve — see Figure 6.16B. Finally, if the inhibitor *only* interacts with the enzyme-substrate complex, this is termed uncompetitive inhibition. This results in a depression of V_{max} and a decrease in the K_m value; i.e., the enzyme becomes more sensitive to the antagonism but operates with a lower V_{max} value — see

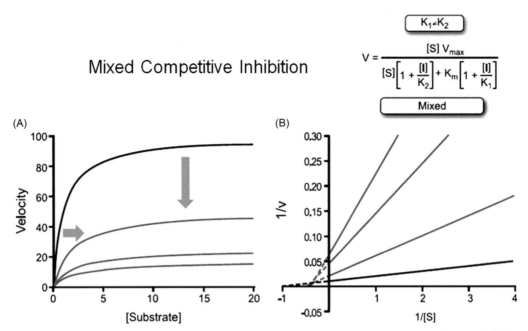

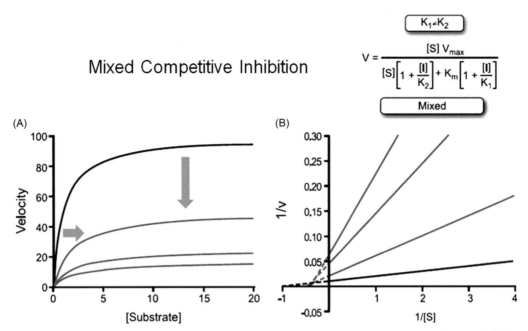

FIGURE 10.13 **Mixed enzyme inhibition.** Mixed inhibitors increase the K_m and decrease V_{max}. In this case, the inhibitor has affinities for both E and ES but they are not equal.

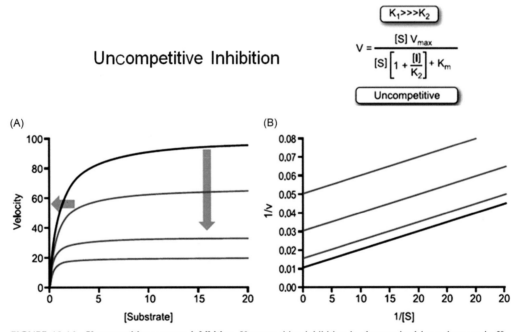

FIGURE 10.14 **Uncompetitive enzyme inhibition.** Uncompetitive inhibition is characterized by a decrease in K_m and a decreasing V_{max}. In this case the enzyme inhibitor binds only to the ES complex.

Figure 10.14. This is similar to some allosteric receptor antagonists (see Figure 7.21B).

It is more than academically interesting to know the mode of enzyme inhibition, because this can dictate the quantitative relationship between how much inhibitor is in the target compartment and how enzyme inhibition is produced. The molecular quantitative parameter that determines the potency of the enzyme inhibition is the equilibrium dissociation constant of the inhibitor-enzyme complex (K_I), but the observed inhibition may be modified by the concentration of substrate present in the form of the IC_{50} (concentration of inhibitor producing 50% inhibition of a given rate of enzyme reaction for a given substrate concentration). In terms of the safety pharmacology profile of hepatic enzymes, this refers to the drugs that the patient is taking for therapy. Figure 10.15 shows

Enzyme Inhibitors

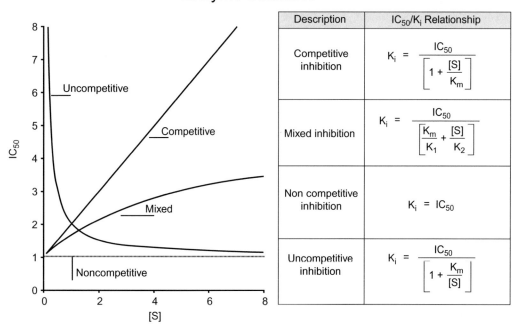

Description	IC_{50}/K_i Relationship
Competitive inhibition	$K_i = \dfrac{IC_{50}}{\left[1 + \dfrac{[S]}{K_m}\right]}$
Mixed inhibition	$K_i = \dfrac{IC_{50}}{\left[\dfrac{K_m}{K_1} + \dfrac{[S]}{K_2}\right]}$
Non competitive inhibition	$K_i = IC_{50}$
Uncompetitive inhibition	$K_i = \dfrac{IC_{50}}{\left[1 + \dfrac{K_m}{[S]}\right]}$

FIGURE 10.15 Relationship between the observed inhibition of enzymes (IC_{50}) and the molecular equilibrium dissociation constant of enzyme inhibitors as a function of substrate concentration. For drug-drug interactions, this deflects the potency of an enzyme inhibitor producing an interaction as a function of the concentration of the second drug used in therapy. For competitive interactions, as the dosage of the second drug increases, the effect of the drug causing a DDI through enzyme inhibition diminishes. To a lesser extent this is true of mixed enzyme inhibitors up to a limiting value. For noncompetitive enzyme inhibitors, the concentration of the second drug is immaterial. For uncompetitive enzyme antagonists, as the concentration of the second drug increases, the effect of the enzyme inhibitor actually increases.

the relationship between the observed potency of inhibition (IC_{50}) and the molecular K_I for enzyme inhibitors with different mechanisms of action. It can be seen that the potency of a competitive inhibitor decreases with increasing substrate concentration as expected (similar to IC_{50} values of competitive antagonists — see Figure 8.10A). This linear relationship becomes curvilinear with mixed enzyme inhibition and non-existent for noncompetitive inhibitors. Thus, the potency of non-competitive enzyme inhibitors is constant in the face of a range of substrate concentrations (similar to non-competitive receptor antagonists — see Figure 8.10B).

An interesting profile is seen with uncompetitive antagonists, where there is an inverse relationship between the substrate concentration and the potency of the enzyme inhibitor. This is because the substrate must be bound to the enzyme for inhibition to occur, i.e., the substrate creates the protein species sensitive to the inhibition. In terms of drug-drug interactions, this can lead to some different observations. For instance, for a putative hepatic competitive enzyme inhibition leading to a drug-drug interaction, increasing the dosage of one of the drugs will reduce the metabolism of the other. In contrast, for an uncompetitive type of interaction, increasing the

dosage of one of the drugs might actually *increase* the drug-drug interaction effect for the other.

In general, enzyme inhibition is measured by subjecting a steady-state ongoing enzyme reaction (operating at a substrate concentration near the K_m value) to a range of concentrations of the putative enzyme inhibitor and determining an IC_{50} much like the antagonism of a functional receptor assay (as shown in Figure 8.9). In the case of hepatic enzymes, human microsomes can be used as the particular cytochrome P450 enzyme in the enzyme mileu and can be functionally isolated in the mix through addition of specific substrates; some of the more common preferred substrates are shown in Table 10.4. It should be noted that enzymes such as CYP3A4 can use a variety of substrates (as would be required for a general protection mechanism), and there are cases where some molecules block the interaction of CYP3A4 with some substrates but not others. For example, the antihistamine aztemisole has an IC_{50} value of 3 nM for CYP3A4 with a substrate of benzoquinone, but has a 10-fold higher IC_{50} value and produces only partial blockade of the enzyme when benzoresorcinol is the substrate [21]. Therefore, in many cases cytochrome P450 interactions with a list of drugs that a given patient might be taking concurrently is a precaution taken to detect possible substrate-dependent drug-drug interactions. For compounds that are progressed to higher orders of development, K_I values are obtained through the comparison of inhibition profiles of a range of concentrations (as depicted in Figures 10.11 to 10.15). A higher throughput approach can be gained through measurement of IC_{50} values for compounds at two substrate concentrations – see Figure 10.16. In this scheme, competitive, mixed, non-competitive and

uncompetitive compounds can rapidly be identified. In general, an IC_{50} value >10 μM is optimal for compound progression.

In addition to the potency of a potential enzyme inhibitor being relevant to possible drug-drug interactions, the real time kinetics, specifically the reversibility, of the interaction is important. If the inhibition is extremely persistent (i.e., pseudoirreversible or irreversible through an aylkylation reaction), then the inhibition is referred to as a time-dependent inhibition. This is because the potency of the inhibitor literally depends upon the time of exposure. Also, if the irreversible reaction is due to an enzymatic mechanism (perhaps the metabolically relevant reaction), then this is referred to as mechanism-based inhibition. Time-dependent (mechanism-based) inhibition can be a serious safety issue that goes beyond simple drug-drug interaction when the possible inhibitor is present because it can cause lasting harm; i.e., in essence the compound becomes an irreversible poison. Figure 10.17A shows the time-dependent inhbition of CYP2C9 by erythromycin; it can be seen that the potency of erythromycin as an enzyme inhibitor continues to increase even after 40 to 50 hours of incubation time. Figure 10.17B shows an example of irreversible inhibition of CYP2B6 by the antiplatelet drug clopidogrel; the formation of the alkyl bond indicates a chemical reaction that will not come to an equilibrium until all of the clopidogrel reacts with water or enzyme protein.

While a reliable K_I cannot be measured for an irreversible enzyme inhibition, the effects can be quantified by measuring the rates of inactivation of various concentrations of enzyme inhibitor, much like the alkylation of receptors by irreversible receptor antagonists – see Figure 6.29. Thus, the rate of inactivation of the enzyme by various concentrations of inhibitor can be measured and plotted as a function of concentration. The result is a curvilinear plot with a midpoint giving the concentration

TABLE 10.4 Preferred Substrates for Some Common Cytochrome P450 Enzymes

CYP	Preferred Substrate
1A2	Phenacetin-O-de-ethylation
2A6	Coumarin-7-hydroxylation
	Nicotine C-oxidation
2B6	Efavirenz hydroxylase
	Bupropion hydroxylation
2C8	Taxol 6-hydroxylation
2C9	Tolbutamide methyl-hydroxylation
	S-warfarin 7 hydroxylation
	Diclenofac 4'-hydroxylation
2C19	S-methphenytoin 4'-hydroxylation
	Dextromethorphan O-demethylation
2D6	(+)-Bufuralol 1'-hydroxylation
	Dextromethorphan O-demethylation
2E1	Chlorzoxazone 6-hydroxylation
3A4/5	Midazolam-hydroxylation
	Testosterone 6β-hydroxylation

FIGURE 10.16 **Screening scheme to detect enzyme inhibition.** The difference in antagonist potency with changes in substrate concentration can be used to identify competitive, mixed, non-competitive and uncompetitive enzyme inhibition.

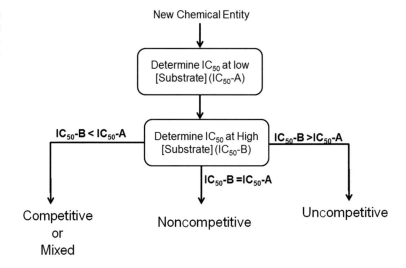

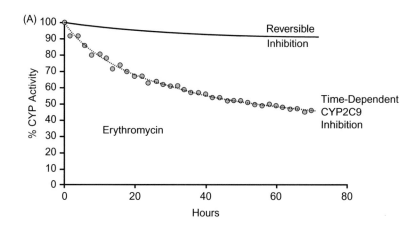

FIGURE 10.17 **Irreversible enzyme inhibition.** (A) Effect of equilibration time on potency of inhibitors of CYP2C9. While the IC_{50} of a reversible inhibitor would not change after approximately a 2 to 3 hour incubation, the potency of the time-dependent CYP2C9 inhibitor erythromycin increases over a period of 60 hours; i.e., a steady state is not attained. Data from [22]. (B) Molecular mechanism of the irreversible blockade of CYP2B6 by clopidogrel. Redrawn from [23].

of enzyme inhibitor for 50% maximal rate of enzyme inactivation (denoted K_I) and a maximum giving the maximal rate of enzyme inactivation (denoted K_{inact}). Clearly an irreversible inhibition is a less than ideal situation, since the only way the body can regain control is to synthesize more enzyme, i.e., compounds producing irreversible inhibition damage the ability of the liver to function as a protecting organ. However, irreversible inhibition must be considered within the context of a steady state of enzyme concentration. Specifically, all proteins are synthesized and degraded at various rates leading to steady-state levels for normal function. Therefore, the real impact of time-dependent enzyme inhibition is felt when the rate of the removal of active enzyme significantly approaches the rate of enzyme synthesis, and so yields a deficit steady-state concentration. Figure 10.18 shows the rate conditions of normal tissue and one where an irreversible enzyme inhibitor removes active enzyme; a ratio "R" is defined, which characterizes the possible deficit in enzyme steady-state levels. The equation for this deficit is given as:

$$R = \frac{K_{inact}\left[\frac{[I]/K_I}{[I]/K_I + 1}\right] + K_{degrad}}{K_{degrad}} \quad (10.7)$$

where K_{inact} is the maximal rate of irreversible inactivion of the enzyme by the inhibitor [I], K_I is the concentration of enzyme inhibitor producing 50% irreversible enzyme

inhibition and K_{degrad} is the natural rate of degradation of native enzyme in the tissue. A regulatory guideline suggests that R values greater than 1.1 constitute values of concern that need to be addressed in the development process. Figure 10.18 shows the effect of various values for K_{inact} on R for a given enzyme of constant K_{degrad}. In general, regulatory agencies suggest that new candidate molecules be tested for time-dependent inhibition of the most common cytochrome P450 enzymes (i.e., CYP1A, CYP2B6, CYP2C9, CYP2C19, CYP2D6, CYP3A4).

Another source of possible hepatic drug-drug interaction stems from the fact that the liver is an adaptable organ which regulates its function in accordance to chemical stress. Thus, some drugs induce liver enzymes to increase the metabolism of other drugs (or in the case of self-induction, a compound may increase the synthesis of the enzyme that metabolizes it). This induction can be at the level of transcription activation of the gene (e.g., CYP1A, CYP2C9, CYP3A4), stabilization of mRNA (CYP3E1, CYP3A4), or protein (CYP3E1), or activation of nuclear receptors (e.g., androstane CAR receptor, pregnane X receptor PXR, peroxisome proliferator-activated receptor PPAR). Enzyme effects are initiated within 24 hours, increase over 3–5 days and can take 1–3 weeks to wane after the drug is withdrawn. Effects can be observed *in vitro* through incubation of human hepatocytes for periods of 24 to 72 hours and then

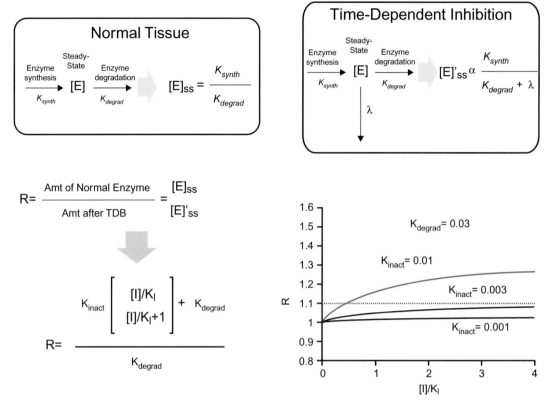

FIGURE 10.18 Gauging the impact of time-dependent enzyme inhibition. Normal tissue box depicts a steady-state enzyme level ($[E]_{ss}$) determined by the rate of enzyme production (K_{syn}) and rate of natural enzyme degradation (K_{degrad}). In the case of time-dependent inhibition, an added removal of enzyme is caused by an irreversible enzyme inhibitor with the rate depicted as λ. The new steady-state enzyme concentration is denoted $[E]'_{ss}$. A term R is derived which represents the ratio of normal to enzyme-inhibited steady-state enzyme levels. Graph shows a system with a fixed natural rate of enzyme degradation ($K_{degrad} = 0.03$) and the value of R for three enzyme inhibitors of varying rates of irreversible enzyme inhibition ($K_{inact} = 0.01, 0.003, 0.001$) as a function of enzyme inhibitor concentration. Curve in red indicates a case where $R > 1.1$, a common regulatory limit for concern.

measuring enzyme function or mRNA levels after cell lysis. Hepatic induction is caused by a number of drugs, e.g., phenobarbital and other barbiturates, anticonvulsants, carbamazepine, phenytoin, polycyclic hydrocarbons, glucocorticoids, and rifampin. In general, it is suggested that tests be done to determine any effects on prominent hepatic enzymes such as CYP3A4, CYP1A2, CYP2C9, CYP2C19, CYP2C8, UGT, CYP2A6, and CYP2E1. It is not clear how tranferable are predictions of hepatic enzyme induction from animal studies to humans, as the effects are often species dependent and also, with the exception of nuclear receptor activation, seen at doses higher than those used therapeutically. However, the effects can be dramatic; such as the near obliteration of the bioavailability of felodipine (from 15% to 1%) in patients concurrently treated with hepatic enzyme-inducing anticonvulsants [24].

10.2.2 Direct Hepatotoxicity

In addition to drug-drug interactions, hepatically-mediated toxicity can be observed through direct effects on liver cells (replicating HepG2 cells and/or metabolically competent primary rat hepatocytes). This is encountered frequently, since the liver is the first line of defense against foreign chemical invasion, and compounds often reach this organ in the highest concentrations. In addition to the standard measures of cytotoxicity (*vide infra*), human liver cells can be used to monitor hepatically-unique toxic effects such as steatosis (accumulation of triglycerides in hepatic cells; e.g., aspirin, tetracyline, amiodarone, alcohol. valproic acid), phospholipidosis — a lysosomal storage disorder leading to accumulation of lipids in cells (e.g., chloroquine, sertraline, fluoxetine, amitriptylene) — intrahepatic cholestasis (impairment of bile formation leading to jaundice; e.g., cyclosporin A, rifamycin, glyburide, troglitazone), and general lysosomal trapping (drug accumulation in the lysosomes.

In addition to cellular assays of hepatic function, animal models of liver function are very useful in determining possible hepatic toxicity. While dose-dependent hepatoxic effects are readily predictable, idiosyncratic hepatic toxicity is much more difficult to define. One

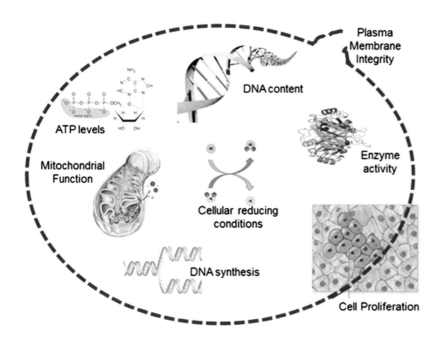

FIGURE 10.19 Cell viability can be assessed from a number of standpoints through monitoring functions such as mitochondrial function (ATP levels), plasma membrane integrity, DNA content and function, cell proliferation, reductive capacity of the cytosol, and enzyme activity (see text).

technique that has been employed is to use a state of chemically-induced inflammation to cause a hypersensitivity of the liver to subthreshold doses of xenobiotics in order to uncover idiosyncratic hepatotoxicity. For example, non-toxic doses of the Gram-negative bacterial source lipopolysaccharide potentiate the toxicity of carbon tetrachloride, monocrotaline, cocaine, aflatoxin B1, and the non-steroidal anti-inflammatory drugs diclofenac and sulindac in rats, and it has been proposed that such sensitization to toxicity leads to a model that is more applicable to the detection of rare idiosyncratic effects [25].

At this point it also is relevant to consider species variation, as many of the safety studies discussed involve animals as predictors of effects in humans. The availability of microsomes and hepatocytes from animal species as well as humans provides direct comparisons which can be used to identify appropriate species for safety testing of new compounds. For example, the HIV-1 attachment inhibitor BMS-378806 is metabolized by microsome preparations from human, monkey, and rat but not from dogs, thereby indicating that the dog would be an inappropriate species for extensive pharmacokinetic study of this compound [26]. Allometric scaling (see Chapter 9.7.1) can be useful to identify species which, at least from a pharmacokinetic standpoint, metabolize a compound in a manner different from that found in humans. For example, allometric scaling with the anticancer compound CS-023 shows uniform pharmacokinetic handling in mice, rats, rabbits, dogs and humans but aberrant pharmacokinetics in the monkey [27]. Subsequent studies have shown that this species had an abnormally high renal tubular reabsorption not seen in any other species.

10.3 CYTOTOXICITY

While the liver is a prime target for toxic effects, it is also important to determine whether new drug candidates cause directly harmful effects in all cells. There are now a number of simple *in vitro* assays used to assess cellular viability in the presence of new molecules. Toxic effects can be caused by a number of mechanisms, thus it is important to observe as many indicators of cellular competency as possible; i.e., changes in cell number, nuclear condensation, total nuclear intensity, cell permeability, mitochondrial membrane potential, cytochrome C release, etc. Some of these are shown schematically in Figure 10.19. One of the most sensitive indicators of cellular state is mitochondrial function. The mitochondria produce >90% of the energy required by a cell in the form of ATP by oxidative phosphorylation. One of the oldest simple tests for mitochondrial function is the MTT test, which uses a change in color of a yellow substrate for mitochondrial reductase (MTT, 3-(4,5-dimethylthiazol-2-yl)-2,5-diphenyltetrazolium bromide) to the purple product formazan; impairment of this reaction (no color change) indicates a low level mitochondrial function. A more sophisticated test utilizes the Crabtree effect. Specifically, cells are grown in a high glucose medium under hypoxic or anaerobic conditions where most of their energy derives from glycolysis rather than mitochondrial oxidative phosphorylation; this reduces the cell sensitivity to mitochondrial toxicants. When glucose is removed and substituted with galactose, the cell has an increased reliance on mitochondrial oxidative phosphorylation for production of ATP. The effects of compounds on cell death under both of these conditions can be used to detect compound-induced mitochondrial impairment of function. For example, the ATPase inhibitor oligomycin has little effect on ATP content in glucose-media HepG2 cells but greatly diminishes ATP in galactose-media cells, indicating drug-induced mitochondrial dysfunction [28]. This type of assay can be an early indicator of compounds that cause mitochondrial damage.

General cell viability can be assessed through incorporation and binding neutral red dye into lysosomes; this is a common reaction in healthy cells. A diminution in the ability of cells to do this in the presence of a compound suggests that the compound reduces cell viability. Membrane integrity is also an important component of cell viability. For example, the stable enzyme lactic dehydrogenase is released into the cell culture medium with membrane damage thus giving an assay of membrane integrity. Similar assays utilize fluorescent dyes that do not normally cross the cell membrane to assess membrane integrity; i.e., when cells become fluorescently labeled, then membrane integrity has been compromised. Another measure of cell viability monitors the reducing environment within the cell cytosol. For example, cell health can be measured through observation of the fluorescence of analogs of resazurin which in healthy cells is reduced to a highly fluorescent colored metabolite resorufin; a decrease in this reaction indicates a reduction of the reducing power of the cell and this is linked to a loss of cell viability. If imaging is used, cell viability assays can yield multiple indices of viability through the use of different dye compounds. Thus, a single assay can be used to determine changes in nuclear morphology, cell proliferation, plasma membrane integrity, and mitochondrial function.

Finally, direct toxic effects can be caused by molecules that produce chemically reactive intermediates, particularly in tissues such as the liver, skin, and blood cells [29]. These electrophilic species can alkylate proteins and DNA to cause lasting damage. For example, it is possible that the high incidence of agranulocytosis seen with the antipsychotic compound clozapine is due to the formation of a reactive nitrenium ion [30]. Cells possess chemical trapping agents such as glutathione (GSH) that go on to form stable molecules with the reactive species, therefore hepatic cells can be used to identify reactive species through their interaction with fluorescent GSH analogs such as Dansyl-GSH [31].

10.4 MUTAGENICITY

Drug-induced mutagenicity, whereby a drug induces mutation of DNA transcription products, can be a devastating liability since such effects can lead to cancer. Also, the effects may not be detected until very late in the drug development process. In fact, their detection may require use of the drug in very large populations, larger than those practical for any Phase III clinical trial. Therefore, early *in vitro* prediction of such effects can be extremely important. One general test that has been used is an *in vitro* genetic toxicology test to determine mutagenic properties of a compound called the *Ames test*. Devised by a group led by Bruce Ames in the 1970s at Berkeley, California, it employs *Salmonella tryphimurium* modified to maximize the probability of mutation (see Figure 10.20A). Whereas normal bacteria can synthesize histidine and thus live in non-histidine-containing media, the Ames test uses bacteria modified such that they cannot synthesize histidine and cannot live in media that do not contain this amino acid. In addition, the

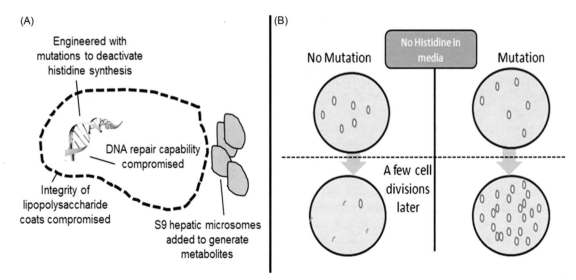

FIGURE 10.20 The Ames test. This assay utilizes bacteria modified to optimize drug-induced mutation. When mutation has occurred, the bacterium may revert to a form that can survive in histidine-free medium; when this is observed, it is assumed that mutation has taken place. Under conditions of no mutation, the bacteria will die in histidine-free medium.

lipopolysaccharide coat of the bacteria is compromised to maximize compound entry, the DNA repair capability of the bacterium is reduced, and S9 fraction microsomes are added to the medium to maximize the formation of metabolites. Often, mutation will convert these bacteria back to a form that can synthesize histidine enabling them to live in histidine-free medium. This produces a simple test whereby candidate molecules are added to these bacteria cultured in histidine-free medium; if the bacteria grow, then it is assumed that the compound has caused a mutation (see Figure 10.20B). While this has been used as a valuable predictor of mutation, it should be noted that it is not infallible. For example, dioxin (2,3,7,8-tetrachlorodibenzo-p-dioxin) is one of the most virulent sources of immunotoxicity, along with reproductive and endocrine disorders and tumor production, yet it produces no effects in the Ames test.

10.5 hERG ACTIVITY AND *TORSADES DE POINTES*

Hydrophobic drugs have been shown to have affinity for calcium channels and, notably, potassium channels, and this latter activity is a clear liability. Specifically, blockade of the hERG potassium channel can lead to cardiac QTc prolongation and a condition called *Torsades de Pointes*; a potentially fatal cardiac arrhythmia which is characterized by a rapid onset (see Figure 10.21). A number of rapid *in vitro* tests have been proposed to screen for this activity, such as blockade of rubidium efflux, but

technology has progressed to the point where the preferable high-throughput direct electrophysiological measurement of potassium channel blockade is now commonly available. These studies can then be followed up with experiments in perfused Langendorf hearts, in anesthetized animals for QTc prolongation, and by chronic study in conscious animals using telemetry. In general, an IC_{50} value for hERG inhibition should exceed $10-50\,\mu M$, although the magnitude of this margin will be linked to the therapeutic potency of the compound. Prolongation of the QT interval in electrocardiogram studies is the indicator of possible *Torsades de Pointes*, with prolongation of >6 ms predicting possible effect, 16−20 ms probable effects, and >21 ms almost definite effects. There have been a number of approved drugs withdrawn from the market due to a risk of *Torsades de Pointes* (see Table 10.5).

10.6 AUTONOMIC RECEPTOR PROFILING

Effects on receptors and ion channels also account for major drug liabilities. In most cases, such as effects on receptors, the untoward effects are a direct result of receptor activation (or blockade). While many batteries of tests can be rapidly done with receptor binding, it is critical that receptor function is also tested, since it could be argued that binding is superfluous if functional antagonism can be measured. The outcomes of the two types of assay can be quite different; a ligand that binds to α-adrenoceptors (as seen in a binding assay) may produce

Blockade of the hERG Channel

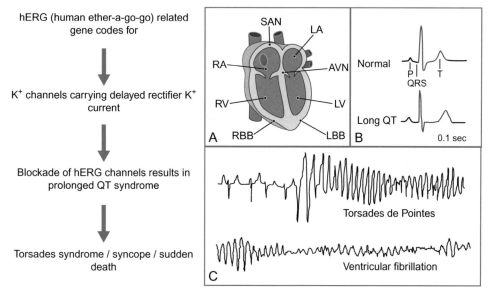

FIGURE 10.21 Schematic diagram showing sequence of events beginning with the blockade of the hERG potassium channel in the heart that causes QT interval prolongation that eventually can lead to a potentially fatal arrhythmia called *torsades de pointes*.

TABLE 10.5 Approved Drugs Withdrawn because of hERG Activity and Risk of *Torsades de Points*

Drug	IC_{50} hERG Channel Inhibition
Terodiline	450 nM
Terfenadine	204 nM
Sertindole	3 nM
Astemizole	0.9 nM
Levomethadyl	3 μM
Cisapride	15 nM
Droperidol	32 nM

From [32].

hypotension if it has no efficacy and hypertension if it does; the functional assay yields the relevant data. Table 10.6 shows some cardiovascular side effects commonly associated with some 7TM receptors [32]. In some cases, the receptor activity belies effects that are not obvious. For example, muscarinic m3 receptor activity has been associated with type 2 diabetes [33]. Promiscuous receptor activity is a potential problem with drugs, therefore rapid *in vitro* tests on panels of receptors known to be associated with toxic effects can be done on candidate chemical scaffolds. Table 10.7 shows a short list of "repeat offenders" in the receptor world that have been associated with a range of toxic effects in humans. Other promiscuous targets are the pregnane X-receptor, a nuclear receptor associated with regulation of cytochrome P450 enzymes. Induction of PXR can have large effects on metabolism, drug-drug interactions, multidrug resistance, and transport mechanisms. While the ratios of relative activity of new compounds on various autonomic receptors can be used to predict hazard and risk of untoward receptor-mediated reactions, they only serve as guidelines. For example, the 36-fold difference between the therapeutic receptor activity of pergolide for dopamine receptors vs. the 5-HT$_{2B}$ receptor (a cardiac safety hazard) coupled with the apparent 47-fold safety margin for the therapeutic C_{max} and ED_{50} required for *in vivo* 5-HT$_{2B}$ interaction did not predict the observed valvular heart disease liability of this drug (causing it to be withdrawn) [34]. Similarly, Bosentan, a drug for pulmonary hypertension, has a very large ratio of activity between the therapeutically relevant receptor (endothelin) and processes for the production of toxic bile salts (8106-fold) and the C_{max} is 255-fold less than that required for the bile effect but *in vivo* studies showed a bile salt hazard which required a black box warning for this drug [34]. These types of data underscore the importance of general *in vivo* studies in the pharmacological safety determination process.

10.7 GENERAL PHARMACOLOGY

In addition to *in vitro* assessments of cell viability, hepatic function, hERG liability, and receptor activity, it is essential to determine the possible effects of a new compound on normal physiology [35]. This is done in a series of *in vivo* animal studies. Figure 10.22 shows a general view of the types of studies usually required by regulatory agencies; these involve the three vital systems of CNS, cardiovascular, and respiratory, although other organ effects need to be monitored as well. Barring any observation of serious effects in these acute studies, chronic studies in a wider variety of systems are initiated. These can be divided into exploratory toxicology (estimates of toxicity when compound is given over a relative short chronic period of two weeks) and the much more extensive GLP (good laboratory practice) standard studies required by regulatory bodies done in parallel with clinical studies (see Figure 10.23) [36]. These studies span 28 days of repeat dosing in two species, as well as chronic three to 12 month experiments in two species and 18−24 month carcinogenic studies.

10.8 CLINICAL TESTING

The final, but most expensive and labor-intensive, step in the drug discovery process is the testing of candidates in humans in a clinical trial setting. This is done in phases of increasing intensity and rigor. Phase I clinical trials explore the first-time exposure to humans to measure tolerance and safety in human volunteers. These trials consist of rising dose studies to determine maximum tolerated dose via the expected route of administration. In addition, pharmacokinetic studies may include multiple dosing in preparation for the next step in the process; namely, Phase II trials. At this stage there may be patient involvement to more accurately reflect the targeted population (e.g., geriatric, healthy patients' tolerance of toxic cancer drugs), or to detect special effects such as differences in tolerance (e.g., schizophrenic patients are 200 times more tolerant of the side effects of haloperidol than are healthy volunteers).

Should a candidate demonstrate positive effects in Phase I trials, then Phase II trials (initial clinical study for treatment efficacy and continued study of safety) are initiated. These trials are divided into two separate stages: Phase IIa trials are limited to determine some degree of efficacy, while Phase IIb trials are more extensive and expensive including a larger number of patients (100−200). At this stage, biochemical and physiological indices of efficacy are sought in a double-blind (neither patient nor clinicians know which group receives drug and which receives a placebo) setting. In addition to a placebo arm, the Food and Drug Administration

TABLE 10.6 Some Cardiovascular Targets Associated with Adverse Drug Effects

Target		Possible Adverse Drug Effects	
adenosine A1	bradycardia	AV-block	renal vasoconstriction
adenosine A2a	hypotension	coronary vasodilation	platelet aggregation
adenosine A3	mediator release		
α_{1a}-adrenoceptor	hypertension	orthostatic hypotension	inotropy
α_{1b}-adrenoceptor	orthostatic hypotension		
α_{2a}-adrenoceptor	hypertension	possible hyperglycemia	
α_{2b}-adrenoceptor	hypertension	cardiac ischemia	vasoconstriction
central ↓ blood pressure			
α_{2c}-adrenoceptor	hypertension	cardiac ischemia	skeletal muscle blood flow
β_1-adrenoceptor	cardiac inotropy	heart rate	ventricular fibrillation
bronchospasm			
β_2-adrenoceptor	fascil. cardiac arrest	impairs cardiac performance	
angiotensin AT_1	hypertension	cell proliferation, migration	tubular Na^+ resorption
bradykinin B_1	nociception	inflammation	cough
bradykinin B_2	nociception	inflammation	cough
CGRP	hypocalcemia	hypophosphatemia	
Ca^{2+} channel	hypotension		
dopamine D_1	induces dyskinesia	vasodilatation, schizophrenia	↓ coordination
endothelin ET_a	vasoconstriction	cell proliferation	aldosterone secretion
endothelin ET_b	vasoconstriction	cell proliferation	bronchoconstriction
histamine H_3	↓ memory, sedation	vasodilatation	↓ GI motility
muscarinic m1	Δblood pressure	↓ GI secretion	
muscarinic m2	vagal effects	Δblood pressure	tachycardia
muscarinic m3	vagal effects, salivation	Δblood pressure, dry mouth	↓ ocular accommodation
muscarinic m4	vagal effects, salivation	Δblood pressure	facilitates D1 stimulation
NE transporter	adrenergic hyperreactivity	facilitates α-activation	
nicotinic Ach	autonomic functions	palpitations, nausea, sweating	tremor, ganglionic function
NPY_1	venous vasoconstriction	↓ gut motility, gastric emptying	anxiogenic
K^+ channel (hERG)	cardiac QTc prolongation		
K^+ channel [ATP]	hypotension, hypoglycemia		
$5-HT_{2b}$	cardiac valvulopathy		
$5-HT_4$	facilitates GI transit	mechanical intestinal allodynia	
Na^+ channel (site 2)	cardiac arrhythmia		
thromboxane $_{a2}$	vascular constriction	bronchial constriction	allergic inflammation, platelet aggregation
vasopressin V_{1a}	vasopressor		
vasopressin V_{1b}	vasopressor, anxiogenic		

Taken from [32].

TABLE 10.7 Some General Seven Transmembrane Receptors Noted for Producing Toxic Effects

General Tox	GI Tox	CV Tox	CV Tox
5-HT$_{2A}$	5-HT$_{1A}$	5-HT$_4$	Muscarinic m3
5-HT$_{2B}$	5-HT$_{1p}$	α_{1A}-adrenoceptor	Muscarinic m4
α_{1A}-adrenoceptor	5-HT$_{2A}$	α_{1B}-adrenoceptor	Nicotinic Ach
α_{1B}-adrenoceptor	5-HT$_{2B}$	α_{2A}-adrenoceptor	NPY$_1$
α_{2A}-adrenoceptor	5-HT$_3$	α_{2B}-adrenoceptor	Thromboxane A2
Adenosine 2 A	5-HT$_4$	α_{2C}-adrenoceptor	Vasopressin V$_{1a}$
Adenosine A1	α_{2A}-adrenoceptor	Adenosine 2 A	Vasopressin V$_{1b}$
β_1-adrenoceptor	α_{2B}-adrenoceptor	Adenosine A1	
β_2-adrenoceptor	α_{2C}-adrenoceptor	Adenosine A3	
Bradykinin B2	CCK2	Angiotensin AT1	
Cannabinoid CB1	Dopamine D2	β_1-adrenoceptor	
Dopamine D2	δ-opioid	β_2-adrenoceptor	
Histamine H1	EP2	Bradykinin B1	
μ opioid	EP3	Bradykinin B2	
Muscarinic m1	Gastrin	Cannabinoid CB1	
Purinergic P2Y1	Histamine H2	CGRP	
μ opioid	Dopamine D2		
Motilin	Endothelin A		
Muscarinic m2	Endothelin B		
Muscarinic m3	Histamine H3		
SST1	Muscarinic m1		
VIP	Muscarinic m2		

GI = gastrointestinal. CV = cardiovascular.

(FDA) often requires a positive control arm (known drug, if available). If the positive control arm fails to show efficacy, the trial is a failure.

Phase III clinical trials are critical and require full-scale treatment in several medical centers. The design of these trials compares the test candidate to known treatment and placebo in a double-blind manner. The dosage used in these trials is critical, as these determine regulatory decisions and marketing. The number of patients can be several hundred to thousands, and assessments of drug interactions are made at this stage. A number of new drug candidates fail at this stage since it can be more difficult to detect significant therapeutic benefit, usually because of the background noise in the patient sample. Whereas efforts are made to make the patient population as uniform as possible to detect safety hazards in the early clinical stages of testing, Phase III utilizes real patient populations which can be diverse and have variable pharmacological characteristics [37]. Thus, a true therapeutic effect may be much more difficult to determine in this setting (see Figure 10.24).

While new drugs are approved after completion of successful Phase III trials, there is yet another stage beyond drug approval. Thus, Phase IV clinical trials consist of post-marketing surveillance. At this point, adverse effects are monitored and additional long-term large-scale studies of efficacy are undertaken. Additional indications are monitored at this stage as well, and pharmacoeconomic data also are obtained to convince health-care payers that the new drug offers significant benefit over existing therapy (time to recovery, quality of life). With regard to pharmacological safety, while dose-dependent hazards can usually be identified by animal testing, idiosyncratic safety hazards depend on stochastic opportunity (encountering rare conditions) and therefore depend on populations both in terms of size and type. Thus, idiosyncratic toxicity is

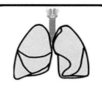

CNS
- Motor Activity
- Behavior
- Coordination
- Sensory/Motor Reflexes
- Body Temperature
- Tremor
- Learning and Memory
- Auditory Function
- Startle Reflex
- Grip Strength
- Nociception
- Electroencephalography
- Anxiety Test
- Visual Function

Respiratory
- Respiratory Rate
- Tidal Volume
- pO_2, pCO_2, pH
- Airway Resistance
- Compliance

Supplemental Systems
- Gastrointestinal
  - Transit Time, Gastric emptying, Secretion
- Renal/Genitourinary
  - Urine volume, total protein, Clearance, GFR, Na^+, K^+, Cl^- Electrolytes, BUN
- Blood
  - Platelet aggregation, bleeding time
- Immunological

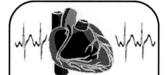

Cardiovascular
- BP & Heart Rate
- Cardiac Output
- Left Ventricular P
- Contractility
- ECG
- Repolarization (APD)
- hERG (I_{Kr}) assay
- Conduction
- QT interval (telemetry)

FIGURE 10.22 Summary of *in vivo* studies done to ensure pharmacological safety for a new compound.

Discovery → Preclinical Development → Clinical Phase I/II → Clinical Phase III/IV

Exploratory (non GLP) Toxicology
- *In vitro* screens
- *In silico* screens
- Cytotoxicity
- Immunotoxicity
- Hepatotoxicity
- Embryotoxicity

Single and repeat dose- range finding studies in 2 species

Regulatory (GLP) toxicology
- Safety pharmacology
- Genotoxocity (in vitro and in vivo)
- 28 day repeat dose toxicity and recovery in 2 species

- 3-12 mo chronic toxicity in 2 species
- 24 mo carcinogenicity in 2 species

- Reproductive toxicity in 1 species covering:
- Fertility, implantation
- Fetal development
- Pre-post natal effects

FIGURE 10.23 Late-stage long-term safety studies of a new drug candidate. The IND (Investigational New Drug) application is filed after the preclinical development stage and the NDA (New Drug Application) after the clinical phase IV stage.

often the product of a succession of unlikely events. These are difficult to detect in animal studies because they usually have too few numbers, and these effects are often species dependent and involve genetic variation. These rare events show how nearly impossible it is to design a clinical trial to detect them. For example, the non-steroidal anti-inflammatory drug diclofenac produces hepatotoxicity in 6 out of every 100,000 patients; an extremely serious event resulting in lethal jaundice. Similarly, the serious cardiovascular effects causing the withdrawal of Vioxx were seen in 1 in 133927 patients. Figure 10.25 shows the number of patients required to be registered in a clinical trial to detect rare events. From this figure it can be seen that a study with greater than 160,000 patients would need to be done to detect an untoward event with incidence of 1 in 1000 (e.g., myocardial infarction) which has in itself a background incidence of 6 per 1000 [38].

10.9 SUMMARY AND CONCLUSIONS

- Safety pharmacology is concerned with the safety margin for a new drug (i.e., nature of the dose-limiting adverse event, the therapeutic indication and the intended patient population), whether the toxicity is reversible and has a biomarker and its mechanism.
- The liver is a primary site for observing safety issues from two points of view: compromise of the liver as a metabolizing organ for drugs with resulting drug-drug interactions and also direct hepatic cytotoxicity.
- The reversibility of hepatic enzyme inhibition is important for assessing progress of candidate drug molecules.
- There are numerous *in vitro* cellular markers for cell viability that can indicate cytotoxicity.
- Mutagenicity can be predicted in many cases with the Ames test, and hERG channel inhibition can predict serious lethal cardiotoxicity.
- Activity on autonomic receptors should be carried out in functional receptor assays where possible.
- Idiosyncratic toxic effects are difficult to detect in preclinical and clinical studies and often appear in the post-marketing usage of drugs.

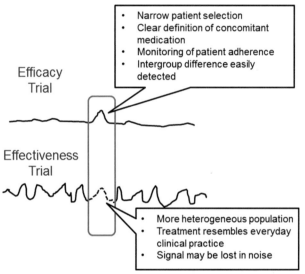

FIGURE 10.24 Signal-to-noise ratios in clinical trials. Whereas Phase I and II trails are designed with a maximally uniform baseline in order to detect events, Phase III trials are done in real patients where the baseline is variable and small events may be difficult to detect above noise levels. Redrawn from [37].

FIGURE 10.25 Detecting rare events in clinical trials. Given a background incidence for an untoward event (x-axis), the ordinate axis gives the number of patients required for detection of rare events with varying drug-related incidence (given next to each curve). Redrawn from [38].

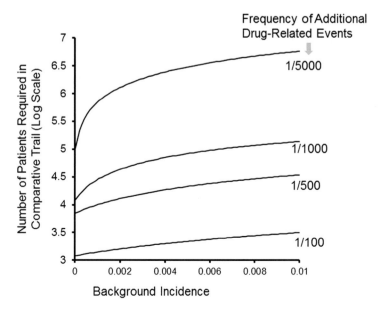

REFERENCES

[1] Tang Z, Taylor MJ, Lisboa P, Dyas M. Quantitative risk modeling for new pharmaceutical compounds. Drug Disc Today 2005;22:1520−6.

[2] Teague SJ, Davis AM, Leeson PD, Oprea TJ. The design of lead-like combinatorial libraries. Angew Chem Int Ed 1999;38:3743−8.

[3] King FD, Brown AM, Gaster LM, Kaumann AJ, Medhurst AD, Parker SG, et al. (+ −)-3-amino-6-carboxamido-1,2,3,4-tetrahydrocarbazole: a conformationally restricted analog of 5-carboxamidotryptamine with selectivity for the serotonin 5-HT1D receptor. J Med Chem 1993;36:1918.

[4] Yanagisawa T, Wakabayashi S, Tomiyama T, Yasunami M, Takase K. Synthesis and anti-ulcer activities of sodium alkylazulene sulfonates. Chem Pharm Bull 1988;36:641.

[5] Giudici D, Ornati G, Briatico G, Buzzetti F, Lombardi P, di Salle E. 6-Methylenandrosta-1,4-diene-3,17-dione (FCE 24304): a new irreversible aromatase inhibitor. J Steroid Biochem 1988;30:391.

[6] Bhat B, Seth M, Bhaduri AP. Indian J Chem 1981;20B:703.

[7] Krapcho J, Turk C, Cushman DW, Powell JR, DeForrest JM, Spitzmiller ER, et al. Angiotensin-converting enzyme inhibitors. Mercaptan, carboxyalkyl dipeptide, and phosphinic acid inhibitors incorporating 4-substituted prolines. J Med Chem 1988;31:1148.

[8] Sham HL, Kempf DJ, Molla A, Marsh KC, Kumar GN, Chen C-M, et al. ABT-378, a highly potent inhibitor of the human immunodeficiency virus protease. Antimicrob Agents Chemother 1998;42:3218.

[9] Proudfoot JR. Drugs, leads, and drug-likeness: an analysis of some recently launched drugs. Bioorg Med Chem Lett 2002;12:1647−50.

[10] Shargel L, Yu ABC, Wu-Pong S. Applied biopharmaceutics and pharmacokinetics. New York: McGraw-Hill; 2004. p. 510

[11] Velaparthi U, Liu P, Balasubramanian B, Carbonia J, Attar R, Gottardis M, et al. Imidazole moiety replacements in the 3-(1 H-benzoyl[d]imidazole-2-yl)pyridine-2-(1 H)-one inhibitors of insulin-like growth factor receptor-1 (IGF-1 R) to improve cytochrome P450 profile. Bioorg Med Chem Lett 2007;17:3072−6.

[12] Kramer JA, Sagartz JE, Morris DL. The application of discovery toxicology and pathology towards the design of safer pharmaceutical lead candidates. Nat Rev Drug Disc 2007;6:636−50.

[13] Valentin J-P, Bialecki R, Ewart L, Hammnod T, Leishmann D, Lindgren S, et al. A framework to assess the translation of safety pharmacology data to humans. J Pharmacol Toxicol Meth 2009;60:152−8.

[14] Genschow E, Spielmann H, Scholz G, Seiler A, Brown N, Piersma A. The EVAM international validation study on in vitro embryotoxicity tests: results of the definitive phase and evaluation of prediction models. European Center for the Validation of Alternative Methods. Altern Lab Anim 2002;30:151−76.

[15] Klabunde T, Evers A. GPCR antitarget modeling: pharmacophore models for biogenic amine binding GPCRs to avoid GPCR-mediated side effect. Chem Bio Chem 2005;6:876−89.

[16] Kazius J, Bursi R. Derivation and validation of toxicophores for mutagenicity prediction. J Med Chem 2005;48:312−20.

[17] Ayrton A, Morgan P. Role of transport proteins in drug absorption, distribution and excretion. Xenobiotica 2001;31:469−97.

[18] Wienkers T, Heath G. Predicting in vivo drug interactions from in vitro drug discovery data. Nat Rev Drug Discov 2005;4:825−33.

[19] Copeland RA. Evaluation of enzyme inhibitors in drug discovery. 2nd ed. Hoboken: Wiley; 2013 pp 1−344

[20] Choi. YH, Lee BK, Lee MG. Pharmacokinetic interaction between itraconazole and metformin in rats: competitive inhibition of metabolism of each drug by each other via hepatic and intestinal CYP3A1/2. Br J Pharmacol 2010;161:815−29.

[21] Stresser DM, Blanchard AP, Turner SD, Erve JCL, Dandeneau AA, Miller VP, et al. Substrate-dependent modulation of CYP3A4 catalytic activity: analysis of 27 test compounds with fluorometric substrates. Drug Metab Dispos 2000;28:1440−8.

[22] McGinnity DF, Berry AJ, Kenny JR, Grime K, Riley RJ. Evaluation of time-dependent cytochrome P450 inhibition using cultured human hepatocytes. Drug Metab Disp 2006;34:1291−300.

[23] Richter T, Murdter TE, Heinkele G, Pleiss J, Tatzel S, Schwab M, et al. Potent mechanism-based inhibition of human CYP2B6 by clopidogrel and ticlopidine. J Pharmacol Exp Ther 2004;308:189−97.

[24] Capewell S, Critchley JAJH, Freestone S, Pottage A, Prescott LF. Reduced felodipine bioavailability in patients taking anticnvulsants. Lancet 1988;332:480−2.

[25] Roth RA, Ganey PE. Intrinsic versus idiosynchratic drug-induced hepatotoxicity − two villains or one?. J Pharmacol Exp Ther 2010;332:692−7.

[26] Yang Z, Zadjura L, D'Arienzo CD, Marino A, Santone K, Klunk L, et al. Preclinical pharmacokinetics of a novel HIV-1 attachment inhibitor BMS-378806 and prediction of its human pharmacokinetics. Biopharm Drug Disp 2005;26:387−402.

[27] Shibayama T, Matsushita Y, Kurihara A, Hirota T, Ikeda T. Prediction of pharmacokinetics of CS-023 (RO4908463), a novel parenteral carbapenem antibiotic, in humans using animal data. Xenobiotica 2007;37:91−102.

[28] Marroquinynes J, Dykens JA, Jamieson JD, Will Y. Circumventing the Crabtree effect: replacing media glucose with galactose increases susceptibility of HepG2 cells to mitochondrial toxicants. Toxicol Sci 2007;97:539−47.

[29] Smith DA, Obach RS. Metabolites and safety: what are the concerns, and how should we address them? Chem Res Toxicol 2006;19:1570−9.

[30] Uetrecht J, Zahid N, Tehim A, Fu JM, Rakhit S. Structural features associated with reactive metabolite formation in clozapine analogues. Chemico-Biol Inter 1997;104:117−29.

[31] Gan J, Harper TW, Hsueh M-M, Qu Q, Humphreys WG. Dansyl glutathione as a trapping agent for the quantitative estimation and identification of reactive metabolites. Chem Res Toxicol 2005;18:896−903.

[32] Whitebread S, Hamon J, Bojanic D, Urban L. In vitro safety pharmacology profiling: an essential tool for drug development. Drug Disc Today 2005;10:1421−33.

[33] Silvetre JS, Prous J. Research on adverse drug events: Muscarinic m3 receptor binding affinity could predict the risk of antipsychotics to induce type 2 diabetes. Meth Find Exp Clin Pharmacol 2005;27:289−304.

[34] Muller PY, Milton MN. The determination and interpretation of the therapeutic index in drug development. Nat Rev Drug Disc 2012;11:751−63.

[35] Pugsley MK, Authier S, Curtis MJ. Principles of safety pharmacology. Br J Pharmacol 2008;154:1382−99.

[36] Rang HP. Assessing drug safety. In: Rang HP, editor. Drug discovery and development. London: Churchill Livingstone, Elsevier. p. 229−242.

[37] Eichler H-G, Abadie E, Breckenridge A, Flamion B, Gustafsson LL, Leufkens H, et al. Bridging the efficacy-effectiveness gap: a regulator's perspective on addressing variability of drug-response. Nat Rev Drug Disc 2011;10:495−507.

[38] Eichler H-G, Pignatti F, Flamion B, Leufkens H, Breckenridge A. Balancing early market access to new drugs with the need for benefit/risk data: a mounting dilemma. Nat Rev Drug Disc 2008;7:818−27.

Chapter 11

The Drug Discovery Process

Success is the ability to go from failure to failure with no lack of enthusiasm...

— Winston Churchill (1874–1965)

I am interested in physical medicine because my father was. I am interested in medical research because I believe in it. I am interested in arthritis because I have it...

— Bernard Baruch, 1959

...new techniques may be generating bigger haystacks as opposed to more needles ...

— D.F. Horrobin, 2000

11.1 Some Challenges for Modern Drug Discovery

11.2 Target-Based Drug Discovery

11.3 Systems-Based Drug Discovery

11.4 *In vivo* Systems, Biomarkers, and Clinical Feedback

11.5 Types of Therapeutically Active Ligands: Polypharmacology

11.6 Pharmacology in Drug Discovery

11.7 Chemical Sources for Potential Drugs

11.8 Pharmacodynamics and High-Throughput Screening

11.9 Drug Development

11.10 Clinical Testing

11.11 Summary and Conclusions

References

11.1 SOME CHALLENGES FOR MODERN DRUG DISCOVERY

The identification of primary biological activity at the target of interest is just one of a series of requirements for a drug. The capability to screen massive numbers of compounds has increased dramatically over the past 10–15 years, yet no corresponding increase in successfully launched drugs has ensued. As discussed in Chapter 9, there are required pharmacokinetic properties and absence of toxic effects that must be features of a therapeutic entity. As more attention was paid to absorption, distribution, metabolism, and excretion (ADME) properties of chemical screening libraries, toxicity, lack of therapeutic efficacy, and differentiation from currently marketed drugs have become the major problems. As shown in Figure 11.1, the number of new drug entities over the years has decreased. This particular representation is normalized against the increasing costs of drug discovery and development, but it does reflect some debilitating trends in the drug discovery process. Undue reliance on robotic screening using simplistic single gene target approaches (inappropriate reliance on the genome as an instruction booklet for new drugs) coupled with a de-emphasis of pharmacological training may have combined to cause the current deficit in new drugs [2]. The lack of success in drug discovery is reflected in the number of drugs that have failed in the transition from Phase II clinical trials (trial in a small number of patients designed to determine efficacy and acute side effects) to Phase III clinical trials (larger trials meant to predict effects in overall populations and determine overall risk-to-benefit ratio of a drug); see Figure 11.2. While 62 to 66% of new drugs entering Phase I passed from Phase II to Phase III in the years 1995 to 1997, this percentage fell to 45% in 2001–2002 [3]. In view of the constantly increasing number of new drugs offered for clinical trial, this suggests that the quality of molecules presented to the clinic is diminishing compared to that seen 10 years ago.

At the heart of the strategies for drug discoveries are two fundamentally different approaches; one focusing on the target, in which a molecule is found to interact with a

T. P. Kenakin: A Pharmacology Primer, Fourth edition. DOI: http://dx.doi.org/10.1016/B978-0-12-407663-1.00011-9
© 2014 Elsevier Inc. All rights reserved.

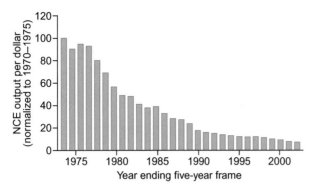

FIGURE 11.1 Histograms show the number of new drugs (normalized for the cost of drug discovery and development in the years they were developed) as a function of the years they were discovered and developed. Adapted from [1].

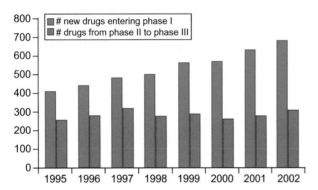

FIGURE 11.2 Histograms showing the number of new drug entities entering Phase I clinical development (blue bars) and, concomitantly, the number entering Phase III development, as a function of year. Adapted from [2].

single biological target thought to be pivotal to the disease process, and one focusing on the complete system. It is worth considering these separately.

11.2 TARGET-BASED DRUG DISCOVERY

A target-based strategy for drug discovery has also been referred to as a *reductionist approach*. The term originates in physics, where it describes complex matter at the level of fundamental particles. In drug discovery, *target-based* refers to the fact that the responsible entity for a pathological process or disease is thought to be a single gene product (or small group of defined gene products) and is based on the premise that isolation of that gene product in a system is the most efficient and least ambiguous method of determining an active molecule for the target. Reductionist approaches are best suited for "me too" molecules with well-validated targets when the first in class already exists. They also are well suited to Mendelian diseases such as cystic fibrosis and sickle cell anemia, where the inheritance of a single gene mutation can be linked to the disease.

Reductionist systems most often are recombinant ones with the target of interest (for example, human G protein coupled receptor [GPCR] expressed in a surrogate cell). The nature of the cell is thought to be immaterial, since the cell is simply a unit reporting activation of the target of interest. For example, belief that peptic ulcer healing is facilitated by blockade of histamine H2 receptor-induced acid secretion suggests a reductionist system involving antagonism of histamine response in surrogate cells transfected with human histamine H2 receptors. In this case, refining primary activity when the target-based activity disease relationship has been verified is a useful strategy. It can also be argued that considerable value may be mined in this approach, since "first in class" often is not "best in class."

Focusing in on a single target may be a way of treating a disease, but not necessarily of curing it. The interplay of multiple genes and the environment leads to complex diseases such as diabetes mellitus, coronary artery disease, rheumatoid arthritis, and asthma. To consider this latter disease, it is known that bronchial asthma is the result of airway hyper-reactivity that itself is the result of multiple system breakdowns involving allergic sensitization, failure of neuronal and hormonal balance to airway smooth muscle, and hyper-reactivity of smooth muscle. Bronchial spasm can be overcome by a system override such as powerful β-adrenergic muscle relaxation, providing a life-saving treatment, but this does not address the origins of the disease, nor does it cure it. The divergence in Phase II from Phase III studies shown in Figure 11.2 is cited as evidence that the target approach is yielding molecules, but that they may be the wrong molecules for curing (or even treating) the disease.

Whereas in physics, the path from the fundamental particle to the complex matter is relatively linear (reductionism requires linearity and additivity), in biology it often is extremely nonlinear. This can be because of system-specific modifications of genes and highly complex interactions at the level of the cell integration of the genes. This can lead to some impressive disconnections; for example, the principal defect in type I diabetes is well known but targeted approaches have still been unable to cure the disease. In theory, pathways can be identified in disease processes, critical molecules in those pathways identified, prediction of the effects of interference with the function of those molecules determined, and the effect of this process on the disease process observed. However, this simple progression can be negated if many such pathways interact in a nonlinear manner during the course of the disease. In fact, in some cases the design of a surrogate system based on the target may be counterproductive. For example, for anticancer drugs, the test system tumors are sometimes chosen or genetically manipulated for sensitivity to drugs. This can make the models overpredictive of drug activity in wild-type tumors where multiple pathways may be affected by numerous accumulated mutations

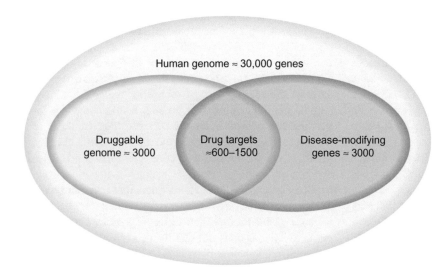

FIGURE 11.3 Venn diagram indicating the human genome and the subsets of genes thought to mediate disease and those that are druggable (thought to be capable of influence by small molecules, i.e., proteins). The intersection of the subsets comprises the set that should be targeted by drug discovery. Adapted from [5].

and/or chromosomal abnormalities used to maintain their phenotype. A classic example of where a single target fails to emulate the properties of diseases is in the therapy of psychiatric disorders. These diseases have a shortage of validated targets (it is unlikely that there are single gene lesions accounting for psychiatric disorders), and the high-throughput screening systems bear little resemblance to the *in vivo* pathology. Genetic approaches in psychiatry are problematic since the effects of "nurture" and epigenetic changes (identical genotypes yielding different phenotypes) are prevalent. In addition, animal models cannot be transposed to Phase I and Phase II clinical testing. In the clinic, placebo effects can approach 60% (in anxiety and depression studies), and inappropriate inclusion of patients clouds the interpretation of data. In general, it is extremely difficult to use a single gene product as a target for psychiatric diseases, making a reductionist approach in this realm impractical [4].

The preclinical process of drug discovery can roughly be divided into three stages. The first is the *discovery phase*, which involves the identification of a valid therapeutic target (i.e., receptor), the development of a pharmacological assay for that target, and the screening of large numbers of molecules in the search for initial activity. The next is the *lead optimization phase*, where chemical analogs of the initial lead molecule are made and tested in either the screening assay or a related assay thought to reflect the therapeutically desired activity. From this stage of the process comes the optimized lead molecule that has sufficient activity and also no obvious non-druglike properties that would preclude development to a candidate for clinical study. In this phase the pharmacokinetic properties of the candidates are of particular interest. The third phase is the *clinical development phase*, where the main issue is choice of an appropriate representative of the lead series to be tested in the clinic. In terms of strategies for drug development, the latter two

steps are common to all modes, that is, screening and lead optimization are required. However, the target validation step is unique to target-based drug discovery.

Once a target-based approach is embarked upon, the choice of target is the first step. In biological systems, there are generally four types of macromolecules that can interact with druglike molecules: proteins, polysaccharides, lipids, and nucleic acids. As discussed in Chapter 1, by far the richest source of targets for drugs is proteins. The sequencing of the human genome was completed in April 2003, and the outcome predicts that, of the estimated 30,000 genes in the human genome, approximately 3,000 code for proteins that bind druglike molecules [5]. Of the estimated 3,000 to 10,000 disease-related genes [6,7], knockout studies (animals bred to be devoid of a specific naturally occurring gene) indicate that 10% of these genes have the potential to be disease modifying. From these estimates, it can be proposed that there are potentially 600–1,500 small molecule drug targets as yet undiscovered (see Figure 11.3) [5].

11.2.1 Target Validation and the Use of Chemical Tools

A detailed discussion of the science of target validation is beyond the scope of this book, but some of the general concepts will be illustrated by example. Evidence of the relevance of a target in a given disease can be pharmacologic and/or genetic. For example, the chemokine receptor CCR5 has been described as the critical target for M-tropic HIV entry into healthy cells (*vide infra*). It is useful to examine the data supporting this idea as an illustration of how these lines of evidence converge to validate a target. One line of evidence to support this is co-location of the target with sensitivity to the disease. Thus, it is known that CCR5 receptors must be present on the cell membrane for HIV infection to occur [8,9]. Similarly, removal of CCR5 from the cell membrane *in vitro* leads to resistance to M-tropic HIV [10]. Another line of evidence is *in vitro* data which show that ligands for CCR5, such as natural chemokines and chemokine small molecule antagonists, interfere with HIV infection [11–15]. This effect extends *in vivo*, where it has been shown that individuals with high levels of circulating chemokines (ligands for CCR5) have a decreased progression to AIDS [16,17]. Similarly, patients with herpes virus 6 (HHV-6) have increased levels of chemokine, and this leads to suppression of HIV replication [18].

Genetic evidence can be powerful for target validation. For example, an extremely useful finding from genetic evidence are data to indicate the effects of a long-term absence of the target. For CCR5, this is the most compelling evidence to show that this protein is the target for HIV. Specifically, individuals with a mutation leading to lack of expression of operative CCR5 receptors (Δ32 CCR5 allele) are highly resistant to HIV infection. These individuals are otherwise completely healthy, indicating that a drug therapy to render this target inoperative should not be detrimental to the host [19–23]. Often these types of data are obtained in genetically modified animals, for example, a knockout mouse where genetic therapy leaves the mouse devoid of the target from birth. In the case of CCR5, the knockout mouse is healthy, indicating the benign consequences of removal of this receptor [24]. Complementary genetic evidence also is available to show that AIDS patients possessing a CCR5 promoter ($-$2450A/G leading to high cellular expression levels of CCR5) have a highly accelerated progression toward death [25]. In general, the data for CCR5 serve as an excellent example of where pharmacological and genetic evidence combine to thoroughly validate a therapeutic target.

Genetic knockout animals can also be used to identify pathways relevant to pathological phenotypes. For example, a number of inbred strains of mice develop lesions and lipid plaques when they are fed a diet that promotes hyperlipidemia. However, knockout mice lacking the major carrier of plasma cholesterol, apolipoprotein E, spontaneously form plaques on a *normal* diet, thereby implicating a role for cholesterol in cardiovascular disease. Gene knockout animals can be used to explore phenotypes resulting from the removal of a given target. Thus, central nervous system (CNS)-target expression of regulator of G protein Gi protein (RGS-I) $G_q\alpha$ protein leads to tremulousness, decreased body mass, heightened response to the 5-HT$_{2C}$ receptor agonist RO60–0175 (which induces anorexia), and convulsions to the 5-HT$_{2A}$ receptor agonists 2,5-dimethoxy-4-iodoamphetamine and muscarinic agonist pilocarpine (at concentrations that are ineffective in normal mice) [26].

Another approach to target validation is through chemical tool compounds. A reductionist view of drug discovery is premised on the fact that a single gene product (or small collection of identifiable gene products) is responsible for a given disease. There are numerous untestable assumptions made in this process, and if unchecked, the final test becomes a very expensive one; namely, the clinical testing of a drug molecule. A large part of the expense of this process results from the fact that the test molecule must be a drug, that is, there are numerous criteria that a molecule must pass to be become a "drug" candidate, and this constitutes much effort and expense *en route* to the final testing of the reductionist hypothesis. The use of chemical tools that may not qualify as drug candidates may substantially reduce the effort and expense of this process, that is, use of a molecule with target activity that does not qualify as a drug *per se* to test the disease target-link hypothesis. Such hypothesis testing molecules may be parenterally administered (obviating the need for oral absorption) and the results assessed on a timescale that may avoid longer-term toxicity problems. For example, the natural product staurosporine, not a drug in its own right, provided useful information regarding tyrosine kinase inhibition in cancer leading to the anticancer drug imatinib (inhibitor of BCR-ABL tyrosine kinase). A classic example of tool compound validation (although unintended) is the progression of histamine H2 receptor antagonists for the treatment of ulcer. In this case, the data obtained with the ultimately unsuitable compounds burimamide and metiamide led to the clinically useful drug cimetidine. Chemical tools have intrinsic advantages over genetic approaches since the latter can adequately answer questions of removal of gene function, but not gain of function. Chemical tools can approach both loss and gain of function. To determine whether the addition of gene activity is involved in disease, an agonist of the gene product is required, a role that can be fulfilled by a chemical tool. This has led to the terms *chemical genetics* or *chemical genomics* for the use of molecules to determine the relevance of gene products in disease. A shortcoming of this approach is that molecules are usually not exquisitely selective (as genetic knockouts are), leading to some ambiguity in the analysis of results.

The requirement for target validation can be a serious limitation of target-based strategies. In addition to being a high resource requirement (estimates suggest three years and US $390 million per target), target validation has intrinsic hazards in terms of equating the data with a conclusion that the given target is the causative factor of (or even intimately related to) a disease. One of the mainstays of target validation is the observation of animal health and behavior after the gene controlling the target of interest is knocked out. However, a problem with this strategy is the different genomic background that the organism is exposed to when the gene is eliminated from birth as opposed to when it is eliminated by a drug in adult life. Removing the gene from birth may bring into effect compensating mechanisms that allow the organism to survive; these may not be operative (or there may not be enough time for them to compensate) in adult life upon sudden elimination of the target. For example, while it is known that humans containing the Δ32 CCR5 mutation, which prevents cell surface expression of CCR5, are otherwise healthy, it still is not certain that elimination of CCR5 with CCR5-based HIV entry inhibitors to adult AIDS patients will not cause abnormalities in chemotaxis. The induction of compensatory mechanisms can substantially be overcome by the construction of conditional knockouts, whereby inducible promoters are used to produce tissue-dependent and/or time-dependent knockout after animal development.

In general, systems achieve robustness with redundancy (i.e., several isoenzymes catalyze the same reaction), making the interaction with a single target of questionable value. Also, the use of mouse knockouts brings in obvious questions as to species-dependent differences between humans and mice ("mice are not men," [27]). Animal studies in general have been shown not to be infallible predictors of clinical activity in humans. For example, preclinical studies in animals indicated that antagonists of the neurokinin NK_1 receptor attenuate nociceptive responses; studies with nonsteroidal anti-inflammatory drugs (NSAIDs) indicate that this should be a predictor of analgesic activity in humans. However, unlike NSAIDs, the NK_1 activity in animals does not transfer into an analgesic activity in humans [28].

It is prudent to not treat target validation as a single answer type of experiment, that is, if the appropriate data indicate that the target is "validated," then no further examination is required. As with all hypothesis testing, theories cannot be proven correct, only incorrect. The fact that data are obtained to support the notion that a given target is involved in a disease does not prove that interference with that target will influence the disease. Target

validation is an ongoing process that really does not end until the drug is tested in the actual disease state in patients with a properly controlled clinical trial.

Finally, another consideration in target selection and subsequent prosecution of a biological target is random variation in gene expression leading to slightly modified proteins; these could be devastating to drug activity. An antagonist of the chemokine receptor CCR5 can be a very potent antagonist of HIV entry. However, the HIV viral coat protein undergoes frequent mutation so, in essence, there are a multitude of targets involved. As seen in Figure 11.4, the potency of the CCR5 antagonist SCH 351125 for various strains of HIV varies with clade, indicating the effects of genetic mutation of the viral coat recognition protein [29]. It can be seen that there is considerable variability due to polymorphism (a 20-fold range of potency of the antagonist on USA clade B, and a 500-fold difference from Russian HIV clade G). Thus it can be seen that the therapeutic systems for which a given drug is required to have activity may differ considerably from the available test system used to develop the drug. Receptor polymorphisms can also create subpopulations of patients for drugs. For example, β_2-adrenoceptor agonists are widely used for acute opening of constricted airways in asthma. However, polymorphism in human β_2-adrenoceptors can cause reductions in clinical efficacy, because some mutations render the receptor much less sensitive to β_2-agonists (see Figure 11.5) [30].

11.2.2 Recombinant Systems

Once a target is validated to a point where it is thought worthy of pharmacological pursuit, a pharmacological assay to screen molecules for potential biological activity must be either found or engineered. Historically, receptor activity has been monitored in isolated tissues from

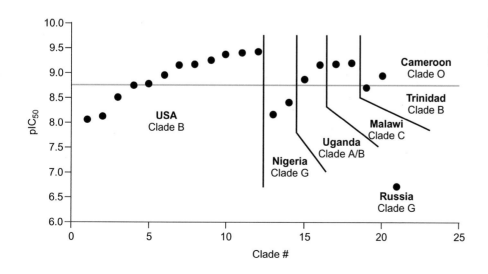

FIGURE 11.4 The activity of maraviroc (pIC_{50} values) in clades of HIV from various regions of the world. Drawn from [29].

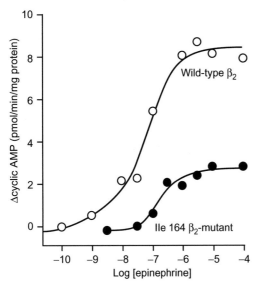

FIGURE 11.5 β-adrenoceptor-mediated cyclic AMP increases to epinephrine in transfected CHW-cells expressing wild-type β_2-adrenoceptors (open circles) and Ile164 β_2-mutant receptors. Redrawn from [30].

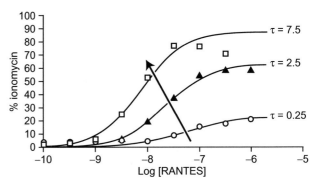

FIGURE 11.6 Calcium transient responses to chemokine agonist RANTES activating CCR5 receptors transduced into U2OS cells with the BacMam virus system. Three expression levels for receptor are shown. Data fit to the operational model with common values for $K_A = 50$ nM: $\tau = 0.25$ (open circles), $\tau = 2.5$ (filled triangles), and $\tau = 7.5$ (open squares) corresponding to increases in receptor expression levels of 1:10:30. Data courtesy of C. Watson, Discovery Research, GlaxoSmithKline.

animals; these systems necessitated extrapolations across species and were less than optimal (see Chapter 1). However, with the advent of technologies that enable the surrogate expression of human genes in cultured cells, a completely new paradigm of therapeutic drug discovery was born. Presently, host cells in culture can be transfected with human cDNA for biological targets. These cells then can be subjected to large-scale exposure to molecules, and the physiological functions controlled by the particular targets can be monitored for changes in physiological activity. One of the most versatile technologies for this is baculovirus expression vectors engineered to contain mammalian cell-active promoter elements. Baculoviruses, while able to replicate in insect cells, cannot do so in mammalian cells to cause infection, making them safe for use in laboratories. The virus has little to no cytopathic effect and can readily be manipulated to accommodate large pieces of foreign DNA [31]. This technology is extremely convenient, in that the level of receptor (or other transduced protein) can be controlled by the amount of virus added to the cells in culture. For example, Figure 11.6 shows the effect of transduction of U2OS cells with increasing amounts of baculovirus containing DNA for CCR5 receptors. Modeling the responses to RANTES (regulated on activation, normal T cell expressed and secreted) in this system indicates that there is a 30-fold functional increase in the receptor expression in this experiment. Such ability to control receptor levels is extremely valuable in the lead optimization process to assess the affinity of agonists (see Chapter 8) and relative efficacy with the operational model.

In general, the use of recombinant systems is very valuable in a target-based approach to drug discovery. However, while the versatility of such systems is

extremely powerful, it should be recognized that the numerous interconnections of cellular pathways and the influence of cellular milieu on signaling targets may make the reconstruction of therapeutic physiological systems impractical. This can be illustrated by examining the possibilities involved in constructing a GPCR recombinant system (Figure 11.7). In the case of GPCRs, the immediate reacting partner for the receptor is a G-protein, or in the case of pleiotropic receptors, a collection of G-proteins. In this latter scenario, it may not be evident exactly which single or combination of G-proteins is therapeutically relevant, and construction of a recombinant system theoretically could bias a test system to an irrelevant G-protein. Similarly, the relative stoichiometry of the reactants (receptors and G-proteins) is important in determining the primary signaling characteristics of a functional system. The physiologically relevant stoichiometry may not be known. In this regard, as well as relative stoichiometry, the absolute stoichiometry may be important in terms of controlling the overall sensitivity of the system to agonism or production of constitutive activity to demonstrate inverse agonism. Finally, it should be noted that a recombinant test system most likely will not have the pathophysiological tone that diseased tissues have, thereby leading to possible dissimulations between the test and therapeutic system. For these reasons, it is evident that attempts at absolute recreation of therapeutic systems for drug testing most likely will be futile.

11.2.3 Defining Biological Targets

In a target-based system, the chemical end point is clearly defined; that is, a molecule with a desired (agonism, antagonism) activity on the biological target. In some cases, the target may be clearly defined – as for the

Receptor genotype

Receptor phenotype

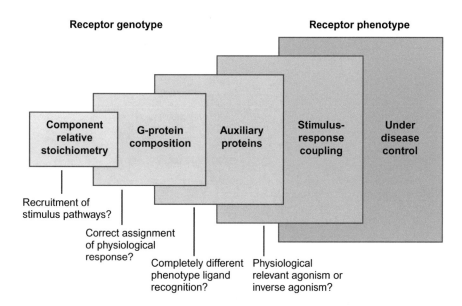

Component relative stoichiometry

G-protein composition

Auxiliary proteins

Stimulus-response coupling

Under disease control

Recruitment of stimulus pathways?

Correct assignment of physiological response?

Completely different phenotype ligand recognition?

Physiological relevant agonism or inverse agonism?

FIGURE 11.7 **Schematic diagram of the layers of construction of a recombinant GPCR cell assay system.** The correct receptor must be transfected into the cell containing the correct G-proteins in the physiologically relevant stoichiometries. The absolute levels of receptor and G-protein will control the sensitivity (with respect to low-level agonism of low-efficacy agonists and/or constitutive activity for inverse agonists). At each step, the recombinant system may differ from the therapeutically relevant natural system. Finally, the therapeutic system is under pathological control, whereas the recombinant system does not have this property.

BCR-ABL kinase inhibitor Gleevec, which inhibits a constitutively active kinase known to be present only in patients with chronic myelogenous leukemia. In other cases, the endogenous players for a biological target may not be known, yet a synthetic molecule with activity on the target still may be thought to be of value (orphan receptors). Also, there are combinations of biological targets that could themselves become new phenotypic targets (i.e., homodimers, heterodimers) and combinations of targets and accessory proteins that could constitute a new target. It is worth considering all these ideas in the context of the definition of a therapeutically relevant biological target.

Targets that have no known endogenous ligands are known as "orphan" receptors, and there are still many such receptors in the genome. A process of "de-orphanization," either with techniques such as reverse pharmacology (*in silico* searches of databases to match sequences with known receptors) or with ligand fishing with compound collections and tissue extracts, has been implemented over the past 10 years, yielding a list of newly discovered pairings of ligands and receptors (see Table 11.1). As chemical tools for such receptors are discovered, they can be used in a chemical genomic context to associate these receptors with diseases.

Once an endogenous ligand for a target is known, there may still be physiological mechanisms that create texture with that target which may not be captured in a recombinant system. Biological phenotype overrides genotype, as a single gene can be expressed in different host cells and take on different functions and sensitivities to molecules. One such mechanism is homo- or heterodimerization of receptors.

For proteins such as tyrosine kinase receptors, dimerization (the association of two receptors to form a new

species in the membrane) is a well-known mechanism of action [33]. Increasingly, this has also been shown for GPCRs, and evidence suggests that this phenomenon may be relevant to drug discovery [34]. The relevance comes from the acquisition of new drug-sensitive phenotypes for existing receptors upon dimerization. These new phenotypes can take the form of increased sensitivity to agonists. For example, recombinant systems containing transfected angiotensin II receptors can be insensitive to angiotensin (subthreshold level of receptor expression) until bradykinin receptors are co-transfected into the system. When this occurs, the angiotensin response appears (angiotensin sensitivity increases through the formation of an angiotensin—bradykinin receptor heterodimer); see Figure 11.8A [35]. Such heterodimerization may have relevance to the observation that an increased number of bradykinin receptors and angiotensin—bradykinin receptor heterodimers are present in women with pre-eclampsia (a malady associated with abnormal vasoconstriction) [36]. Similarly, chemokines show a 10- to 100-fold increased potency on a heterodimer of CCR2 and CCR5 receptors than with either receptor alone [37]. Oligomerization can be especially prevalent among some receptor types such as chemokine or opioid receptors. A historical mystery in the opioid field had been the question of how only three genes for opioid receptors could foster so many opioid receptor phenotypes in tissues (defined as $\mu 1$, $\mu 2$, $\delta 1$, $\delta 2$, $\kappa 1$, $\kappa 2$, $\kappa 3$), until it became clear that opioid receptor heterodimerization accounted for the diversity. This latter receptor family illustrates another possible therapeutic application of dimerization, namely the acquisition of new drug sensitivity. For example, the agonist 6'-guanidinoaltrindole (6'-GNTI) produces no agonist response at δ-opioid receptors and very little at κ-opioid receptors. However, this agonist produces powerful responses on the heterodimer

TABLE 11.1 De-Orphanized Receptors for Cardiovascular Function

Orphan Receptor	Ligand	Cardiovascular Effect
UT (GPR14, SENR)	Urotensin II	Vasoconstriction, cardiac inotropy
Mas	Angiotensin (1-7)	Anti-diureses, vasorelaxation
GPR66 (TGR1, FM3)	Neuromedin U	Regional vasoconstriction, inotropy
APJ	Apelin	Vasoconstriction, cardiac inotropy
PTH2	TIP-39	Renal vasodilatation
GPR10 (GE3, UHR-1)	Prolactin rel. peptide	Regulation of BP
OXR (HFGAN72)	Orexin A,B	Regulation of BP
GPR103 (HLWAR77)	RF-amides	Regulation of BP
TA	Trace amines (tyramine)	Vasoconstriction
GPR38	Motilin	Vasodilatation
GHS-R	Ghrelin	Vasodilatation
LGR7,8	Relaxin	Cardiac inotropy, vasodilatation
CRF1/2	Urocortin	Vasodilatation
edg-1 (LPB1)	Sphingosine-1-phosphate	PLC, MAPK activation
edg-2,4,7 (LPA1−3)	Lysophosphatidic acid	DNA synthesis
G2A	Lysophosphatidylcholine	Macrophage function
P2Y12 (SP1999)	ADP	Platelet aggregation
HM74/-A	Nicotinic acid	Lipid lowering, anti-lipolytic
GOR40	Medium chain fatty acids	Insulin regulation
AdipoR1,R2	Adiponectin	Fatty acid metabolism

From [32].

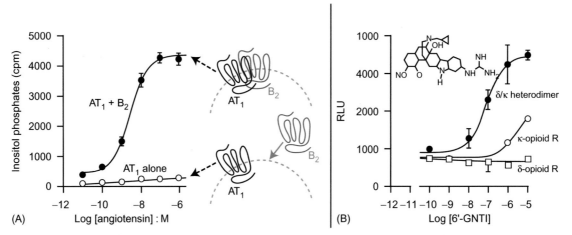

FIGURE 11.8 Acquisition of drug phenotype with receptor heterodimerization. (A) Cells transfected with a subthreshold level of angiotensin I receptor (no response to angiotensin; open circles) demonstrate response to the same concentrations of angiotensin upon co-transfection of bradykinin 1 receptors (filled circles). Redrawn from [35]. (B) The opioid agonist 6′-guanidinonaltrindole (6′-GNTI) produces no response in human embryonic kidney cells transfected with δ-opioid receptors (open squares) and little response on cells transfected with κ-opioid receptors (open circles). However, co-transfection of δ- and κ-opioid receptors produces a system responsive to 6′-GNTI (filled circles). Redrawn from [38].

TABLE 11.2 Homo- and Hetero-dimeric Receptors

A. Homo-Oligomers

adenosine A1	histamine H_2	somatostatin $SSTR_{1B}$
AT_1 angiotensin II	luteinizing horm./hCG	somatostatin $SSTR_{1C}$
β_2-adrenoceptor	melatonin MT_1	somatostatin $SSTR_{2A}$
bradykinin B_2	melatonin MT_2	thyrotropin
chemokine CCR2	muscarinic Ach M_2	vasopressin V_2
chemokine CCR5	muscarinic Ach M_3	IgG hepta
chemokine CXCR4	μ-opioid	gonadotropin rel. horm.
dopamine D_1	-opioid	metabotropic $mGluR_1$
dopamine D_2	κ-opioid	metabotropic $mGluR_2$
dopamine D_3	serotonin $5\text{-}HT_{1B}$	Ca^{2+} sensing
histamine H_1	serotonin $5\text{-}HT_{1D}$	$GABA_{B(2)}$
$GABA_{B(1)}$	somatostatin $SSTR_{1A}$	

B. Hetero-Oligomers

$5\text{-}HT_{1B}$	plus	$5\text{-}HT_{1D}$	$SSTR_{2A}$	plus	$SSTR_{1B}$
adenosine A_1	plus	dopamine D_1	$SSTR_{1A}$	plus	μ-opioid
adenosine A_1	plus	$mGluR_1$	$SSTR_{1A}$	plus	$SSTR_{1C}$
adenosince A_1	plus	purinergic $P2Y_1$	$SSTR_{1B}$	plus	dopamine D_2
adenosine A_2	plus	dopamine D_2	T1R1 a.a. taste	plus	T1R3 a.a. taste
angiotensin AT_1	plus	angiotensin AT_2	T1R2 a.a. taste	plus	T1R3 a.a. taste
CCR2	plus	CCR5	-opioid	plus	κ-opioid
dopamine D_2	plus	dopamine D_3	μ-opioid	plus	-opioid
$GABA_{B(1)}$	plus	$GABA_{B(2)}$	-opioid	plus	β_2-adrenoceptor
muscarinic M_2	plus	muscarinic M_3	k-opioid	plus	β_2-adrenoceptor
melatonin MT_1	plus	melatonin MT_2			

From [34].

of δ- and κ-opioid receptors (see Figure 11.8B) [38]. Interestingly, the responses to 6′-GNTI are blocked by antagonists for either δ- or κ-opioid receptors. Moreover, 6′-GNTI produces analgesia only when administered into the spinal cord, demonstrating that the dimerization is organ specific, and that reductions in side effects of agonists (and antagonists) may be achieved through targeting receptor dimers. In the case of 6′-GNTI, reduced side effects with spinal analgesia is the projected drug phenotype.

The systematic study of drug profiles on receptor dimers is difficult, although controlled expression of receptor levels through technologies such as the baculovirus expression system (see Figure 11.6) provides a practical means to begin to do so. The study of receptor association also is facilitated by technologies such as bioluminescence resonance energy transfer (BRET) and fluorescence resonance energy transfer (FRET) [39]. BRET monitors energy transfer between a bioluminescent donor and a fluorescent acceptor (each on a C-terminal tail of a GPCR) as the two are brought together through dimerization. This technique requires no excitation light source and is ideal for monitoring the real-time interaction of GPCR interaction in cells. FRET enables observation of energy transfer between two fluorophores bound in close proximity to each other. The change in energy is dependent upon the distance between the donor and acceptor fluorophores to the sixth power, making the method sensitive to very small changes in distance (see Figure 11.36). When the fluorophores are placed on the C-terminal end of GPCRs, interaction between receptors can be detected. As homo- and hetero-dimerization is studied, the list of receptors observed to utilize this mechanism is growing; Table 11.2 shows a partial list of the receptors known to form dimers with themselves (Table 11.2A) or other receptors (Table 11.2B). The list of phenotypes associated with these dimerization processes is also increasing. With the emergence of receptor dimers as possible therapeutic targets have developed parallel ideas about dimerized ligands (see Section 11.5).

Drug targets can be complexes made up of more than one gene product (i.e., integrins, nicotinic acetylcholine ion channels). Thus, each combination of targets could be considered a target in itself [40]. Some of these phenotypes may be the result of protein-protein receptor interactions [41−43]. For example, the human calcitonin receptor has a distinct profile of sensitivity to and selectivity for various agonists. Figure 11.9A shows the relative potency of the human calcitonin receptor to the agonists human calcitonin and rat amylin; it can be seen that human

calcitonin is a 20-fold more potent agonist for this receptor than is rat amylin [41]. When the antagonist AC66 is used to block responses, both agonists are uniformly sensitive to blockade ($pK_B = 9.7$; Figure 11.9B). However, when the protein RAMP3 (receptor activity modifying protein type 3) is co-expressed with the receptor in this cell, the sensitivity to agonists and antagonists completely changes. As seen in Figure 11.9C, the rank order of potency of human calcitonin and rat amylin reverses, such that rat amylin is now threefold more potent than human calcitonin. Similarly, the sensitivity of responses to AC66 is reduced by a factor of seven when amylin is used as the agonist ($pK_B = 8.85$; Figure 11.9D). It can be seen from these data that the phenotype of the receptor changes when the cellular milieu into which the receptor is expressed

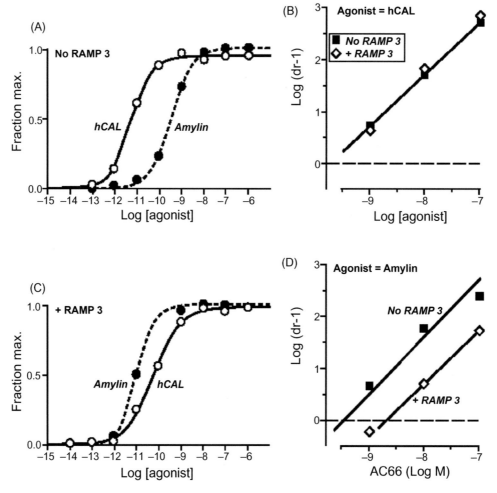

FIGURE 11.9 **Assumption of a new receptor phenotype for the human calcitonin receptor upon co-expression with the protein RAMP3.** (A) Melanophores transfected with cDNA for human calcitonin receptor type 2 show a distinct sensitivity pattern to human calcitonin and rat amylin; hCAL is 20-fold more potent than rat amylin. (B) A distinct pattern of sensitivity to the antagonist AC66 also is observed; both agonists yield a pK_B for AC66 of 9.7. (C) Co-expression of the protein RAMP3 (receptor activity modifying protein type 3) completely changes the sensitivity of the receptor to the agonists. The rank order is now changed such that amylin has a threefold greater potency than human calcitonin. (D) This change in phenotype is carried over into the sensitivity to the antagonist. With co-expression of RAMP3, the pK_B for AC66 changes to 8.85 when rat amylin is used as the agonist. Data redrawn from [41].

changes. RAMP3 is one of a family of proteins that affect the transport, export, and drug sensitivity of receptors in different cells. The important question for the drug development process is this: If a given receptor target is thought to be therapeutically relevant, what is the correct phenotype for screening? As can be seen from the example with the human calcitonin receptor, if a RAMP3 phenotype for the receptor is the therapeutically relevant phenotype, then screening in a system without RAMP3 co-expression would not be useful.

11.3 SYSTEMS-BASED DRUG DISCOVERY

With a target-based approach, the activity of molecules interacting with the previously identified target of interest can readily be assessed. As discussed previously, such an approach requires a linear relationship between targets and cellular activity. If pathways interact in a complex and nonlinear fashion, then redundancy and feedback effects may make predictions from single targets difficult and erroneous. A major criticism of target approaches is that they stray from a relatively tried and true successful historical strategy in drug research, whereby discovery relied upon proven physiology and/or pathophysiology and appropriate models. Another more pragmatic criticism of target-based strategies is that, while they yield drugs for targets, this activity does not necessarily translate to overall clinical utility (see Figures 11.1 and 11.2).

An alternative to target-based strategies is referred to as *systems-based drug discovery*. The study of the assembled cellular system has evolved into "systems biology," whereby natural cells are used for screening, and complex outputs, ranging from secreted cellular products to genomic data, are utilized to measure system responses to drugs. The term originated in engineering, where it describes a theoretical framework for controlling a complicated system, for example, flying an airplane. The assembly of genes into living cells creates an infinitely richer pallet for potential intervention:

Move over human genome, your day in the spotlight is coming to a close. The genome ... contains only the recipes for making proteins ... it's the proteins that constitute the bricks and mortar of cells and that do most of the work.
— Carol Ezzell, *Scientific American*, April 2002.

Systems approaches may yield more abundant opportunities for drug discovery. In organs under the control of pathological mechanisms, genes can interact to provide multifactorial phenotypes; this can greatly expand the possible targets for drugs. Therefore, the study of the same target in its therapeutic environment can enrich the recognition possibilities for new drugs, in essence increasing the biological space of that target [40].

There is a fundamental difference between the target-based approach, where a very large number of compounds are screened against one target, versus a systems approach, where a smaller number of compounds (but perhaps higher-quality, more druglike molecules) are screened in a system that has many targets. Systems can have a great many (possibly hundreds) small molecule intervention sites and be engineered to incorporate many disease-relevant pathways. The output of such systems can be extremely complex and requires high-throughput genomic tools and technologies to process. The development of sophisticated computing tools as well as the advancement of genetic technology has facilitated the construction of biological systems for screening and the study of structure-activity relationships. Specifically, the use of the short interfering RNA (siRNA) duplex molecules that can be used to silence specific genes in the cell allows the observation of their relevance to total cellular function (Figure 11.10A). This approach is vulnerable to biological redundancy in the system, but overexpression of targets in the cell also can be used in conjunction with siRNA approaches to identify and characterize pathways. Analysis of multiple readouts of cellular function then acts as a fingerprint for the particular silenced portion of a pathway; as multiple histograms viewed from the top and color-coded for response, these outputs form a heatmap for cell function that can be used to compare control conditions and the effects of drugs (Figure 11.10B).

In general, systems allow the identification of unknown (and previously hidden) drug activity and/or can add texture to known drug activity. This can lead to the identification of new uses for existing targets, identification of new targets (so-called "therapeutic target space," involving discovery of a molecular phenotype in a system and subsequent determination of the molecular target), and determination of an entry point into signaling cascades that may be amenable to drug intervention (optimize efficacy and minimize side effects). Comparison of normal and diseased samples can be used to determine disease-specific signaling as a target for drug intervention. The complexity of the system's response output allows discrimination of subtle drug activities. For example, Figure 11.11 shows three levels of output from a system and the results observed for three hypothetical compounds. Compound A is inactive in the system, whereas compounds B and C block different points on the integrated pathways' cascades. The first level of output (i.e., second messenger production) does not indicate activity in any of the three ligands. It can be seen that the second level of output does not discriminate between the activity seen for compounds B and C, whereas the third (and more complex) level of output shows them to be different. In general, systems are designed to provide maximally complex outputs in different contexts (different milieu of cellular activating agents) to yield complex heatmap fingerprints

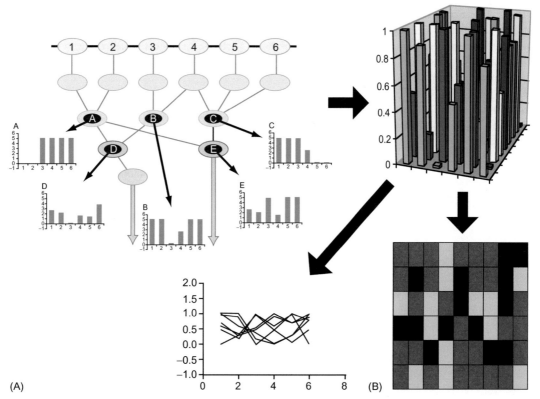

(A)

FIGURE 11.10 Study of integrated cellular pathways. (A) The activation of six extracellular targets is represented by histograms. Selective inhibition of various points along the pathways (by application of siRNA) yields characteristic patterns for the activity histograms. The letters on the sets of histograms refer to the effect of blocking the corresponding letter's intersecting point of the pathway. (B) A collection of such histograms are combined into a three-dimensional array. Multiple readouts of such arrays can be made either by showing lines for related sets of readings (for example, readings obtained for the same cellular context) or by coding the height of the various histograms with colors to form a heatmap. These two-dimensional representations become characteristic fingerprints for a given biological activity in the system.

FIGURE 11.11 Levels of complexity for response readouts of cellular systems. Extracellular targets (light blue boxes) activate intracellular networks to produce biological response. Histograms show the activity of three hypothetical compounds (coded green, blue, and red). The green compound is inactive, blue blocks an intracellular target (green pentangle labeled with oval marked B), and the red compound blocks another intracellular target (blue hexagram labeled with oval marked C). If the response is read at a primary level of response (for example, levels of intracellular second messenger), the three compounds all appear to be inactive. Readings farther down the cellular cascade detect one active compound (output level 2) and even farther down, detect the other active compound and differentiate the activity of the two active compounds (output level 3).

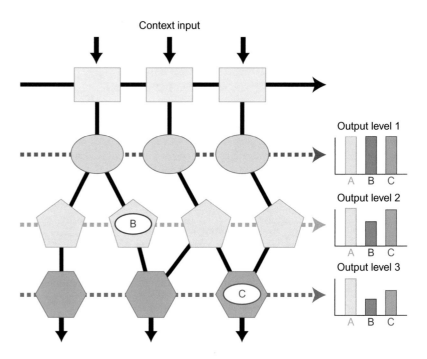

Anti-Inflammatory Testing (Arthritis/Asthma)

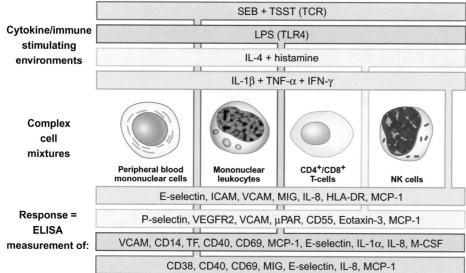

FIGURE 11.12 An example of a cellular system designed to study inflammatory processes related to asthma and arthritis. Multiple readouts (ELISA [enzyme-linked immunosorbent assay] measurements) from four cell types are obtained under conditions of four contexts (mixture of stimulating agents). This results in a complex heatmap of basal cellular activities that can be affected by compounds. The changes in the heatmap (measured as ratios of basal to compound-altered activity) are analyzed statistically to yield associations and differences.

of drug activity. Statistical methods such as multidimensional scaling are then used to associate similar profiles (define functional similarity maps) and determine differences. This gives added levels of power to screening systems and subsequent lead optimization assays. In general, integrated systems can be used to correlate functional responses with mechanistic classes of compounds, identify secondary activities for molecules, provide insight into the mechanism of action of compounds that give clinical activities, and characterize pathways and correlate them with functional phenotypes [44,45].

Cellular screening systems can be developed with primary human cells cultured in biologically relevant contexts; the outputs of these systems are focused sets of biologically relevant parameters (gene transcription, protein production). For example, vascular endothelium cells in different contexts, defined by stimulation with different proinflammatory cytokines, are used to screen for drugs of possible use in inflammatory diseases such as rheumatoid arthritis (Figure 11.12). Cellular outputs can be enhanced by overexpression to constitutively active levels. For asthma (TH2-mediated inflammation), arthritis, and autoimmune diseases (TH1-mediated disease), and transplantation (T cell driven) and cardiovascular disease-related (monocyte and endothelial cell driven) inflammatory responses, four complex cell systems can be utilized [44]. With this approach, the NF-kB signaling pathway, phosphatidylinositol 3-kinase (PI3K/Akt pathway) and RAS/mitogen-activated protein kinase (MAPK) pathways can be used to model proinflammatory activity. Measurement of surface proteins such as VCAM-1, ICAM-1, and E-selectin (vascular adhesion molecules for leukocytes); MIG/CXCL9 and IL-8/CXCL8 (chemokines that mediate

selective leukocyte recruitment); platelet-endothelial cell adhesion molecule 1/CD31 (controls leukocyte transmigration); and HLA-DR (MHC class II; the protein responsible for antigen presentation) are then used to monitor drug effect. Figure 11.12 shows the components of the system.

Integrated systems are useful to differentiate intracellular targets such as kinases; the kinome is large and the targeted ATP binding sites are very similar. In this regard, systems can show texture where there is none in isolated systems. For example, general tyrosine kinase inhibitors with poor target specificity such as AG126 and genisten; nonspecific JAK inhibitors ZM39923, WHI-P131, and AG490; and the nonselective 5-lipoxegenase inhibitors AA861 and NGDA are quite dissimilar when tested in an integrated system [44]. Systems also are useful in detecting off-target or secondary activities. For example, differences can be seen between Raf1 inhibitors BAY 43−9006, GW5074, and ZM336372 and also between casein kinase inhibitors apigenin, DRB (5,6-dichloro-1-b-D-ribofurnaosylbenzimidazole), and TBB (4,5,6,7-tetrabromo-2-aza-benzimidazole). The selective p38 MAPK inhibitors PD169316 and SB2033580 have similar potency for the primary target p38a. However, testing in an integrated system reveals significant differences between the two drugs consistent with newly detected inhibition of P-selectin expression and strong inhibition of VCAM-1, E-selectin, and IL-8 for SB203580, consistent with an off-target activity for this compound.

Systems also can reveal similarity in functional responses by mechanistically distinct drugs. For example, the activity of the mTOR antagonist rapamycin correlates with that of general PI-3 kinase inhibitors LY294002 and

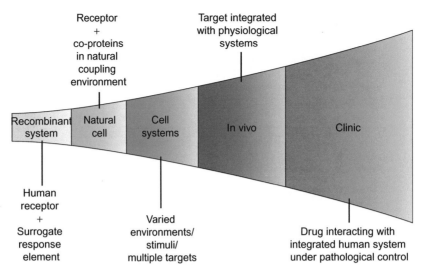

FIGURE 11.13   Increasing complexity of drug development from *in vitro* cellular systems to the clinic.

wortmannin. Similarly, nonsteroidal fungal estrogen receptor agonists zearalenone and β-zearalenol cluster activity with many p38 MAPK inhibitors. In fact, some striking mechanistic dissimilarities show like behavior in integrated systems. For example, phosphodiesterase IV inhibitors Ro-20−1724 and rolipram cluster with glucocorticoids dexamethasone, budesonide, and prednisolone; both classes of drug have shown involvement in suppression of leukocyte function.

Studying established drugs in systems can yield new biological insights into mechanisms. For example, statins targeting HMG-CoA reductase for lipid lowering show anti-inflammatory effects (reduction in the leukocyte activation antigen CD69), activity shared by other HMG-CoA inhibitors. Subsequent studies have shown that the integrated activity is the consequence of HMG-CoA inhibition and not an off-target activity. Interestingly, experiments in systems-based assays have shown different ranking of potency from isolated target potency. Specifically, the anti-inflammatory potency of statins in an integrated cellular system is cerivastatin >> atorvastatin >> simvastatin > lovastatin->> rosuvastatin >> pravastatin. However, the most potent target-based HMg-acetyl CoA (cholesterol-lowering) compounds are atorvastatin and rosuvastatin.

Clearly, as testing of candidate molecules progresses toward the clinical therapeutic end point, the complexity increases. Thus, complications ensue along the journey from biochemical studies (isolated receptors, enzymes), through recombinant cellular systems, to natural whole systems. The next level of complexity beyond these involves assays in context and *in vivo* systems (Figure 11.13). It should be noted that, while the veracity of data to the true clinical profile for a molecule increases as the testing enters into these realms, so too do the resource requirements and risk. For this reason, a paramount need in drug discovery is the collection of quality data, capable of predicting failure in these expensive systems as early as possible in the drug discovery process. It is worth discussing some unique applications of complex conditions in testing systems for drug screening and also the determination of surrogate markers for prediction of successful therapeutic activity.

11.3.1 Assays in Context

Cellular context refers to the physiological conditions present for the particular tissue of interest in a therapeutic environment. It can be important in determining the effects of drugs and, therefore, how drugs are screened and tested. For example, the signaling molecule TGF-β helps prevent the malignant transformation of cells in the breast epithelium. However, if the cells are already transformed, TGF-β enhances blood vessel formation and tumor-cell invasiveness, thereby *promoting* tumor growth and dispersion [46]. Context can be especially important *in vivo*, and this may be critical to the therapeutic use of new drugs. Some context can be discerned with knockout animals or under special physiological conditions. For example, the role of β-adrenoceptors, bradykinin B₂, prostanoid EP₂, and dopamine D₃ receptors in the control of blood pressure becomes evident only if physiological stress is applied (i.e., salt loading or exercise). For these reasons, it is important that cell models mimic conditions *in vivo* and incorporate environmental effects and cell-cell interactions.

Through "context-dependent" biological effect, increased breadth of function can be detected; additional discrimination (context-dependent activity) can be obtained by changing conditions. For example, as discussed previously, PDE-IV inhibitors and glucocorticoids

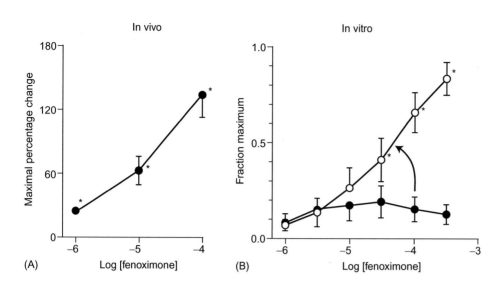

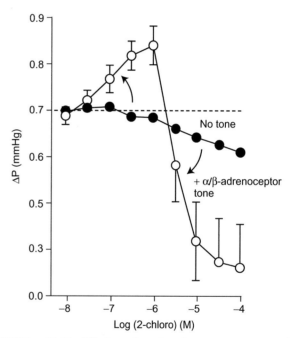

FIGURE 11.14 **Cardiovascular responses to the PDE inhibitor fenoximone in different contexts.** (A) *In vivo* effects of fenoximone in anesthetized dogs; ordinates reflect positive inotropy. Redrawn from [47]. (B) *In vitro* effects of fenoximone in guinea pig untreated isolated left atria (filled circles) and atria in the presence of subthreshold β-adrenoceptor stimulation with prenalterol (open circles). Redrawn from [48].

cluster in leukocyte-dependent systems; however, they can be differentiated in lipopolysaccharide systems under different cell stimuli. For drugs that produce an effect by modifying signaling, context can be critical. For example, the phosphodiesterase inhibitor fenoximone produces positive cardiac inotropy and can be useful for congestive heart failure; the positive inotropic effects can be observed *in vivo* [47] in a working myocardium under hormonal and transmitter control (Figure 11.14A). However, in an isolated heart *in vitro* with no such neural tone, fenoximone has no visible effect (Figure 11.14B). Fenoximone blocks the degradation of intracellular cyclic AMP, therefore increased inotropy is observed only under conditions where cyclic AMP is being produced by transmitter tone. These conditions can be simulated by adding a very low concentration of weak β-adrenoceptor agonist (in this case, prenalterol). Figure 11.14B shows the positive inotropic effect to fenoximone observed in the presence of subthreshold levels of prenalterol [48]. This defines a possible context for assays designed to potentiate cyclic AMP levels; namely, the presence of a subthreshold of β-adrenoceptor agonism. Similarly, adenosine receptors mediate renal vascular tone but mainly through the modification of the existing renal tone. Figure 11.15 shows the relative lack of effect of the adenosine agonist 2-chloroadenosine on vascular tone in a perfused kidney *in vitro*. In a different context, namely, subthreshold α-adrenoceptor vasoconstriction with methoxamine and vasodilation with forskolin (elevated cyclic AMP), 2-chloradenosine vascular effects become evident (Figure 11.15). In this case, a context of physiological vascular tone increases the effect of the modifying adenosine agonism [49].

The interplay of levels of low intrinsic efficacy compounds with levels of physiological tone is very important. For example, the effects of β-adrenoceptor partial agonist-antagonists pirbuterol, prenalterol, and pindolol

FIGURE 11.15 **Effects of adenosine receptor agonist 2-chloroadenosine on vascular perfusion pressure of isolated perfused rat kidneys.** Minor effects seen in untreated kidneys (filled circles) and pronounced vasoconstriction, while vasodilatation in kidneys co-perfused with subthreshold concentrations of α-adrenoceptor vasoconstrictor methoxamine and vasodilatory activation of adenylyl cyclase with forskolin (open circles). Redrawn from [49].

are quite different in conditions of high basal and low basal physiological tone (as altered by types of anesthesia; Figure 11.16) [50]. It can be seen that the partial agonist with the highest intrinsic efficacy (pirbuterol) produces elevated heart rate under conditions of low basal tone, and has little effect on heart rate when anesthesia produces high basal tone (Figure 11.16A). Prenalterol has a lower intrinsic efficacy and produces less tachycardia under conditions of low tone and a slight bradycardia

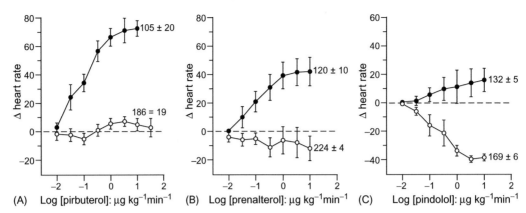

FIGURE 11.16 *In vivo* effects of β-adrenoceptor partial agonists of differing intrinsic efficacy. Changes in heart rate (increases in beats/min) shown in anesthetized cats. Chloralose-pentobarbital anesthesia (filled circles) yields low basal heart rates, while urethane-pentobarbital anesthesia (open circles) yields high basal heart rates. Responses to (in order of descending relative intrinsic efficacy) (A) pirbuterol, (B) prenalterol, and (C) pindolol. Redrawn from [50].

with high tone (Figure 11.16B). Finally, the very low intrinsic efficacy β-adrenoceptor partial agonist pindolol produces very little tachycardia with high tone and, in fact, there is profound bradycardia in conditions of high tone (Figure 11.16C). Such changes in the effects of drugs with low levels of intrinsic efficacy make prediction of therapeutic response *in vivo* difficult without data obtained in cellular context.

11.4 *IN VIVO* SYSTEMS, BIOMARKERS, AND CLINICAL FEEDBACK

Pharmacological hypotheses are the most rigorously tested in all of biological science; a potential drug molecule must emerge through the entire drug discovery and development process and be tested in humans to give a desired therapeutic effect before the initial hypothesis beginning the process can be negated or not. In keeping with the notion that systems are more predictive of eventual therapeutic worth than isolated target assays, the next step in complexity is *in vivo* models of normal physiological function and disease (Figure 11.13). Historically, drug discovery was based on animal models and natural cell systems. On one hand, the differences between species (humans and animals) was a hurdle and potential stopping point for the development of drugs for humans in such systems. On the other hand, it could be argued that testing was done in systems of proven physiology and pathology; the system was more like what the drug would encounter when it was used in the therapeutic environment. *In vivo* systems also allow observation of what a small drug molecule usually is designed to do; namely, perturb the diseased state to cause it to return to a normal state, or at least to alleviate symptoms.

The relevant phenotype for complex multifaceted diseases such as obesity, atherosclerosis, heart failure, stroke,

behavioral disorders, neurodegenerative diseases, and hypertension can be observed only *in vivo*. Historically, *in vivo* animal testing has led to the initiation of some classical treatments for disease. For example, the mode of action of the antihypertensive clonidine and subsequent elucidation of presynaptic α_2-adrenoceptors resulted from *in vivo* experimentation. Similarly, the demonstration of an orally active angiotensin converting enzyme (ACE) inhibitor showing reduced blood pressure in spontaneously hypertensive rats led to the emergence of captopril and other clinically active ACE inhibitors for hypertension. While investigation of drug effect is more complicated *in vivo*, there are tools and techniques that can be used to better derive this information. Thus, protein-specific antibodies, gene knockouts and knockins, RNA interference, and imaging techniques can provide rich information on *in vivo* processes and validation of pathways. *In vivo* experimentation can show integrated response from multiple sources, reveal unexpected results, determine therapeutic index (ratio between efficacious and toxic concentrations), help assess the importance of targets and processes identified *in vitro*, and assess pharmacokinetics and help predict clinical dosing. These obvious advantages come with a price tag of high resource requirements (Figure 11.13).

While the obvious value of *in vivo* animal models is clear, there also are instances, especially in cases of inflammatory arthritis, CNS behavior, and tumor growth, where they have failed to be predictive of useful clinical activity in humans [51]. For example, leukotriene B_4 (LTB_4) antagonists showed activity in animal models of inflammatory arthritis yet failed to be useful in rheumatoid arthritis [52]. Similarly, dopamine D_4 antagonists showed activity in animal behavior models previously predictive of dopamine D_2 antagonists in schizophrenia. However, testing of dopamine D_4 antagonists showed no efficacy in humans [53].

The ultimate *in vivo* model is humans in a controlled clinical environment, and there are considerable data to show that even complex models fail to predict clinical utility [40,54]. Increasingly it is becoming evident that the complexities of disease states modify, cancel, and change target-based drug effects, sometimes in unpredictable ways. Clinical data are extremely valuable in the assessment of both the drug in question and understanding of the relationship between the target and the disease state. Therefore, clinical feedback of these data is an essential part of the drug discovery process. The emerging field that relates to the use of clinical data in the drug discovery process is *translational medicine*. The metaphor used to describe the translational medicine process of information utilization from the clinic is that of a highway. The insights and information gained have led to the idea that, whereas in the past the drug discovery process was a one-way highway (from the bench to the clinic), it now needs to be a two-way highway, where the learnings in the clinic should be applied directly to the criteria used early on in discovery. Furthermore, the lanes of this highway need to be expanded, and much more information from the clinic needs to be considered earlier.

The next question, then, is, what is the nature of the tools available to obtain such clinical data. Imaging techniques can be used to gain insight into drug activity in a non-invasive manner. Similarly, surrogate end points (from the Latin *surrogare*: to substitute) are increasingly used, especially in cancer research, where monitoring of effects such as cell cycle, mitotic spindle separation, apoptosis, angiogenesis, and tumor invasion are relevant to the assessment of clinical value. Thus, readings of tumor shrinkage and time to disease progression can be better predictors of long-term survival. Another increasingly valuable avenue of efficacy assessment is through biomarkers; these are especially useful in the treatment of diseases requiring long-term administration of drugs. The impact of drugs on cellular processes requires metabolite data predictive of subtle changes in molecular networks not accessible in target studies. In cancer, serum biochemical tumor markers can be useful predictors of outcome. Biomarkers are especially useful in cases where the precise mechanism of the drug is known. This can open the possibility of restricting clinical testing to those patients expressing the marker. In cancer patients, this includes HER2b overexpression I breast cancer (Herceptin), BCR-ABL translocation in chronic myeloid leukemia (Gleevec), and expression of CD20 in non-Hodgkin's lymphoma (Rituximab) [55]. In general, a biomarker can be a physiological byproduct (i.e., hypotension, platelet aggregation) or a biochemical substance (tumor markers). In this latter case, serum cholesterol or glycated hemoglobin can be useful biomarkers for statin therapy, control of diabetes, or antihypertensive treatment. A biomarker can also be a change in image (i.e., positron emission tomography). Thus, functional imaging can be used to visualize mitosis, apotosis,

inflammation, structural changes in tumor regression, and blood flow. Immunohistology also can be used to furnish predictive markers of success of a given treatment.

A practical problem that can be encountered in the use of biomarkers is the optimal identification of the ideal biomarker for a given treatment. There can be a number of biochemical changes seen with a given drug treatment, some of which may simply be coincidental and not a direct consequence of the treatment. One approach to the identification of the best biomarker is through receiver operated characteristic (ROC) curve analysis first implemented during the second world war as a tool to aid radar operators identify enemy airplanes (as opposed to birds or other harmless flying objects). Two pieces of data are plotted; on the abscissal axis is 1 − fraction of truly negative events correctly identified as negative (CNF) and on the ordinate axis is the fraction of truly positive events correctly identified as positive (CPF). Values on a diagonal line of unit slope are consistent with random chance (the observation gives no insight into the process). The best predictor yields values with the greatest possible positive slope (see Figure 11.17); therefore, a number of biomarkers can be compared in this way to identify the best predictor.

11.5 TYPES OF THERAPEUTICALLY ACTIVE LIGANDS: POLYPHARMACOLOGY

In addition to diversity in biological targets, there is emerging diversity in the types of chemicals that can be used therapeutically to interact with these targets. Before the advent of widespread functional high-throughput screening (HTS), the majority of new therapeutic entities could be classed as full agonists, partial agonists, or antagonists. Since the screening mode used to discover these often was orthosterically based (i.e., displacement of a radioligand in binding), the resulting leads usually were correspondingly orthosteric. With HTS in functional mode, there is the potential to cast a wider screening net to include allosteric modulators. The changing paradigm of biologically active molecules found in HTS is shown in Figure 11.18. With the use of the cellular functional machinery in detecting biologically active molecules comes the potential to detect allosteric antagonists (modulators) where $\alpha < 1$ or potentiators ($\alpha > 1$). As discussed in Chapter 7, there are fundamental differences between orthosteric and allosteric ligands that result in different profiles of activity and different therapeutic capability (see Section 7.3). As more allosteric ligands are detected by functional HTS, the ligand-target validation issues may become more prominent. In general, the requirement of target presence in the system to demonstrate an effect is the first, and most important, criterion to be met. In cases where sensitivity of the effect to known target antagonists is not straightforward, demonstration of the

FIGURE 11.17 **Receiver operation characteristic (ROC) curve analysis**. Abscissae: 1 − fraction of truly negative events correctly identified as negative (CNF). Ordinates: Fraction of truly positive events correctly identified as positive (CPF). Values on the dotted horizontal straight line can occur by random chance and yield no useful predictive data. The further skewed the relationship is toward the ordinate axis the better the predictive power of the value being measured.

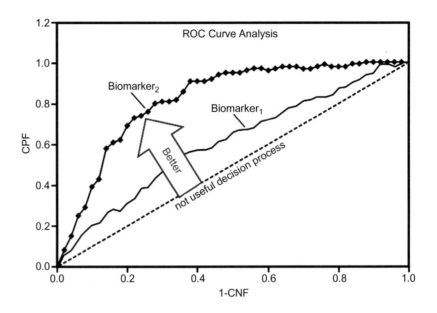

FIGURE 11.18 The use of new screening techniques employing functional assays promises a richer array of biologically active molecules that will not only mimic natural endogenous ligands for the targets but also will modify existing physiological activity.

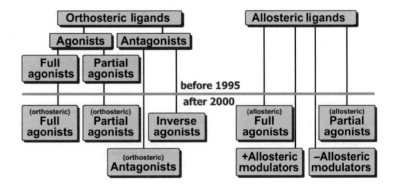

target effect, when the target is transfected into a range of host cells, is a useful confirmation.

Another variation on a theme for biological targets involves a concept known as *polypharmacology*; namely ligands with activity at more than one target within the same concentration range. The unique therapeutic profiles of such molecules rely upon the interplay of activities at multiple biological targets. Polypharmacological ligands make positive use of the generally observed phenomenon that many drugs, although designed to be selective, often have numerous other activities. Thus, drugs should be considered to be selective but not specific (where specific means the molecule possesses only one single activity at all concentration ranges). For example, Figure 11.19 shows the numerous activities found for the α_2-adrenoceptor antagonist yohimbine (Figure 11.19A) and the antidepressant amitryptylene (Figure 11.19B).

There are increasing numbers of examples of clinically active drugs in psychiatry that have multiple target activities. For example, olanzapine, a useful neuroleptic, has highly unspecific antagonist activity at 10 different neurotransmitter receptors. Similarly, there are numerous antidepressant drugs where multiple inhibitory effects on transport processes (norepinephrine, serotonin, dopamine) may be of therapeutic utility; see Figure 11.20. Additionally some antipsychotic drugs have numerous activities; for example, the atypical antipsychotic clozapine has activity at histamine H_4, dopamine D_2, dopamine D_4, 5-HT_{2A}, 5-HT_{2C}, and 5-HT_6 receptors. In addition, its major metabolite, desmethylclozapine, is an allosteric modulator of muscarinic receptors. This phenomenon is not restricted to the CNS; there is evidence that multiple activities may be an important aspect of kinase inhibitors in oncology as well. The unique value of the antiarrhythmic drug amiodarone is its activity on multiple cardiac ion channels [56].

Introducing multiple activities into molecules can be a means of maximizing possible therapeutic utility. Figure 11.21 shows the theoretical application for activity at two types of receptors; namely, α- and β-adrenoceptors. Depending on the dominant activities, molecules from a program designed to yield dual α- and β-adrenoceptor ligands could be directed toward a range of therapeutic applications. Chemical strategies can introduce multiple

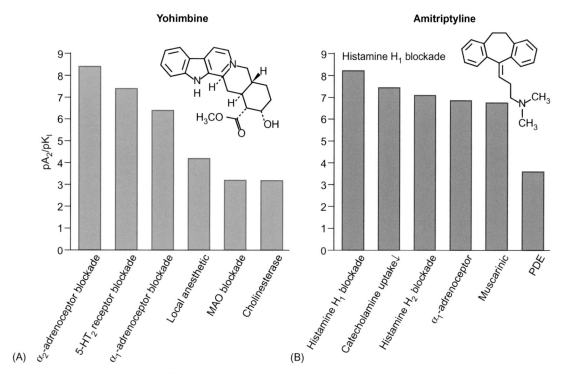

FIGURE 11.19 Multiple receptor effects (ordinates denote pK values for antagonism or receptor occupancy) of (A) yohimbine and (B) amitriptylene.

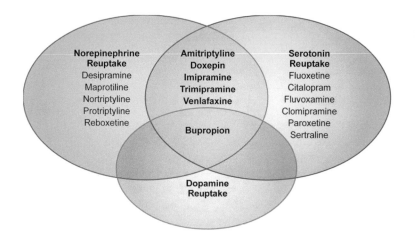

FIGURE 11.20 Mixture of activities of known antidepressants as inhibitors of amine transport processes (norepinephrine, serotonin, and dopamine).

activities into a single molecule range by dimerization of structures known to possess a single activity to form structures which possess multiple activities. The linkage of known active chemical structures for multiple activity has been described as a strategy, but an even more obvious amalgam of structures, joined with a linker, can be used to target receptor homo- and hetero-dimers [57]. Dimeric ligands can show increased potency. For example, a dimer of the 5-HT$_{1B}$ receptor ligand sumitryptan, used for the treatment of migraine, shows a 100-fold increase in potency over monomeric sumitryptan [58]. Dimerization of ligands is a way to introduce mixtures of activity. One example of this is a dimeric linking of a δ-opioid antagonist (naltrindole) and κ$_1$-opioid agonist (ICI-199,441) to

yield a molecule of greater potency *and* mixed activity [59]; see Figure 11.22. Dimeric ligands need not be obvious amalgams of active structures. For example, in view of clinical data suggesting that a mixture of histamine and leukotriene antagonism was superior to either single agent in asthma, and the finding that the antihistamine cyproheptadine was a weak antagonist of LTD$_4$, a molecule based on cyptroheptadine that was modified with features from the endogenous leukotriene agonist LTD$_4$, yielded a molecule with better activity in asthma [60]; see Figure 11.23. Dual activity also has been designed from knowledge of similar substrates. The treatment of hypertension with the ACE inhibitor captopril is established. The enzyme neutral endopeptidase (NEP) is a metalloprotease that degrades atrial

FIGURE 11.21 Venn diagram consisting of the various possible activities (agonism and antagonism) on two receptor subtypes (α- and β-adrenoceptors). Letters label the areas of intersection denoting joint activity; the table shows possible therapeutic application of such joint activity.

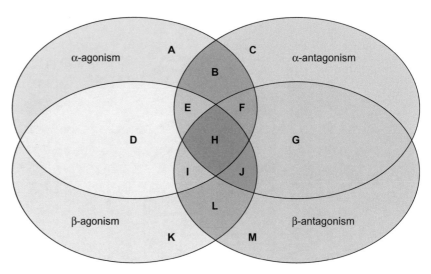

	α-Adrenoceptors	β-Adrenoceptors	Possible Indication
A	Full agonist		
B	Partial agonist		Shock, trauma
C	Antagonist		Hypertension
D	Full agonist	Full agonist	
E	Partial agonist	Full agonist	Acute cardiac decompensation
F	Partial agonist	Antagonist	Nasal decongestion, glaucoma, shock, cardiopulmonary resuscitation
G	Antagonist	Antagonist	Hypertension
H	Partial agonist	Partial agonist	Lipolysis
I	Full agonist	Partial agonist	
J	Antagonist	Partial agonist	Asthma, hypertension, congestive heart failure
K		Full agonist	Asthma
L		Partial agonist	Asthma
M		Antagonist	Hypertension, angina, glaucoma

natriuretic factor, a peptide known to cause vasodilatation and oppose the action of angiotensin. These activities led to the postulate that a combined ACE-NEP inhibitor would be efficacious in hypertension, and one approach to this utilizes the notion that these two enzymes cleave similar dipeptide fragments. From this, a constrained antiphenylalanine dipeptide mimetic designed to mimic a low-energy conformation of the His-Leu portion of angiotensin bound to ACE, and the Phe-Leu portion of leu-enkephalin bound to NEP, were used to produce a dual inhibitor of both ACE and NEP (Figure 11.23). This formed the basis for the synthesis of a potent ACE-NEP inhibitor of nanomolar potency (Figure 11.23).

One of the practical problems involved with ligands yielding polypharmacology is that their therapeutic profiles of action often can be tested effectively only *in vivo*. For example, debilitating concomitant tachycardia seen with beneficial increases in cardiac performance is a common finding for standard β-adrenoceptor agonist catecholamines such as isoproterenol (see Figure 11.24A). However, the β-adrenoceptor agonist dobutamine produces much less tachycardia for the same increased cardiac performance. This interesting

differentiation has been shown to be due to a low-level pressor effect of dobutamine (which opposes tachycardia through a reflex vagal stimulation) caused by weak α-adrenoceptor agonism [61]; blockade of α-adrenoceptors *in vivo* greatly reduces the difference between isoproterenol and dobutamine (see Figure 11.24B). This inotropic (over chronotropic selectivity) cannot be seen in isolated organs, only in the *in vivo* system. In this case, the whole animal is needed to detect the beneficial properties of dobutamine polypharmacology (α + β-agonism).

11.6 PHARMACOLOGY IN DRUG DISCOVERY

The drug discovery process can be envisioned in four interconnected phases;

1. The acquisition of chemicals to be tested for biological activity.
2. The determination of the activity of those chemicals on biological systems (pharmacodynamics).

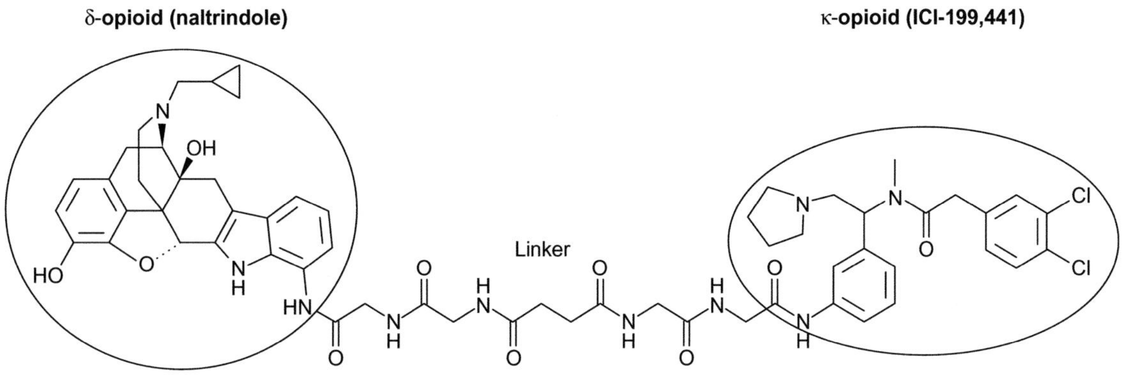

FIGURE 11.22 Dimeric antagonist formed by oligoglycyl-based linkage of two opioid receptor subtype antagonists naltrindole and ICI-199,441. From [59].

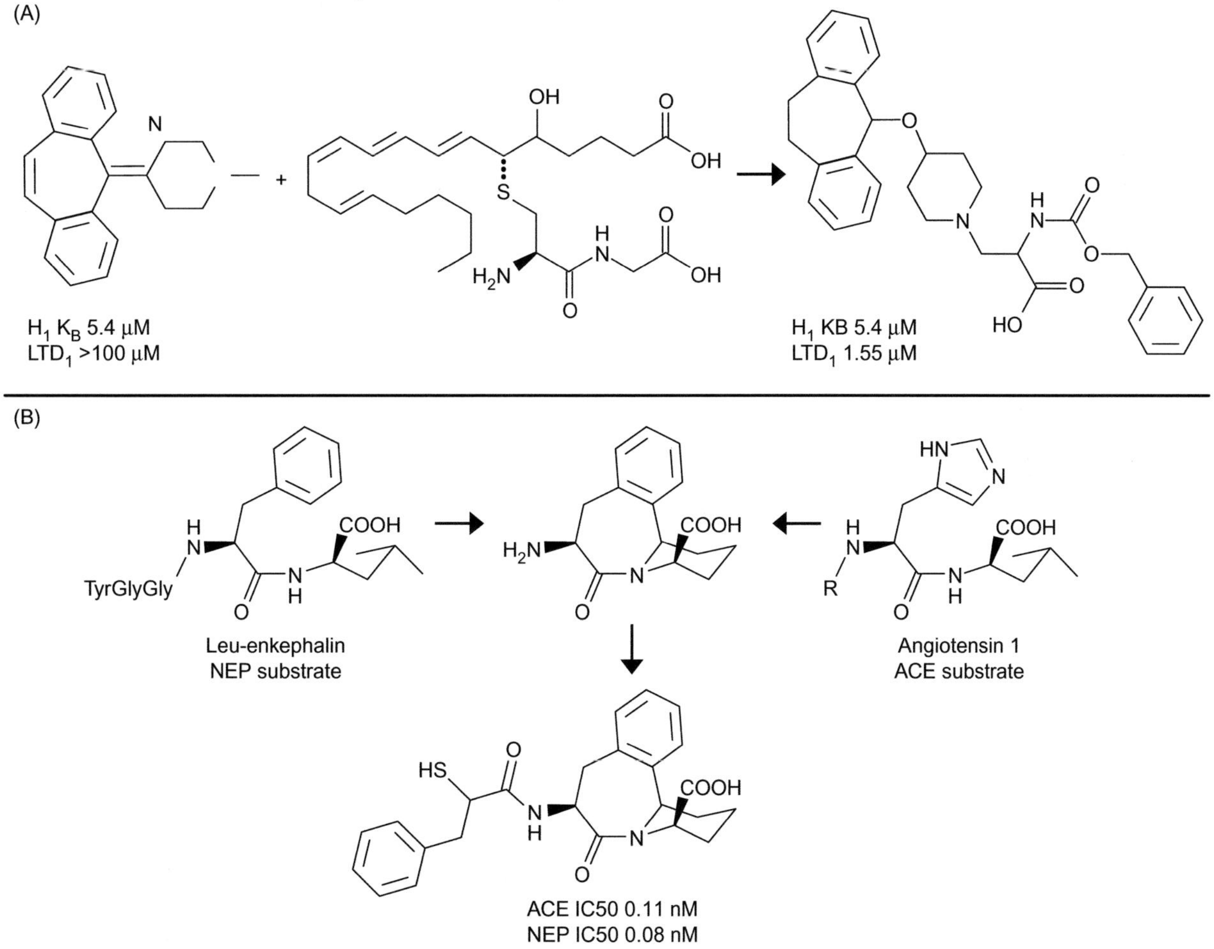

FIGURE 11.23 **Design of multiple ligand activity**. (A) Dual histamine H_1 receptor and leukotriene receptor antagonist incorporating known antihistaminic properties of cyproheptadine and LTD_4 (data from [60]). (B) Joint ACE-NEP inhibitor formed from incorporating similarities in substrate structures for both enzymes. From [57].

3. The formulation of the most active of these for therapeutic testing in humans (pharmaceutics).
4. The determination of adequate delivery of the active drug to diseased tissues (pharmacokinetics).

Each phase of this collection of processes is interconnected with the others, and failure in any one of them can halt the development process. Discussion of pharmaceutical drug form is beyond the scope of this book and will

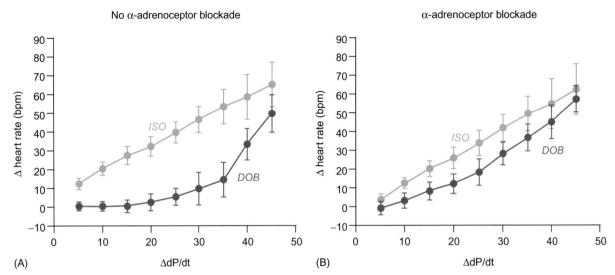

FIGURE 11.24 **Changes in heart rate (ordinates) for agonist-induced changes in cardiac inotropy (changes in rate of ventricular pressure) in anesthetized cats**. Responses shown to isoproterenol (blue circles) and dobutamine (red circles). (A) Response in normal cats shows inotropic selectivity (less tachycardia for given changes in inotropy) for dobutamine over isoproterenol. (B) The inotropic selectivity of dobutamine is reduced by previous α-adrenoceptor blockade by phentolamine. From [61].

not be discussed. Pharmacokinetics is discussed fully in Chapter 9. The remainder of this chapter will be devoted to the molecules that provide new drug entities and the methods utilized to detect biological activity in them.

11.7 CHEMICAL SOURCES FOR POTENTIAL DRUGS

A starting point to this process is the definition of what the therapeutic end point of the drug discovery process will be; namely, a drug. There are certain properties that molecules must have to qualify as therapeutically useful chemicals. While in theory, any molecule possessing activity that can be introduced into the body compartment containing the therapeutic target could be a possible drug, in practice, therapeutically useful molecules must be absorbed into the body (usually by the oral route), distribute to the biological target in the body, be stable for a period of time in the body, be reversible with time (excreted or degraded in the body after a reasonable amount of time), and be nontoxic. Ideally, drugs must be low molecular weight bioavailable molecules. Collectively, these desired properties of molecules are often referred to as "druglike" properties. A useful set of four rules for such molecules has been proposed by Lipinski and coworkers [62]. Molecules that fulfill these criteria generally can be considered possible therapeutically useful drugs, providing they possess target activity and few toxic side effects. Specifically, these rules state that "druglike" molecules should have less than five hydrogen-bond donor atoms, a molecular mass of <500 Da, and high lipophilicity (Clog P > 5), and

that the sum of the nitrogen and oxygen atoms should be <10. Therefore, when estimating the potential therapeutic drug targets, these properties must be taken into consideration.

There are numerous chemical starting points for drugs. Historically, natural products have been a rich source of molecules. As discussed in Chapter 1, the *Ebers Papryus,* is one of the earliest documents recording ancient medicine. Similarly, the Chinese *Materia Medica* (100 B.C.), the *Shennong Herbal* (100 B.C.), the *Tang Herbal* (659 A.D.), the Indian *Ayurvedic* system (1000 B.C.), and books of Tibetan medicine *Gyu-zhi* (800 A.D.) all document herbal remedies for illness. Some medicinal substances have their origins in geographical exploration. For example, tribes indigenous to the Amazon River had long been known to use the bark of the *Cinchona officinalis* to treat fever. In 1820, Caventou and Pelletier extracted the active antimalarial quinine from the bark, which provided the starting point for the synthetic antimalarials chloroquine and mefloquine. Traditional Chinese herbal medicine has yielded compounds such as artemisinin and derivatives for the treatment of fever from the *Artemisia annua.* The anticancer vinca alkaloids were isolated from the Madagascar periwinkle *Catharanthus roseus.* Opium is an ancient medicinal substance described by Theophrastus in the third century B.C., which was used for many years by Arabian physicians for the treatment of dysentery and "relief of suffering" (as described by Sydenham in 1680) in the Middle Ages. Known to be a mixture of alkaloids, opium furnished therapeutically useful pure alkaloids when Serturner isolated morphine in 1806, Robiquet isolated codeine in 1832, and Merck isolated papaverine in 1848. At present, only

5−15% of the 25,000 species of higher plants have been studied for possible therapeutic activity. Of prescriptions in the United States written between 1959 and 1980, 25% contained plant extracts or active principals.

Marine life can also be a rich source of medicinal material. For example, the C-nucleosides spongouridine and spongothymidine isolated from the Caribbean sponge *Cryptotheca crypta* possess antiviral activity. Synthetic analogs led to the development of cytosine arabinoside, a useful anticancer drug. Microbes also provide extremely useful medicines, the most famous case being penicillin from *Penicillium chrysogenum*. Other extremely useful bacterially-derived products include the fungal metabolites, the cephalosporins (from *Cephalosporium cryptosporium*), aminoglycosides and tetracyclines from *Actinomycetales*, immunosuppressives such as the cyclosporins and rapamycin (from *Streptomyces*), cholesterol-lowering agents mevastatin and lovastatin (from *Penicillium*), and anthelmintics and antiparasitics such as the ivermectins (from *Stroptomyces*). As with plants, less than 1% of potential bacterial and less than 5% of fungal sources have been explored for their medicinal value. In general, the World Health Organization estimates that 80% of the world's population relies on traditional medicine with natural products.

From this perspective, natural products appear to be a great future source of drugs. However, teleologically, there may be evolutionary pressure against biological activity of natural products. Thus, while millions of years of selective pressure has evolved molecules that specifically interact with physiological receptors (i.e., neurotransmitters, hormones) with little "cross talk" to other targets, it can be argued that those same years exerted a selective evolutionary pressure to evolve receptors that interact only with those molecules and not the myriad of natural products to which the organism has been exposed. In practical terms, natural products as drugs or starting points for drugs have certain inherent disadvantages as well. Specifically, these tend to be expensive, not chemically tractable (structurally complex and difficult to derivatize), and involve difficult and expensive scale-up procedures (active species tend to be minor components of samples). Natural products also often contain a larger number of ring structures and more chiral centers and have sp^3 hybridization bridgehead atoms present. Natural products are often high in steric complexity and, containing few nitrogen, halogen, and sulfur atoms and being oxygen rich with many hydrogen donors, natural products often are very prone to enzymatic reactions. In addition, a practical problem in utilizing such pharmacophores is the unpredictable novelty and intellectual property that may result. In spite of these shortcomings, between the years 1981 and 2002, of the 67% of 877 synthetic new chemical entities, 16.4% utilized pharmacophores derived directly from natural products.

Another approach to the discovery of drugs is "rational design." The basis for this strategy is the belief that detailed structural knowledge of the active site to which the drug binds will yield corresponding information that can guide the design of molecules to interact with it. One of the best-known examples, yielding rich dividends, is the synthesis of the ACE inhibitor captopril from a detailed analysis of the enzyme's active site. Similar design of small molecules to fit specific binding loci of enzymes was accomplished for HIV protease (nelfinavir) and Relenza for the prevention of influenza. Other rational design approaches utilize dual pharmacophores from other active drugs to combine useful therapeutic activities. This approach offers the advantage that the dual biological activity will be absorbed, metabolized, and excreted in a uniform manner, that is, the activity profile of the drug will not change through the varying ratios of two simultaneously dosed drugs. This also gives medicinal chemists a place to start. For example, ICS 205-903, a novel and potent antagonist of some neural effects of serotonin in migraine, was made by utilizing the structure of cocaine, a substance known to have seriously debilitating central effects but also known to block some of the neural effects of serotonin with the serotonin structure [63]. The result was a selective serotonin antagonist devoid of the disadvantages of cocaine (Figure 11.25A). Similarly, a β-adrenoceptor blocker with vasodilating properties has been made by combining the structure of the β-blocker propranolol with that of a vasodilator (Figure 11.25B). The idea of introducing dual or multi-target activities into molecules is discussed in Section 11.5.

There are numerous natural substances that have useful therapeutic properties as well as other undesirable properties. From these starting points, medicinal chemists have improved on nature. For example, while extremely useful in the treatment of infection, penicillin is not available by the oral route; this shortcoming is overcome in the analog ampicillin (Figure 11.26A). Similarly, the obvious deleterious effects of cocaine have been eliminated in the local anesthetic procaine (Figure 11.26B). The short activity and weak steroid progesterone is converted to a stronger, long-acting analog (+)-norgestrel through synthetic modification (Figure 11.26C). Catecholamines are extremely important for sustaining life and have a myriad of biological activities. For example, norepinephrine produces a useful bronchodilation that has utility in the treatment of asthma. However, it also has a short duration of action, is a chemically unstable catechol, and it produces debilitating tachycardia, vasoconstriction, and digital tremor. Synthetic modification to salbutamol eliminated all but the tremorogenic side effects to produce a very useful bronchodilator for the treatment of asthma (Figure 11.26D).

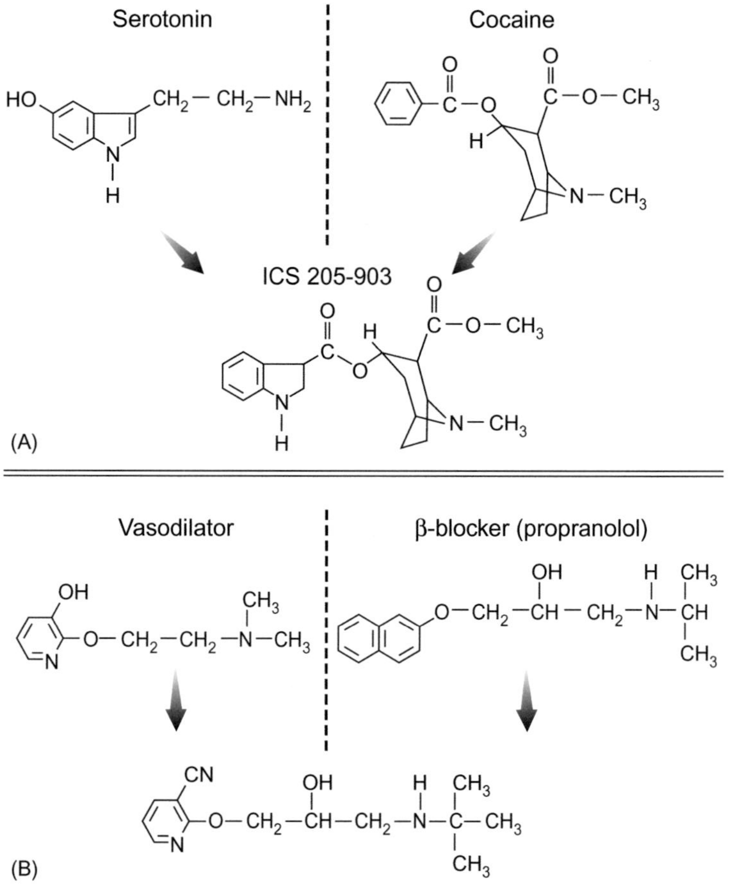

FIGURE 11.25 Examples of drug design through hybridization: combination of two structural types to produce a unique chemical entity. (A) Design of ICS 205–903 [2]. (B) Compound with vasodilating and β-blocking properties [64].

(A)

(B)

It can be argued that drugs themselves can be extremely valuable starting points for other drugs in that, by virtue of the fact that they are tolerated in humans, they allow the observation of their other effects. Some of those effects ("side effects") may lead to useful therapeutic indications. For example, the observed antiedemal effects of the antibacterial sulfanilamide in patients with congestive heart failure led to the discovery of its carbonic anhydrase inhibitor activity and the subsequent development of the diuretic furosemide (Figure 11.27A). Similarly, the antidiabetic effects of the antibiotic carbutamide led to the development of the antidiabetic tolbutamide (Figure 11.27B). Some of the early antihistamines were found to exert antidepressant and antipsychotic properties; these led to modern psychopharmaceuticals. The immunosuppressant activity of the fungal agent ciclosporin also was exploited for therapeutic utility.

Endogenous substances such as serotonin, amino acids, purines, and pyrimidines all have biological activity and also are tolerated in the human body. Therefore, in some cases these can be used as starting points for synthetic drugs. For example, the amino acid tryptophan and neurotransmitter serotonin were used to produce selective ligands for 5-HT$_{5A}$ receptors and a selective somatostatin3 antagonist, adenosine A2b receptor antagonists

from adenine, and a selective adenosine 2A receptor agonist from adenosine itself (Figure 11.28).

Major pharmaceutical efforts revolve around the testing of large chemical libraries for biological activity. Assuming that most drugs must have a molecular weight of less than 600 (due to desired pharmacokinetic properties, as discussed in Chapter 9), there are wide ranges in the estimates of the number of molecules that exist in "chemical space," that is, how many different molecules can be made within this size limit? The estimates range from 10^{40} to 10^{100} molecules, although the need for activated carbon centers for the construction of carbon-carbon bonds in synthetic procedures reduces the possible candidates for synthetic congeners. In spite of this fact, the number of possibilities is staggering. For example, in the placement of 150 substituents on mono to 14-substituted hexanes there are 10^{29} possible derivatives. Considering a median value of 10^{64} possible structures in chemical space clearly indicates that the number of possible structures available is far too large for complete coverage by chemical synthesis and biological screening. It has been estimated that a library of 24 million compounds would be required to furnish a randomly screened molecule with biological activity in the nanomolar potency range. While combinatorial libraries have greatly increased the

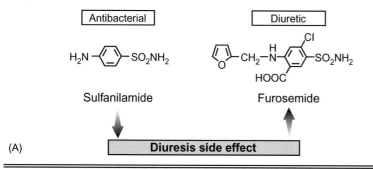

(A)   Penicillin   Ampicillin

FIGURE 11.26 Examples of chemical modification of active drugs that have either unwanted effects (cocaine, norepinephrine) or suboptimal effects (penicillin, progesterone) to molecules with useful therapeutic profiles.

(B)   Cocaine   Procaine

(C)   Progesterone   (+)-norgestrel

(D)   Norepinephrine   Salbutamol

Antibacterial	Diuretic

Sulfanilamide   Furosemide

FIGURE 11.27 Examples of case where the side effects of drugs used for another indication led to the discovery and development of a new therapeutic entity for another disease.

(A)   **Diuresis side effect**

Antibacterial	Antidiabetic

Carbutamide   Tolbutamide

(B)   **Antidiabetic side effect**

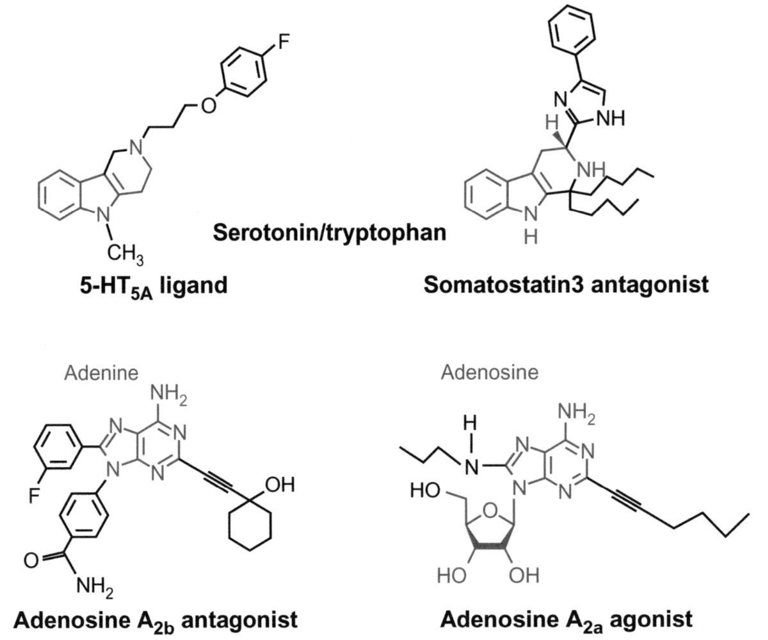

FIGURE 11.28 Examples of natural substances (shown in red) that have been chemically modified to yield therapeutically useful selective drugs.

productivity of medicinal chemists (i.e., a single chemist might have produced 50 novel chemical structures in a year 10 years ago, but with the availability of solid and liquid phase synthesis and other combinatorial techniques, a single chemist can produce thousands of compounds in a single month at a fraction of the cost of previous techniques), 24 million compounds per lead is still considerably larger than the practical capability of industry.

One proposed reason for the failure of many high-throughput screening campaigns is the lack of attention to "druglike" (namely, the ability to be absorbed into the human body and having a lack of toxicity) properties in the chemical library. The non-druglike properties of molecules lead to biological activity that cannot be exploited therapeutically. This is leading to improved drug design in chemical libraries incorporating features to improve "druglike properties." One difficulty with this approach is the multifaceted nature of the molecular properties of druglike molecules; that is, while druglike chemical space is simpler than biological target space, the screens for druglike activity are multimechanism based and difficult to predict. Thus, incorporating favorable druglike properties into chemical libraries can be problematic. Also, different approaches can be counter-intuitive to the incorporation of druglike properties. Thus, the rational design of drugs tends to increase molecular weight and lead to molecules with high hydrogen bonding and unchanged lipophilicity; this generally can lead to reduced permeability. A target permeability for druglike molecules (which should have aqueous solubility minimum of $>52\,\mu g/ml$) should achieve oral absorption from a dose of >1 mg/kg. High-throughput screening approaches tend to increase molecular weight, leave hydrogen bonding unchanged from the initial hit, and increase lipophilicity; this can lead to decreases in aqueous solubility with concomitant decrease in druglike properties. Ideas centered on the concept of druglike properties have caused a change in the types of molecules made for screening libraries. It has been seen that drugs often resemble their screening hit molecular origins (see zofenopril, Figure 11.29). For this reason, candidates for new drug libraries are pre-selected to have druglike properties in anticipation of better pharmacokinetics. Thus, physiochemical rules for library candidates have been reported in the literature (see [65], Figure 11.29).

The assumption made in estimations of the number of molecules that would be required to yield biologically active molecules is that potential drugs are randomly and uniformly distributed throughout chemical space. Analysis of known drugs and biologically active structures indicates that this latter assumption probably is not valid. Instead, drugs tend to cluster in chemical space, that is, there may be as little as 10,000 druglike compounds in pharmacological space [66]. The clustering of druglike molecules in chemical space has led to the concept of "privileged structures" from which medicinal chemists may choose for starting points for new drugs. A *privileged structure* is defined as a molecular scaffold with a range of binding properties that yield potent and selective ligands for a range of targets through modification of functional groups. Privileged structures can be a part of already known drugs, such as the dihydropyridines

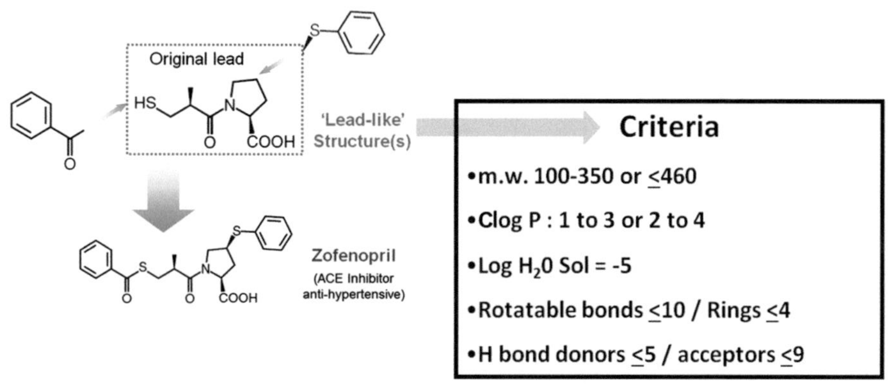

FIGURE 11.29 Relationship of the chemical structure of the ACE inhibitor antihypertensive drug zofenopril to the molecule found in a high-throughput screen that led to its discovery and development. In panel on right are physicochemical rules for candidate library molecules to retain druglike activity. (Data from [65].)

(known as *calcium channel blockers*). In this case, inhibitors of platelet aggregation (platelet activating factor [PAF] inhibitors) and neuropeptide Y type 1 receptor ligands have been made from the dihydropyridine backbone (Figure 11.30). Privileged structures also can simply be recurring chemical motifs such as the indole motif shown in Figure 11.31 and shared by marketed drugs and investigational ligands. Similarly, the 2-tetrazole-biphenyl motif is found in the angiotensin2 receptor antagonist losartan and GHS receptor ligand L-692,429 (Figure 11.32A), and a wide range of biologically active structures is based in spiropiperidines (Figure 11.32B).

11.8 PHARMACODYNAMICS AND HIGH-THROUGHPUT SCREENING

The history of medicine and pharmacology abounds with anecdotes of serendipitous drug discovery. Perhaps the most famous example of this is the discovery of penicillin by Fleming in 1928. This led to the systematic screening of hundreds of microorganisms for antibiotics. However, even in those early discovery efforts, the value of screening was appreciated. For example, though Ehrlich's invention of salvarsan for syphilis has many serendipitous elements, it was nevertheless the result of a limited screening of 600 synthetic compounds.

Without prior knowledge of which chemical structure will be active on a particular target, a wide sampling of chemical space (i.e., diverse choice of chemical structures) must be made to detect biological activity. This is done through so-called *high-throughput screening* (HTS), whereby a robust biological assay is used to test as large a sample of chemical compounds as possible. Usually robotic automation is employed in this process. Presently, sophisticated liquid-handling devices, extremely sensitive detection devices, and automated assay platforms allow testing of several thousands of compounds in very small volumes (<10 μL). The ideal HTS is generic (i.e., can be used for a wide range of targets utilizing formats in which any receptor can be transfected and subsequently

expressed), robust (insensitive to assumptions), relatively low cost with a low volume (does not require large quantities of substance), amenable to automation (has a simple assay protocol), ideally is nonradioactive, and has a high tolerance to solvents such as DMSO. Some requirements of functional screening assays are given in Table 11.3.

One of the most negative aspects of drug screening is that basically it is a one-way experiment. The single direction stems from the fact that, while activity guides structure-activity relationships, much less use can be made of lack of activity. This is because there are numerous reasons why a compound may not show activity; that is, there are more defined reasons why a molecule is active on a biological target than reasons why it lacks activity [66]. For example, lack of aqueous solubility accounts for a substantial number of potentially false negatives in the screening process.

A major consideration in screening is the detection capability of the screen for both false negatives (lack of detection of an active drug) and propensity to find false positives (detection of a response to the compound not due to therapeutic activity of interest). Ostensibly, false positives might not be considered a serious problem in that secondary testing will detect these and they do not normally interfere with the drug discovery process. However, they can be a serious practical problem if the hit rate of a given HTS is abnormally high due to false positives and the major resource for decoding (following up initial hits) becomes limiting. In this regard, binding assays generally have a lower false positive rate than do functional assays. Also, the false positive rate in functional assays where the exposure time of the assay to the compounds is short (i.e., such as calcium transient studies) is lower than in assays such as reporter assays where the time of exposure is of the order of 24 hr. On the other hand, binding studies require confirmation of primary activity in a functional assay to identify therapeutic activity.

A more serious problem is that of false negatives, since there is no way of knowing which compounds are active but not detected by the assay. In this regard, binding assays have the shortcoming of detecting only

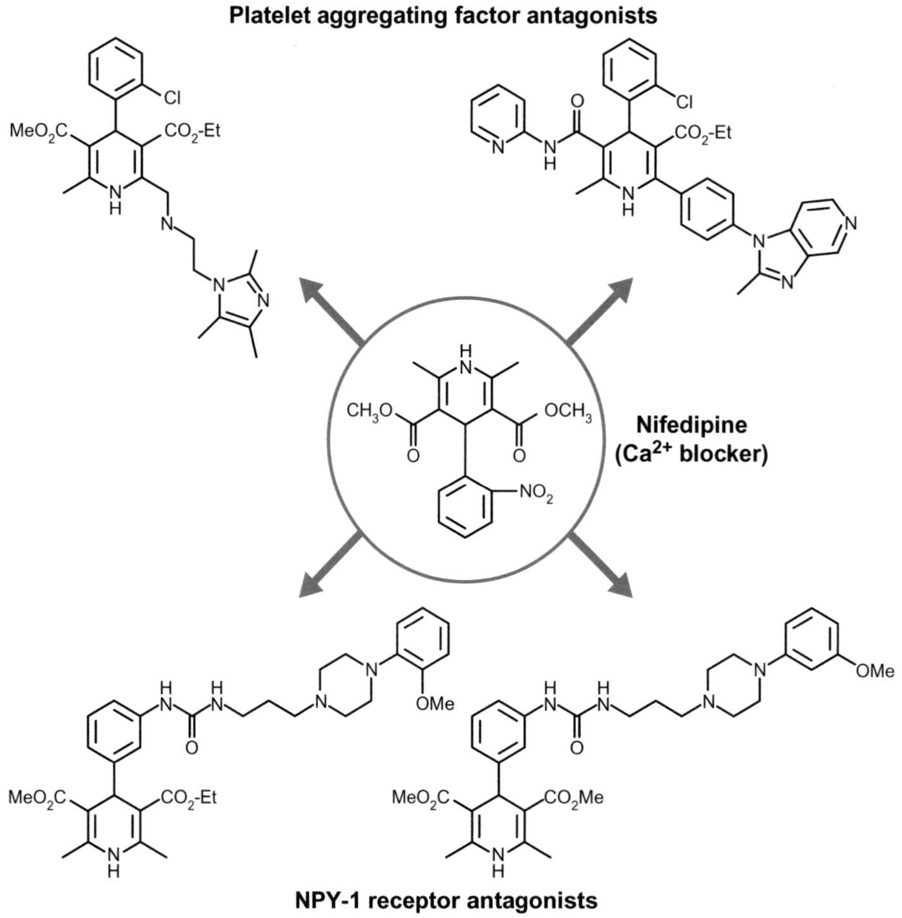

Platelet aggregating factor antagonists

Nifedipine (Ca²⁺ blocker)

NPY-1 receptor antagonists

FIGURE 11.30   Example of a preferred structure, in this case the dihydropyridine scaffold.

compounds that interfere with the binding of the tracer probe. Within this scenario, allosteric compounds that affect the physiological function of the target but otherwise do not interfere with binding of the tracer are not detected. As allosterism is probe dependent (i.e., not all molecules are equally affected by an allosteric ligand; see Chapter 7), the endogenous agonist should be used for screening to detect physiologically relevant activity. For example, the allosteric ligand for muscarinic receptors, alcuronium, produces a 10-fold change in the affinity of the receptor for the natural endogenous agonist acetylcholine but only a 1.7-fold change is observed for the synthetic muscarinic agonist arecoline [67]. Therefore, screening with arecoline may not have detected a physiologically relevant (for acetylcholine, the natural agonist) activity of alcuronium.

There are instances where the screen for biologically active molecules cannot be the ideal and appropriate biological test. For example, the screening process for drugs that block against HIV infection theoretically should involve live HIV. However, there are obvious limitations and constraints with using a virus that can cause AIDS — specifically, the containment required with such virulent

species is not compatible with HTS. Therefore, a surrogate screen must be done. In this case, a receptor screen of the protein recognition site for HIV, namely the chemokine receptor CCR5, can be used to screen for drugs that block HIV infection. What then is required is a secondary assay to ensure that the ligands that block CCR5 also block HIV infection.

The complex protein-protein interactions involved in HIV entry strongly suggest that the blockade of these effects by a small molecule requires an allosteric mechanism; that is, a specific orthosteric hindrance of a portion of the protein interface will not be adequate to block HIV infection. Therefore, the surrogate screen for HIV blockers would be a surrogate allosteric screen. As noted in Chapter 7 and discussed previously, allosteric effects are notoriously probe dependent, and therefore there is the possibility that the HTS will detect molecules devoid of the therapeutically relevant activity; that is, they will block the binding of the probe for screening but not HIV. This also means that the screen may miss therapeutically relevant molecules by using a therapeutically irrelevant allosteric probe. Figure 11.33 shows how the use of a surrogate probe for biological testing can

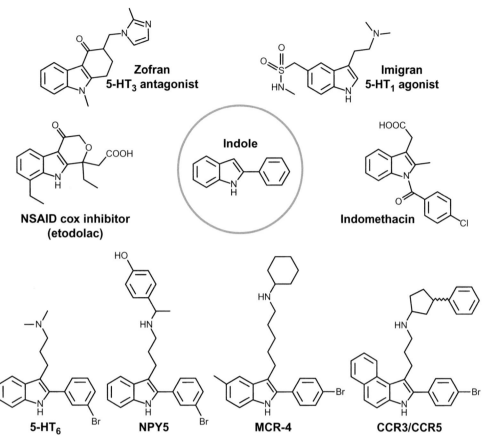

FIGURE 11.31 The preferred indole structure forms the basis of a number of selective ligands for receptors.

deviate from therapeutic relevance [13]. Initially, a molecule with potent blocking effects on the surrogate probe (radioactive chemokine binding) was shown to also be a potent antagonist of HIV infection (ordinate scale as the IC_{95} for inhibition of HIV infection; see data point for compound A in Figure 11.33). In efforts to optimize this activity through modification of the initial chemical structure, it was found that the chemokine-blocking potency could be retained while HIV activity was lost (see data point for compound B in Figure 11.33). In this case, alteration of the chemical structure caused a twofold decrease in chemokine antagonist potency and a disproportionate 3020-fold decrease in HIV antagonist potency. These compounds clearly show the independence of chemokine binding and HIV binding effects in this molecular series.

The major requirements for a screen are high sensitivity and a large signal-to-noise ratio for detecting the effect. This latter factor concerns the inherent error in the basal signal and the size of the window for producing the biological effect. A large detection window for response (i.e., difference between basal response and maximal agonist-stimulated response) is useful but not necessary if the random error intrinsic to the measurement of biological effect is low. A smaller maximal detection window, but with a concomitant lower random error in measurement, may be preferable. Since the vast majority of compounds will be exposed to HTS only once, it is critical that the assay used for screening has a very high degree of sensitivity and accuracy. These factors are quantified in a statistic called the Z' factor [68].

The Z' factor calculates a number that is sensitive to the separation between the mean control values for HTS (background) and mean of the positive sample as well as the relative standard deviations of both of those means. In validating a screen, a number of negative controls (background signal) and positive controls (wells containing a ligand that gives a positive signal) are run; this process yields a mean value. A positive control mean signal (μ_{c+}) (for example, the maximal response to an agonist for the target receptor), with accompanying standard deviation (denoted σ_{c+}) and negative control signal (background noise, no agonist) denoted μ_{c-} (with σ_{c-}), are generated with a standard positive control drug (i.e., full agonist for the receptor). The bandwidth of values 3 σ units either side of the mean is designated the *data variability band*, and the width of the spread between the two means (+3 σ units) is denoted the *separation band* (or dynamic range) of the screen. It is assumed that 3 σ units represent a 99.73% confidence that a value outside this

2-tetrazole-biphenyls

(A)

L-692,429
GHS agonist

Losartan
AG2 agonist

Spiropiperidines

Chemokine antagonist   **Cholecystokinin antagonist**   **GHS-R1a agonist**

(B) **Somatostatin agonist**   **NK1 antagonist**   **Orphanin FG antagonist**

FIGURE 11.32 Examples of preferred structures (2-tetrazole-biphenyls, panel A; and spiropiperidines, panel B) yielding selective ligands for receptors.

TABLE 11.3 Requirements for a Functional Screening Assay

Minimal

1. Cell line with appropriate receptor is available.
2. There is some means of detecting when there is a ligand-receptor interaction taking place.
3. Agonist and selective antagonist are available.
4. Agonist is reversible.

Optimal

1. There is a commercial cell line available.
2. Response should be sustained, not transient.
3. Response should be rapid.

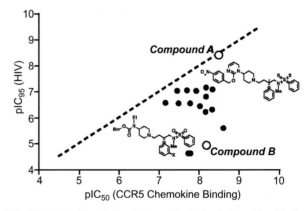

FIGURE 11.33 Correlation between blockade of chemokine binding to CCR5 (abscissae as pK_i values) and 95% inhibition of HIV infection as pIC_95 (ordinates) for a series of CCR5 antagonists. It can be seen that compound A is nearly equiactive as a blocker of chemokine binding (pK_i = 8.5) and HIV infection (pIC_95 = 8.4; ratio of affinities = 1.3), whereas structural analogs (filled circles) clearly differentiate these activities. For the structure B shown, the chemokine-blocking activity has been somewhat retained (pK_i = 8.2), whereas the HIV-blocking activity largely has been lost (pIC_95 = 4.9; ratio of affinities = 3020). Data drawn from [13].

limit is different from the mean (see Chapter 12 for further discussion). An optimum screen will have a maximum dynamic range and minimum data variability band (see Figure 11.34A). It can be seen that problems can occur with either a large intrinsic standard error of measurement (Figure 11.34B) or small separation band (Figure 11.34C). Interestingly, an efficient and accurate

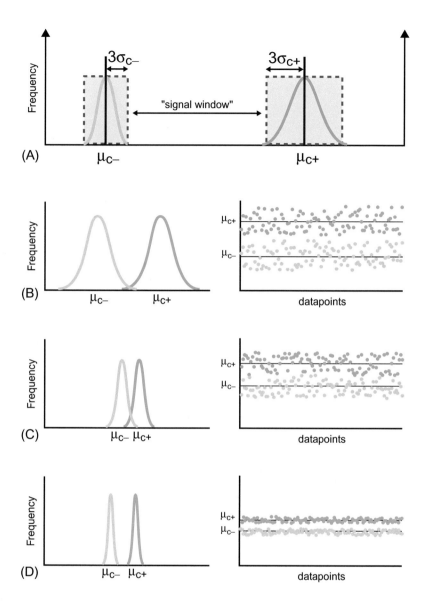

FIGURE 11.34 **Representation of Z′ values**. (A) Shaded areas represent distribution of values for control readings (no drug) and the distribution for readings from the system obtained in the presence of a maximal concentration of standard active drug. The signal window for this assay is the separation between the distributions at values 3 × the standard deviation of the mean away from the mean. (B) A representation of an assay with a low Z′ value. Though there is a separation, the scatter about the mean values is large and there is no clear window between the lower and upper values. (C) An assay with a low signal window. This assay has a low Z′ value. (D) An assay with a low signal window but correspondingly low error leading to a better Z′ value.

HTS can be achieved with a low separation band (contrary to intuition) if the data variability band is very small (see Figure 11.34D). The Z′ factor (a control drug of known high activity for the assay target) calculates these effects by subtracting the difference between the means from the sum of the difference of the standard deviations of the means divided by the difference between the means:

$$Z' = \frac{|\mu_{c+} - \mu_{c-}| - (3\sigma_{c+} + 3\sigma_{c-})}{|\mu_{c+} - \mu_{c-}|} = 1 - \frac{(3\sigma_{c+} + 3\sigma_{c-})}{|\mu_{c+} - \mu_{c-}|}. \quad (11.1)$$

Table 11.4 shows the range of possible Z′ values with comments on their meaning in terms of high-throughput screening assays.

The calculation of Z′ values for experimental compounds can yield valuable data. Values of Z′ for test compounds are calculated in the same way as Z′ values except the μ_{c+} and σ_{c+} values are the signals from the

test compounds (denoted μ_s and σ_s for test sample) and μ_{c-} and σ_{c-} from the assay with no test compounds run (i.e., controls for noise, denoted μ_c and σ_c for controls). While the Z′ indicates the robustness and detection capability of the screen (calculated with known active compounds), a value of Z′ for a set of unknown compounds also can test other factors related to the screen, such as the concentration at which the compounds are tested and/ or the chemical makeup of the compound set. For example, Figure 11.35A shows a screen with an excellent Z′ value (Z′ = 0.7), and Z′ values for a set of test compounds run at two concentrations; it can be seen that the higher concentration yields a higher signal and variation (possibly due to toxic effects of the high concentration). This, in turn, will lead to a lower Z′ factor. Similarly, Figure 11.35B shows distributions for two chemical libraries; it can be seen that there is a clear difference in the quality of the assay with these two sets of compounds,

TABLE 11.4 Z' Values and High-Throughput Screening Assays

Z' Value	Description of Assay	Comments
Z' = 1	No variation ($\sigma = 0$) or infinite band of separation	Ideal assay
$1 > Z' > 0.5$	Large dynamic range	Excellent assay
$0.5 > Z' > 0$	Small dynamic range	Adequate assay
0	No band of separation, σ_{c+} and σ_{c-} touch	Dubious quality
<0	No band of separation, σ_{c+} and σ_{c-} overlap	Impossible for screening

From [68].

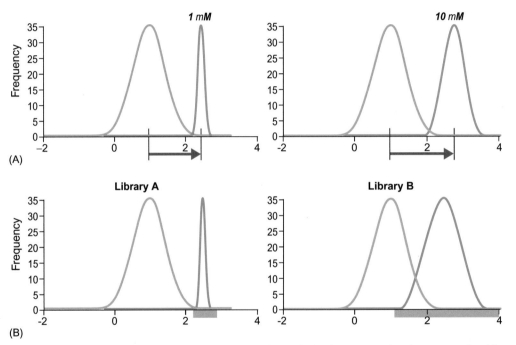

FIGURE 11.35   Distributions for various screens. (A) The larger distribution represents inactive compounds, while the smaller one shows a small sample with values greater than the mean of the total compound library. Distributions are shown for two concentrations tested from this library. It can be seen that, while the mean of the higher concentration is slightly farther away from the control distribution, the error is also much greater, leading to a lower Z' value. (B) The results of single concentration of two compound libraries are shown. It can be seen that library A has a smaller standard error about the mean and therefore is a higher-quality library for potentially active molecules.

indicating a possible inherent property of one of the chemical scaffolds leading to variability in the screen. In effect, the quality of the compound set can be quantified for this assay with a value of Z' [68].

Of major importance for HTS is sensitivity to weak ligands. As discussed in Chapter 2, functional systems generally amplify responses, as the signal is measured distal to the agonist-receptor interaction. For this reason, agonist screens utilizing end organ response are preferred (i.e., melanophore function, reporter assays). In contrast, the sensitivity of antagonist screening can be controlled by adjustment of the magnitude of the agonism used to detect the blockade. At least for competitive ligands, the lower

the amount of stimulation to the receptor the system, the more sensitive it will be to antagonism. This effect is inversely proportional to the window of detection for the system. On one hand, as large a window of agonist response as possible is preferred to maximize signal-to-noise ratios. On the other hand, too large a window may require a strong agonist stimulation that, in turn, would create insensitivity to antagonism. This can be offset by screening at a higher concentration of antagonist, but this can introduce obfuscating factors such as toxic effects of high concentrations of weakly active compounds. Thus, for antagonist screening, it becomes a trade-off of strength of agonist stimulation against concentration of antagonist.

The process of tracking screening hits and determining which chemical series is likely to produce a fruitful lead involves the verification of activity within a series of related structures. While the absolute potency of the hit is clearly important, it is recognized that factors such as selectivity, favorable physicochemical properties, absence of toxophores (pharmacophores leading to toxicity: *vide infra*), and the capability for the rapid production of chemical analogs are also very important features of lead molecules. For this reason, the concept of "ligand efficiency" has been used to evaluate the worth of screening hits. This idea converts ligand affinity to the experimental binding energy per atom (so-called *Andrews binding energy* [69]) to normalize the activity of ligand to its molecular weight [70]. It has been estimated that a maximum affinity per atom for organic compounds is -1.5 kcal mol^{-1} per nonhydrogen atom (Δg [free energy of binding] $= -RT \ln K_d$/number of nonhydrogen atoms) [71].

Before discussion of the drug discovery process following lead identification, it is relevant to discuss variations on the theme of hit identification. Screening has traditionally been based on finding a defined primary biological activity, that is, receptor-based agonism or antagonism of physiological effect. Such an approach presupposes that all potentially useful receptor activity will be made manifest through these effects. However, some receptor activities may not be mediated through G-protein activation. For example, the CCK antagonist D-Tyr-Gly-[(Nle^{28,31},D-Trp^{30})cholecystokinin-26-32]-phenethyl ester actively induces receptor internalization without producing receptor activation [72]. This suggests that screening assays other than simple agonism and/or antagonism may be useful for the detection of ligand activity.

A similar idea involves the modification of screening assays for the detection of special ligands. For example, certain inhibitors of enzyme function trap the enzyme in dead end complexes that cannot function; this is referred to as *interfacial inhibition* [73]. Thus, inhibitors such as brefeldin A and camptothecin target a transient kinetic intermediate that is not normally present in a nonactivated protein. Screening assays designed to detect these types of inhibitor have a small concentration of substrate in the medium to produce the enzyme transition state (the target of the interfacial inhibitor). Similarly, topoisomerase assays have been designed to identify transient trapping of catalytic-cleavage complexes. Interestingly, such inhibitors may offer an added measure of selectivity since they are active only when both partners of a physiological interaction are present and target only this interaction.

This has particular relevance to allosteric modification of receptors. As described in Chapter 7, the fraction of receptor bound to an agonist [A], expressed in terms of the presence of an allosteric modulator [B], is given as:

$$\frac{[AR]}{[R_{tot}]} = \frac{[A]/K_A(1 + \alpha[B]/K_B)}{[B]/K_B(\alpha[A]/K_A + 1) + [A]/K_A + 1}. \quad (11.2)$$

This leads to the following expression for the observed affinity (expressed as equilibrium dissociation constant of the ligand-receptor complex) of the modulator:

$$K_{obs} = \frac{K_B([A]/K_A + 1)}{\alpha[A]/K_A + 1}. \quad (11.3)$$

It can be seen from Equation 11.3 that the concentration of the probe molecule ($[A]/K_A$) affects the observed affinity of the modulator. This can have practical consequences, especially when allosteric potentiators are the desired chemical target. Just as an allosteric potentiator will increase the affinity of the probe molecule (agonist, radioligand), the reciprocal also is true; namely, that the agonist will increase the affinity of the receptor for the modulator. This can be used in the screening process to make an assay more sensitive to potentiators. For example, for a potentiator that increases the affinity of the agonist 30-fold ($\alpha = 30$), the observed affinity of the modulator will increase by a factor of 15.5 when a small concentration of agonist ($[A]/K_A = 1$) is present in the medium. Such modification of screening assays can be used to tailor detection for specific types of molecules (for further discussion see Section 7.4.3).

In general, there are certain changes that need to be made to convert a conventional high-throughput screen into one that is aimed at the discovery of allosteric modulators. These are:

1. Screening must be done in context with the co-binding ligand. For agonists, the optimal concentration is one that yields approximately 30% maximal response (EC$_{30}$). In addition, the endogenous ligand must be used as the co-binding ligand whenever possible.

2. Some allosteric modulators are known to have extraordinarily long time requirements for complete equilibration, therefore as long a pre-incubation period as possible should be employed in the screening assay.

3. Some allosteric effects (i.e., PAMs) can be quite small yet therapeutically relevant (i.e., 2–3 -fold increased sensitivity) therefore the assay must be robust and reproducible. In addition, statistical power analysis (see Chapter 12) should be employed to optimize the replications needed to detect a significant effect.

Finally, as a corollary to the screening process, there are thermodynamic reasons for supposing that any ligand that has an affinity for a biological target may also change that target in some way (i.e., have efficacy). This is because the energetics of binding involve the same forces responsible for protein conformation, that is, as discussed in Section 1.10 in Chapter 1, a ligand will bias the natural conformational ensemble of the receptor. This can be simulated with a probabilistic model of receptor function [74,75] described in Chapter 3. One of the main predictions of this model is that the same molecular forces that control ligand affinity also control efficacy, and thus they are linked. Under these circumstances, the binding of a ligand may well have thermodynamic consequences that result in a receptor species with different reactive properties towards the cell; that is, the ligand may also have efficacy. As discussed in Chapter 2, this efficacy may not be a conventional stimulation of cellular pathway but rather may involve a changing behavior of the receptor toward the cell, such as a change in the ability to be phosphorylated, internalized, or otherwise altered. The important point is that the theory predicts an efficacy that may not be observed experimentally until the correct pharmacological assay is used, that is, all possible "efficacies" of ligands should be looked for in ligands that bind to the receptor. This can be demonstrated by simulation using the probabilistic model.

Figure 11.36 shows calculated values (see Equations 3.33 and 3.34 in Chapter 3) for affinity (ordinates) and efficacy (abscissae) for 5000 simulated ligands; the probabilities are random, but it can be seen that there is a correlation between affinity and efficacy. The calculations show that the energy vectors that cause a ligand to associate with the protein also will cause a shift in the bias of protein conformations, that is, the act of binding will cause a change in the nature of the protein ensemble. This suggests that if a ligand binds to a receptor protein, it will in some way change its characteristics toward the system. This has implications in screening, since it suggests that all compounds with measured affinity should be

tested for all aspects of possible biological activity, not just interference with the binding of an endogenous agonist [76]. This, in turn, indicates that a screen that detects fundamental changes in the receptor protein might be an effective method of detecting molecules that bind to the receptor. For example, resonance techniques such as FRET and BRET take advantage of the fact that energy-sensitive probes alter their wavelength of emission when their relative proximity changes; if two such probes are engineered into a receptor protein, then a change in the conformation of the protein alters the relative positions of the probes and the conformation change can be detected (see Figure 11.37). For example, cyan (CFP) and yellow (YFP) variants of green fluorescent protein allow the transfer of energy from light-excited CFP to YFP (for FRET). In a variant technique, CFP is replaced by light-emitting luciferase (BRET); this approach reduces the background signal but also causes a loss of sensitivity [77]. Replacement of YFP with small fluorescein-derivative FlAsh binds to short cysteine-containing sequences to allow the use of a label much smaller than GFPs [78]. A screen that can detect generic binding of any molecule to the receptor through BRET or FRET then allows the reduction of potential molecules from the order of millions to perhaps a few thousand. This is a much more manageable number in which to pursue specific activities that may be therapeutically relevant (Figure 11.37). This is an alternative to presupposing the therapeutically relevant receptor coupling (i.e., cyclic AMP) and screening on that basis. For example, the β-blocker propranolol does not produce elevation of cyclic AMP and thus would not be detected as an agonist in a cyclic AMP assay. However, in assays designed to detect ERK (extracellular signal-related kinase) activation, propranolol is an active ERK agonist [79]. These data underscore the importance of the assay in drug detection.

11.9 DRUG DEVELOPMENT

Once hits have been identified, they must be confirmed. The test data obtained from a screen form a normal distribution. One criterion for determining possible active molecules is to retest all initial values >3σ units away from the mean; this will capture values for which there is >99.3% probability that they are significantly greater than the mean of the population (see Figure 11.38). The distribution of the apparently active compounds, when retested, will have a mean centered on the 3σ value for the distribution of the total compound set. It can be seen that 50% of these will retest as active (be greater than 3σ units away from the initial total compound set mean). Therefore the compounds that retest will have a 99.85% probability of having values greater than the mean of the original data set. The criteria for retest may

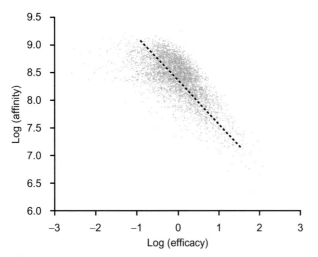

FIGURE 11.36 Simulation for 5000 theoretical ligands with calculated efficacy (Equation 3.33) and affinity (Equation 3.32). It can be seen that efficacy and affinity are correlated, suggesting that all ligands that have been shown to bind to a receptor should be extensively tested for possible efficacy effects on the receptor directly, through agonist effects on the receptor, or through changes in constitutive behavior of the receptor itself. Redrawn from [77].

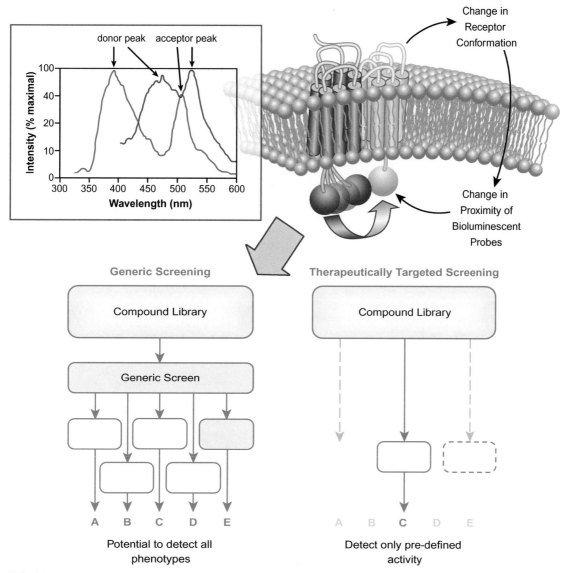

FIGURE 11.37 "Generic" screening using bioluminescence resonance energy transfer (BRET), which detects changes in receptor conformation through ligand binding. Two probes are placed on the receptor protein, which have a characteristic bioluminescence signal that changes when the distance between them is altered. Changes in receptor conformation cause a change in the relative position of the probes, which then causes a change in the luminescence signal. This type of assay detects all compounds that bind to the receptor and cause a conformational change; as discussed in the context of the probabilistic model of receptor function, this could essentially entail all compounds that bind to the receptor (see Chapter 3). This detection is based on the principle that the ligand-bound receptor is thermodynamically different from the unliganded receptor. Secondary testing of the subset of binding molecules (a much smaller set than the original library) can then sort compounds with respect to function. A contrasting approach uses a therapeutically relevant screen, where a specific receptor coupling pathway is chosen for detection, and depends on the assumption that the pathway is all that is required for therapeutic activity. With this approach, ligands with unknown potential may not be detected, and the strategy may not be successful if the chosen pathway is the incorrect one.

be governed by practical terms. If the hit rate is inordinately high then it may be impractical to test all hits that give values $>3\sigma$ units from the mean; a lower (having a greater probability of retest) number of "hits" ($>4\sigma$ or 5σ units away from the mean) may need to be tested to reduce the retest load.

Another important concept in the process of early confirmation of lead activity is ligand-target validation.

The first, and most obvious, criterion for selective target interaction is that the ligand effect is observed in the host cell only when the target is present. Thus, in a cell-based assay using cells transfected with receptor, the response to a putative agonist should be observed only in the transfected cell line and not in the host cell line (or at least a clearly different effect should be seen in the host cell line; see Figure 11.39).

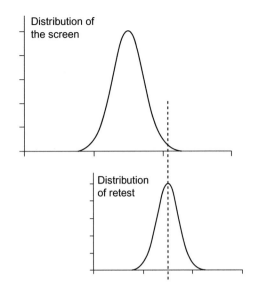

FIGURE 11.38 Confirmation of initial hits in the HTS. Top panel shows the distribution of values from a single test concentration of a high-throughput screen. The criteria for activity and subsequent retest are all values >3 standard error units away from the mean (dotted line). The process of retesting will generate another distribution of values, half of which will be below the original criteria for activity.

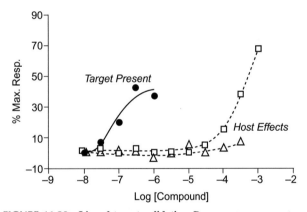

FIGURE 11.39 Ligand-target validation. Dose-response curves to a putative agonist for a therapeutic target on cell lines transfected with the target receptor (filled circles) and on cell lines not transfected with the target receptor (dotted lines, open squares, and open triangles). The open symbol curves reflect nonspecific and nontarget-related effects of the compound on the host cell line. The clear differentiation between the target curves and the host curves indicate a specific effect on the therapeutically relevant target.

There are two general types of observable biological response: agonism and antagonism. There are common issues for all drug discovery programs where pharmacology plays a central role; it is worth considering these. Table 11.5 shows some of the major issues that drug discovery teams deal with throughout a discovery-development program. Two of the first tasks for these teams are to define the lead criterion for success and the critical path designed to get there. Table 11.6 shows some example lead criteria in terms of chemistry, pharmacology, and pharmacokinetics. A critical path can

evolve throughout a program being more concerned with discovery, quantification, and optimization of primary target activity in the early stages and more on required druglike properties of molecules (pharmacokinetics) and issues of safety pharmacology in later stages. One important aspect of a critical path is the type of assay that controls progress; a clear simple readout is required. In contrast, assays that do not necessarily control compound progress (so-called "texture" assays that more fully describe a compound but do not furnish critical data for progression) should not be on the critical path, since these types of data tend to obscure development. Also, the proper placement of assays is important because progression assays placed early on in the path may preclude exploration of chemical scaffolds that will later define flexible structure-activity relationships that can be used to optimize pharmacokinetics and/or eliminate safety issues. However, if these assays are placed too near the end of the critical path (i.e., near the point where the structure-activity relationships are defined in detail), then a "dead end" may be reached whereby a progression-stopping activity may be encountered without sufficient options for alternate structures.

11.10 CLINICAL TESTING

The final, but most expensive and labor-intensive, step in the drug discovery process is the testing of candidates in humans in a clinical trial setting. This is done in phases of increasing intensity and rigor. Phase I clinical trials explore the first time exposure to humans to measure tolerance and safety in human volunteers. These trials consist of rising dose studies to determine maximum tolerated dose via expected route of administration. In addition, pharmacokinetic studies may include multiple dosing in preparation for the next step in the process; namely, Phase II trials. At this stage there may be patient involvement to more accurately reflect targeted populations (i.e., geriatric, healthy patients to toxic cancer drugs) to detect special effects such as differences in tolerance (i.e., schizophrenics are 200 times more tolerant of the side effects of haloperidol than are healthy volunteers).

Should a candidate demonstrate positive effects in Phase I trials, then Phase II trials (initial clinical study for treatment efficacy and continued study of safety) are initiated. These trials are divided into two separate stages: Phase IIa trials are limited to determine some degree of efficacy, while Phase IIb trials are more extensive and expensive including a larger number of patients (100−200). At this stage, biochemical and physiological indices of efficacy are sought in a double-blind (neither patient nor clinicians know which group receives drug and which receives a placebo) setting. In addition to a placebo arm, the Food and Drug Administration (FDA)

TABLE 11.5 Issues at Various Stages of Drug Discovery and Development

A. Early Discovery Phase

- Accomplish target validation (is this worth the effort?).
- Identify biological reagents and assay design for screening.
- Lead optimization.
- Animal orthologues of target.
- Develop animal models for efficacy.
- Design critical path and lead criteria.
- Create information technology system for data analysis and data visualization tools.
- Run the screen; identify hits and assess chemical tractability.

B. Lead Optimization Phase

- Identify tractable scaffold candidate for chemistry.
- Synthesize numerous analogs for enhancement of activity and selectivity.
- Identify structure–activity relationship for primary activity and selectivity.
- Explore all facets of scaffold for intellectual property protection and follow-up.
- Explore possible spin-offs for other indications.
- Attain activity with druglike properties to achieve candidate selection (first time in humans).

C. Clinical Development Phase

- Define NOAEL (no observed adverse effect level) and MRSD (maximum recommended starting dose) for clinical trial.
- Synthesize numerous analogs for enhancement of activity and selectivity for follow-up candidate(s).
- Explore other clinical indications.

TABLE 11.6 Lead Criteria

Chemical

- Novel active structures (activity not due to impurity).
- Search prior art and correct analysis of hit composition.
- Demonstrable SAR (activity can be quantified and associated with specific changes in chemical structure).
- Druglike physicochemical properties, stable, fulfillment of "Lipinski rules," and good solubility.
- Chemically tractable scaffolds, not complex (amenable to analog synthesis).

Biological

- Confirmed pharmacology for determination of affinity, efficacy, target geography, and kinetics of interaction with target in system-independent manner.
- Demonstrable interaction with target (pharmacological validation with no effect in absence of target).
- Selective for target with acceptable liability.
- Defined genetic polymorphisms (<2% population).

Preferred Features

- There is a number of tractable hit series.
- There is good permeation potential (log P_{APP} value > -5.0 desirable).
- Blood-brain barrier entry potential, usually desirable – see Chapter 9.
- No evidence of induction or binding to CYP450s – see Chapter 9.
- *In vitro* metabolic stability (i.e., S9 metabolism <50% at 1hr) – see Chapter 9.
- There are sites available to modify pharmacokinetics that do not affect primary activity *in vivo*, a generally good pharmacokinetic profile.
- There is low protein binding.
- No genotoxicity evident.
- There is 100-fold separation between potency at primary target and cytotoxicity.

Strategic

- Existence of acceptable intellectual property (IP) (determined IP position and competitive landscape).
- Target is therapeutically relevant (strong association between target and disease in literature), not associated with toxicology.

often requires a positive control arm (known drug, if available). If the positive control arm fails to show efficacy, the trial is a failure.

Phase III clinical trials are critical and require full-scale treatment in several medical centers. The design of these trials compares the test candidate to known treatment and placebo in a double-blind manner. The dosage used in these trials is critical, as these determine regulatory decisions and marketing. The number of patients can be several hundred to thousands, and assessments of drug interactions are made at this stage.

While new drugs are approved after completion of successful Phase III trials, there is yet another stage beyond drug approval. Thus, Phase IV clinical trials consist of postmarketing surveillance. At this point, there is monitoring of adverse effects and additional long-term large-scale studies of efficacy. There is monitoring of additional indications at this stage as well. Pharmacoeconomic data also are obtained to convince healthcare payers that the new drug offers significant benefit over existing therapy (time to recovery, quality of life).

11.11 SUMMARY AND CONCLUSIONS

- There is evidence to suggest that, while more drugs are being discovered, there is no commensurate increase in the number of novel treatments for disease.
- A major approach to discovery is target based, whereby a single biological target is identified (and validated) as a primary cause of disease. Ligands that produce a defined action at the target (i.e., agonism, antagonism) are therefore expected to alleviate the disease in the therapeutic situation.
- Recombinant systems are the main tools of target-based approaches. These can be manipulated, but information is lacking for complete modeling of therapeutic systems.
- Biological targets may consist of single entity proteins, complexes of receptors (dimers), or receptors plus accessory proteins. Mixtures of gene products can produce unique phenotypic biological targets.
- An alternative approach involves testing of new drug entities on whole cell systems and measuring effects on integrated cellular pathways. Favorable phenotypic responses are identified with this approach, which may better produce alteration of multicomponent disease processes.
- An added complexity, but one that may better predict therapeutic activity, is the testing of drugs in assays with different contexts (i.e., basal stimulation).
- Testing *in vivo* can further produce therapeutic model systems. Certain multicomponent disease conditions can be adequately modeled only *in vivo*.

- The ultimate model is the human in the clinical situation. Translational medicine with noninvasive imaging techniques and biomarkers now are able to furnish valuable information that can be used in the initial discovery process to produce better-defined drugs.
- As well as complex biological targets, complex chemical targets (drugs with multiple activity, pro-drugs) can be used to produce therapeutically useful phenotypic responses.
- The drug discovery process can be divided into four subsets: acquisition of chemical drug candidates, pharmacodynamic testing of large numbers of compounds (screening), optimization of pharmacokinetic properties, and optimization of pharmaceutical properties.
- Potential chemical structures for drug testing can originate from natural products, design from modeling the active site of the biological target, modification of natural substances, hybridization of known drugs, or random screening of chemical diversity.
- There is evidence to suggest that druglike structures exist in clusters in chemical space (privileged structures); identification of these can greatly enhance success in screening.
- Large-scale sampling of chemical space can be achieved with high-throughput screening. This process involves the design of robust but sensitive biological test systems and the statistical sifting of biological signals from noise. The Z' statistic can be useful in this latter process.
- Surrogate screening (utilizing similar but not exact therapeutically relevant targets) can lead to dissimulation in screening data, especially for allosteric molecules. For this reason, frequent reality testing with a therapeutically relevant assay is essential.
- The importance of the definition of lead criteria and critical paths is discussed as well as the differences involved in following single- and multiple-variate structure-activity relationships.

REFERENCES

[1] Booth B, Zemmel R. Prospects for productivity. Nat Rev Drug Disc 2004;3:451–6.

[2] Williams M. A return to the fundamentals of drug discovery. Curr Opin Invest Drugs 2004;5:29–33.

[3] Walker MJA, Barrett T, Guppy LJ. Functional pharmacology: the drug discovery bottleneck? Drug Disc Today 2004;3:208–15.

[4] Spedding M, Jay T, Cost de Silva J, Perret L. A pathophysiological paradigm for the therapy of psychiatric disease. Nat Rev Drug Disc 2005;4:467–76.

[5] Hopkins AL, Groom CR. The druggable genome. Nat Rev Drug Disc 2002;1:727–30.

[6] Claverie J-M. What if there were only 30,000 human genes? Science 2001;291:1255−7.

[7] Drews J. Drug discovery: a historical perspective. Science 2000;287:1960−4.

[8] Luster AD. Mechanisms of disease: Chemokines − chemotactic cytokines that mediate inflammation. N Eng J Med 1998;338:436−45.

[9] Zaitseva M, Blauvelt A, Lee S, Lapham CK, Klaus-Kovtun V, Mostowski H, et al. Expression and function of CCR5 and CXCR4 on human langerhans cells and macrophages: implications for HIV primary infection. Nature Medicine 1997;3:1369−75.

[10] Cagnon L, Rossi JJ. Downregulation of the CCRS beta-chemokine receptor and inhibition of HIV-1 infection by stable VA1-ribozyme chimeric transcripts. Antisense Nucleic Acid Drug Dev 2000;10:251−61.

[11] Baba M, Nishimura O, Kanzaki N, Okamoto M, Sawada H, Iizawa Y, et al. A small-molecule, nonpeptide CCR5 antagonist with highly potent and selective anti-HIV-1 activity. Proc Natl Acad Sci USA 1999;96:5698−703.

[12] Cocchi F, De Vico AL, Garzino-Demo A, Arya SK, Gallo RC, Lusso P. Identification of RANTES, MIP-1α, and MIP-1β as the major HIV-suppressive factors produced by CD8$^+$ T cells. Science 1995;270:1811−5.

[13] Finke PE, Oates B, Mills SG, MacCoss M, Malkowitz L, Springer MS, et al. Antagonists of the human CCR5 receptor as anti-HIV-1 agents. Part 4: synthesis and structure: activity relationships for 1-[N-(Methyl)-N-(phenylsulfonyl)amino]-2-(phenyl)-4-(4-(N-(alkyl)-N-(benzyloxycarbonyl)amino)piperidin-1-yl)butanes. Bioorg Med Chem Lett 2001;11:2475−9.

[14] Mack M, Luckow B, Nelson PJ, Cihak J, Simmons G, Clapham PR, et al. Aminooxypentane-RANTES induces CCR5 internalization but inhibits recycling: a novel inhibitory mechanism of HIV infectivity. J Exp Med 1998;187:1215−24.

[15] Simmons G, Clapham PR, Picard L, Offord RE, Rosenkilde MM, Schwartz TW, et al. Potent inhibition of HIV-1 infectivity in macrophages and lymphocytes by a novel CCR5 antagonist. Science 1997;276:276−9.

[16] Garzino-Demo A, Moss RB, Margolick JB, Cleghorn F, Sill A, Blattner WA, et al. Spontaneous and antigen-induced production of HIV-inhibitory-chemokines are associated with AIDS-free status. Proc Natl Acad Sci USA 1999;96:11986−91.

[17] Ullum H, Lepri AC, Victor J. Production of beta-chemokines in human immunodeficiency virus (HIV) infection: Evidence that high levels of macrophage in inflammatory protein-1-beta are associated with a decreased risk of HIV progression. J Infect Dis 1998;177:331−6.

[18] Grivel J-C, Ito Y, Faga G, Santoro F, Shaheen F, Malnati MS, et al. Suppression of CCR5 − but not CXCR4 − tropic HIV-1 in lymphoid tissue by human herpesvirus 6. Nature Med 2001;7:1232.

[19] Dean M, Carrington M, Winkler C, Huttley GA, Smith MW, Allikmets R, et al. Genetic restriction of HIV-1 infection and progression to AIDS by a deletion allele of the CKR5 structural gene. Science 1996;273:1856−62.

[20] Huang Y, Paxton WA, Wolinsky SM, Neumann AU, Zhang L, He T, et al. The role of a mutant CCR5 allele in HIV-1 transmission and disease progression. Nature Med 1996;2:1240−3.

[21] Liu R, Paxton WA, Choe S, Ceradini D, Martin SR, Horuk R, et al. Homozygous defect in HIV-1 coreceptor accounts for resistance of some multiply-exposed individuals to HIV-1 infection. Cell 1996;86:367−77.

[22] Paxton WA, Martin SR, Tse D, O'Brien TR, Skurnick J, VanDevanter NL, et al. Relative resistance to HIV-1 infection of CD4 lymphocytes from persons who remain uninfected despite multiple high-risk sexual exposures. Nature Med 1996;2:412−7.

[23] Samson M, Libert F, Doranz BJ, Rucker J, Liesnard C, Farber CM, et al. Resistance to HIV-1 infection in Caucasian individuals bearing mutant alleles to the CCR-5 chemokine receptor gene. Nature 1996;382:722−5.

[24] Cook DN, Beck MA, Coffman TM, Kirby SL, Sheridan JF, Pragnell IB, et al. Requirement of MIP-1α for an inflammatory response to viral infection. Science 1995;269:1583−5.

[25] Knudsen TB, Kristiansen TB, Katsenstein TL, Eugen-Olsen J. Adverse effect of the CCR5 promoter -2459A allele on HIV-1 disease progression. J Med Virol 2001;65:441.

[26] Neubig RR, Siderovski DP. Regulators of G-protein signaling as new central nervous system drug targets. Nat Rev Drug Disc 2002;1:187−96.

[27] Mestas J, Hughes CC. Of mice and not men: differences between mouse and human immunology. J Immunol 2004;172:2731−8.

[28] Hill R. NK1 (Substance P) receptor antagonists: Why are they not analgesic in humans? Trends Pharmacol Sci 2000;21:244−6.

[29] Strizki JM, Xu S, Wagner NE, Wojcik L, Liu J, Hou Y, et al. SCH-C (SCH 351125), an orally bioavailable, small molecule antagonist of the chemokine receptor CCR5, is a potent inhibitor of HIV-1 infection in vitro and in vivo. Proc Natl Acad Sci USA 2001;98:12718−23.

[30] Brodde O-E, Leineweber K. β₂-adrenoceptor gene polymorphisms. Pharmacogenet Genom 2005;15:267−75.

[31] Kost TA, Condreay JP. Recombinant baculoviruses as mammalian cell gene-delivery vectors. Trends Biotechnol 2002;20:173−80.

[32] Douglas SA, Ohlstein EH, Johns DG. Techniques: cardiovascular pharmacology and drug discovery in the 21st century. Trends Pharmacol Sci 2004;25:225−33.

[33] Heldin CH. Dimerization of cell surface receptors in signal transduction. Cell 1995;80:213−23.

[34] George SR, O'Dowd BF, Lee SP. G-protein-coupled receptor oligomerization and its potential for drug discovery. Nat Rev Drug Disc 2002;1:808−20.

[35] AbdAlla S, Lother H, Quitterer U. At1-receptor heterodimers show enhanced G-protein activation and altered receptor sequestration. Nature 2000;407:94−8.

[36] AbdAla S, Lother H, el Massiery A, Quitterer U. Increased AT(1) receptor dimers in preeclampsia mediate enhanced angiotensin II responsiveness. Nature Med 2001;7:1003−9.

[37] Mellado M, Rodríguez-Frade JM, Vila-Coro AJ, Fernández S, Martín de Ana A, Jones DR, et al. Chemokine receptor homo- or heterodimerization activates distinct signaling pathways. EMBO J 2001;20:2497−507.

[38] Wildoer M, Fong J, Jones RM, Lunzer MM, Sharma SK, Kostensis E, et al. A heterodimer-selective agonist shows in vivo relevance of G-protein coupled receptor dimers. Proc Natl Acad Sci USA 2005;102:9050−5.

[39] Milligan G, Ramsay D, Pascal G, Carrillo JJ. GPCR dimerization. Life Sci 2003;74:181−8.

[40] Kubinyi H. Drug research: Myths, hype, and reality. Nat Rev Drug Disc 2003;2:665−8.

[41] Armour SL, Foord S, Kenakin T, Chen W-J. Pharmacological characterization of receptor activity modifying proteins (RAMPs) and

the human calcitonin receptor. J Pharmacol Toxicol Meth 1999;42:217—24.

[42] Foord SM, Marshall FH. RAMPS: accessory proteins for seven trans-membrane domain receptors. Trends Pharmacol Sci 1999;20:184—7.

[43] Fraser NJ, Wise A, Brown J, McLatchie LM, Main MJ, Foord SM. The amino terminus of receptor activity modifying proteins is a critical determinant of glycosylation state and ligand binding of calcitonin-like receptor. Mol Pharmacol 1999;55:1054—9.

[44] Kunkel EJ, Dea M, Ebens A, Hytopoulos E, Melrose J, Nguyen D, et al. An integrative biology approach for analysis of drug action in models of human vascular inflammation. FASEB J 2004;18:1279—301.

[45] Kunkel EJ, Plavec I, Nguyen D, Melrose J, Rosler ES, Kao LT, et al. Rapid structure-activity and selectivity analysis of kinase inhibitors by BioMap analysis in complex human primary cell-based models. ASSAY Drug Dev Technol 2004;2:431—41.

[46] Siegel PM, Massague J. Cytostatic and apoptotic actions of TGF-β in homeostasis and cancer. Nature Rev Cancer 2003;3:807—21.

[47] Dage RC, Roebel LE, Hsieh CP, Weiner DL, Woodward JK. The effects of MDL 17,043 on cardiac inotropy in the anesthetized dog. J Cardiovasc Pharmacol 1982;4:500—12.

[48] Kenakin TP, Scott DL. A method to assess concomitant cardiac phosphodiesterase inhibition and positive inotropy. J Cardiovasc Pharmacol 1987;10:658—66.

[49] Kenakin TP, Pike NB. An in vivo analysis of purine-mediated renal vasoconstriction in rat isolated kidney. Br J Pharmacol 1987;90:373—81.

[50] Kenakin TP. Drug and organ selectivity: similarities and differences. In: Test B, editor. Advances in drug research, Vol. 15. New York: Academic Press; 1985. p. 71—109.

[51] Littman BH, Williams SA. The ultimate model organism: progress in experimental medicine. Nat Rev Drug Disc 2005;4:631—8.

[52] Polmar S, Diaz-Gonzalez F, Dougados M, Ortiz P, del-Miguel G. Limited clinical efficacy of a leukotriene B4 receptor (LTB₄) antagonist in patients with active rheumatoid arthritis (RA). Arthritis Rheum 2004;50:S239.

[53] Tarazi FI, Zhang K, Baldessarini RJ. Review: Dopamine D4 receptors: Beyond schizophrenia. J Recept Sig Transduct Res 2004;24:131—47.

[54] Milne GM. Pharmaceutical productivity: the imperative for new paradigms. Annu Rep Med Chem 2003;38:383—96.

[55] Sikora K. Surrogate endpoints in cancer drug development. Drug Disc Today 2002;7:951—6.

[56] Baczko I, El-Reyani NE, Farkas A, Virág L, Iost N, Leprán I, et al. Antiarrhythmic and electrophysiological effects of GYK-16638, a novel N-(phenoxyalkyl)-N-phenylalkylamine, in rabbits. Eur J Pharmacol 2000;404:181—90.

[57] Morphy R, Rankovic Z. Designed multiple ligands: An emerging drug discovery paradigm. J Med Chem 2005;48:6523—43.

[58] Perez M, Pauwels PJ, Fourrier C, Chopin P, Valentin J-P, John GW, et al. Dimerization of sumitryptan as an efficient way to design a potent, centrally and orally active 5-HT1B agonist. Bioorg Med Chem Lett 1998;8:675—80.

[59] Daniels DJ, Kulkarni A, Xie Z, Bhushan RG. A bivalent ligand (KDAN-18) containing δ-antagonist and κ-agonist pharmacophores bridges δ₂ and κ₁ opioid receptor phenotypes. J Med Chem 2005;48:1713—6.

[60] Zhang M, van de Stolpe A, Zuiderveld O, Timmermans H. Combined antagonism of leukotrienes and histamine produces predominant inhibition of allergen-induced early and late phase airway obstruction in asthmatics. Eur J Med Chem 1997;32:95—102.

[61] Kenakin TP, Johnson SF. The importance of α-adrenoceptor agonist activity of dobutamine to inotropic selectivity in the anesthetized cat. Eur J Pharmacol 1985;111:347—54.

[62] Lipinski C, Lombardo F, Dominy B, Feeney P. Experimental and computational approaches to estimate solubility and permeability in drug discovery and development settings. Adv Drug Deliv Rev 2001;23:3—25.

[63] Richardson BP, Engel G, Donatsch P, Stadler PA. Identification of serotonin M-receptor subtypes and their specific blockade by a new class of drugs. Nature 1985;316:126—31.

[64] Baldwin JJ, Lumma Jr. WC, Lundell GF, Ponticello GS, Raab AW, Engelhardt EL, et al. Symbiotic approach to drug design: antihypertensive β-adrenergic blocking agents. J Med Chem 1979;22:1284—90.

[65] Hann MM, Oprea TI. Pursuing lead likeness concept in pharmaceutical research. Curr Opin Chem Biol 2004;8:255—63.

[66] Lipinski CA. Druglike properties and the causes of poor solubility and poor permeability. J Pharmacol Tox Meth 2000;44:235—49.

[67] Jakubic J, Bacakova I, El-Fakahany EE, Tucek S. Positive cooperativity of acetylcholine and other agonists with allosteric ligands on muscarinic acetylcholine receptors. Mol Pharmacol 1997;52:172—9.

[68] Zhang J-H, Chung TDY, Oldenburg KR. A simple statistical parameter for use in evaluation and validation of high throughput screening assays. J Biomolecular Screening 1999;4:67—72.

[69] Andrews PR, Craik DJ, Martin JL. Functional group contributions to drug-receptor interactions. J Med Chem 1984;27:1648—57.

[70] Hopkins AL, Groom CR, Alex A. Ligand efficiency: a useful metric for lead selection. Drug Disc Today 2004;9:430—1.

[71] Kuntz ID, Chen K, Sharp KA, Kollman PA. The maximal affinity of ligands. Proc Natl Acad Sci USA 1999;96:9997—10002.

[72] Roettger BF, Ghanekar D, Rao R, Toledo C, Yingling J, Pinon D, et al. Antagonist-stimulated internalization of the G protein-coupled cholecystokinin receptor. Mol Pharmacol 1997;51:357—62.

[73] Pommier Y, Cherfils J. Interfacial inhibition of macromolecular interactions: nature's paradigm for drug discovery. Trends Pharmacol Sci 2005;26:138—45.

[74] Onaran HO, Costa T. Agonist efficacy and allosteric models of receptor action. Ann N Y Acad Sci 1997;812:98—115.

[75] Onaran HO, Scheer A, Cotecchia S, Costa T. A look at receptor efficacy. From the signaling network of the cell to the intramolecular motion of the receptor. In: Kenakin TP, Angus JA, editors. The pharmacology of functional, biochemical, and recombinant systems handbook of experimental pharmacology, Vol. 148. Heidelberg: Springer; 2000. p. 217—80.

[76] Kenakin TP, Onaran O. The ligand paradox between affinity and efficacy: can you be there and not make a difference? Trends Pharmacol Sci 2002;23:275—80.

[77] Marullo S, Bouvier M. Resonance energy transfer approaches in molecular pharmacology and beyond. Trends Pharmacol Sci 2007;28:362—5.

[78] Hoffmann C, Gaietta G, Bünemann M, Adams S, Oberdorff-Maass S, Behr B, et al. A FLASH-based approach to determine G protein-coupled receptor activation in living cells. Nat Methods 2005;2:171—6.

[79] Azzi M, Charest PG, Angers S, Rousseau G, Kohout T. β-arrestin-mediated activation of MAPK by inverse agonists reveals distinct active conformations for G-protein-coupled receptors. Proc Natl Acad Sci USA 2003;100:11406—11.

Statistics and Experimental Design

To call in the statistician after the experiment is done may be no more than asking him to perform a postmortem examination: he may be able to say what the experiment died of...

— Indian Statistical Congress, Sankya (ca 1938)

12.1 Structure of This Chapter
12.2 Introduction
12.3 Descriptive Statistics: Comparing Sample Data
12.4 How Consistent is Experimental Data with Models?
12.5 Comparison of Samples to "Standard Values"
12.6 Experimental Design and Quality Control
12.7 Chapter Summary and Conclusions
References

12.1 STRUCTURE OF THIS CHAPTER

This chapter is divided into three main sections. The first is devoted to methods, ideas, and techniques aimed at determining whether a set of pharmacological data is internally consistent, that is, to what extent a given value obtained in the experiment will be obtained again if the experiment is repeated. The second section is devoted to methods and techniques aimed at determining to what extent the experimentally observed value is externally consistent with literature, other experimental data sets, or values predicted by models. This second section is divided into two subsections. The first deals with comparing experimental data to models that predict values for the entire population (i.e., curve fitting, etc.) and the second subsection is concerned with differences, between either experimentally determined data or an experimentally determined data set and values, from the literature. Finally, some ideas on experimental design will be discussed in the context of improving experimental techniques.

12.2 INTRODUCTION

Statistics in general is a discipline dealing with ideas on descriptions of data, implications of data (in relation to general pharmacological models), and questions such as what effects are real, and what effects are different? Biological systems are variable. Moreover, often they are living. What this means is that they are collections of biochemical reactions going on in synchrony. Such systems will have an intrinsic variation in their output, due to the variances in the rates and set points of the reactions taking place during the natural progression of their function. In general, this will be referred to as biological "noise" or variation. For example, a given cell line kept under culture conditions will have a certain variance in the ambient amount of cellular cyclic AMP present at any instant. Pharmacological experiments strive to determine whether or not a given chemical can change the ambient physiological condition of a system and thus demonstrate pharmacological activity. The relevant elements in this quest are the level of the "noise" and the level of change in response of a system imparted by the chemical, that is, the signal-to-noise ratio.

12.3 DESCRIPTIVE STATISTICS: COMPARING SAMPLE DATA

In general, when a pharmacological constant or parameter is measured, it should be done so repeatedly to give a measure of confidence in the value obtained, that is, how likely is it that if the measurement were repeated it would yield the same value. There are various statistical tools available to determine this; an important tool and concept in this regard is the Gaussian distribution.

T. P. Kenakin: A Pharmacology Primer, Fourth edition. DOI: http://dx.doi.org/10.1016/B978-0-12-407663-1.00012-0
© 2009 Elsevier Inc. All rights reserved.

12.3.1 Gaussian Distribution

When an experimental value is obtained a number of times, the individual values will symmetrically cluster around the mean value with a scatter that depends on the number of replications made. If a very large number of replications are made (i.e., > 2000), the distribution of the values will take on the form of a Gaussian curve. It is useful to examine some of the features of this curve, since it forms the basis of a large portion of the statistical tools used in this chapter. The Gaussian curve for a particular population of N values (denoted x_i) will be centered along the abscissal axis on the mean value where the mean (η) is given by:

$$\eta = \frac{\sum\limits_{i} x_i}{N} \tag{12.1}$$

The measure of variation in this population is given by the standard deviation of the population (σ):

$$\sigma = \sqrt{\frac{\sum (x_i - \eta)^2}{N}} \tag{12.2}$$

The ordinates of a Gaussian curve are the relative frequency that the particular values on the abscissae are encountered. The frequency of finding these values for a particular value diminishes the farther away it is from the mean. The resulting curve is shown in Figure 12.1A. The abscissal axis is divided into multiples of σ values; thus, $+1$ or -1 refers to values that are within one standard deviation either greater than or less than the mean. It is useful to consider the area under the curve at particular points along the abscissae, since this gives a measure of the probability of finding a particular value within the standard deviation limits chosen. For example, for a standard Gaussian curve, 68.3% of all the values reside within one standard deviation unit of the mean. Similarly, 95.5% of all the values lie within two σ units, and 99.7% of the values within three σ units (see Figure 12.1A). Most statistical tests used in pharmacology are parametric (i.e., they require the assumption that the distribution of the values being compared are from a normal distribution). If enough replicates are obtained, a normal distribution of values will be obtained. For example, Figure 12.1B shows a collection of 58 replicate estimates of the pK_B of a CCR5 antagonist TAK 779 as an inhibitor of HIV infection. It can be seen that the histograms form a relatively symmetrical array around the mean value. As more values are added to such collections, they take on the smoother appearance of a Gaussian distribution (Figure 12.1C). It should be noted that the requirements of normal distribution are paramount for the statistical tests that are to be described in this chapter. As discussed in Chapter 1, while pK_I, pEC_{50}, and pK_B estimates are normally distributed because they are derived from logarithmic axes on curves, the corresponding IC_{50}, EC_{50}, and K_B values are not (Figure 1.17) and thus cannot be used in parametric statistical tests.

12.3.2 Populations and Samples

Populations are very large collections of values; in practice, experimental pharmacology deals with samples (much smaller collections) of a population. The statistical

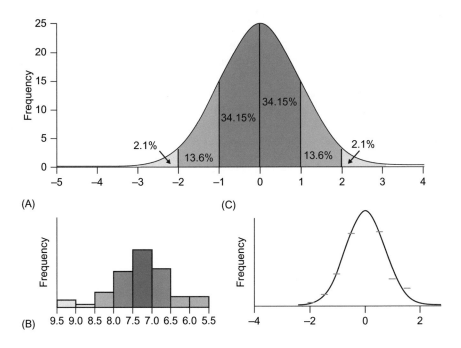

FIGURE 12.1 Normal distributions. (A) Gaussian distribution showing the frequency of values in a population expressed as a function of distance away from the value from the mean of the population. Percentage values represent areas in the strips of curve, that is, between 0 and 1 represents the area within one standard deviation unit from the mean. (B) Histogram showing the pK_B of an antagonist (TAK 779, an antagonist of HIV infection) divided into bins composed of 1 SEM unit away from the mean value. (C) The histogram is an approximation of a Gaussian normal distribution shown in panel B.

tools used to deal with samples differ somewhat from those used to deal with populations. When an experimental sample is obtained, the investigator often wants to know about two features of the sample: central tendency and variability. *Central tendency* refers to the most representative estimate of the value, while *variability* defines the confidence that the estimate is a true reflection of that value. Central tendency estimates can be the median (value that divides the sample into two equal halves) or the mode (most commonly occurring value). These values (especially the median) are not affected by extreme values (outliers). However, the most common estimate of central tendency in experimental work is the mean (x_m), defined for a set of n values as:

$$x_m = \frac{\sum_i x_i}{n} \qquad (12.3)$$

The estimate of variability for a sample mean is the standard error of the mean:

$$s_x = \sqrt{\frac{\sum (x_i - x_m)^2}{(n-1)}} \qquad (12.4)$$

Alternatively, this frequently-used quantity can be calculated as:

$$s_x = \sqrt{\frac{n \sum x^2 - (\sum x)^2}{n(n-1)}} \qquad (12.5)$$

There are instances where deviations, as measured by the standard error, are scaled to the magnitude of the mean to yield the coefficient of variation. This is calculated as:

$$C.V. = 100 \times \text{standard deviation/mean.} \qquad (12.6)$$

A frequently asked question is, are two experimentally derived means equal? In fact, this question really should be stated, "Do the two experimentally derived samples come from the same population?" Hypothesis testing is used to answer this question. This process is designed to disprove what is referred to as the *null hypothesis* (i.e., the condition of no difference). Thus, the null hypothesis states that there is no difference between the two samples (i.e., that they both come from the same population). It is important to note that experiments are designed to disprove the null hypothesis, not prove the hypothesis correct. Theoretically speaking, a hypothesis can never be proven correct since failure to disprove the hypothesis may mean only that the experiment designed to do so is not designed adequately. There could always be a yet-to-be-designed experiment capable of disproving the null hypothesis, thus it is a Sisyphean task to prove it "correct." However, the danger of overinterpreting failure to disprove the null hypothesis cannot be overemphasized; as put by the statistician

Finney (1955) "…failure to disprove that certain observations do not disprove a hypothesis does not amount to proof of a hypothesis…"

This concept is illustrated by the example shown in Table 12.1. Shown are three replicate pEC_{50} values for the agonist human calcitonin obtained from two types of cells; wild-type HEK 293 cells and HEK 293 cells enriched with $G_{\alpha s}$-protein. The respective pEC_{50} values are 7.47 ± 0.15 and 8.18 ± 0.21. The question is whether or not these two estimates come from the same population.

That is, is there a statistically significant difference between the sensitivity of cells enriched and not enriched with $G_{\alpha s}$-protein to human calcitonin? To go further toward answering this question requires discussion of the concepts of probability and the t-distribution.

Statistical tests do not declare anything with certainty; they only assess the probability that the result is true. Thus, values have a "level of confidence" associated with them. Within the realm of hypothesis testing, where the verisimilitude of a data set to predictions made by two hypotheses is examined, a probability is obtained. As discussed previously, the approach taken is that the data must disprove the null hypothesis (stating that there is no difference). For example, when testing whether a set of data is consistent with or disproves the null hypothesis, a level of confidence of 95% states that the given hypothesis is disproved but that there is a 5% chance that this result occurred randomly. This means that there is a small (5%) chance that the data

TABLE 12.1 T-Test for Differences Between Experimental Means

pEC_{50} values for human calcitonin in wild-type HEK 293 cells (x_2) and HEK 293 cells enriched with $G_{\alpha s}$-protein (x_1).

x_1	x_2
7.9	7.5
8.2	7.3
8.3	7.6
$\sum x_1 = 24.4$	$\sum x_2 = 22.4$
$\sum x_1^2 = 198.54$	$\sum x_2^2 = 167.3$
$x_{m1} = 8.13$	$x_{m2} = 7.47$
$s_{x1} = 0.21$	$s_{x2} = 0.15$
$s_p^2 = 0.033$	
difference $= 0.67$	
$SE_{(difference)} = 0.149$	
$t = 4.47$	
d.f. $= 4$	

Data from [1].

supported the hypothesis but that the experiment was unable to discern the effect. This type of error is termed a *type I error* (rejection of a true hypothesis erroneously) and often is given the symbol α. Experimenters preset this level before the experiment (i.e., $\alpha = 0.05$ states that the investigator is prepared to accept a 5% chance of being incorrect). Statistical significance then is reported as $p < 0.05$, meaning that there is less than a 5% probability that the experiment led to a type I error. Another type of error (termed *type II error*) occurs when a hypothesis is erroneously accepted (i.e., the data appear to be consistent with the null hypothesis), but, in fact, the samples do come from separate populations and are indeed different.

So how does one infer that two samples come from different populations when only small samples are available? The key is the discovery of the t-distribution by Gosset in 1908 (publishing under the pseudonym of Student) and the development of the concept by Fisher in 1926. This revolutionary concept enables the estimation of σ (standard deviation of the population) from values of standard errors of the mean and thus to estimate population means from sample means. The value t is given by:

$$t = (X_m - \eta)/SE_x, \tag{12.7}$$

where SE_x is the standard deviation and η is the mean of the population. Deviation of the estimated mean from the population mean in SE_x units yields values that then can be used to calculate the confidence that given sample means come from the same population. Returning to the data in Table 12.1 (two sample means x_{m1} and x_{m2} of size n_1 and n_2, respectively), the difference between the two means is $(x_{m1} - x_{m2}) = 0.67$ log units. A standard error of this difference can be calculated by:

$$S.E._{difference} = s_p^2(1/n_1 + 1/n_2)^{1/2}, \tag{12.8}$$

where s_p^2 is the pooled variance, given as:

$$s_p^2 = \frac{(n_1 - 1)s_{x1}^2 + (n_2 - 1)s_{x2}^2}{n_1 + n_2 - 2}. \tag{12.9}$$

For the example shown in Table 12.1, $S.E._{difference} = 0.15$. The value of t is given by:

$$t = (X_{m1} - X_{m2})/S.E._{difference}. \tag{12.10}$$

For the example shown in Table 12.1, the calculated t is 4.47. This value is associated with a value for the number of degrees of freedom in the analysis; for this test the degree of freedom (df) is $n_1 + n_2 - 2 = 4$. This value can be compared to a table of t values (Appendix I) to assess significance. There are t values for given levels of confidence. Referring to Appendix I, it can be seen that for df = 4, the value for t at a level of significance of 95% is 2.132. This means that if the calculated value of t is less than 2.132, then there is a greater than 5% chance that the two samples came from the same population (i.e., they are

not different). However, as can be seen from Table 12.1, the calculated value of t is 2.776, indicating that there is less than a 5% chance ($p < 0.05$) that the samples came from the same population.

In fact, a measure of the degree of confidence can be gained from the t calculation. Shown in Appendix I are columns for greater degrees of confidence. The value for df = 4 for a 99% confidence level is 3.747, and it can be seen that the experimentally calculated value is also greater than this value. Therefore, the level of confidence that these samples came from different populations is raised to 99%. However, the level of confidence in believing that these two samples came from separate populations does not extend to 99.5% (t = 4.604). Therefore, at the 99% confidence level, this analysis indicates that the potency of human calcitonin is effectively increased by enrichment of $G_{\alpha s}$-protein in the cell.

A measure of variability of the estimate can be gained from the standard error, but it can be seen from Equations 12.4 and 12.5 that the magnitude of the standard error is inversely proportional to n; that is, the larger the sample size, the smaller will be the standard error. Therefore, without prior knowledge of the sample size, a reported standard error cannot be evaluated. A standard error value of 0.2 indicates a great deal more variability in the estimate if n = 100 than if n = 3. One way around this shortcoming is to report n for every estimate of mean ± standard error. Another, and better, method is to report confidence intervals of the mean.

12.3.3 Confidence Intervals

The confidence interval for a given sample mean indicates the range of values within which the true population value can be expected to be found and the probability that this will occur. For example, the 95% confidence limits for a given mean are given by:

$$c.l._{95} = x_m + s_x(t_{95}), \tag{12.11}$$

where s_x is the standard error and the subscripts refer to the level of confidence (in this case, above 95%). Values of t increase with increasing levels of confidence, therefore the higher the level of confidence required for defining an interval containing the true value from a sample mean, the wider the confidence interval. This is intuitive since it would be expected that there would be a greater probability of finding the true value within a wider range. The confidence limits of the mean pEC_{50} value for human calcitonin in wild-type and $G_{\alpha s}$-protein-enriched HEK 293 cells are shown in Table 12.2. A useful general rule (but not always explicitly accurate, especially for small samples; see Section 12.6.1) is to note that if the mean values are included in the 95% confidence limits of the other mean (if $p < 0.05$ is the predefined level of significance in the experiment), then the means probably are from the same population. In general, reporting variability as confidence limits eliminates

TABLE 12.2 Confidence Intervals for the Means in Table 12.1

	x_{m1}			x_{m2}		
	Lower c.l	Mean	Greater c.l	Lower c.l	Mean	Greater c.l
95%	7.55	8.13 to	8.71	7.05	7.47 to	7.89
98%	7.34	8.13 to	8.92	6.91	7.47 to	8.03
99%	7.16	8.13 to	9.10	6.78	7.47 to	8.16
99.5%	6.95	8.13 to	9.31	6.63	7.47 to	8.31

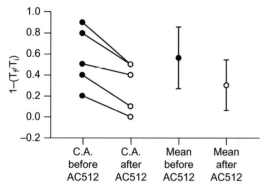

FIGURE 12.2 Paired experimental data. Values of constitutive calcitonin receptor activity $(1 - (T_f/T_i)$ units) in transiently transfected melanophores. Five separate experiments are shown. Points to the left indicate the basal level of constitutive activity before (filled circles) and after (open circles) addition of 100 nM AC512 (calcitonin receptor inverse agonist); lines join values for each individual experiment. Points to the right are the mean values for constitutive activity in control (filled circles) and after AC512 (open circles) for all five experiments (bars represent standard errors of the mean). Data shown in Table 12.3.

TABLE 12.3 Paired T-Tests
Changes in Constitutive Calcitonin Receptor Responses with 100 nM AC512. Values are levels of constitutive activity $(1 - (T_f/T_i))$ for four individual transfection experiments (denoted x_1); x_2 are the constitutive receptor activity values after exposure to AC512 in the same experiment.

x_1	x_2	d
0.8	0.5	−0.3
0.5	0.4	−0.1
0.2	0	−0.2
0.9	0.5	−0.4
0.4	0.1	−0.3
		$\sum d = -1.3$
		$\sum d^2 = 0.39$
		$d_m = -0.26$
		$n = 5$
		$s_{dm} = 0.05$
		$t = -5.10$
		$df = 4$

$d = x_1 - x_2$.

ambiguity with respect to the sample size since the limits are calculated with a t value that itself is dependent upon degrees of freedom (the sample size).

While statistical tests are helpful in discerning differences in data, the final responsibility in determining difference remains with the researcher. While a given statistical test may indicate a difference, it will always do so as a probability, that is, 95% confidence that a given value is different. This means that there is always a 5% chance that this conclusion is incorrect, that is, there is a 5% chance of error in this conclusion. Therefore, statistics furnish confidence limits only for conclusions, and the individual researcher must take responsibility for applying those limits to particular research problems.

12.3.4 Paired Data Sets

The previous discussion is concerned with two samples independently and randomly chosen from populations. A more powerful test of difference can be gained if paired data are used, that is, if the data can be associated. This is because the variance between subsamples is lower than the variance between independent samples. For instance,

the effect of a drug on the body weight of rats can be determined by weighing the rats before dosage of the drug, and then again after the treatment. Each rat becomes its own control and variation is reduced. Figure 12.2 shows the effects of an inverse agonist AC512 on constitutive activity of melanophores transfected with human calcitonin receptor. In this scenario, paired data are important because constitutive activity from transient transfection with receptor cDNA can be quite variable. Therefore, the effects of a drug that affects the magnitude of the constitutive activity (such as an inverse agonist) must be paired to the original basal value of constitutive activity. The data for the inverse agonist AC512 shown in Figure 12.2 are given in Table 12.3 and show the observed constitutive receptor activity as a value of visible light transmittance $(1 - $ (final light transmittance/original light transmittance)) obtained with five separate transient transfections of receptor. It can be seen that the results are variable (mean value for $1 - (T_f/T_i) = 0.56 \pm 0.29$). After treatment with 100 nM AC512 for 60 min, the resulting mean transmittance value of the five experiments is 0.3 ± 0.23.

In the example shown in Figure 12.2, an unpaired t-test finds these samples are not significantly different from each other ($t = 1.21$, df = 8). However, it can be seen from the individually graphed changes for each preparation that there was a consistent fall in constitutive activity for every one of the five preparations (Figure 12.2). Examining the differences for each (difference where $d = x_1 - x_2$) indicates a mean difference of -0.26 ($1 - (T_f/T_i)$ units). The fact that the change can be associated with each individual experiment eliminates the obfuscating factor that the different preparations each started from different values of constitutive activities. The ability to pair the values greatly strengthens the statistical analysis. The value of t for paired data is given by:

$$t = d_m/s_{dm}, \qquad (12.12)$$

where s_{dm} is given by:

$$s_{dm} = \sqrt{\frac{\sum (d_i - d_m)^2}{n(n-1)}}. \qquad (12.13)$$

As can be seen from the analysis in Table 12.3, the paired t-test indicates that the effect of AC512 on the constitutive activity is significant at the 99% level of confidence ($p < 0.01$ that AC512 is an inverse agonist and does decrease the constitutive receptor activity of calcitonin receptors).

12.3.5 One-Way Analysis of Variance

A comparison of two or more means can be made with a one-way analysis of variance (ANOVA). This tool compares sample variability between groups to the sample variability within groups; the data are grouped and the question is asked, "is there a significant difference between any of the means of the groups?" An example of this procedure is shown in Table 12.4. In this example, as discussed previously, the magnitude of the inverse agonism observed for an

TABLE 12.4 One-Way Analysis of Variance
Differences in constitutive calcitonin receptor activity in four separate receptor transfection experiments (x_1 to x_4). Four readings of activity taken for each transfection.

A. Data			
x_1	x_2	x_3	x_4
0.1	0.08	−0.03	0
0.15	0	0.03	0.07
0.04	−0.05	0.08	0.08
0.15	0.02	−0.02	0.02
$\sum x = 0.44$	0.05	0.06	0.17
$n = 4$	4	4	4
$\sum x^2 = 0.0566$	0.0093	0.0086	0.0117
	$\sum ((\sum x)^2/n) = 0.1$		$\sum (\sum x^2) = 0.0862$
	$\sum (\sum x) = 0.72$		

B. Calculations				
	SSq	df	MSq	V_{ratio}
Between groups	A	$a - 1$	s^2_c	
Within groups	C	$N - a$	s^2	$F = s^2_c/s^2$
Total	B	$N - 1$		

$N = $ total number of x values, $a = $ number of groups
where

$$A = \sum \left[\frac{(\sum x)^2}{n} \right] - \frac{[\sum (\sum x)]^2}{\sum n} \qquad B = \sum (\sum x^2) - \frac{[\sum (\sum x)]^2}{\sum n}$$

$$C = A - B \qquad s^2_c = \frac{A}{a-1} \qquad s^2 = \frac{C}{N-a}$$

inverse agonist is dependent upon the amount of constitutive receptor activity present in the system. Therefore, this system effect must be controlled between experiments if comparisons of drug activity are to be made on different test occasions. Table 12.4 shows four basal readings of light transmittance in melanophores ($1 - (T_f/T_i)$ values) after transient transfection of the cells with cDNA for calcitonin receptor activity. The basal readings are indicative of constitutive receptor activity. This same experiment was repeated four times (four separate test occasions with four basal readings in each) and the question asked, "was there a significant difference in the levels of constitutive receptor activity on the various test occasions?" Histograms of the mean basal readings for the four test occasions are shown in Figure 12.3. It can be seen that there is an apparently greater constitutive activity on test occasion 1 but the standard errors are great enough to cast doubt on the significance of this apparent difference. Analysis of variance is used to calculate a value for F, a variance ratio, which then is compared to a table, such as is done with t-tables, for given degrees of freedom. The data and calculations are shown in Table 12.4, where it can be seen that the analysis indicates no significant difference in the readings at the $p < 0.05$ level (tables of F values given in the Appendix). A useful statistic in this analysis is the standard error of the difference between two of the groups. The standard error of the difference between two of the means in the data set x_{m1} and x_{m2} (difference $= |x_{m1} - x_{m2}|$) is:

$$s_d = \left(\frac{s_{i1}^2}{n_1} + \frac{s_{i2}^2}{n_2} \right)^{1/2} \qquad (12.14)$$

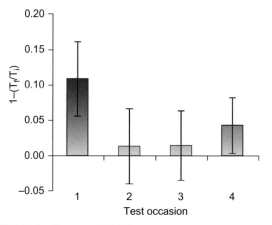

FIGURE 12.3 One-way ANOVA. One-way analysis of variance of basal rates of metabolism in melanophores (as measured by spontaneous dispersion of pigment due to G_s-protein activation) for four experiments. Cells were transiently transfected with cDNA for human calcitonin receptor ($8\,\mu g/mL$) on four separate occasions to induce constitutive receptor activity. The means of the four basal readings for the cells for each experiment (see Table 12.4) are shown in the histogram (with standard errors). The one-way analysis of variance is used to determine whether there is a significant effect of test occasion (any one of the four experiments is different with respect to level of constitutive activity).

where s_i^2 is given by:

$$s_i^2 = \frac{n \sum x^2 - (\sum x)^2}{n(n-1)}. \qquad (12.15)$$

For the data shown in Table 12.4, the difference between the two extreme means of constitutive activity is 0.098 ± 0.04 ($1 - (T_f/T_i)$) units. It can be seen from the general rule $t \cdot s_x \pm$ either mean ($x_{m1} = 0.11 \pm 0.05$, $x_{m2} = 0.013 \pm 0.05$) that this difference is not significant at the $p < 0.05$ level ($t = 3.182$ at $df = 3$). This also can be seen from the fact that $t \cdot s_d$ is $>$ the difference.

12.3.6 Two-Way Analysis of Variance

Data also can be ordered in two ways and the question asked, "is there a difference in the means of data sets when analyzed according to either criterion of ordering?" For example, in cellular functional assays, a convenient practical method of obtaining dose-response curve data on a 96-well cell culture plate is to test a range of concentrations in one row of the plate (i.e., a 12-point dose-response curve). In robotic systems, it is possible that there could be a systematic position effect with respect to rows on a plate (dependent on which row is used to obtain the data for the curve) or which plate in the collection of plates is used for the data. A two-way analysis of variance can be done to test whether such an effect exists. For this analysis, the data are arranged in a table according to one criterion by row and by one column. For example, Table 12.5 shows a set of 32 pEC_{50} values for a calcitonin receptor agonist (human calcitonin) in a functional melanophore experiment. The rows of data correspond to the row of the 96-well plate where the agonist was placed to obtain the value. This will test the possible effect of row position on the plate on the magnitude of the pEC_{50}. The columns are four separate plates to test if the position of the plate in the queue had an effect on the value of the pEC_{50}. The type of data obtained is shown in Figure 12.4. The analysis is shown in Table 12.6, where it can be seen that there was no effect either from the standpoint of the rows ($F_R = 1.02$, $df = 7, 21$) or from plate position (columns, $F_c = 0.56$, $df = 3, 21$).

12.3.7 Regression and Correlation

Two major categories of research are *experimental*, where one variable is manipulated to influence another, and *correlational*, where neither variable is manipulated and only the relationship between variables is quantified. Correlations can be useful to determine relationships between variables, but it should be noted that only experimental research can determine a true causal relationship. In fact, quite erroneous conclusions can be drawn from observing correlations and assuming they are due to a causal relationship. For example, Figure 12.5A shows an apparent inverse correlation between

TABLE 12.5 Two-Way Analysis of Variance pEC_{50} for human calcitonin obtained in culture plates arranged by row (row of the 96-well plate yielding the data) and plate number (columns); see Figure 12.4

x_1	x_2	x_3	x_4	R_{sum}	R_{sum}^2
9.1	8.6	9.5	9.2	36.4	1325.0
8.7	9.2	9.2	8.2	35.3	1246.1
9.5	8.4	9.2	9.4	36.5	1332.3
9.4	8.5	8.9	9.1	35.9	1288.8
8.8	9.3	9	8.6	35.7	1274.5
8.4	9	9.1	8.9	35.4	1253.2
8.5	8.4	8.5	9.2	34.6	1197.2
8.7	8.4	8.9	9.6	35.6	1267.4
$C = 71.1$	69.8	72.3	72.2		

$c = 4$ $T = 285.4$

$r = 8$ $\sum x^2 = 2550.1$

$\sum R^2 = 10184.28$ $N = 32$

Two-Way Analysis of Variance: Calculations

	SSq	df	MSq	V_{ratio}
Between rows	A	$r - 1$	s^2_R	$F_R = s^2_R/s^2$
Within columns	B	$c - 1$	s^2_c	$F_c = s^2_c/s^2$
Residuals	E	$(r-1)(c-1)$	s^2	
Total	D	$N - 1$		

R = sum of rows.
c = number of columns. R = sum of values in each row.
r = number of rows. C = sum of values in each column.
$T = \Sigma$ all values.

$A = \sum R^{2/c} - T^{2/N}$ $B = \sum C^{2/r} - T^{2/N}$
$C = \sum x^2 - T^{2/N}$ $E = D - (A + B)$

the instance when houses in a given neighborhood are painted and house value; that is, it appears that painting your house will actually decrease its value! This correlation is really the product of two other causal relationships; namely, the fact that as a house ages the probability that it will require painting increases and the fact that the value of a house decreases as it gets older (Figure 12.5A). Taking out the common variable of age and plotting the probability of painting and value leads to the surprising, but not causal, relationship. What the correlation really means is that the houses that are being repainted are in fact older and of less value. This is a type of "reverse Simpson's effect" (i.e., Simpson's paradox, in which the association between two variables is confounded by a strong association with a third variable to obscure the original effect).

The correlation between variables can be quantified by a correlation coefficient (denoted r); considering two samples x and y, r is given by:

$$r = \frac{S_{xy}}{\sqrt{S_x^2 S_y^2}} \tag{12.16}$$

where:

$$S_{xy} = \sum xy_1 - \frac{(\sum x_i)(\sum y_i)}{n_i} \tag{12.17}$$

$$S_x^2 = \sum x_i^2 - \frac{(\sum x)^2}{n_i} \tag{12.18}$$

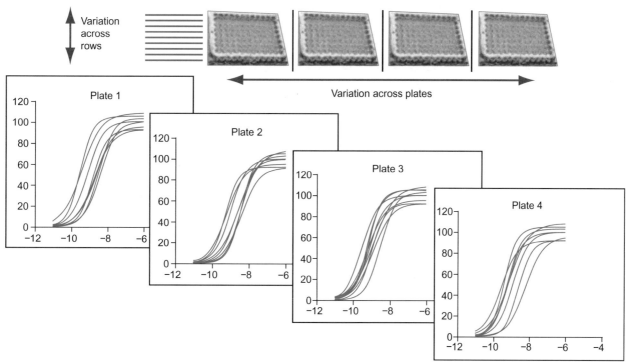

FIGURE 12.4 **Two-way analysis of variance.** Arrangement of data in rows and columns such that each row of the cell culture plate (shown at the top of the figure) defines a single dose-response curve to the agonist. Also, data are arranged by plate in that each plate defines eight dose-response curves and the total data set is composed of 32 dose-response curves. The possible effect of location with respect to row on the plate and/or which plate (order of plate analysis) can be tested with the two-way analysis of variance.

TABLE 12.6 Results of the Two-Way Analysis of Variance for Data Shown in Figure 12.4 and Table 12.5

	SSq	df	MSq	F
Between rows	0.66	7	0.09	0.56
Between columns	0.51	3	0.17	1.02
Residual	3.52	21	0.17	
Total	4.69	31		

and:

$$S_y^2 = \sum y_i^2 - \frac{\left(\sum y\right)^2}{n_i} \qquad (12.19)$$

The correlation coefficient ranges between 1 and −1; a perfect positive correlation has $r = 1$; no correlation at all, $r = 0$; and a perfect negative correlation, $r = -1$. Some examples of correlations are shown in Figure 12.5B.

A measure of the significance of a relationship between two variables can be gained by calculating a value of t:

$$t = r \cdot \sqrt{\frac{(n-2)}{(1-r^2)}}, \quad df = n - 2 \qquad (12.20)$$

12.3.8 Detection of Single Versus Multiple Populations

Often it is important in pharmacological experiments to discern whether or not one or more than one population of biological targets (i.e., receptors) mediate an effect or whether one or more properties of a drug are being observed. One approach to this problem is through population analysis. Under ideal circumstances, a frequency histogram of the data set (as a function of intervals that are some multiple of the standard error) will indicate whether the sample is normally distributed around the mean. Figure 12.6A shows a data set of 59 pEC_{50} values for an agonist in a series of transient transfection experiments (i.e., each experiment consists of transfecting the cells with cDNA for the receptor, therefore a certain intrinsic variability for this process is expected). The data set (mean $pEC_{50} = 8.7 \pm 0.36$) appears to be normally distributed as seen by the frequency histogram. In contrast, another set of 59 pEC_{50} values yields an ambiguous distribution (Figure 12.6B) with no clear normality around the mean. This often is the case with small data sets; that is, there are too few data to clearly evaluate the distribution by sorting into bins and observing the frequency distribution. A more sensitive method is to plot the cumulative frequency of the value as a function of the

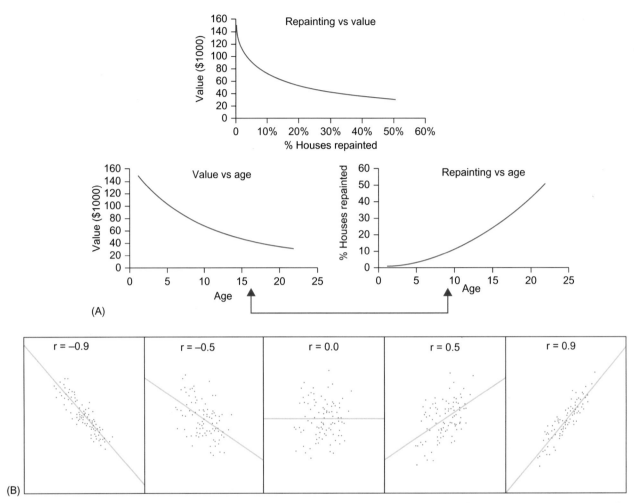

FIGURE 12.5 Misleading correlations. (A) Correlation between percent of houses that are repainted and house value; it can be seen that the relationship is inverse (i.e., painting a house will decrease its value). This correlation comes from two other correlations showing that the value of a house decreases as it ages and the fact that, as a house ages, there is greater probability that it will need to be repainted. (B) Some correlations. A very good negative correlation has r = −0.9; a weak negative correlation, r = −0.5; no correlation, r = 0; a weak positive correlation, r = 0.5; and strong positive correlation, r = 0.9.

value itself. Figure 12.6C shows the cumulative frequency distribution of the data shown in Figure 12.6A. It can be seen that the curve (it will be some form of sigmoidal curve) is consistent with one population of values (it is unimodal). In contrast, the cumulative frequency distribution curve for the data in Figure 12.6B clearly shows two phases, thereby suggesting that the data sample may come from two populations.

12.4 HOW CONSISTENT IS EXPERIMENTAL DATA WITH MODELS?

Experiments yield samples of data that can be likened to the tip of the iceberg, that is, showing a little of what a given system or drug can do. The general aim of experimental pharmacology is to extend this to reveal the complete iceberg and define the model for the complete behavior of

the system. Thus, the sample is used to fuel models, and the verisimilitude of the result assessed to determine whether or not the complete population has been described. Once this is the case, then predictions of other behaviors of the system are made and tested in other experiments.

12.4.1 Comparison of Data to Models: Choice of Model

One of the most important concepts in pharmacology is the comparison of experimental data to models, notably to models describing dose-response curves. The aim is to take a selected sample of data and predict the behavior of the system generating that data over the complete concentration range of the drug, that is, to predict the population of responses. Nonlinear curve fitting is the technique used to do this.

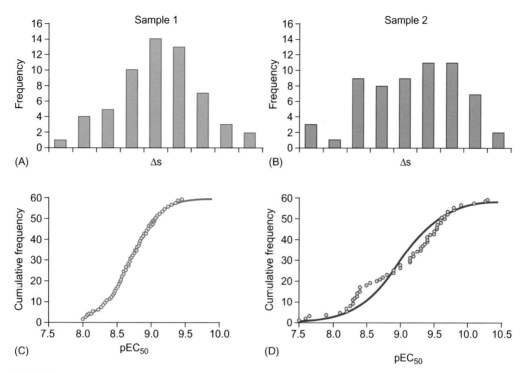

FIGURE 12.6 **Distribution of 59 pEC$_{50}$ values.** (A) Frequency of pEC$_{50}$ values displayed as a function of binning by increments of $0.5 \times$ standard error (mean pEC$_{50}$ = 8.7 ± 0.36). (B) Another data set with an equivocal (with respect to single or bimodal) distribution (mean pEC$_{50}$ = 9.0 ± 0.67). (C) Cumulative distribution curve for the data set shown in panel A. The data are best fit by a single phase curve. (D) Cumulative distribution curve for the data set shown in panel B. In this case, a single phase curve clearly deviates from the data, which indicates bimodality.

The process of curve fitting utilizes the sum of least squares (denoted SSq) as the means of assessing "goodness of fit" of data points to the model. Specifically, SSq is the sum of the differences between the real data values (y_d) and the value calculated by the model (y_c) squared to cancel the effects of arithmetic sign:

$$SSq = \sum (y_d - y_c)^2 \qquad (12.21)$$

There are two approaches to curve fitting. The first uses empirical models that may yield a function that closely fits the data points but has no biological meaning. An example of this was given in Chapter 3 (Figure 3.1). A danger in utilizing empirical models is that nuances in the data points that may be due to random variation may be unduly emphasized as true reflections of the system. The second approach uses parameters rooted in biology (i.e., the constants have biological meaning). In these cases, the model may not fit the data quite as well. However, this latter strategy is preferable since the resulting fit can be used to make predictions about drug effect that can be experimentally tested.

It is worth considering hypothesis testing in general from the standpoint of the choice of models one has available to fit data. On the surface, it is clear that the more complex a model is (more fitting parameters), the

greater the verisimilitude of the data to the calculated line, that is, the smaller will be the differences between the real and predicted values. Therefore, the more complex the model is, the more likely it will accurately fit the data. However, there are other factors that must be considered. One is the physiological relevance of the mathematical function used to fit the data. For example, Figure 12.7 shows a collection of responses to an agonist. A physiologically relevant model to fit these data is a variant of the Langmuir adsorption isotherm, that is, it is likely that these responses emanate from a binding reaction, such as that described by the isotherm which is followed by a series of Michaelis−Menten-type biochemical reactions that also resemble the adsorption isotherm. Therefore, a model such as that described by an equation rooted in biology would seem to be pharmacologically relevant. The fit to such a model is shown in Figure 12.7A. However, a better mathematical fit can be obtained by a complex mathematical function of the form:

$$Response = \sum_{n=4}^{n=1} a^n e^{-(([A]-b_n)/c_n)} \qquad (12.22)$$

While better from a mathematical standpoint, the physiological relevance of Equation 12.22 is unknown.

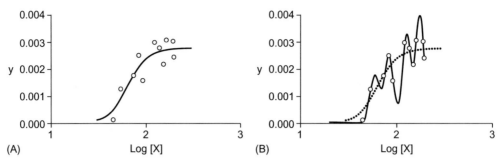

FIGURE 12.7 Fitting dose-response data. (A) Data points fit to Langmuir adsorption isotherm with $E_{max} = 0.00276$, $n = 4.36$, and $EC_{50} = 65$. (B) Data fit to empirical model of the form $y = (600^{-1})e^{-((x-60)2/80)} + (400^{-1})e^{-((x-85)2/400)} + (320^{-1})e^{-((x-130)2/300)} + (280^{-1})e^{-((x-180)2/800)}$.

Also, the more complex a fitting function is, the greater the chance that problems in computer curve fitting will ensue. Fitting software generally uses a method of least squares to iteratively come to a best fit, that is, each parameter is changed stepwise and the differences between the fit function and real data are calculated. The best fit is concluded when a "minimum" in the calculated sum of those differences is found. The different fitting parameters often have different weights of importance in terms of the overall effect produced when they are changed, therefore "local minima" can occur, where further changes in parameters do not appear to produce further changes in the sum of the differences, but these minima may still fall short of the overall minimum value that could be attained if further iteration were allowed. The likelihood of encountering such local minima (which in turn leads to incorrect fitting of functions to data) increases as the model used to fit the data becomes more complex (has many fitting parameters). Therefore, complex models with many fitting parameters can lead to practical problems in computer fitting of data. A sampling of mathematical fitting functions is given in the Appendix for application to fitting data to empirical functions.

Local minima will rarely be observed if the data have little scatter, if an appropriate equation has been chosen, and if the data are collected over an appropriate range of x values. One way to check whether or not a local minimum has been encountered in curve fitting is to observe the effect of making large changes in one of the variables on the sum of squares. If there is a correspondingly large change in the sum of squares, it is possible that a local minimum is operative; ideally, the sum of squares should converge to the same value with any changes in the values of parameters.

Another criterion for goodness of fit is to assess the residual distribution; that is, how well does the model predict values throughout the complete pattern of the data set? Some models may fit some portions of the data well but not other portions, and thus the residuals (differences between the calculated and real values) will not be uniformly distributed over the data set. Figure 12.8 shows a set of data fit to an empirical model (Equation 3.1) and the Langmuir

adsorption isotherm; inspection of the fit dose-response curves does not indicate a great difference in the goodness of fit. However, an examination of the residuals, expressed as a function of the concentration, indicates that while the adsorption isotherm yields a uniform distribution along the course of the data set (uniform distribution of values greater than and less than zero), the empirical fit shows a skewed distribution of errors (values at each end positive and values in the middle negative). A uniform distribution of the residual errors is desired, and models that yield such balanced residuals statistically are preferred.

Finally, complex models may be inferior for fitting data purely in statistical terms. The price of low sums of differences between predicted and real values obtained with a complex model is the loss of degrees of freedom; this results in a greater $(df_s - df_c)$ value for the numerator of the F-test calculation and a greater denominator value, since this is SSq_c divided by df_c (see the following section on hypothesis testing). Therefore, it is actually possible to decrease values of F (leading to a preference for the more simple model) by choosing a more complex model (*vide infra*).

12.4.2 Curve Fitting: Good Practice

There are practical guidelines that can be useful for fitting pharmacological data to curves:

1. All regions of the function should be defined with real data. In cases of sigmoidal curves, it is especially important to have data define the baseline, maximal asymptote, and mid-region of the curve.
2. In usual cases (slope of curve is unity), the ratio of the maximum to the minimum concentrations should be on the order of 3200 (approximately 3.5 log units).
3. The middle of the concentration range should be as near to the location parameter (i.e., EC_{50}, IC_{50}) of the curve as possible.
4. The spacing of the concentration intervals should be equal on a logarithmic scale (i.e., threefold increments).

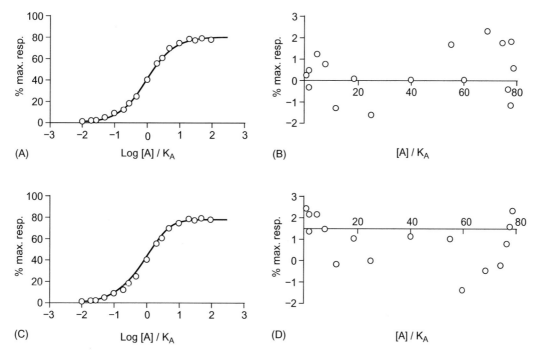

FIGURE 12.8   Residual distribution as a test for goodness of fit.   (A) Data points fit to a physiologically appropriate model (Langmuir isotherm). (B) Residuals (sum of squares of real data points minus calculated data points) expressed as a function of the x value on the curve. It can be seen that the residuals are relatively symmetrically centered around the mean of the residual value over the course of the data set. (C) Same data fit to a general mathematical function (Equation 3.1). (D) The residuals in this case group below the mean of the residuals, indicating a nonsymmetrical fitting of the values.

5. Ideally, there should be > 4 data points for each estimated parameter. Under this guideline, a three-parameter logistic function should have 12 data points. At the least, the number of data points and number of parameters should be > 3.

6. An inspection of the residuals should indicate no systematic deviation of the calculated curve from the data points.

7. It is better to have more points at different x values than many replicates of x; this leads to higher precision in estimating parameters.

8. If the fit is poor and it is suspected that the full concentration range of data has not been tested, the top and/or bottom of the fit may be constrained if no data are available in these regions. If control data from other sources are available, these may be used to constrain maxima and/or minima.

9. The scales of the various parameters should be comparable. Large differences in scale can lead to problems in fitting convergence.

In general, there are rules associated with curve fitting that should be kept in mind when interpreting the curves:

1. The estimates of errors given by nonlinear curve-fitting programs are not estimates of biological variability but rather estimates of errors in fitting the data to the line; the magnitude of these errors depends on the model and the data. The estimation of biological error is gained from repeated experimentation.

2. Correlations between parameters are not favorable and can lead to difficulty in making unique estimates of the parameters.

3. Simple models (fewer parameters) are more robust, but more complex models will usually provide a better fit.

There can be confusion regarding the number of replicate data points used for a curve fit. Replicates are independent (and therefore considered separately) when the source of error for each data point is the same. For example, separate wells in a cell culture plate each containing a collection of cells are independent in that if the error in one of the wells is inordinately high there is no *a priori* reason to assume that the error in other wells also will be as high. Replicate values are not independent when a measurement is repeated many times for the same biological sample (e.g., three readings of radioactivity of tube containing radioligand). Similarly, three replicate readings of a response of a given preparation to the same concentration of agonist are not independent. In these cases the mean of the readings should be taken as a single value.

12.4.3 Outliers and Weighting Data Points

There are occasions when one or more data points do not appear to fit the observed dose-response relationship for an agonist or an antagonist. In this situation, the errant data point(s) can be either weighted or rejected. One common method is to weight the ordinate values according to the square of their value ($1/Y2$ method). The rationale for this approach is the expectation that the distance a given point (y_d) is away from a calculated regression line (y_c) is larger for ordinate values of greater magnitude, therefore scaling them reduces this differential. Under these circumstances, the sum of least squares for assessment of goodness of fit (Equation 12.21) is:

$$SSq = \sum \left(\frac{(y_d - y_c)}{y_d}\right)^2 = \sum \frac{(y_d - y_c)^2}{y_{d^2}}. \quad (12.23)$$

A useful method of weighting is through the use of an iterative reweighted least squares algorithm. The first step in this process is to fit the data to an unweighted model; Table 12.7 shows a set of responses to a range of concentrations of an agonist in a functional assay. The data are fit to a three-parameter model of the form:

$$\text{Response} = \text{Basal} + \frac{\text{Max} - \text{Basal}}{1 + 10^{(\text{LogEC}_{50} - \text{Log}[A])^n}}. \quad (12.24)$$

The fit is shown in Figure 12.9. It can be seen from this figure that the third from the last response point appears to be abnormally higher than the rest of the data set. The next step is to calculate an estimate of the scale of the error (referred to as υ):

$$\upsilon = \frac{\text{median}(|\theta_i - \text{median}(\theta_i)|)}{0.6745} \quad (12.25)$$

TABLE 12.7 Iterative Least Squares Weighting

[Conc] (μM)	Response	Calculated[1]	Residual (θ_i)	$|\theta_I - \text{Median}(\theta_i)|$	Weighting
0.01	2	0.8	−1.2	1.2	0.99
0.03	8	5.2	−2.8	2.8	0.94
0.1	28	28	0	0	1.00
0.3	59	62.6	3.6	3.6	0.90
1	95	77.9	−17.1	17.1	0
3	78	80.4	2.4	2.4	0.96
10	80	80.8	0.8	0.8	1.00
		Median	Residual = 2.4		
			$\upsilon = 3.56$		

[1]*Calculated from model.*
Residual = Calculated − Experimental data.
Weighting calculated with Equation 12.26.

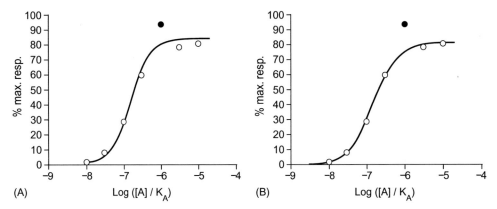

FIGURE 12.9 Outliers. (A) Dose-response curve fit to all of the data points. The potential outlier value raises the fit maximal asymptote. (B) Iterative least squares algorithm weighting of the data points (Equation 12.25) rejects the outlier, and a refit without this point shows a lower fit maximal asymptote.

where θ is the residual error of the point i from the point calculated with the model. The median of these residuals is found and subtracted from the rest of the residuals. The median of the absolute value of these differences is found and divided by 0.6745 to yield the estimate of υ (see Table 12.7). The weighting for each point i is then calculated by:

$$W_i = \left[1 - \left[\frac{(\theta_i / \upsilon)}{B} \right]^2 \right]^2 \quad \text{if } |\theta_i| / \upsilon \leq B \qquad (12.26)$$

where B is a tuning constant with a default value of 4.685. The weighting factors (w_i) for each data point are calculated with Equation 12.26 with the caveat that:

$$W_i = 0 \quad \text{if } |\theta_i| / \upsilon > B. \qquad (12.27)$$

As seen in Table 12.7, the θ_i value for the errant response value obtained for 1 μM agonist (93% versus a calculated value of 77.9%) leads to a value for θ_i / υ of 4.97. Since this value is greater than the default for B, the weighting for this point is zero and the point is removed. Figure 12.9 shows the weighted fit (calculated in Table 12.7) for the same data. It can be seen that the weighting factor for the third from last data point was zero, thereby eliminating it from the fit.

Extreme cases of weighting lead to rejection of outlier points (weighting = 0). This raises scientific issues as to the legitimate conditions under which a data point can be eliminated from the analysis (see Section 12.6.1); is the

rejection of a point due to a truly aberrant reading or just cosmetics for a better fit? This becomes a practical issue with automated curve-fitting procedures for large data sets. For example, in a screening campaign for agonist activity, all single concentrations of compounds that satisfy a criterion for activity (i.e., produce a response above basal noise level at a single concentration) are retested in a dose-response mode to determine a dose-response curve and potency. Under these circumstances, there are a large number of curves to be fit and robotic procedures often are employed. Figure 12.10A shows instances where the curves are continued into regions of concentration that may produce toxic or secondary effects (bell-shaped dose-response curves). Elimination of the low values in these data sets allows a curve to be fit. It should be noted that no value judgment is made (i.e., the bell-shaped dose-response curve may in fact reflect true dual agonist activity that should be noted). The elimination of the point allows only an empirical estimation of potency as a guide for more detailed testing. In other cases, the outlier may be bounded by data (Figure 12.10B). In this case, fitting the curve to all of the data points clearly gives a non-representative curve, and elimination of the outlier at least summarizes the potency of the agonist empirically. In cases of possible "cosmetic" elimination of outliers, it should be noted that, for rough indications of agonist potency, the elimination of a single apparent outlier may make little difference to the essential parameters estimated by the curve (see Figure 12.11). The important idea to

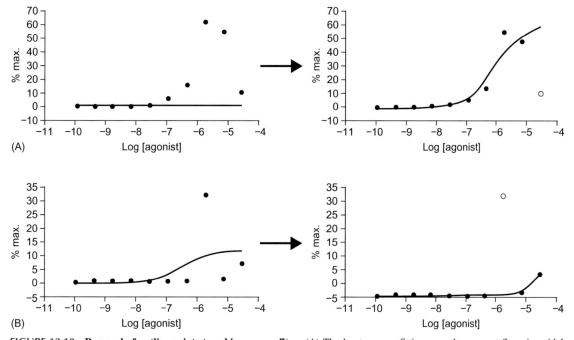

FIGURE 12.10 **Removal of outlier points to achieve curve fits.** (A) The least squares fitting procedure cannot fit a sigmoidal curve to the data points due to the ordinate value at 20 μM. Removal of this point allows an estimate of the curve. (B) The outlier point at 2 μM causes a capricious and obviously errant fit to the complete data set. Removal of this point indicates a clearer view of the relationship between concentration and response.

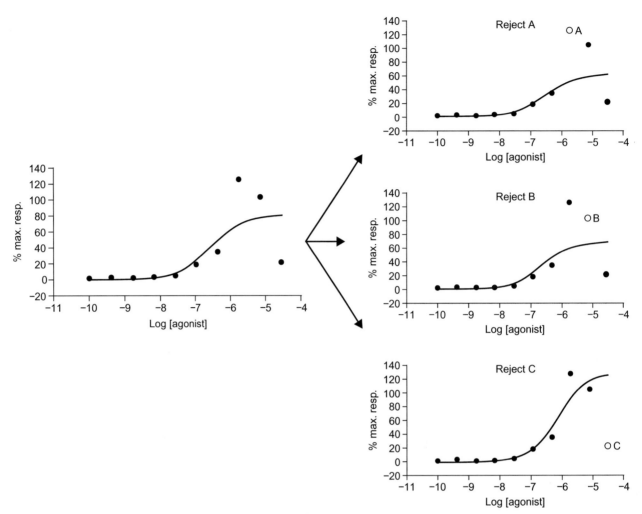

FIGURE 12.11   **Rejection of outliers for curve fitting.**   The curve shown in the left-hand panel ($E_{max} = 81.8\%$; $pEC_{50} = 5.4$) can be refit, eliminating a single data point. Eliminating point A leads to $E_{max} = 61\%$, $pEC_{50} = 5.46$; point B, $E_{max} = 68.4\%$, $pEC_{50} = 5.3$; and point C, $E_{max} = 130\%$, $pEC_{50} = 5.8$.

note is whether or not one or more outliers lead the curve-fitting procedure to pass over a possibly valuable agonist activity because of SSq issues. At least in automated procedures, the bias is to err to fitting the data points to obtain parameters that can be confirmed with repeat testing.

12.4.4 Overextrapolation of Data

Another important issue in the determination of possible drug activity is the observation of incomplete curves. This is especially important in the confirmation of weak activity since the concentrations needed to delineate the complete curve may not be run in the experiment (either through the design of the experiment or because of solubility constraints). For example, apparent curves such as those shown in Figure 12.12A are obtained. The question is, how can a unique parameter characterizing

the potency of such compounds be calculated? Computer curve-fitting procedures will utilize the existing points and fit a curve. The estimated parameters (E_{max}, n) from such fits can be used to estimate potency (pEC_{50}), but the magnitude of the E_{max} estimate directly affects the potency estimate. Figure 12.12A shows data with a maximal reading at 48% of the system maximal response. Curve-fitting procedures yield a fit with an estimated E_{max} value of 148%. It should first be noted that E_{max} values $> 100\%$ should be suspect if the E_{max} value for the system has been determined with a powerful standard agonist. In contrast, another data set (by virtue of the shape of the existing pattern of dose-response) is fit to a much lower E_{max} value (57%). A general practical guideline is to accept fits where the difference between the actual data point and estimated E_{max} value is $< 25\%$ and where the fitted E_{max} is $\leq 100\%$ if this value is known.

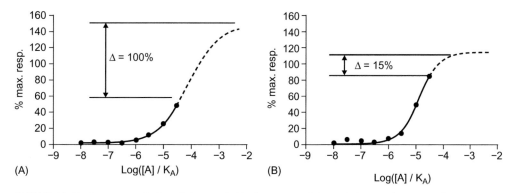

FIGURE 12.12 **Overextrapolation of data.** (A) Nonlinear curve-fitting techniques estimate an ordinate maximal asymptote that is nearly 100% beyond the last available data point. (B) The curve-fitting procedure estimates a maximal asymptote much closer to the highest available data point. A useful rule is to reject fits that cause an estimated maximal asymptote that is > 25% of the value of the highest available data point.

12.4.5 Hypothesis Testing: Examples with Dose-Response Curves

A very important concept in statistical comparison is the idea of *hypothesis testing*. The object of this inferential statistical tool is to compare groups, taking into account variability, to ascertain whether or not the differences between groups are greater than those predicted by chance. In general, hypothesis testing consists of a procedure whereby SSq values are calculated for two models, one more complex (more fitting parameters) than the other. The default is to choose the simplest model if possible, that is, as put by the Franciscan Friar William of Occam (1280−1349): "When you have competing theories which make the same predictions ... the one that is simplest is better." The two SSq estimates are used to calculate a value for the statistic F (variance ratio), which, in turn, is compared to statistical tables to determine significance at various levels of confidence (see the Appendix for F tables). If the value of F indicates significance, then this constitutes evidence to support the notion that the more complex model better fits the data and therefore should be used.

A common problem in pharmacology is answering the question, "when can a molecule be considered to have biological activity?" For activity to be confirmed, there must be a clear pattern of biological response with increasing concentration of drug, that is, a clear concentration-response relationship. If a drug has weak effects on the biological system, such a dose relationship may not seem obvious. Consider the following problem. A range of concentrations of a possible agonist is tested on a functional pharmacological receptor system. The result is a very low level of response that may be a true dose-response relationship or, alternatively, simply represent random noise. Hypothesis testing can be used to discern the difference. The two models to which the data can be compared are

one of random noise and one describing a sigmoid dose-response relationship. The model for random noise is the mean of all the responses. For example, Figure 12.13 shows a set of low-level responses to a possible agonist. The simplest model for these data is a straight line mean of all the responses (random noise level) shown by the dotted line:

$$\text{Simple Model} = y_m = \left(\sum y\right)/n. \tag{12.28}$$

The responses are values of y, and n is the number of responses. A calculated SSq value will have associated with it a value for the degrees of freedom. If there are no fitting parameters involved in applying the model, the number of degrees of freedom will be n; for the data in Figure 12.13, $df_s = 10$.

A more complex model for these data is a four-parameter logistic function of the form:

$$\text{Comple Model} = y_c = \text{Basal} + \frac{E_{max} - \text{Basal}}{1 + 10^{-(\text{LogEC}_{50} + \text{Log[A]})^n}} \tag{12.29}$$

where the concentration of the agonist is [A], E_{max} refers to the maximal asymptote response, EC_{50} refers to the location parameter of the curve along the concentration axis, basal is the response value in the absence of drug, and n is a fitting parameter defining the slope of the curve. The data points in Figure 12.13 fitted to Equation 12.29 provide an estimate of SSq_c (sum of squares for the complex model). This SSq_c has associated with it a value for the degrees of freedom equal to the number of data points, n, the number of parameters used to fit the data points minus k, the number of defined parameters. In this case there are four parameters (E_{max}, n, basal, and EC_{50}); therefore, df = 6. The data and calculations are shown in Table 12.8.

TABLE 12.8 Hypothesis Testing: F-Test Calculations for F for data shown in Figure 12.13.

[Conc] (nM)	Response (y_d)	$\Sigma(y_d - y_m)^2$	Fit Response	$\Sigma(y_d - y_c)^2$	
0.11	0.30	2.51	0.50	0.04	
0.46	1.20	0.47	0.50	0.48	Max = 5.2
1.83	1.00	0.78	0.52	0.23	EC_{50} (nM) = 40
7.32	1.30	0.34	0.57	0.53	n = 1
29.30	−0.36	5.05	0.78	1.30	basal = 0.30
117.00	1.64	0.06	1.45	0.04	
469.00	1.50	0.15	2.92	2.02	
1860.00	5.27	11.49	4.44	0.69	
7500.00	5.10	10.35	5.19	0.01	
30,000.00	4.10	4.92	5.42	1.74	
		$SSq_s = 31.19$		$SSq_c = 5.34$	

$$y_m = 2.10$$

$$F = 7.26$$

Simple Model = $y_m = (\sum y)/n$
$df_s = n$

Complex Model:

$$y_c = Basal + \frac{E_{max} - Basal}{1 + 10^{(LogEC_{50} - Log[A])^n}}$$

$df_c = n - k$ where k = the number of parameters used to fit the data.

$$F = \frac{(SSq_s - SSq_s)/(df_s - df_c)}{(SSq_c)/df_c}.$$

A variance ratio known as the F statistic then is calculated by:

$$F = \frac{(SSq_s - SSq_c)/(df_s - df_c)}{(SSq_c)/df_c}. \quad (12.30)$$

This value is identified in F tables for the corresponding df_c and df_s. For example, for the data in Figure 12.13, F = 7.26 for df = 6, 10. To be significant at the 95% level of confidence (5% chance that this F actually is not significant), the value of F for df = 6, 10 needs to be > 4.06. In this case, since F is greater than this value, there is statistical validation for usage of the most complex model. The data then should be fitted to a four-parameter logistic function to yield a dose-response curve.

Another potential application of this method is to determine whether or not a given antagonist produces dextral parallel displacement of agonist dose-response curves with no diminution of maximum response or change in slope. There are pharmacological procedures, such as Schild analysis, for which it is relevant to know if the data can be fit by dose-response curves of common

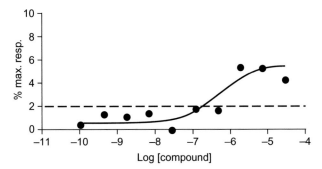

FIGURE 12.13 A collection of 10 responses (ordinates) to a compound resulting from exposure of a biological preparation to 10 concentrations of the compound (abscissae, log scale). The dotted line indicates the mean total response of all the concentrations. The sigmoidal curve indicates the best fit four-parameter logistic function to the data points. The data were fit to $E_{max} = 5.2$, n = 1, $EC_{50} = 0.4$ μM, and basal = 0.3. The value for F is 9.1, df = 6, 10. This shows that the fit to the complex model is statistically preferred (the fit to the sigmoidal curve is indicated).

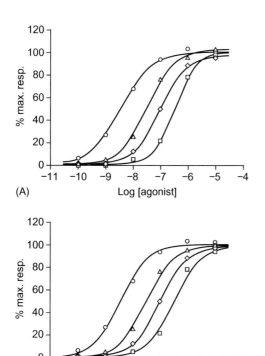

(A) Log [agonist]

(B) Log [agonist]

FIGURE 12.14 **Data set comprising a control dose-response curve; curves obtained in the presence of three concentrations of antagonist.** (A) Curves fit to individual logistic functions (Equation 12.4), each to its own maximum, K value, and slope. (B) Curves fit to the average maximum of the individual curves (common maximum) and average slope of the curves (common n) with only K fit individually. The F value for the comparison of the two models is 2.4, df = 12, 18. This value is not significant at the 95% level, therefore there is no statistical support for the hypothesis that the more complex model of individual maxima and slopes is required to fit the data. In this case, a set of curves with common maximum and slope can be used to fit these data.

maximal response and slope. For example, Figure 12.14 shows data points for a control dose-response curve and a family of curves obtained in the presence of a range of antagonist concentrations. The data are first fitted to the most complex model, specifically a three-parameter logistic equation where E_{max}, n, and EC_{50} values are specific for each curve (curves are fit to their own maximum and slope). An estimate of SSq_c (sum of squares for the complex model) then is obtained with a three-parameter logistic function equation fit. This SSq_c will have degrees of freedom (df_c) for the four six-point dose-response curves shown in Figure 12.14 of df_c = number of data points − the number of constants used to fit the model. For the complex model, there are four values for max, n, and K; therefore, df_c = 24 − 12 = 12. This complete procedure then is repeated for a model where the maxima and slopes of the curves are the average of the individual maxima and slopes. This is a simpler model, and the resulting sum of squares is denoted SSq_s. The degrees of freedom for the SSq_s (df_s) is number of data points − the common max, common slope, and four fitted values for EC_{50}; thus,

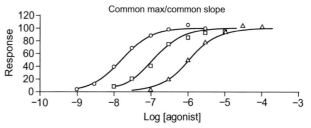

	SSq	AIC	n	K
Individual fits	102	66.1	23	9
Common maxima	211	73.0	23	7
Common slope/maxima	119	65.4	23	5

Common max/common slope

Log [agonist]

FIGURE 12.15 **Aikake's information criteria (AIC) calculations.** Lower panel shows three dose-response curves that can alternately be fit to a three-parameter logistic such that each curve is fit to its own particular value of maximum and slope ("individual fits"), or with common maxima but individual slopes ("common maxima"), or with common maxima and slope. The IAC values (Equation 12.31) for the fits are shown in the table above the figure. It can be seen that the lowest value corresponds to the fit with common maxima and slope, therefore this fit is preferred.

df_s = 24 − 6 = 18. The value for F for comparison of the simple model (common maximum and slope) to the complex model (individual maxima and slopes) for the data shown in Figure 12.14 is F = 2.4. To be significant at the 95% level of confidence (5% chance that this F actually is not significant), the value of F for df = 12, 18, needs to be > 2.6. Therefore, since F is less than this value, there is no statistical validation for usage of the most complex model. The data then should be fit to a family of curves of common maximum and slope and the individual EC_{50} values used to calculate values of dose ratio (DR).

The same conclusion can be drawn from another statistical test for model comparison; namely, through the use of Aikake's information criteria (AIC) calculations. This is often preferred, especially for automated data fitting, since it is simpler than F-tests and can be used with a wider variety of models. In this test, the data are fit to the various models and the SSq determined. The AIC value then is calculated with the following formula:

$$AIC = n \cdot \ln\left[\frac{SSq}{n}\right] + 2 \cdot K + \left[\frac{2 \cdot K \cdot (K+1)}{(n-K-1)}\right] \quad (12.31)$$

where n is the number of total data points and K is the number of parameters used to fit the models. The fit to the model with the lowest AIC value is preferred. A set of dose-response curves is shown in Figure 12.15; as with the previous example, the question is asked, can these data points be fit to a model of dose-response curves with common maximum and slope? The AIC values for the various models for the data are given in the table shown in Figure 12.15. It can be seen that the model of common slope and maximum has the lowest AIC value, therefore this model is preferred.

12.4.6 One Curve or Two? Detection of Differences in Curves

There are instances where it is important to know the concentration of a drug, such as a receptor antagonist, which first produces a change in the response to an agonist. For example, a competitive antagonist will produce a twofold shift to the right of an agonist dose-response curve when it is present in the receptor compartment at a concentration equal to the K_B. A tenfold greater concentration will provide a tenfold shift to the right. With an antagonist of unknown potency, a range of concentrations usually is tested, and there can be ambiguity about small differences in the dose-response curves at low antagonist concentrations. Hypothesis testing can be useful here. Figure 12.16 shows what could be two dose-response curves: one control curve and one possibly shifted slightly to the right by an antagonist. An alternative interpretation of these data is that the

antagonist did nothing at this concentration and what is being observed is random noise around a second measurement of the control dose-response curve. To resolve this, the data are fitted to the most simple model (a single dose-response curve with one maximum, slope, and location parameter EC_{50} for all 12 data points) and then refitted to a more complex model of two dose-response curves with a common maximum and slope but different location parameters EC_{50}. Calculation of F then can be used to resolve whether the data fit better to a single curve (indicating noise around the control curve and no antagonism) or to two separate curves (antagonist produces a low level of receptor blockade). For the data shown in Figure 12.16, the value for F indicates that a statistically significant improvement in the fit was obtained with two dose-response curves as opposed to one. This indicates, in turn, that the antagonist had an effect at this concentration.

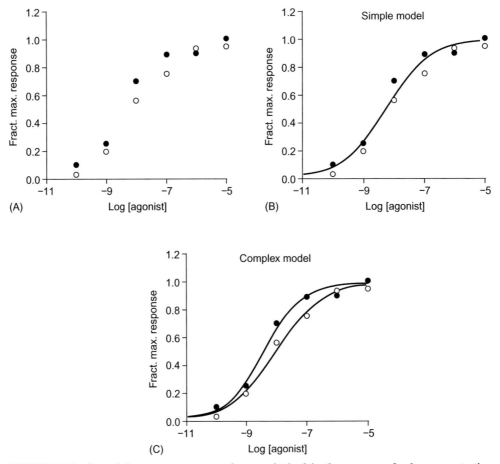

FIGURE 12.16 Control dose-response curve and curve obtained in the presence of a low concentration of antagonist. (A) Data points. (B) Data fit to a single dose-response curve. $SSq_s = 0.0377$. (C) Data fit to two parallel dose-response curves of common maximum. $SSq_c = 0.0172$. Calculation of F indicates that a statistically significant improvement in the fit was obtained by using the complex model (two curves; $F = 4.17$, $df = 7, 9$). Therefore, the data indicate that the antagonist had an effect at this concentration.

12.4.7 Asymmetrical Dose-Response Curves

As noted in Chapter 1, the most simple and theoretically sound model for drug-receptor interaction is the Langmuir adsorption isotherm. Other models, based on receptor behavior (see Chapter 3), are also available. One feature of all these models (with the exception of some instances of the operational model) is that they predict symmetrical curves. A symmetrical curve is one where the half-maximal abscissal point (EC_{50}, concentration of x that yields 50% of the maximal value of y) and the inflection point of the curve (where the slope is zero) are the same; see Figure 12.17A. However, many experimentally derived dose-response curves are not symmetrical because of biological factors in the system. Thus, there

can be curves where the EC_{50} does not correspond to the point at which the slope of the curve is zero; see Figure 12.17B. Attempting to fit such data to symmetrical functions leads to a lack of fit on either end of the data set. For example, Figure 12.18A shows an asymmetrical data set fit to a symmetrical Langmuir isotherm. The values $n = 0.65$ and $EC_{50} = 2.2$ fit the upper end of the curve, whereas a function $n = 1$ and $EC_{50} = 2$ fits the lower end; no single symmetrical function fits the entire data set. There are a number of options, in terms of empirical models, for fitting asymmetrical data sets. For example, the Richards function can be used [2]:

$$y = \frac{E_{max}}{1 + 10^{m(Log[A]+pEC_{50})^s}}. \tag{12.32}$$

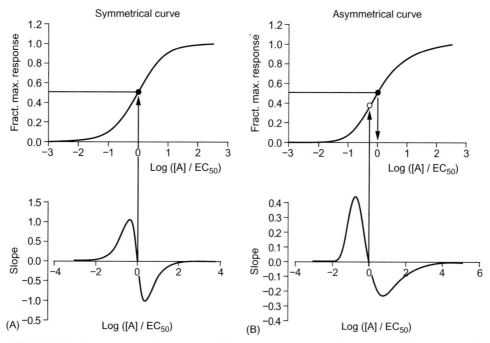

FIGURE 12.17 **Symmetrical and asymmetrical dose-response curves.** (A) Symmetrical Hill equation with $n = 1$ and $EC_{50} = 1.0$. Filled circle indicates the EC_{50} (where the abscissa yields a half-maximal value for the ordinate). Below this curve is the second derivative of the function (slope). The zero ordinate of this curve indicates the point at which the slope is zero (inflection point of the curve). It can be seen that the true EC_{50} and the inflection match for a symmetrical curve. (B) Asymmetrical curve (Gompertz function with $m = 0.55$ and $EC_{50} = 1.9$). The true EC_{50} is 1.9, while the point of inflection is 0.36.

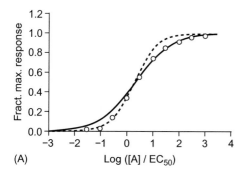

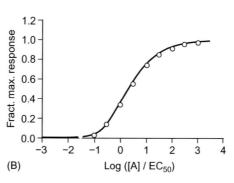

FIGURE 12.18 **Asymmetrical dose-response curves.** (A) Dose-response data fit to a symmetrical Hill equation with $n = 0.65$ and $EC_{50} = 2.2$ (solid line), or $n = 1$ and $EC_{50} = 2$ (dotted line). It can be seen that neither symmetrical curve fits the data adequately (B) Data fit to the Gompertz function with $m = 0.55$ and $EC_{50} = 1.9$.

In this model, the factor s introduces the asymmetry. Alternatively, a modified Hill equation can be used [3]:

$$y = \frac{E_{max}}{1 + 10^{(Log[A]+pEC_{50})^p}} \,. \quad (12.33)$$

The introduction of the p factor yields asymmetry. Finally, the Gompertz function can be used [4]:

$$y = \frac{E_{max}}{e^{10 \cdot m(Log[A]+pEC_{50})}} \,. \quad (12.34)$$

For this model, the factor m introduces asymmetry. The asymmetrical data set shown in Figure 12.18A is fit well with the Gompertz model.

In general these models are able to fit asymmetrical data sets but require the use of added parameters (thereby reducing degrees of freedom). Also, some of the parameters can be seriously correlated (see discussion in [5−7]). Most importantly, these are empirical models with no correspondence to biology.

12.4.8 Comparison of Data to Linear Models

There are instances where data are compared to models that predict linear relationships between ordinates and abscissae. Before the widespread availability of computer programs allowing nonlinear fitting techniques, linearizing data was a common practice because it yielded simple algebraic functions and calculations. However, as noted in discussions of Scatchard analysis (Chapter 4) and double reciprocal analysis (Chapter 5), such procedures produce compression of data points, abnormal emphasis on certain data points, and other unwanted aberrations of data. For these reasons, nonlinear curve fitting is preferable. However, in cases where the pharmacological model predicts a linear relationship (such as Schild regressions;

see Chapter 6), there are repeated questions asked in the process:

1. Is the relationship linear?
2. Do two data sets form one, two, or more lines?

It is worth discussing these questions with an example of each.

12.4.9 Is a Given Regression Linear?

There are instances where it is important to know whether a given regression line is linear. For example, simple competitive antagonism should yield a linear Schild regression (see Chapter 6). A statistical method used to assess whether or not a regression is linear utilizes analysis of covariance. A prerequisite for this approach is that there must be multiple ordinates for each value of the abscissae. An example of this method is shown in Figure 12.19, where a Schild regression for the α-adrenoceptor antagonist phentolamine is shown for blockade of norepinephrine responses in rat anococcygeus muscle. Saturation of neuronal catecholamine uptake is known to produce curvature of Schild regressions and resulting aberrations in pK_B estimates, therefore this method can be used to determine whether the regression is linear (with a slope less than unity) or curved; the conclusions regarding the relationship between the intercept and the pK_B differ for these two outcomes. The data for this example are given in Table 12.9. The calculations for this procedure are detailed in Table 12.10A. As can be seen in Table 12.10B, the value for F_2 is significant at the 1% level of confidence, indicating that the regression is curved ($p < 0.05$).

Curvature in a straight line can be a useful tool to detect departures from model behavior. Specifically, it is easier for the eye to detect deviations from straight lines than from curves (i.e., note the detection of excess protein in the binding curve in Figure 4.4 by linearization of the

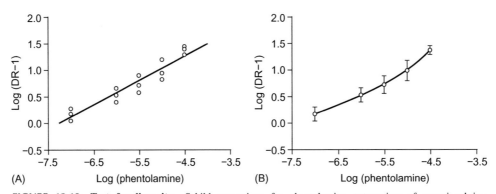

FIGURE 12.19 **Test for linearity.** Schild regressions for phentolamine antagonism of norepinephrine responses in rat anococcygeus muscle. Ordinates: log (DR − 1). Abscissae: logarithms of molar concentrations of phentolamine. (A) Individual log (DR − 1) values plotted and a best fit straight line passed through the points. (B) Joining the means of the data points (shown with SEM) suggests curvature. The statistical analysis of these data is shown in Table 12.9. Data redrawn from [8].

TABLE 12.9 Schild Regression Data for Phentolamine Blockade of Norepinephrine Responses in Rat Anococcygeus Muscle (Data shown in Figure 12.19.)

Log [Phent.]	Log (DR − 1)	T
−7	0.25	0.4
−7	−0.05	
−7	0.2	
−6	0.53	1.53
−6	0.3	
−6	0.7	
−5.5	0.71	2.19
−5.5	0.57	
−5.5	0.91	
−5	1	3.12
−5	0.82	
−5	1.3	
−4.5	1.7	4.25
−4.5	1.1	
−4.5	1.45	
$\sum x = -84.00$	$\sum y = 11.49$	$\sum T_i^2/n_i = 11.70$
$\sum x^2 = 481.50$	$\sum y^2 = 12.19$	
$n = 20$	$\sum xy = -58.75$	
$k = 5$		

T = sum of each replicate log (DR − 1) value.
Data from [8].

TABLE 12.10 Test for Linearity

A: Procedure

	SSq	df	Mean Sq	Var. Ratio
Due to regression	A	1	s_1^2	
Deviation of means	D	$k-2$	s_2^2	$F_1 = s_1^2/s_3^2$
Within-assay residual	B	$n-k$	s_3^2	$F_2 = s_2^2/s_3^2$
Total	C	$n-1$		

B: Calculations:

	SSq	df	Mean Sq	Var. Ratio
Due to regression	0.86	1	0.855	
Deviation of means	4.24	3	1.414	26.19
Within-assay residual	0.49	15	0.033	43.29
Total	5.59	19		

$$A = \frac{\left[\sum xy - \frac{\sum x \sum y}{n}\right]^2}{\sum x^2 - \left(\frac{\sum x}{n}\right)^2} \qquad B = \sum y^2 - \sum T_i^2/n_i$$

$$C = \sum y^2 - \frac{(\sum y)^2}{n} \qquad D = C - A - B$$

12.4.10 One or More Regression Lines? Analysis of Covariance

There are methods available to test whether or not two or more regression lines statistically differ from each other in the two major properties of lines in Euclidean space; namely, position (or elevation) and slope. This can be very useful in pharmacology; an example will be given for the comparison of Schild regressions (see Chapter 6).

A Schild regression for an antagonist in a given receptor preparation is equivalent to a fingerprint for that receptor and antagonist combination. If the receptor population is uniform (i.e., only one receptor is interacting with the agonist) and the antagonist is of the simple competitive type, then it should be immaterial which agonist is used to produce the receptor stimulation. Under these circumstances, all Schild regressions for a given antagonist in a given uniform preparation should be equivalent for blockade of all agonists for that receptor. However, if there is receptor heterogeneity and the antagonist does not have equal affinity for the receptor types, then unless the agonists used to elicit response all have identical efficacy for the receptor types, there will be differences in the Schild regressions for the antagonist when different agonists are used. Before the advent of recombinant systems, natural cells and/or tissues were the only test systems available, and often these contained mixtures of receptor subtypes. Therefore, a test of possible receptor heterogeneity is to use a number of agonists to elicit response and block these with a single antagonist; this is a common practice for

binding curve). An example of this is detection of cooperativity in binding. Specifically, a bimolecular interaction between a ligand and a receptor predicts a sigmoidal binding curve (according to the Langmuir adsorption isotherm) with a slope of unity if there is no cooperativity in the binding. This means that the binding of one ligand to the receptor population does not affect the binding of another ligand to the population. If there is cooperativity in the binding (as, for example, the binding of oxygen to the protein hemoglobin), then the slope of the binding curve will deviate from unity. Figure 12.20 shows a series of binding curves with varying degrees of cooperativity ($n = 0.8$ to 2). While there are differences between the curves, they must be compared to each other to detect them. In contrast, if the binding curves are linearized (as, for example, through the Scatchard transformation; see Chapter 4), then the deviations readily can be seen. This is because the eye is accustomed to identifying linear plots (no cooperativity, $n = 1$) and therefore can identify nonlinear regressions with no required comparison.

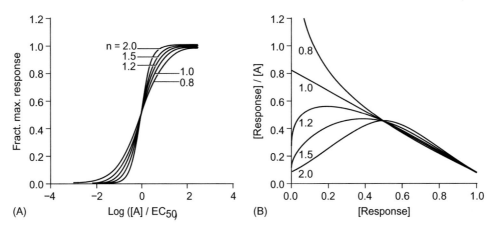

FIGURE 12.20 Use of linear transformation to detect deviation from model behavior. (A) A series of binding curves with various levels of cooperativity in the binding. Numbers next to the curves show the value of the slope of the binding curve according to the equation $[AR] = B_{max}[A]^n/([A]^n + K^n)$. (B) Scatchard transformation of the curves shown in panel A according to the equation $[AR]/[A] = (B_{max}/K) - ([AR]/K)$ (Equation 4.5). Numbers are the value of the slope of the binding curves. Cooperativity in binding occurs when $n > 1$.

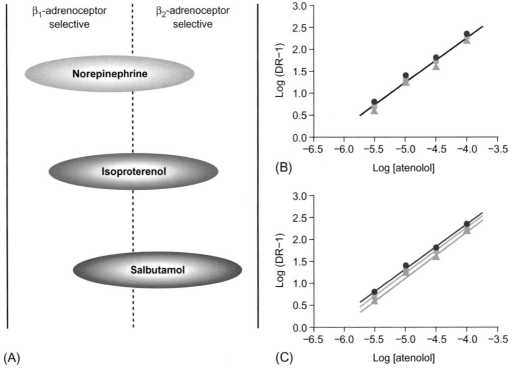

FIGURE 12.21 Analysis of straight lines to detect receptor heterogeneity. (A) Schematic diagram depicts the relative affinity and efficacy of three agonists for two subtypes of β-adrenoceptor. Norepinephrine is relatively β_1-adrenoceptor selective, while salbutamol is relatively β_2-adrenoceptor selective. (B) Schild regression for blockade of β-adenoceptor-mediated relaxation of guinea pig tracheae using the three agonists: salbutamol (purple circles), isoproterenol (green triangles), and norepinephrine (yellow circles). Data points fit to a single regression. (C) Regression for each agonist fit to a separate regression. Analysis for these data is given in Tables 12.12B and 12.13B. In this case, the data best fit three separate regressions, indicating there is a difference in the antagonism produced by atenolol and therefore probably a heterogeneous receptor population mediating the responses.

identifying mixtures of receptor populations. Conformity of Schild regressions suggests no receptor heterogeneity; a useful way to compare Schild regressions is with analysis of co-variance of regression lines.

Figure 12.21 shows three sets of log (DR − 1) values for the β_1-adrenoceptor antagonist atenolol in guinea pig tracheae; the data points were obtained by blocking the effects of the agonists norepinephrine, isoproterenol, and

TABLE 12.11 Analysis of Co-variance of Regression Lines Data for Figure 12.15: Schild analysis for atenolol in guinea pig trachea

Log [Phentol.]	Norepi	Iso	Salb
−5.5	0.8	0.7	0.6
−5	1.4	1.29	1.25
−4.5	1.8	1.75	1.6
−4	2.35	2.3	2.2
$\Sigma x_i = -19$	$\Sigma y_i = 6.35$	6.04	5.65
$\Sigma x_i^2 = 91.5$	$\Sigma y_i^2 = 11.36$	10.51	9.32
	$\Sigma xy_i = -28.90$	−27.38	−25.55

norepi. = norepinephrine; Iso. = isoproterenol; salb. = salbutamol; phentol. = phentolamine.

TABLE 12.12A Analysis of Co-variance of Regression Lines (Comparison of Slopes)

	SSq	df	Mean Sq
Due to common slope	A	1.00	
Differences between slopes	B	$k - 1$	C
Residual	D	$n - 2k$	E

$F = C/E, df = (k - 1), (n - 2k).$

$$s_x^2 = \sum X_i^2 - \frac{\left(\sum x\right)^2}{n_i} \qquad s_y^2 = \sum y_i^2 - \frac{\left(\sum y\right)^2}{n_i}$$

$$s_{xy} = \sum xy_i - \frac{\left(\sum x\right)_i \left(\sum y\right)_i}{n_i} \qquad A = \frac{\left[\sum\limits_k^{i=1}(s_{xy})_i\right]^2}{\sum\limits_k^{i=1}(s_x^2)_i}$$

$$B = \sum\limits_k^{i=1}\frac{(s_{xy})_i^2}{(s_x^2)_i} - A \qquad C = \frac{B}{(k - 1)}$$

$$D = \sum\limits_k^{i=1}(s_y^2)_i - \sum\limits_{s_x^2}^{k}\frac{(s_{xy})^2}{(s^2)_i} \qquad E = \frac{D}{(n - 2k)}$$

TABLE 12.12B Calculations: Analysis of Data in Figure 12.15 (Analysis of Co-variance of Slopes)

	SSq	df	Mean Sq
Due to common slope	3.98	1	
Differences between slopes	0.001	2	0.0006
Residual	0.03	6	0.0042

$$F = 0.13$$
$$df = 2, 6$$

TABLE 12.13A Analysis of Co-variance of Regression Lines (Comparison of Position)

	S_x^2	S_{xy}	S_y^2	SSq	df	Mean Sq
Within groups	A	B	C	D	$n - k - 1$	E
Total	F	G	H	I		
Between groups				J	$k - 1$	K

$F = K/E, df = (k - 1), (n - k - 1).$

$$A = \left(\sum X^2\right)_{total} = \sum_{i=1}^{k}\frac{\left(\sum X\right)_i^2}{n_i}$$

$$B = \left(\sum X^2\right)_{total} = \sum_{i=1}^{k}\frac{\left(\sum x\right)_i \left(\sum y\right)_i}{n_i}$$

$$D = C - \frac{(B)^2}{A}$$

$$C = \left(\sum y^2\right)_{total} = \sum_{i=1}^{k}\frac{\left(\sum y\right)_i^2}{n_i}$$

$$E = \frac{D}{n - k - 1}$$

$$F = \left(\sum x^2\right)_{total} = \frac{\left(\sum x\right)_{total}^2}{n_{total}}$$

$$G = \left(\sum xy\right)_{total} = \frac{\left(\sum x\right)_{total}\left(\sum y\right)_{total}}{n_{total}}$$

$$I = C - \frac{(G)^2}{F}$$

$$J = |D - 1|$$

$$H = \left(\sum y^2\right)_{total} = \frac{\left(\sum y\right)_{total}^2}{n_{total}} \qquad K = \frac{J}{k - 1}$$

salbutamol. These were chosen because they have differing efficacy for β_1- versus β_2-adrenoceptors (see Figure 12.21). If a mixture of two receptors mediates responses in this tissue, then responses to the selective agonists should be differentially sensitive to the β_1-adrenoceptor-selective antagonist. In the example shown in Figure 12.21, it is not immediately evident if the scatter around the abscissal values is due to random variation or if there is indeed some dependence of the values on the type of agonist used. The data for Figure 12.21 are shown in Table 12.11. The procedure for determining possible differences in slope of the regressions is given in Table 12.12A; for the data set in Figure 12.21, the values are given in Table 12.12B. The resulting F value indicates that there is no statistical difference in the slopes of the Schild regressions obtained with each agonist.

The procedure for determining possible differences in position of regression lines is given in Table 12.13A. In contrast to the analysis for the slopes, these data indicate that there is a statistical difference in the elevation of these regressions (F = 9.31, df = 2, 8; see Table 12.13B). This indicates that the potency of the antagonist varies with the type of agonist used in the analysis. This, in turn, indicates that the responses mediated by the agonists are not due to activation of a homogeneous receptor population.

TABLE 12.13B Analysis of Co-variance of Position (Calculations for Data Shown in Figure 12.15)

	S_x^2	S_{xy}	S_y^2	SSq	df	Mean Sq
Within groups	3.75	3.86	4.01	0.03	8.00	0.003
Total	3.75	3.86	4.07	0.09		
Between groups				0.06	2.00	0.03

F = 9.31

df = 2,8

12.5 COMPARISON OF SAMPLES TO "STANDARD VALUES"

In the course of pharmacological experiments, a frequent question is, does the experimental system return expected ("standard") values for drugs? With the obvious caveat that "standard" values are only a sample of the population that have been repeatedly attained under a variety of circumstances (different systems, different laboratories, different investigators), there is a useful statistical test that can provide a value of probability that a set of values agree or do not agree with an accepted standard value. Assume that four replicate estimates of an antagonist affinity are made (pK_B values) to yield a mean value (see Table 12.14): A value of t can be calculated that can give the estimated probability that the mean value differs from a known value with the formula:

$$t_{calculated} = \frac{|\text{known value} - x_m|}{s}\sqrt{n} \quad (12.35)$$

where x_m is the mean of the values. For the example shown in Table 12.14, t = 2.36 (df = 3). Comparison of

this value to the table in Appendix I indicates that there is 95% confidence that the mean value obtained in the experimental system is not different from the accepted standard value of pK_B = 7.4. Therefore, there is a 95% level of certainty that the experimental value falls within the accepted normal standard for this particular antagonist in the experimental system.

12.5.1 Comparison of Means by Two Methods or in Two Systems

Another frequent question considers whether the mean of a value measured by two separate methods differs significantly. For example, does the mean pK_B value of an antagonist measured in a binding experiment differ significantly from its affinity as an antagonist of agonist function? The value of t for the comparison of the mean values x_{m1} and x_{m2} can be calculated with the following equation:

$$t_{calculated} = \frac{(x_{m1} - x_{m2})}{s_{pooled}}\sqrt{\frac{n_1 n_2}{n_1 + n_2}} \quad (12.36)$$

where:

$$s_{pooled} = \sqrt{\frac{s_1^2(n_1 - 1) + s_2^2(n_2 - 1)}{n_1 + n_2 - 2}} \quad (12.37)$$

and s_1^2 and s_2^2 are given by Equation 12.4.

Table 12.15 shows the mean of four estimates of the affinity of an antagonist measured with radioligand binding and also in a functional assay. Equation 12.36 yields a value for t of 2.29. For $n_1 + n_2 - 2$ degrees of freedom, this value of t is lower than the t for confidence at the 95% level (2.447; see Appendix table of t values). This

TABLE 12.14 Experimental Estimates of Antagonist Affinity: Comparison to Standard Value

pK_B	Standard
7.6	Value = 7.4
7.9	
8.1	
7.5	t = 2.36
	df = 3
mean = 7.775	
s = 0.28	

TABLE 12.15 Comparing Two Mean Values to Evaluate Method/Assay

Binding pK_I	Function pK_B
8.1	7.6
8.3	7.7
7.9	7.9
7.75	7.5
mean = 8.01	7.68
s = 0.24	0.17
s_{pooled} = 0.21	
t = 2.29	
df = 6	

indicates that the estimate of antagonist potency by these two different assay methods does not differ at the 95% confidence level. It should be noted that the preceding calculation for pooled standard deviation assumes that the standard deviation for both populations is equal. If this is not the case, then the degrees of freedom are calculated by:

$$\text{degrees of freedom} = \left[\frac{s_1^2/n_1 + s_2^2/n_2}{\frac{(s_1^2/n_1)^2}{n_1 + 1} + \frac{(s_2^2/n_2)^2}{n_2 + 1}} \right] - 2 \quad (12.38)$$

12.5.2 Comparing Assays/Methods with a Range of Ligands

One way to compare receptor assays is to measure a range of agonist and antagonist activities in each. The following example demonstrates a statistical method by which two pharmacological assays can be compared. Table 12.16 shows the pK_B values for a range of receptor antagonists for human α_{1B} adrenoceptors carried out with a filter binding assay and also with a scintillation proximity assay (SPA). The question asked is, does the method of measurement affect the measured affinities of the antagonists? The relevant measurement is the difference between the estimates made in the two systems (defined as $x_{1i} - x_{2i} = d$):

$$t_{\text{calculated}} = \frac{d_m}{s_d} \sqrt{n} \quad (12.39)$$

TABLE 12.16 Multiple Values to Compare Methods pK_B values for human α_{1B}-adrenoceptor antagonists obtained in binding studies with SPA and filter binding[1]

	pK$_I$	pK$_I$	Difference
Prazosin	10.34	10.27	0.0049
5-CH3 Urapidil	7.05	7.32	0.0729
Yohimbine	6.1	6.31	0.0441
BMY7378	7.03	7.06	0.0009
Phentolamine	7.77	7.91	0.0196

mean = 0.03.
s = 0.03.
t = 2.12.
df = 5

[1]Data from [9].

where d_m is the mean difference and s_d is given by:

$$t_{\text{calculated}} = \frac{d_m}{s_d} \sqrt{n}$$

$$s_d = \frac{\sqrt{\sum (d_i - d)^2}}{n - 1}. \quad (12.40)$$

As seen in Table 12.16, the values for α_{1B}-adrenoceptor antagonists obtained by filter binding and SPA do not differ significantly at the $p < 0.05$ level. This suggests that there is no difference between the two methods of measurement.

12.6 EXPERIMENTAL DESIGN AND QUALITY CONTROL

12.6.1 Detection of Difference in Samples

In a data set it may be desirable to ask the question, is any one value significantly different from the others in the sample? A t statistic (for $n - 1$ degrees of freedom where the sample size is n) can be calculated which takes into account the difference of the magnitude of that one value (x_i) and the mean of the sample (x_m):

$$t_{n-1} = \frac{(x_m - x_i)}{s \sqrt{((1/n) + 1)}} \quad (12.41)$$

where s is the standard error of the means. This can be used in screening procedures where different compounds are tested at one concentration and there is a desire to detect a compound that gives a response significantly greater than basal noise. As samples get large, it can be seen that the square root term in the denominator of Equation 12.39 approaches unity and the value of t is the deviation divided by the standard error. In fact, this leads to the standard rule where values are different if they exceed $t \cdot s$ limits (i.e., for t_{95}; these would be the 95% confidence limits; see Section 12.3.3). This notion leads to the concept of control charts (visual representation of confidence intervals for the distribution) whereby the scatter and mean of a sample are tracked consecutively to detect possible trends of deviation. For example, in a drug activity screen, a standard agonist is tested routinely for quality control and the pEC_{50} noted chronologically throughout the screen. If, on a given day, the pEC_{50} of the control is outside the 95% confidence limits of the sample means collected throughout the course of the screen, then the data collected on that day are suspect and the experiment may need to be repeated. Figure 12.22A shows such a chart where the definitions of a warning limit are the values that exceed 95.5% (>2 s units) of the confidence limits of the mean, and action (removal of the data) applies to values > 99.7% (three s units) c.l. of the

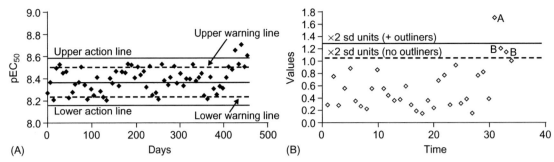

FIGURE 12.22 Control charts and outliers. (A) pEC_{50} values (ordinates) run as a quality control for a drug screen over the days on which the screen is run (abscissae). Dotted lines are the 95% c.l. (upper and lower warning lines) and the solid lines the 99.7% c.l. (upper and lower action lines). Data points that drift beyond the action lines indicate significant concern over the quality of the data obtained from the screen on those days. (B) The effect of significant outliers on the criteria for rejection. For the data set shown, the inclusion of points A and B lead to a c.l. for 95% confidence that includes point B. Removal of point A causes the 95% limits to fall below point B, causing them to be suspect as well. Thus, the presence of the data to be possibly rejected affects the criteria for rejection of other data.

mean. Caution should be included in this practice since the presence of outliers themselves alter the outcome of the criteria for the test, in this case the standard mean and standard error of that mean. Figure 12.22B shows a collection of data where inclusion of the outlier significantly alters the mean and standard error, to the extent that the decision to include or exclude two other data points is affected. This effect is more serious with smaller samples and loses importance as sample size increases.

Another method that may be employed to test whether single data points should be included in a sample mean is the Q-test. This simple test determines the confidence with which a data point can or cannot be considered as part of the data set. The test calculates a ratio of the gap between the data point and its nearest neighbor and the range of the complete data set:

$$Q_{calculated} = gap/range \qquad (12.42)$$

If Q is greater than values from a table yielding Q values for 90% probability of difference, then the value may be removed from the data set ($p < 0.10$). An example of how this test is used is given in Table 12.17. In this case, the pK_B value of 8.1 appears to be an outlier with respect to the other estimates made. The calculated Q is compared to a table of Q values for 90% confidence (Table 12.17B) to determine the confidence with which this value can be accepted into the data set. In the case shown in Table 12.17, $Q < 0.51$; therefore, there is $< 90\%$ probability that the value is different. If this level of probability is acceptable to the experimenter, then the value should remain in the set.

Scientifically, the question of outliers is a difficult one. On the one hand, they could be due to high random biological and/or measurement variation and therefore legitimately rejected. On the other hand, they might be the most interesting data in the set and indicative of a

TABLE 12.17 Q-Test for Rejection of Data Point

Table A pK_B Values	Gap	Table B Q @ 90%	n
7.5		0.76	4
7.6	0.1	0.64	5
7.6	0	0.56	6
7.7	0.1	0.51	7
7.8	0.1	0.47	8
7.8	0	0.44	9
8.1	0.3	0.41	10
Range = 0.06			
Q = 0.5			
n = 7			

rare but important effect. For instance, in a psychological cognition test, outliers may represent a rare but real cognitive problem leading to a fractal change in the test score. As with hypothesis testing, the ultimate responsibility lies with the investigator.

12.6.2 Power Analysis

There is an increasing appreciation of the importance of power analysis in the drug discovery process. This method enables decisions to be made regarding the size of the experimental sample needed to make accurate and reliable judgments, and also the estimation of the likelihood that the statistical tests will find differences of a given magnitude. The size of the sample is important

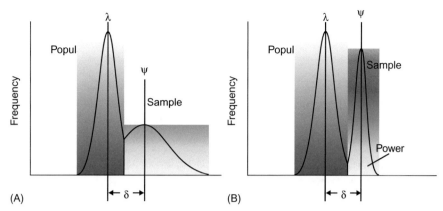

FIGURE 12.23 Power analysis. The desired difference is > 2 standard deviation units ($\lambda - \psi = \delta$). The sample distribution in panel A is wide, and only 67% of the distribution values are $> \delta$. Therefore, an experimental design that yields the sample distribution shown in panel A will have a power of 67% to attain the desired end point. In contrast, the sample distribution shown in panel B is much less broad, and 97% of the area under the distribution curve is $> \delta$. Therefore, an experimental design yielding the sample distribution shown in panel B will gave a much higher power (97%) to attain the desired end point. One way to decrease the broadness of sample distributions is to increase the sample size.

since too small a sample will be useless (the result will be too imprecise for definitive conclusions to be drawn) and too large a sample leads to diminishing returns and wasted resources. These ideas can be dealt with in sampling theory and power analysis.

Essentially, the decision regarding the sample size involves this question: How large does a sample need to be to accurately reflect the characteristics of the population? For example, the question could be stated, "is the potency of a given agonist in a recombinant assay equal to the known potency of the same agonist in a secondary therapeutic assay?" The true value of the potency in the recombinant system, denoted λ, is estimated by choosing a sample of n values from the population. The mean observed potency of the agonist in this sample is denoted ψ. Unless the sample size is nearly infinite, the value λ will not equal ψ since λ was obtained by random sampling. The magnitude of the difference is referred to as the *sampling error*. The larger the value of n, the lower the sampling error. Computer calculation of power curves can yield guidelines for the sample needed to find a defined difference between the population and the sample (if there is one), the probability that this difference is real, and the likelihood that the defined sample size will be successful in doing so, that is, find the minimal sampling error.

Statistical power can be illustrated with a graphical example. There are three principal components to power analysis: (1) Define the magnitude of the difference δ that one wishes to detect, (2) quantify the error in measuring the values, and (3) choose the power (make the experimental choice of defining the probability that the experiment will reject the null hypothesis). Assume that the aim of a study is to find values that are greater than 95% of a given population ($p < 0.05$ for difference). The sample of data we obtain will be represented by a normal distribution; the difference we wish to find is denoted δ (see Figure 12.23). We want to know what proportion of the sample distribution is greater than the 95th percentile of the population distribution (shaded area of the sample distribution in Figure 12.23). The proportion of the sample distribution that lies in the defined region (in this case > 95th percentile) is defined as the power to be able to detect the sample value that is greater than the 95th percentile. The sample for a given experiment will yield a distribution of values. In Figure 12.23A, the percentage of the sample distribution greater than the 95th percentile of the population is 67%; therefore, that is the power of the analysis as shown. This means that, with the experiment designed in the present manner, there will be a 67% chance that the defined difference δ will be detected with $> 95\%$ probability. One way to increase the chances of detecting the defined difference δ is to produce a sampling distribution that has a larger area lying to the right of the 95th percentile; Figure 12.23B shows a distribution with 97% of the area (> 95th percentile of the population). This second situation has a much greater probability of finding a value $> \delta$, that is, it has a higher statistical power. It can be seen that this is because the distribution is narrower. One way of getting from the situation shown in Figure 12.23A to the one in Figure 12.23B (narrower sampling distribution) is to reduce the standard error. This can be done by increasing the number of samples (n; see Equation 12.4). Therefore, the power and n are interrelated, thereby allowing researchers to let power define the value of n (sample size) needed to determine a given difference δ with a defined probability.

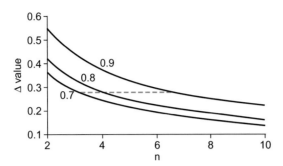

FIGURE 12.24 Power curves. Abscissae are the sample size required to determine a difference between means shown on the ordinate. Numbers next to the curves refer to the power of finding that difference. For example, the lower line shows that a sample size of n = 3 will find a difference of 0.28 with a power of 0.7 (70% of the time) but that the sample size would need to be increased to 7 to find that same difference 90% of the time. The difference of 0.28 has previously been defined as being 95% significantly different.

The number of samples given by power analysis to define a difference δ, the measurement of which has a standard deviation S, is given by:

$$n \geq \frac{2(t_i + t_p)^2 S^2}{\delta^2} \qquad (12.43)$$

where t_i is the t value for significance level desired (in the example in Figure 12.23, this was 95%) and t_p is the level of power (67% for Figure 12.23A and 97% for Figure 12.23B). This latter value (t_p) is given by power analysis software and can be obtained as a "power curve." Figure 12.24 shows a series of power curves giving the sample sizes required to determine a range of differences. From these curves, for example, it can be seen that a sample size of 3 will be able to detect a difference of 0.28 with a power of 0.7 (70% of time) but that a sample size of 7 would be needed to increase this power to 90%. In general, power analysis software can be used to determine sample sizes for optimal experimental procedures.

12.7 CHAPTER SUMMARY AND CONCLUSIONS

- Descriptive statistics quantify central tendency and variance of data sets. The probability of occurrence of a value in a given population can be described in terms of the Gaussian distribution.
- The t-distribution allows the use of samples to make inferences about populations.
- Statistical tests simply define the probability that a hypothesis can be disproven; the experimenter still must assume the responsibility of accepting the risk that there is a certain probability that the conclusion may be incorrect.

- The most useful description of variance is confidence limits since these take into account the sample size.
- While a t-test can be used to determine if the means of two samples can be considered to come from the same population, paired data sets are more powerful to determine difference.
- Possible significant differences between samples can be estimated by one-way and two-way analysis of variance.
- While correlation can indicate relationships, it does not imply cause and effect.
- There are statistical methods to determine the verisimilitude of experimental data to models. One major procedure to do this is nonlinear curve fitting to dose-response curves predicted by receptor models.
- Choosing models that have parameters that can be related to biology is preferable to generic mathematical functions that may give better fits.
- There are statistical procedures available to choose models (hypothesis testing), assess outliers (or weight them), and deal with partial curves.
- Procedures also can be used to analyze straight lines with respect to slope and position, compare sample values to standard population means, compare methods, and detect differences in small samples.
- Power analysis can be used to optimize experiments for detection of difference with minimal resources.

REFERENCES

[1] Watson C, Chen G, Irving PE, Way J, Chen W-J, Kenakin TP. The use of stimulus-biased assay systems to detect agonist-specific receptor active states: implications for the trafficking of receptor stimulus by agonists. Mol Pharmacol 2000;58:1230−8.

[2] Richards FJ. A flexible growth function for empirical use. J Exp Bot 1959;10:290−300.

[3] Boeynaems JM, Dumont JE. Outlines of receptor theory. Amsterdam: Elsevier/North-Holland; 1980.

[4] Gompertz B. On the nature of the function expressive of the law of human mortality. Philo Trans R Soc Lond 1825;36:513−85.

[5] Freund RJ, Litell CR, editors. Non-linear models: SAS system recognition. Cary, North Carolina: SAS Institute; 1991.

[6] Giraldo J, Vivas NM, Vila E, Badia A. Assessing the (a)symmetry of concentration-effect curves: empirical versus mechanistic models. Pharmacol Therap 2002;95:21−45.

[7] Van Der Graaf PH, Schoemaker RC. Analysis of asymmetry of agonist concentration-response curves. J Pharmacol Toxicol Meth 1999;41:107−15.

[8] Kenakin TP, Beek D. The measurement of antagonist potency and the importance of selective inhibition of agonist uptake processes. J Pharmacol Exp Ther 1981;219:112−20.

[9] Gobel J, Saussy DL, Goetiz AS. Development of scintillation-proximity assays for alpha adrenoceptors. J Pharmacol Toxicol Meth 1999;42:2−7.

Chapter 13

Selected Pharmacological Methods

In mathematics you don't understand things. You just get used to them.

— Johann von Neumann (1903–1957)

13.1   Binding Experiments   13.2   Functional Assays

13.1 BINDING EXPERIMENTS

13.1.1 Saturation Binding

Aim: To measure the binding of a radioligand (or ligand that is traceable by other means) to a receptor. The objective is to obtain an estimate of the equilibrium dissociation constant of the radioligand-receptor complex (denoted K_d) and also the maximal number of binding sites (denoted B_{max}).

General Procedure: The receptor preparation is incubated with a range of concentrations of radioligand (to give a measure of total binding), and again in the presence of a high concentration of nonradioactive receptor-selective ligand (present at a concentration of $100 \times K_d$ for the nonradioactive ligand) to give a measure of nonspecific binding (nsb). After a period of equilibration (30 to 90 min), the amount of bound ligand is quantified, and the total binding and nsb are fitted to simultaneous equations to yield a measure of the ligand specifically bound to a receptor.

Procedure:

1. A range of concentrations of radioligand is added to a range of tubes (or wells); an example of such a range of concentrations (in pM) is shown in Table 13.1. A parallel array of tubes is prepared with an added concentration of nonradioactive ligand (to define nsb) at a concentration $100 \times$ the K_d for binding to receptor.

2. The membrane (or cell) preparation is added to the tubes to begin the binding reaction. The reagents are equilibrated for 30–90 min (time required for equilibration must be determined experimentally) and then the amount of bound ligand is quantified (either by separation or reading of scintillation proximity beads). The nsb and total binding are obtained from this experiment as shown (in bound pM).

3. The total binding and nsb are plotted as a function of added radiolabel as shown in Figure 13.1A and fitted simultaneously with nonlinear curve fitting techniques. For the example shown in Figure 13.1A, the data are fitted to:

$$\text{Total binding} = \frac{[A^*]^n B_{max}}{[A^*]^n + K_d{}^n} + k[A^*] \qquad (13.1)$$

and:

$$nsb = k[A^*]. \qquad (13.2)$$

4. The data for Table 13.1, columns A to C, were fitted to Equations 13.1 and 13.2 simultaneously to yield $B_{max} = 6.63 \pm 1.5$ pmoles/mg protein, $n = 0.95 \pm 0.2$, and $K_d = 26.8$ pM ($pK_d = 10.57 \pm 0.3$). The fitted curves are shown in Figure 13.1B along with a dotted line to show the calculated specific binding.

13.1.2 Displacement Binding

Aim: To measure the affinity of a ligand by observing the inhibition of a receptor-bound radioligand (or ligand that is traceable by other means). The objective is to obtain an estimate of the equilibrium dissociation constant of the nonradioactive ligand-receptor complex (alternately denoted K_B or K_i). The pattern of displacement curves

T. P. Kenakin: A Pharmacology Primer, Fourth edition. DOI: http://dx.doi.org/10.1016/B978-0-12-407663-1.00013-2
© 2009 Elsevier Inc. All rights reserved.

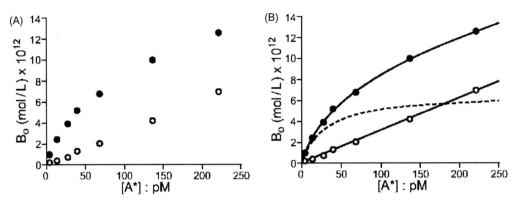

FIGURE 13.1 (A) Human calcitonin receptor binding. Ordinates: pmole ^{125}I-AC512 bound/mg protein. Abscissae: concentration of ^{125}I-AC512 (pM). Total binding (filled circles) and nsb (open circles). (B) Curves fit simultaneously to Equations 13.1 and 13.2. (B_{max} = 6.63 pmoles/mg protein, n = 0.95, K_d = 26.8 pM). Dotted line shows specific binding.

TABLE 13.1 Data for Saturation Binding Curves

A [A*]:M	B nsb	C Total Binding
4.29×10^{-12}	0.16	0.97
1.3×10^{-11}	0.45	2.42
2.7×10^{-11}	0.81	3.87
4.0×10^{-11}	1.29	5.16
6.86×10^{-11}	2.1	6.77
1.37×10^{-10}	4.19	10
2.2×10^{-10}	6.94	12.58

Binding in pmole/mg protein.

also can be used to determine whether or not the antagonism is competitive.

General Procedure: The receptor preparation is incubated with a single concentration of radioligand (this furnishes the B_0 value) in the absence and presence of a range of concentrations of nonradioactive displacing ligand. This is also done in the presence of a high concentration of nonradioactive ligand (present at a concentration of $100 \times K_d$ for the nonradioactive ligand) to give a measure of nonspecific binding (nsb). After a period of equilibration (30 to 90 min), the amount of bound ligand is quantified. The nsb value is subtracted from the estimates of total binding to yield a measure of the ligand specifically bound to a receptor. The resulting displacement curves are fitted to models to yield the equilibrium dissociation constant of the displacing ligand-receptor complex.

Procedure:

1. Choice of radioligand concentration: The optimal concentration is one that is below the K_d for

saturation binding (i.e., [A*] = 0.1 K_d, 0.3 K_d) such that the IC_{50} of the displacement curves will not be significantly higher than the K_B for the antagonist. This will minimize the extrapolation required for determination of the K_i. However, a higher concentration may be required to achieve a useful window of specific binding and sufficient signal-to-noise ratio. The amount of membrane protein also can be adjusted to increase the signal strength with the caveat that too much protein will deplete the radioligand and produce error in the measurements (see Chapter 4, Section 4.4.1). For this example, four radioligand concentrations are chosen to illustrate the Cheng–Prusoff correction for determination of K_B from the IC_{50} values.

2. The chosen concentration of radioligand is added to a set of tubes (or wells). To a sample of these a concentration of a designated nonradioactive ligand used to define nsb is added at a concentration of $100 \times$ the K_d for binding to receptor. Then a range of concentrations of the nonradioactive ligand for which the displacement curve will be determined is added to the sample of tubes containing prebound radioligand; the concentrations for this example are shown in Table 13.2A.

3. The membrane (or cell) preparation is added to the tubes to begin the binding reaction. The reagents are equilibrated for 30–90 min (see considerations of temporal effects for two ligands coming to equilibrium with a receptor in Chapter 4, Section 4.4.2), and then the amount of bound ligand is quantified (either by separation or by reading of scintillation proximity beads). The nsb and total binding are obtained from this experiment, as shown in Table 13.2A (in bound pM). For a radioligand concentration of [A*]/K_d = 0.1, the total binding is shown in Table 13.2A; for three higher concentrations of radioligand, the

TABLE 13.2 Displacement Binding

A: Data for Displacement of Radioligand Binding Curves

[B]:M	$[A^*]/K_d = 0.1$	$[A^*]/K_d = 0.3$	$[A^*]/K_d = 1.0$	$[A^*]/K_d = 3.0$
10^{-14}	17.7	21.87	29.93	37.44
3×10^{-14}	17.65	21.77	29.78	37.33
10^{-13}	17.5	21.43	29.29	36.95
3×10^{-13}	17.14	20.63	28.04	35.93
10^{-12}	16.43	18.91	25	33
3×10^{-12}	15.73	17.09	21	27.86
10^{-11}	15.27	15.8	17.5	21.43
3×10^{-11}	15.1	15.29	15.94	17.65
10^{-10}	15.03	15.09	15.29	15.87
3×10^{-10}	15.01	15.03	15.1	15.3

B: Fitted Parameters to Data Shown in A

$[A^*]/K_d$	IC_{50} (M)	n
0.9	1.1×10^{-12}	0.95
2.7	1.3×10^{-12}	0.97
9	2×10^{-12}	0.92
27	3.9×10^{-12}	0.95

Concentration of displacing ligand in pM. Binding shown as pmole/mg protein. nsb = 15 ± 0.2 pmoles/mg protein.

data are shown in the columns to the right in Table 13.2A.

4. The nsb for this example was shown to be 15.2 ± 0.2 pM/mg protein. This value is subtracted from the total binding numbers or the total binding fit to displacement curves. Total binding with a representation of nsb is used in this example and shown in Figure 13.2A.

5. Nonlinear fitting techniques (for example, to Equation 13.3, which follows) are used to fit the data points to curves. The IC_{50} values from the fit curves are shown in Table 13.2B.

$$\rho^* = \frac{B_0 - \text{basal}}{1 + \left(\dfrac{10^{\text{Log}[B]}}{10^{\text{Log}[IC_{50}]}} \right)^n} + \text{basal} \qquad (13.3)$$

where B_0 is the initial binding of radioligand in the absence of displacing ligand and basal is the nsb.

6. It can be seen that the IC_{50} increases with increasing values of $[A^*]/K_d$ in accordance with simple competitive antagonism. This can be tested by comparison of the data to the Cheng−Prusoff equation (Equation 4.11). The data in Table 13.2B are fitted to:

$$IC_{50} = K_B([A^*]/K_d + 1). \qquad (13.4)$$

The resulting fit is shown in Figure 13.2C. The regression is linear with a slope not significantly different from unity (slope $= 0.95 \pm 0.1$). The intercept yields the K_B value, in this case 1 pM.

7. In cases where the plot of $[A^*]/K_d$ versus IC_{50} is not linear, other mechanisms of antagonism may be operative. If there is a nearly vertical relationship, this may be due to noncompetitive antagonism in a system with no receptor reserve (see Figure 13.2D). Alternatively, if the plot is linear at low values of $[A^*]/K_d$ and then approaches an asymptotic value, the antagonism may be allosteric (the value of α defines the value of the asymptote) or noncompetitive in a system with receptor reserve (competitive shift until the maximal response is depressed; Figure 13.2D).

13.2 FUNCTIONAL ASSAYS

13.2.1 Determination of Equiactive Concentrations on Dose-Response Curves

Aim: Mathematical estimation of concentrations on a dose-response curve that produces the same magnitude of response as those on another dose-response curve. This is

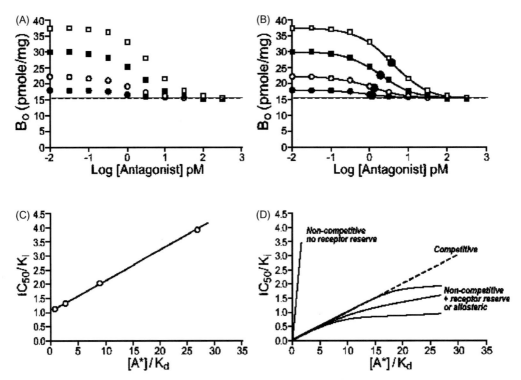

FIGURE 13.2 (A) Displacement of a radioligand by a nonradioactive competitive ligand. Ligand displaces signal to nsb, which, in this case, is 15 pmoles/mg protein. Ordinates: pmole/mg protein bound. Abscissae: concentration of displacing ligand in pM on a logarithmic scale. Data for displacement curves shown for increasing concentrations of radioligand. Curves shown for $[A^*]/K_d = 0.1$ (filled circles), $[A^*]/K_d = 0.3$ (open circles), $[A^*]/K_d = 1.0$ (filled squares), $[A^*]/K_d = 3.0$ (open squares). (B) Nonlinear curve fitting according to Equation 13.3. (C) Cheng–Prusoff correction for IC_{50} to K_B values for data shown in panel B. (D) Theoretical Cheng–Prusoff plots for competitive antagonist (dotted line) and noncompetitive and/or allosteric antagonists in different systems.

a procedure common to many pharmacological methods aimed at estimating dose-response curve parameters.

General Procedure: A function is fitted to both sets of data points and a set of responses is chosen that has data points for at least one of the curves that is within the range of the other curve. A metameter of the fitting function is then used to calculate the concentrations of agonist for the other curve that produces the designated responses from the first curve.

Procedure:

1. Dose-response data are obtained and plotted on a semilogarithmic axis as shown in Figure 13.3A (data shown in Table 13.3A).

2. The data points are fitted to a function with nonlinear fitting procedures. For this example, Equation 13.5 is used:

$$\text{Response} = \text{basal} + \frac{E_{max}[A]^n}{[A]^n + (EC_{50})^n}. \qquad (13.5)$$

The procedure calculates the concentrations from both curves that produce the same level of response. Where possible, one of the concentrations will be defined by real data and not the fitted curve (see Figure 13.3B). The fitting parameters

for both curves are shown in Table 13.3B. Some alternative fitting equations for dose-response data are shown in Figure 13.4.

3. A range of responses (corresponding to real data points) is chosen from the dose-response curves. For this example, the responses from concentrations of curve 1 (3, 10, and 30 nM) and responses from curve 2 (30, 100, and 300 nM) are compared; the corresponding responses are 0.06, 0.145, 0.25, 0.3, and 0.145 $(1 - (T_f/T_i))$ units (melanophore responses).

4. These responses are used for "Response" in the concentration metameter for the fit for the second curve. For example, the response defined by real data for curve 1 at 3 nM is 0.06. The corresponding equiactive concentration from curve 2 is given by Equation 13.6 (following) with response = 0.06; basal = 0; and the values of n', E'_{max}, and EC'_{50} derived from the fit of curve 2 (1, 0.52, and 79 nM, respectively; see Table 13.3B). The calculated equiactive concentration for curve 2 from Equation 13.6 is 10.3 nM:

$$[A] = (EC'_{50}) \left[\frac{(\text{Response} - \text{basal}')}{E'_{max} - \text{response}} \right]^{1/n'} \qquad (13.6)$$

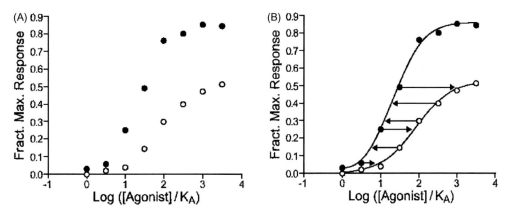

FIGURE 13.3 Determination of equiactive concentrations of agonist. (A) Two dose-responses curves. (B) Concentrations of agonist (denoted with filled and open circles) that produce equal responses are joined with arrows that begin from the real data point and end at the calculated curve.

TABLE 13.3 Estimation of Equiactive Agonist Concentrations

A: Dose-Response Data for Two Curves		
[A]:M	Control Curve 1	Treated Curve 2
10^{-9}	0.025	0
3×10^{-8}	0.06	0.02*
10^{-8}	0.25	0.04*
Designated responses		
3×10^{-8}	0.49	0.145*
10^{-7}	0.755	0.3
3×10^{-7}	0.8	0.4
10^{-6}	0.85	0.47
3×10^{-6}	0.84	0.51

B: Parameters for Fitted Curves	
Curve 1	Curve 2
$E_{max} = 0.86$	$E'_{max} = 0.52$
$EC_{50} = 22$ nM	$EC'_{50} = 79$ nM
$n = 1.2$	$n' = 1$
Basal $= 0$	Basal$' = 0$

C: Equiactive Agonist Concentrations		
Response	[A$_1$]:M	[A$_2$]:M
0.06	**3×10^{-9}**	1.03×10^{-8}
0.145	3.38×10^{-9}	**3.0×10^{-8}**
0.25	**10^{-8}**	7.3×10^{-8}
0.3	7.8×10^{-9}	**10^{-7}**
0.4	1.17×10^{-8}	**3.0×10^{-7}**
0.49	**3.0×10^{-8}**	1.29×10^{-6}

Real data points in bold font; calculated from fitted curves in normal font.

5. The complete set of equiactive concentrations (real data in bold font; calculated data in normal font) is shown in Table 13.3C.

13.2.2 Method of Barlow, Scott, and Stephenson for Measurement of the Affinity of a Partial Agonist

Aim: To measure the affinity of partial agonists.

General Procedure: Full dose-response curves to a full and partial agonist are obtained in the same receptor preparation. It is essential that the same preparation be used as there can be no differences in the receptor density and/or stimulus-response coupling behavior for the receptors for all agonist curves. From these dose-response curves, concentrations are calculated that produce the same response ("equiactive" concentrations); these are used in linear transformations to yield estimates of the affinity of the partial agonist.

Procedure:

1. A dose-response curve to a full agonist is obtained. Shown for this example later (see Table 13.4) are data to the full agonist histamine in guinea pig ileal smooth muscle (responses as percent of the maximal response to histamine).

2. After a period of recovery for the preparation (to avoid possible desensitization) a dose-response curve to a partial agonist is obtained. Data are shown in Table 13.4A for the histamine partial agonist E-2-P (N,N-diethyl-2-(1-pyridyl) ethylamine); response to E-2-P is expressed as a percentage of the maximal response to histamine.

3. Data points are subjected to nonlinear curve fitting; for these data, Equation 13.5 is used to fit the curve with basal = 0. The fitting parameters for histamine and E-2-P are given in Table 13.4B; the curves are shown in Figure 13.5A.

Fitting Function | **Equiactive Concentration (Concentration metameter)**

A

$$\text{Response} = \text{Basal} + \frac{E_{max} - \text{Basal}}{1 + 10^{(\text{Log } EC_{50} - \text{Log } [A])^n}}$$

$$\text{Log } [A] = \text{Log } [EC'_{50}] - \frac{1}{n'} \cdot \text{Log} \left[\frac{E'_{max} - \text{Response}}{\text{Response} - \text{Basal}'} \right]$$

B

$$\text{Response} = \text{Basal} + \frac{E_{max} - \text{Basal}}{1 + \left[\frac{10^{\text{Log } [EC_{50}]}}{10^{\text{Log } [A]}} \right]^n}$$

$$\text{Log } [A] = \text{Log } [EC'_{50}] - \frac{1}{n'} \cdot \text{Log} \left[\frac{E'_{max} - \text{Response}}{\text{Response} - \text{Basal}'} \right]$$

C

$$\text{Response} = \text{Basal} + \frac{E_{max} [A]^n}{[A]^n + (EC_{50})^n}$$

$$[A] = [EC'_{50}] \cdot \left[\frac{(\text{Response} - \text{Basal}')}{(E'_{max} + \text{Basal}' - \text{Response})} \right]^{1/n'}$$

FIGURE 13.4   Metameters for determining equiactive concentrations of agonist.

TABLE 13.4 Method of Barlow, Scott, and Stephenson for Partial Agonist Affinity

A: Data for Dose-Response Curves

[Histamine]:M	Response	[E-2-P]:M	Response
10^{-8}	0.12	10^{-6}	0.04
3×10^{-8}	0.27	3×10^{-6}	0.12
10^{-7}	0.53	10^{-5}	0.26
3×10^{-7}	0.76	3×10^{-5}	0.42
10^{-6}	0.93	10^{-4}	0.53
3×10^{-6}	1.01	3×10^{-4}	0.58
10^{-3}	0.61		

B: Parameters for Fitted Curves

Histamine		E-2-P
$E_{max} = 1.05$		0.62
$EC_{50} = 90$ nM		12.5 μM
$n = 0.95$		0.95

C: Equiactive Agonist Concentrations

Response	[Histamine]: M	1/[Hist]	[E-2-P]: M	1/[E-2-P]
0.12	5×10^{-8}	2×10^7	3×10^{-6}	3.3×10^5
0.26	1.3×10^{-7}	7.7×10^6	10^{-5}	10^5
0.42	2.8×10^{-7}	3.57×10^6	3×10^{-5}	3.3×10^4
0.53	4.4×10^{-7}	2.27×10^6	10^{-4}	10^4
0.58	5.4×10^{-7}	1.85×10^6	3×10^{-4}	3.33×10^3

4. Equiactive concentrations of histamine and E-2-P are calculated (see previous method in Section 13.2.1). For this calculation, responses produced by E-2-P are used since they cover a convenient range to characterize both dose-response curves. The equiactive concentrations are shown in Table 13.4C.

5. A regression of 1/[E-2-P] versus 1/[histamine] is constructed; this is shown in Figure 13.5B. This regression is linear and has a slope of 55.47 ± 0.855 and an intercept of $1.793 \pm 0.132 \times 10^6$ M^{-1}. The K_p estimate (denoted K'_p) is calculated by $K'_p = $ slope/intercept. For this example, $K'_p = 30.9$ μM.

6. This is an estimate of the K_p modified by an efficacy term alternatively depicted as $(1 - \tau_p/\tau_A)$ or $(1 - e_p/e_A)$. Since $\tau_A >> \tau_p$ (also $e_A >> e_p$), it is considered that the K'_p is a fairly accurate description of K_p.

13.2.3 Method of Furchgott for the Measurement of the Affinity of a Full Agonist

Aim: To measure the affinity of full agonists.

General Procedure: Dose-response curves for a full agonist, before and after irreversible inactivation of a portion of the receptor population, are obtained in the same receptor preparation. It is essential that the same preparation be used, as there can be no differences in the stimulus-response coupling behavior of the preparation for both curves. From these dose-response curves, concentrations are calculated that produce the same response ("equiactive" concentrations); these are used in linear transformations to yield estimates of the affinity of the full agonist.

Procedure:

1. A dose-response curve to a full agonist is obtained. Shown are data for the dose-response to the full agonist oxotremorine (responses as a percent of the maximal response to oxotremorine) in Table 13.5A. The dose-response curve is shown in Figure 13.6A.

2. After completion of the determination of the control dose-response curve, the receptor preparation is treated to reduce the number of active receptors. There are numerous methods to do this; a common

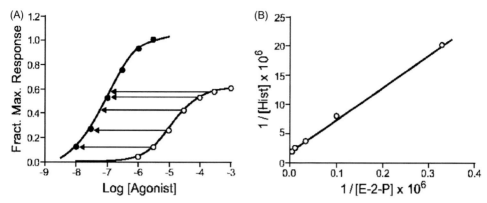

FIGURE 13.5 **The method of Barlow, Scott, and Stephenson for the measurement of the affinity of a partial agonist.** (A) Concentrations of a full agonist (histamine; filled circles) are compared to concentrations of a partial agonist that produce an equal response in the same preparation (E-2-P; (N,N-diethyl-2-(1-pyridyl) ethylamine)); open circles). For this example, real data for the partial agonist were used with fitted data for the full agonist (note arrows). (B) Double reciprocal plot of equiactive concentrations of histamine (ordinates) and E-2-P (abscissae) according to Equation 5.6. The regression is linear with a slope of 55.47 and intercept of $1.79 \times 10^6 \, M^{-1}$.

TABLE 13.5 Method of Furchgott for Measuring Affinity of Full Agonists

A: Data for Dose-Response Curves to Oxotremorine

[A]:M	Response	[A']:M	Response
3×10^{-9}	3.7	10^{-6}	0.0
10^{-8}	21.0	3×10^{-6}	2.0
3×10^{-8}	59.3	10^{-5}	14.0
10^{-7}	90.1	3×10^{-5}	22.2
3×10^{-7}	98.8	10^{-4}	27.0
10^{-6}	100.0	3×10^{-4}	28.0

B: Parameters for Fitted Curves

Control Curve		Alkylated Curve
$E_{max} = 101$		28
$EC_{50} = 2.4 \times 10^{-8}$		10^{-5}
$n = 1.54$		1.5

C: Equiactive Agonist Concentrations

Response	[A']:M	1/[A']	[A]:M	1/[A]
14	10^{-5}	10^5	7.4×10^{-9}	1.35×10^8
22	3×10^{-5}	3.3×10^4	1.1×10^{-8}	9.1×10^7
27	10^{-4}	10^4	1.3×10^{-8}	7.7×10^7

method is through chemical alkylation. For the example shown, the tissue is treated with phenoxybenzamine 10 μM for 12 min. After treatment, the tissue is washed for 60 min with fresh physiological salt solution. It should be noted that there are specific protocols for these treatments, as they are unique for different receptors.

3. The dose-response curve after receptor alkylation is shown in Figure 13.6A (open circles). The same function is used to fit the data as employed for the control curve (for this example, Equation 13.5). The parameters of the fitted dose-response curves are shown in Table 13.5B. Equiactive concentrations of oxotremorine are calculated according to the procedure given in Section 13.2.1.

4. The equiactive concentrations are shown in Table 13.5C. A regression using the reciprocals of these equiactive concentrations is shown in Figure 13.6B. The regression is linear with a slope of 609 ± 11.2 and an intercept of $7.43 \pm 0.68 \times 10^7$. The resulting K_A estimate for oxotremorine according to Equation 5.13 ($K_A =$ slope/intercept) is 8.1 μM.

13.2.4 Schild Analysis for the Measurement of Competitive Antagonist Affinity

Aim: To measure the potency of a competitive antagonist (and/or to determine if a given antagonist is competitive). The objective is to obtain an estimate of the equilibrium dissociation constant of the antagonist-receptor complex (denoted K_B).

General Procedure: A set of dose-response curves to an agonist is obtained, one in the absence of and the others in the presence of a range of concentrations of the antagonist. The magnitude of the displacement of the curves along the concentration axis is used to determine the potency of the antagonist.

Procedure:

1. Dose-response curves to the agonist carbachol are obtained in the presence and absence of the antagonist scopolamine; the data are given in

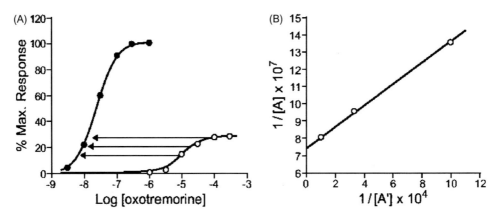

FIGURE 13.6 Measurement of full agonist affinity by the method of Furchgott. (A) Dose-response curve to oxotremorine obtained before (filled circles) and after (open circles) partial alkylation of the receptor population with controlled alkylation with phenoxybenzamine (10 μM 12 min followed by 60 min wash). Real data for the curve after alkylation were compared to calculated concentrations from the fitted control curve (see arrows). (B) Double reciprocal of equiactive concentrations of oxotremorine before (ordinates) and after (abscissae) alkylation according to Equation 5.12. The slope is linear with a slope of 609 and an intercept of 7.4×10^7 M^{-1}.

Table 13.6A. Responses are contractions of rat trachea resulting from muscarinic receptor activation by the agonist (expressed as a percent maximum contraction to carbachol). Columns also show responses obtained in the presence of the designated concentrations of the muscarinic antagonist scopolamine. The antagonist must be pre-equilibrated with the tissue before responses to carbachol are obtained (pre-equilibration period 30 to 60 min).

2. The responses are plotted on a semilogarithmic axis as shown in Figure 13.7A. The curves can be fitted to a four-parameter logistic equation if there are appreciable effects on the basal response, or a three-parameter logistic equation if basal effects are not observed. The curves for the data shown were fitted to a three-parameter logistic equation (Equation 13.5).

3. The data are fitted to curves with individual E_{max}, slope, and EC_{50} values; the parameters for these fitted curves are given in Table 13.6B.

4. The mean maximal response for the five curves is 96.1, and the mean slope is 1.27. The five curves are then refitted to three-parameter logistic functions utilizing the mean maximal response and mean slope. The EC_{50} values for the curves fitted in this manner are shown in Table 13.6B (EC_{50} values in column labeled "Mean").

5. A statistical test is performed to determine whether or not the data may be fitted to a set of curves of common maximal response and slope, or if they must be fitted to individual equations. For this example, Aikake's information criteria are calculated (see Section 12.4.5). The responses calculated by the logistic equations are

subtracted from the actual data points and the result squared; the sum of these deviations becomes the sum of squares for the deviations.

6. The squared deviations between the calculated and actual responses are shown in Table 13.6C (see column labeled "SSq"). The area inside the curve (AIC) values are calculated according to Equation 12.31; the values are shown in Table 13.6C. It can be seen that the fit to the curves with a mean E_{max} and slope gives a lower AIC value; therefore, this model is statistically preferable. It also is the most unambiguous model for simple competitive antagonism, since it fulfills the criteria of parallel dextral displacement of dose-response curves with no diminution of maxima. The calculated curves are shown in Figure 13.7B.

7. The fitted EC_{50} values for the mean curves (Table 13.6B, column labeled "Mean EC_{50}") are used to calculate dose ratios (DR); these are shown in Table 13.6D.

8. The values of log (DR − 1) are plotted as a function of the logarithm of scopolamine concentrations for a Schild plot (see Figure 13.7C).

9. A linear equation is fitted to the data (y = mx + b). The plot shown in Figure 13.7C has a slope of 1.09 with 95% confidence limits of 0.66 to 1.5. Since unity is within the 95% confidence limits of this slope, the data are refitted to a linear model of unit slope (y = x + b).

10. 10 The fit to a linear model of unit slope is shown in Figure 13.7D. The best fit equation is y = x + 9.26. This yields the pK_B for scopolamine of 9.26 with 95% confidence limits of 9.1 to 9.4.

TABLE 13.6 Schild Analysis

A: Data for Scopolamine Antagonism of Responses to Carbachol

[Carbachol]:M	Control	Scopol. 1 nM	Scopol. 3 nM	Scopol. 10 nM	Scopol. 30 nM
10^{-7}	0	0	0		
3×10^{-7}	14.3	8.6	0		
10^{-6}	44.3	19	2.9	0	0
3×10^{-6}	80	48	22.9	11.4	0
10^{-5}	93	77.1	60	32.9	9
3×10^{-5}	98	91.4	82.9	65.7	24
10^{-4}	97.1	94.3	81.4	51	
3×10^{-4}	96	88.6	73		
10^{-3}	97.1	88.6			
3×10^{-3}	94.3				

B: Parameters for Fitted Dose-Response Curves

	E_{max}	N	Individ. EC_{50}	Mean EC_{50}
Control	98	1.46	1.1×10^{-6}	1.1×10^{-6}
1 nM scopol.	97.7	1.17	3.1×10^{-6}	3.0×10^{-6}
3 nM scopol.	95	1.44	7.0×10	7.2×10^{-6}
10 nM scopol.	94	1.2	1.6×10^{-5}	1.7×10^{-5}
30nM scopol.	96	1.1	9.4×10^{-5}	9.1×10^{-5}

C: Aikake's Information Criteria for Assessment of Fitted to Common Slope and Maximum

Model	SSq	K	n	AIC
Individ.	240.64	15	31	125.53
Mean	403.95	7	31	98.46

D: Data for Scopolamine Schild Plot

[Scopol.]:M	Log [Scopol.]	DR	Log (DR − 1)
$10 - ^9$	−9	2.7	0.24
$3 \times 10 - ^9$	−8.5	6.5	0.74
$10 - ^8$	−8	13.6	1.1
$3 \times 10 - ^8$	−7.5	82.7	1.91

"Individ. EC_{50}" refers to EC_{50} values for curve fitted to individual values of E_{max} and slope; "Mean EC_{50}" refers to EC_{50} values from curves fitted to a common E_{max} and slope.

13.2.5 Method of Stephenson for Measurement of Partial Agonist Affinity

Aim: This procedure measures the affinity of a partial agonist by quantifying the antagonism of responses to a full agonist by the partial agonist.

General Procedure: Dose-response curves to a full agonist are obtained in the absence and presence of a range of concentrations of partial agonist. For a single pair of curves (full agonist alone and in the presence of one concentration of partial agonist), a plot of equiactive concentrations of full agonist yields a linear regression; the K_p for the partial agonist can be calculated from the slope of this regression. An extension of this method utilizes a number of these slopes for a more complete analysis. For this method, the individual slopes are used in a metameter of the equation to yield a single linear regression from which the K_p can be calculated much like in Schild analysis.

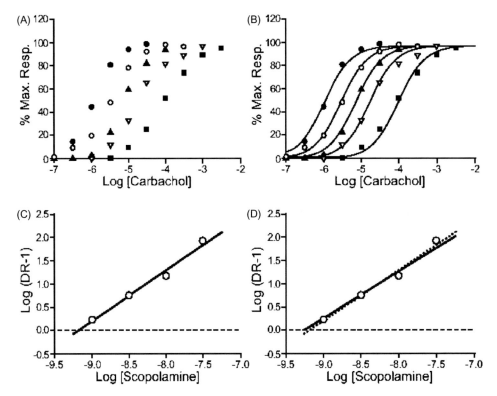

FIGURE 13.7   Schild analysis. (A) Dose-response data showing carbachol responses in the absence (filled circles) and presence of scopolamine 1 nM (open circles), 3 nM (filled triangles), 10 nM (open inverted triangles), and 30 nM (filled squares). (B) Data points fitted to a set of logistic functions with a common maximum and slope. (C) Schild regression for the data shown in panels A and B. Regression is linear with a slope of 1.09 (95% c.l. = 0.66 to 1.5). (D) Schild regression refit to a slope of unity (solid line). Dotted line is regression from panel C.

Procedure:

1. A dose-response curve to a full agonist is obtained. A concentration of partial agonist is equilibrated with the same preparation (30 to 60 min) and then the dose-response curve is repeated in the presence of the partial agonist. The data are fitted to curves (for this example, Equation 13.5) to yield a pair of curves like those shown in Figure 13.8A. For this example, the full agonist is isoproterenol, the partial agonist is chloropractolol, and the response emanates from rat atria containing β-adrenoceptors.

2. Equiactive concentrations of isoproterenol, in the absence [A] and presence [A′] of chloropractolol (100 nM), are calculated according to the general procedure described in Section 13.2.1. These are given in Table 13.7A. A plot of these equiactive concentrations yields a linear regression (according to Equation 6.24; see Figure 13.8B). The x values are the concentrations of isoproterenol [A′] in the presence of chloropractolol, and the y values are the control concentrations of isoproterenol [A].

3. The slope of this regression is given in Table 13.7A (slope = 0.125). The K_p for the partial agonist is given by Equation 6.25 ($K_p = [P] \bullet$ slope/(1 − slope) $\bullet \partial$). The term ∂ represents an efficacy term modifying the estimate of affinity $(1 − (\tau_p/\tau_a))$ in terms of the operational model and $(1 − (e_p/e_a))$ in terms of the classical model. For weak partial agonists and highly efficacious full agonists, this factor approaches unity and the method approximates the affinity of the partial agonist.

Extension of the method: Method of Kaumann and Marano

1. The preceding procedure can be repeated for a number of concentrations of partial agonist (see Figure 13.8C) to provide a wider base of data on which to calculate the partial agonist affinity. Thus, a number of regressions, like that shown in Figure 13.8B, are constructed to yield a number of slopes for a range of partial agonist concentrations. An example is shown in Table 13.7B.

2. The slope values are used in a metameter (log ((1/slope) − 1)) as the y values for the corresponding

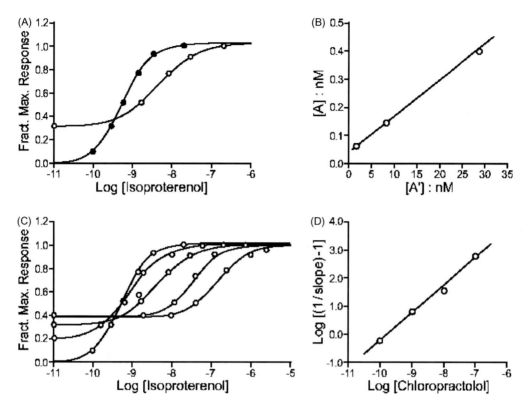

FIGURE 13.8 Method of Stephenson for measurement of partial agonist affinity. (A) Dose-response curves to isoproterenol in the absence (filled circles) and presence of chloropractolol (100 nM; open circles). (B) Regression of equiactive concentrations of isoproterenol in the absence (ordinates) and presence (abscissae) of chloropractolol (100 nM; data from panel A). Regression is linear with a slope of 0.125. (C) Extension of this method by Kaumann and Marano. Dose-response curves to isoproterenol in the absence and presence of a range of concentrations of chloropractolol. (D) Each shift of the isoproterenol dose-response curve shown in panel C yields a regression such as that shown in panel B. A regression of the respective slopes of these regressions is made upon the concentrations of partial agonist (chloropractolol) according to Equation 6.26. The regression is linear with a slope of $0.96 + 0.05$.

log concentrations of the partial agonists (x values) to construct a linear regression according to Equation 6.26. The regression for chloropractolol is shown in Figure 13.8D.

3. This regression is linear with a slope of 0.96 ± 0.05. This slope is not significantly different from unity; thus, the data points are refit to a linear regression with a slope of unity. The intercept of this regression yields an estimate of the pK_p for the partial agonist (as for Schild analysis). For this example, the $pK_p = 7.74 \pm 0.05$ (95% c. l. = 7.6 to 7.9).

13.2.6 Method of Gaddum for Measurement of Noncompetitive Antagonist Affinity

Aim: This method is designed to measure the affinity of a noncompetitive antagonist.

General Procedure: Dose-response curves to a full agonist are obtained in the absence and presence of the noncompetitive antagonist. From these curves, equiactive

concentrations of full agonist are compared in a linear regression (see Section 13.2.1); the slope of this regression is used to estimate the K_B for the noncompetitive antagonist.

Procedure:

1. A dose-response curve is obtained for the agonist. Then the same preparation is equilibrated with a known concentration of noncompetitive antagonist (for 30−60 min, depending on the time needed to reach temporal equilibrium) and a dose-response curve to the agonist repeated in the presence of the antagonist. A hypothetical example is shown in Figure 13.9A; the data are given in Table 13.8A. For this example, the preparation is equilibrated with 100 nM antagonist.

2. The data points are fitted to an appropriate function (Equation 13.5); see Figure 13.9B. From the real data points and calculated curves, equiactive concentrations of agonist in the absence and presence of the antagonist are calculated (see Section 13.2.1). For this example, real data points

---

TABLE 13.7 Method of Stephenson for Affinity of Partial Agonists (+ Method of Lemoine and Kaumann)

A:

Response	[A]	[A']
0.51	5.9×10^{-10}	1.79×10^{-9}
0.76	1.43×10^{-9}	8.3×10^{-9}
0.90	4.0×10^{-9}	2.89×10^{-8}

Slope = 0.125.

$K_p = 1.43 \times 10^{-8}$.

B:

[Chloro]:M	Slope(s)
10^{-8}	0.619
10^{-7}	0.127
10^{-6}	0.023
10^{-5}	0.0018

Slope = 0.96 ± 0.05.

$pK_p = 7.74 \pm 0.05$.

95% c.l. = 7.6 to 7.9.

TABLE 13.8 Gaddum Method for Measuring the Affinity of a Noncompetitive Antagonist

A:

[A]	Control Resp.	Blocked Resp.
10^{-6}	0.08	0.01
3.0×10^{-6}	0.25	0.03
10^{-5}	0.47	0.1
3.0×10^{-5}	0.64	0.15
10^{-4}	0.84	0.29
3.0×10^{-4}	0.9	0.39
10^{-3}	0.89	0.46
3.0×10^{-3}	0.48	
10^{-2}	0.46	

B:

Response	[A']	1/[A']	[A]	1/[A]
0.1	10^{-5}	105	7.0×10^{-7}	1.4×10^{6}
0.15	3×10^{-5}	3.33×10^{4}	1.7×10^{-6}	5.88×10^{5}
0.29	10^{-4}	104	4.3×10^{-6}	2.32×10^{5}
0.39	3×10^{-4}	3.33×10^{3}	7.26×10^{-6}	1.37×10^{5}
0.46	10^{-3}	103	1.02×10^{-5}	9.76×10^{4}

Intercept = 1.01×10^{5}.

Slope = 13.4.

for the blocked curve were used and the control concentrations calculated (control curve $E_{max} = 1.01$, n = 0.9, $EC_{50} = 10\ \mu M$). The equiactive concentrations are shown in Table 13.8B.

3. A regression of 1/[A] where [A] values are the equiactive concentrations for the control curve (no antagonist) upon 1/[A'] (x values) and where [A'] values are the equiactive concentrations in the presence of the antagonist is constructed; this is shown in Figure 13.9C. This regression is linear with a slope of 13.4.

4. The K_B for the noncompetitive antagonist is calculated with Equation 6.36 ($K_B = [B]/(\text{slope} - 1)$). For this example, the calculated K_B for the antagonist is 8.06 nM.

13.2.7 Method for Estimating Affinity of Insurmountable Antagonist (Dextral Displacement Observed)

Aim: This method is designed to measure the affinity of an antagonist that produces insurmountable antagonism (depression of maximal response to the agonist) but also shifts the curve to the right by a measurable amount.

General Procedure: Dose-response curves to a full agonist are obtained in the absence and presence of the antagonist. At a level of response approximately 30% of the maximal response of the depressed concentration-response curve, an equiactive dose ratio for agonist concentrations is measured; this is used to calculate a pA_2.

Procedure:

1. A dose-response curve is obtained for the agonist. Then the same preparation is equilibrated with a known concentration of noncompetitive antagonist (for 30–60 min, depending on the time needed to reach temporal equilibrium) and a dose-response curve to the agonist repeated in the presence of the antagonist. A hypothetical example is shown in Figure 13.10A; the data are given in Table 13.9. For this example, the preparation is equilibrated with 2 μM antagonist.

2. The data points are fitted to an appropriate function (Equation 13.5); see Figure 13.10B. At a response level of 0.3, an equiactive dose ratio of agonist is calculated. The respective concentrations of agonist producing this response are 50 nM (control) and 0.20 μM in the presence of the antagonist. The dose ratio is (DR = 2.0/0.5 = 4).

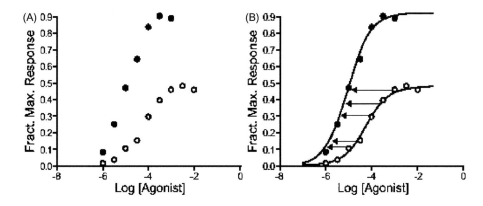

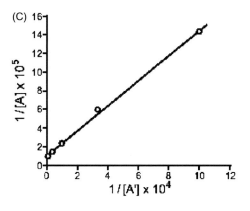

FIGURE 13.9 **Measurement of affinity for noncompetitive antagonists.** (A) Dose-response curve to an agonist in the absence (filled circles) and presence (open circles) of a noncompetitive antagonist. (B) Data points in panel A fitted to dose-response curves. Equiactive concentrations of agonists determined as in Section 13.2.1. Real data points used from curve in the presence of antagonist; equiactive concentrations of agonist from control curve calculated (see arrows). (C) Double reciprocal plot of equiactive concentrations of agonist in the absence (ordinates) and presence (abscissae) of antagonist. Regression is linear with a slope of 13.4.

3. The value for DR is converted to log (DR-1) value, which in this case = 0.48. The pA$_2$ is calculated with the equation

$$pA_2 = -\log[B] + \log(DR - 1), \qquad (13.7)$$

which in this case is $5.7 + 0.48 = 6.18$. This translates into a K$_B$ value of 0.67 μM.

4. This value should be considered an upper limit for the potency of the antagonist as the pA$_2$ corresponds to the pK$_B$ according to Equation 6.37:

$$pK_B = pA_2\log(1 + 2[A]/K_A) \qquad (13.8)$$

for orthosteric insurmountable antagonists, and Equation 7.8:

$$pK_B = pA_2 - \log(1 + 2\alpha[A]/K_A) \qquad (13.9)$$

for allosteric insurmountable antagonists.

It is worth examining the possible magnitudes of the error with various scenarios. The maximal value for [A]/K$_A$ can be approximated assuming a system where response is directly proportional to receptor occupancy. Under these circumstances, response = $0.3 = [A]/K_A/([A]/K_A + 1)$, which in this case is $[A]/K_A = 0.5$. Therefore, the pA$_2$ is pK$_B$ + log (2), that is, the pA$_2$ will overestimate the affinity of the antagonist by a maximal factor of 2. If the insurmountable antagonist is an allosteric antagonist that reduces the affinity of the receptor for agonist ($\alpha < 1$), then

the error will be <2. However, if the modulator increases the affinity of the receptor for the agonist, then the error could be as high as 2α where $\alpha > 1$.

13.2.8 Resultant Analysis for Measurement of Affinity of Competitive Antagonists with Multiple Properties

Aim: This procedure can be used to measure the potency of a competitive antagonist (denoted the *test antagonist*) that has secondary properties that complicate observation of the antagonism.

General Procedure: Schild regressions to a reference antagonist are obtained in the presence of a range of concentrations of the test antagonist. The multiple Schild regressions are plotted on a common antagonist concentration axis and their dextral displacement along the concentration axis used to construct a resultant plot. This plot, if linear with a slope of unity, yields the pK$_B$ of the test antagonist as the intercept.

Procedure:

1. Schild regressions to a reference antagonist are obtained according to standard procedures (see Section 13.2.4) in the absence and presence of a range of concentrations of the test antagonist. In the cases where the test antagonist is present, it is

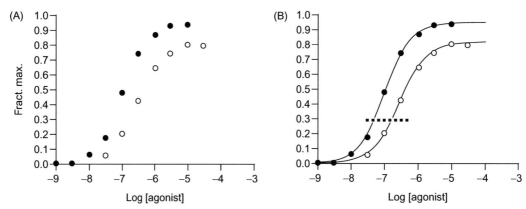

FIGURE 13.10 Calculation of a pA₂ value for an insurmountable antagonist. (A) Concentration-response curve for control (filled circles) and in the presence of 2 μM antagonist (open circles). (B) Data points fitted to logistic functions. Dose ratio measured at response value 0.3 (dotted line). In this case, the DR = (200 nM/50 nM = 4).

TABLE 13.9 Responses in the Absence and Presence of an Insurmountable Antagonist That Causes Dextral Displacement of the Concentration-Response Curve

Conc.	Control Response[1]	Modulated Response[1]
1×10^{-8}	0.06	
3×10^{-8}	0.17	0.05
1×10^{-7}	0.47	0.2
3×10^{-7}	0.73	0.42
1×10^{-6}	0.86	0.64
3×10^{-6}	0.92	0.74
1×10^{-5}	0.93	0.8
3×10^{-5}	0.79	

[1]Fraction of system maximal response.

included in the medium for the control dose-response curve as well as the curves obtained in the presence of the reference antagonist. For this example, the scheme for the dose-response curves used for the construction of regressions I to IV is shown in Table 13.10A. The test antagonist is atropine and the reference antagonist is scopolamine.

2. The Schild regressions for scopolamine, obtained in the absence (regression I) and presence of a range of concentrations of atropine (regressions II to IV) are shown in Figure 13.11A. The data describing these regressions are given in Table 13.10B.

3. The displacement, along the antagonist concentration axis, of the Schild regressions is calculated. To obtain a value for [B′]/[B] (shift along the concentration axis) that is independent of log (DR-1) values, the Schild regressions must be parallel.

The first step is to fit the regressions to a common slope of unity (Figure 13.11B). This can be done if the 95% confidence limits of the slopes of each regression include unity (which is true for this example; see Table 13.10B).

4. The pK_B values for scopolamine from slopes I to IV each fitted to a slope of unity are given in Table 13.10C.

5. The resultant plot is constructed by calculating the shift to the right of the Schild regressions produced by the addition of atropine (pK_B for unit slope regression for scopolamine regressions II to IV divided by the pK_B for scopolamine found for regression I; see Table 13.10C); these yield values of κ for every concentration of atropine added. For example, the κ value for regression II ([atropine] = 3 nM) is $10^{-8.7}/10^{-9.4} = 5$. These values of κ are used in a resultant plot of log (κ − 1) versus the concentration of the test antagonist (atropine) used for the regression. The resultant plot is shown in Figure 13.11C.

6. The resultant regression is linear and has a slope not significant from unity (slope = 0.9 ± 0.07; 95% c.l. = 0.4 to 1.35). A refit of the data points to a linear slope with linear slope yields a pK_B for atropine of 9.05 ± 0.04 (95% c.l. 8.9 to 9.2).

13.2.9 Measurement of the Affinity and Maximal Allosteric Constant for Allosteric Modulators Producing Surmountable Effects

Aim: This procedure measures the affinity and cooperativity constant of an allosteric antagonist. It is used for known allosteric antagonists or molecules that produce a saturable antagonism that does not appear to follow the Gaddum equation for simple competitive antagonism.

TABLE 13.10 Resultant Analysis

A: Concentration Scheme for Resultant Analysis.

Ref. Antagonist Scopol. (M)	Regression I Test Antag. Atropine	Regression II Test Antag. Atropine (M)	Regression III Test Antag. Atropine (M)	Regression IV Test Antag. Atropine (M)
10^{-9}	0			
3×10^{-9}	0	3×10^{-9}		
10^{-8}	0	3×10^{-9}	10^{-8}	3×10^{-8}
3×10^{-8}	0	3×10^{-9}	10^{-8}	3×10^{-8}
10^{-7}	3×10^{-9}	10^{-8}	3×10^{-8}	
3×10^{-7}	10^{-8}	3×10^{-8}		

B: Data Describing Schild Analyses for Scopolamine (I) and Scopolamine and Atropine (II to IV).

Regression	Slope	95% C.I.	Intercept
I	1.3	0.9 to 1.5	11.88
II	1.2	0.9 to 1.4	10.34
III	1.06	0.76 to 1.3	8.77
IV	0.95	0.78 to 1.1	7.5

C: Parameters for Schild Regressions Fitted to Unit Slope and Data for Resultant Regression (log [atropine] versus log ($\kappa - 1$)).

Regression	pK$_B$ from Slope = 1	κ	[Atropine]:M	Log ($\kappa - 1$)
I	9.4 ± 0.1			
II	8.7 ± 0.07	5	$3.00E - 09$	0.6
III	8.29 ± 0.04	12.9	$1.00E - 08$	1.08
IV	7.9 ± 0.02	31.6	$3.00E - 08$	1.49

Test antagonist = atropine. Reference antagonist = scopolamine.
The Schild regression is obtained to the concentrations of scopolamine shown in the left-hand column in the presence of the concentrations of atropine shown in columns labeled "Regression I" to "Regression IV."

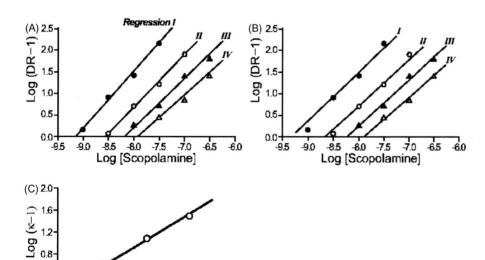

FIGURE 13.11 **Resultant analysis.** (A) Schild regressions for scopolamine in the absence (I, filled circles) and presence of atropine 3 nM (II, open circles), 10 nM (III, filled triangles), and 30 nM (IV, open triangles). (B) Schild regressions shown in panel A fitted to regressions of unit slope. (C) Resultant plot for atropine. Displacements of the Schild regressions shown in panel B furnish values for κ for a regression according to Equation 6.38.

TABLE 13.11 Allosteric Antagonism

A: Dose-Response Data for Gallamine Blockade of Acetylcholine Responses

[A]:M	Control Resp.	[A]:M	1×10^{-5} M Gallamine	[A]:M	3.0×10^{-5} M Gallamine
10^{-9}	3.1	3×10^{-8}	9.38	3×10^{-7}	29.69
10^{-8}	20.3	10^{-7}	25	5×10^{-7}	41
3×10^{-8}	53.1	3×10^{-7}	45	10^{-6}	56.25
10^{-7}	74	10^{-6}	76.56	2×10^{-6}	67.19
2×10^{-7}	85.9				
3×10^{-7}	92.2				
5×10^{-7}	93.7				

[A]:M	1.00×10^{-4} M Gallamine	[A]:M	3×10^{-4} M Gallamine	[A]:M	$5.00E - 04$ Gallamine
5×10^{-7}	25	10^{-7}	3.1	10^{-6}	31.2
10^{-6}	40.6	5×10^{-7}	15.6	2×10^{-6}	46.87
3×10^{-6}	71.87	10^{-6}	31.25	5×10^{-6}	65.62
10^{-5}	87.5	2×10^{-6}	46.87	10^{-5}	78.12
5×10^{-6}	73.44				
10^{-5}	79.69				
3×10^{-5}	89.06				

B: Parameters for Fitted Dose-Response Curves for Acetylcholine

Curve	$EC_{50}(M)$
I	2.94×10^{-8}
II	2.9×10^{-7}
III	7.5×10^{-7}
IV	1.3×10^{-6}
V	2×10^{-6}
VI	2.4×10^{-6}

Common $E_{max} = 97.6$.

Common slope = 1.09.

General Procedure: Dose-response curves are obtained for an agonist in the absence and presence of a range of concentrations of the antagonist. The dextral displacement of these curves (EC_{50} values) is fitted to a hyperbolic equation to yield the potency of the antagonist and the maximal value for the cooperativity constant (α) for the antagonist.

Procedure:

1. Dose-response curves are obtained for an agonist in the absence and presence of a range of concentrations of the antagonist and the data points fitted with standard linear fitting techniques (Equation 13.5) to a common maximum asymptote and slope. An example of acetylcholine responses in the presence of a range of concentrations of gallamine are shown in Table 13.11A. The curves are shown in Figure 13.12A.

2. The EC_{50} values for the fitted curves (see Table 13.11B) are then fitted to a function of the form (variant of Equation 7.2):

$$\frac{EC'_{50}}{EC_{50}} = \frac{(x/B + 1)}{(Cx/B + 1)}, \qquad (13.10)$$

where EC'_{50} and EC_{50} are the location parameters of the dose-response curves in the absence and presence of the allosteric antagonist, respectively; x is the molar concentration of antagonist; and B and C are fitting constants.

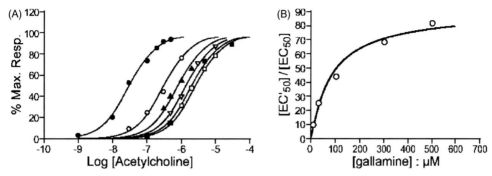

FIGURE 13.12 **Measurement of allosteric antagonism.** (A) Dose-response curves to acetylcholine in the absence (filled circles) and presence of gallamine 10 µM (open circles), 30 µM (filled triangles), 100 µM (open inverted triangles), 300 µM (filled squares), and 500 µM (open squares). Data points fitted to curves with a common maximum and slope. (B) Displacement of dose-response curves shown in panel A used to furnish dose ratios for acetylcholine ([EC$'_{50}$ in the presence of gallamine]/[EC$_{50}$ for control curve]) ordinates. Abscissae are concentrations of gallamine. Line is the best fit according to Equation 13.10.

TABLE 13.12 Responses in the Absence and Presence of an Insurmountable Antagonist that Causes No Dextral Displacement of the Concentration-Response Curve

A: Concentration-Response Curve Data

Agonist Concentration	Control	1×10^{-7} Antagonist	2×10^{-7} Antagonist	5×10^{-7} Antagonist	1×10^{-6} Antagonist	2×10^{-6} Antagonist
1×10^{-8}	0.02					
3×10^{-9}	0.05	0.03	0.04	0.03	0.02	0.02
1×10^{-7}	0.15	0.13	0.12	0.085	0.05	0.03
3×10^{-7}	0.3	0.25	0.22	0.15	0.1	0.05
1×10^{-6}	0.5	0.38	0.32	0.22	0.13	0.06
3×10^{-6}	0.6	0.45	0.37	0.23	0.15	0.07
1×10^{-5}	0.646	0.48	0.39	0.25	0.13	0.06
1×10^{-5}	0.67	0.49	0.4	0.26	0.16	0.07

B: Conversion to Inhibition Curves

Concentration Antagonist	Concentration Agonist 1×10^{-7} Response	Percent Response	Concentration Agonist 1×10^{-5} Response	Percent Response
0	0.15	100	0.64	100
1×10^{-7}	0.13	87	0.48	75
2×10^{-7}	0.12	80	0.39	61
5×10^{-7}	0.09	60	0.25	39
1×10^{-6}	0.05	33	0.13	29
2×10^{-6}	0.03	20	0.07	11

3. The data in Table 13.11B are fitted to Equation 13.10 to yield estimates of $B = 9.5 \times 10^{-7}$ and $C = 0.011$; see Figure 13.12B. These values can be equated to the model for allosteric antagonism (Equation 7.4) to yield a K_B value of 95 nM and a value for α of 0.011.

13.2.10 Method for Estimating Affinity of Insurmountable Antagonist (No Dextral Displacement Observed): Detection of Allosteric Effect

Aim: This method is designed to measure the affinity of a noncompetitive antagonist that produces depression of the maximal response of the agonist concentration-response curve with no dextral displacement.

General Procedure: The response to the agonist is determined in the absence and presence of a range of concentrations of the insurmountable antagonist. The data points may be fitted to logistic functions (for observation of trends; this is not necessary for calculation of IC_{50}).

A concentration of agonist is chosen and the response to that concentration (expressed as a fraction of control) is plotted as a function of the concentration of antagonist to form an inhibition curve. This curve is fitted to a function and the midpoint (IC_{50}) calculated; this is an estimate of the affinity of the insurmountable antagonist. To detect a possible allosteric increase in affinity of the antagonist with agonist concentration, more than one concentration may be chosen for this procedure.

Procedure:

1. Responses to the agonist are obtained in the absence and presence of a range of concentrations of antagonist. A sample set of data is given in Table 13.12 and Figure 13.13A.

2. Data may be fitted to an appropriate function (i.e., Equation 13.5) but this is not necessary for the analysis (see Figure 13.13B).

3. Two concentrations of agonist are chosen for further analysis. These should be two concentrations as widely spread as possible along the concentration axis and with the lowest producing a robust

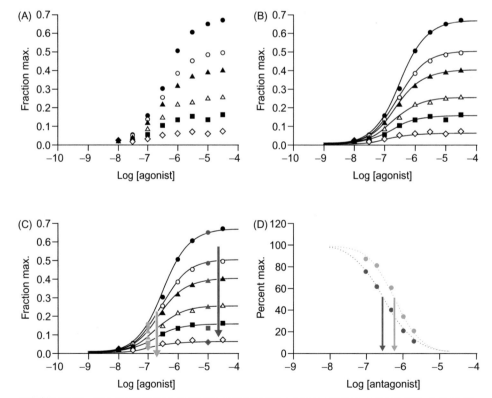

FIGURE 13.13 Measurement of potency of a noncompetitive antagonist that produces little dextral displacement of the agonist concentration-response curve. (A) Data points for control response to agonist (filled circles) and response in the presence of noncompetitive antagonist at concentrations = 0.1 μM (open circles), 0.2 μM (filled triangles), 0.5 μM (open triangles), 1 μM (filled squares), and 2 μM (open diamonds). (B) Logistic function fitted to data points (optional). (C) Response to two specific concentrations of agonist identified (10 μM in red and 100 nM in blue). (D) Effects of antagonist on responses to 10 μM (red) and 100 nM (blue) agonist expressed as a percent of the control response plotted as a function of the concentration of antagonist to yield an inhibition curve (data shown in Table 13.12B). Arrows indicate the IC_{50} values for each curve.

TABLE 13.13 Measurement of Antagonist pIC_{50} and Calculation of pK_B

A: Dose-Response Data for Agonist

[A]	Response
10^{-9}	10
3×10^{-9}	25
10^{-8}	33
3×10^{-8}	55
10^{-7}	72
3×10^{-7}	80
10^{-6}	90
3×10^{-6}	93

B: Response to the Test Concentration of Agonist in the Presence of a Range of Concentrations of the Antagonist

[B]	Response
10^{-8}	86
3×10^{-8}	86
5×10^{-8}	84
10^{-7}	80
3×10^{-7}	65
10^{-6}	43
3×10^{-6}	26
10^{-5}	10

size of response. For this example, responses chosen for agonist concentration were 100 nM (blue, Figure 13.13.C) and 10 μM (red, Figure 13.13.C).

4. The responses to the respective concentrations of agonist are expressed as a percentage of the initial control response (obtained in the absence of antagonist) as a function of the concentration of antagonist. The data for this step are shown in Table 13.12B and the resulting inhibition curves (plot on a semilogarithmic concentration scale) are shown in Figure 13.13D.

5. The inhibition curves are fitted to an appropriate function to allow estimation of the half-maximal value for blockade (IC_{50}). For example, the data from Table 13.12B were fitted to

$$\text{Percent} = 100 - \frac{100[B]^n}{[B]^n + (IC_{50})^n},\qquad (13.11)$$

where the concentration of antagonist is [B], n is a slope-fitting parameter, and IC_{50} is the half-maximal value for blockade. For this example, the

IC_{50} values for the two curves are 0.65 μM (n = 1.15) for 100 nM agonist (blue) and 0.3 μM (n = 1.05) for 10 μM agonist (red).

6. It can be seen from this example that the inhibition curve shifts to the left with increasing concentration of agonist, indicating an allosteric mechanism whereby the modulator blocks receptor signaling but increases the affinity of the receptor for the agonist.

13.2.11 Measurement of pK_B for Competitive Antagonists from a pIC_{50}

Aim: This method allows estimation of the potency of an antagonist that produces dextral displacement of the agonist concentration-response curve. The potency of the antagonist is quantified as the pIC_{50}, defined as the molar concentration of antagonist that produces a 50% inhibition of a defined level of agonist response; this parameter is then used to calculate the equilibrium dissociation constant of the antagonist-receptor complex (in the form of a pK_B).

General Procedure: A dose-response curve to an agonist is obtained and a concentration of agonist that produces between 50% and 80% maximal response chosen for further study. Specifically, the effects of a range of antagonist concentrations on the response produced to the chosen agonist concentration are measured, and the IC_{50} (concentration of antagonist that produces a 50% blockade of the initial agonist response) is measured to yield an inhibition curve. This concentration is then corrected to yield an estimate of the antagonist pK_B.

Procedure:

1. A dose-response curve to the agonist is obtained. Ideally, it should be done as near to the time for analysis of antagonism as possible to negate possible variances in preparation sensitivity. Dose-response data are shown in Table 13.13A (and Figure 13.14A). The data are fitted to a curve; for this example, to Equation 13.12, shown as follows with fitting parameters $E_{max} = 96$, n = 0.7, and $EC_{50} = 20$ nM. The curve is shown in Figure 13.14B.

$$\text{Response} = \frac{E_{max}[A]^n}{[A]^n + EC_{50}^n}\qquad (13.12)$$

2. A target agonist concentration is chosen; for this example, a concentration of 0.3 μM agonist was used, which approximates the concentration that produces an 80% maximal response. The antagonist is tested against the response produced by 0.3 μM agonist.

3. A set of responses to the target agonist concentration is measured in the absence and presence of a

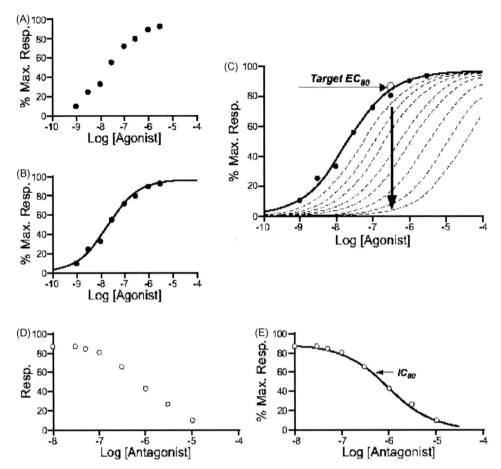

FIGURE 13.14 **Measurement of pA₂ values for antagonists.** (A) Dose-response curve data for an agonist. (B) Curve fitted to data points according to Equation 13.12. (C) Open circle represents EC_{80} concentration of agonist chosen to block with a range of concentrations of antagonist. The antagonist, if competitive, will produce shifts to the right of the agonist dose-response curve as shown by dotted line. The inhibition curve tracks the response to the target concentration of agonist (open circle) as shown by the arrow. (Note: If the antagonism is noncompetitive, the curves will not shift to the right but rather will be depressed. This will still produce diminution of the response to the target agonist concentration and production of an inhibition curve.) (D) Inhibition curve produced by a range of antagonist concentrations (abscissae) producing blockade of response to the target concentration of agonist. (E) Data points fitted to curve according to Equation 13.13. The IC_{50} is shown; the pA_2 of the antagonist is calculated from this value.

range of antagonist concentrations. The fitted agonist response curve is shown in Figure 13.14C. For this example, the repeat test of the target concentration (0.3 μM agonist) gives a response value of 86. The repeat response to the target agonist concentration is shown as the open circle. The addition of the antagonist to the preparation theoretically produces a shift of the agonist dose-response curve shown as the dotted lines. The arrow on Figure 13.14C indicates the expected response to the target concentration of agonist as increasing concentrations of the antagonist are added.

4. The responses to the target concentration of agonist in the presence of a range of concentrations of

the antagonist are given in Table 13.13B and shown in Figure 13.14D.

5. The data points are fitted to a function; for this example, Equation 13.13 is used:

$$\text{Response} = \text{basal} - \frac{\text{Resp}_0[\text{B}]^n}{[\text{B}]^n + IC_{50^n}} \qquad (13.13)$$

where Resp_0 refers to the response produced by the target agonist concentration in the absence of antagonist. For the example, values for the fitted curve are $\text{Resp}_0 = 86$, $n = 0.93$, and $IC_{50} = 1$ μM. The fitted curve is shown in Figure 13.14E.

6. The IC_{50} is used in a version of the Cheng–Prusoff equation for functional assays. Thus, the apparent

K_B (apparent equilibrium dissociation constant for the antagonist-receptor complex) is given by Equation 13.14 (from Equation 11.7):

$$\text{Antilog } pK_B = IC_{50}/((2+([A]/EC_{50})^n)^{1/n} - 1), \quad (13.14)$$

where the values of n and EC_{50} are the values from the control agonist dose-response curve

($n = 0.7$, $EC_{50} = 20$ nM, and [A] = 30 nM). Equation 13.14 yields the molar concentration that occupies 50% of the receptor population (equilibrium dissociation constant of the antagonist-receptor complex). The negative logarithm of this value is the pK_B. For this example ($IC_{50} = 1$ μM), the antilog $pK_B = 48$ nM; the $pK_B = 7.3$.

Chapter 14

Exercises in Pharmacodynamics and Pharmacokinetics

When your work speaks for itself, don't interrupt...

— Henry J. Kaiser (1882–1967)

My work is a game, a very serious game...

— M. C. Escher (1898–1972)

14.1   Introduction
14.2   Agonism
14.3   Antagonism

14.4   *In vitro–In vivo* Transitions and
        General Discovery
14.5   SAR Exercises

14.6   Pharmacokinetics
14.7   Conclusions
References

14.1 INTRODUCTION

The main function of pharmacology in the drug discovery process is to furnish system-independent estimates of the biological activity of molecules. A useful way to look at this is to consider that, as molecules are used in a therapeutic setting, they encounter a myriad of other processes. These "secondary" activities can potentiate, modulate, reduce, or nullify the primary activity and also can initiate completely new activities. Pharmacodynamics is used to identify the primary therapeutically useful activity and to quantify the degree of selectivity a molecule has in a complex system. The following sections discuss several exercises in pharmacodynamics and pharmacokinetics; most of these are actual cases encountered in experimental pharmacology and drug discovery and development. The first class of compounds considered are agonists, molecules that interact with targets in cells to actively produce a change of state of that cell.

14.2 AGONISM

14.2.1 Agonism: Structure-Activity Relationships

Question: A discovery program designed to produce an agonist is in the lead optimization stage; the chemists are actively synthesizing molecules which are subsequently tested in a sensitive cellular response system to yield concentration-response relationships. The pEC_{50} and maximal response values for nine new compounds are shown in Table 14.1. The standard agonist for this target, signifying good activity, is "activone."

1.   Is this assay system a good one to assess structure-activity relationships (SAR) for these agonists? If so, why?
2.   Are there compounds that allow separation of efficacy and affinity effects? Which ones for each?

Answer: It is useful to draw the theoretical concentration-response curves as shown in Figure 14.1A.

T. P. Kenakin: A Pharmacology Primer, Fourth edition. DOI: http://dx.doi.org/10.1016/B978-0-12-407663-1.00014-4
© 2009 Elsevier Inc. All rights reserved.

TABLE 14.1 Agonist Affinity and Efficacy: Agonist Responses for a Series of Agonists with Structure Activity Relationship

	Identifier	R_1	R_2	Maximum	pEC_{50}
1	activone			1	7.1
2	ACS238479	propyl	butyl	0.16	6.52
3	ACS238469	ethyl	methyl	0.34	3.1
4	ACS238481	phenyl	propyl	0.6	5.6
5	ACS238483	cyclohexyl	phenyl	0.5	4.9
6	ACS238484	cyclohexyl	butyl	0.5	6.45
7	ACS238489	butyl	phenyl	0.37	4.9
8	ACS238492	phenyl	phenyl	0.52	4.1
9	ACS238495	phenyl	t-butyl	0.69	6.6
10	ACS238474	propyl	ethyl	0.22	4

Maximum response is calculated as a fraction of the maximal response to agonist ("activone"). The pEC_{50} is the negative log of the molar concentration producing half-maximal response to the agonist.

For all partial agonists, the maximal response is solely dependent on the efficacy of the compound. Also, for all partial agonists, the pEC_{50} is essentially solely dependent upon affinity. Compounds 2, 6, and 9 have the same pEC_{50} (no effect on affinity) but increasing maximal response (Figure 14.1B). Therefore, these changes in structure solely affect efficacy, not affinity. Compounds 8, 5, and 6 have essentially the same maximal response (no effect on efficacy) but increasing affinity (increasing pEC_{50} values); see Figure 14.1C. Therefore, these changes in structure uniquely affect affinity, not efficacy. This is an excellent system to measure agonism, as most of the compounds are partial agonists enabling separate evaluation of changes in structure on efficacy and affinity.

14.2.2 Prediction of Agonist Effect

Question: The data describing two analogues of activone are shown in Table 14.2; which agonist would be predicted to give agonism in most organ systems, agonist 2 or agonist 3? Why?

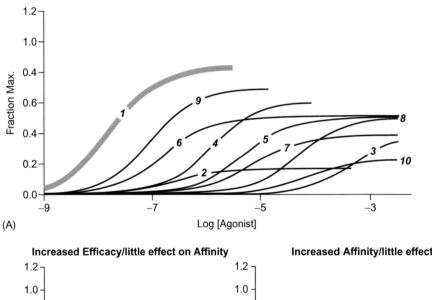

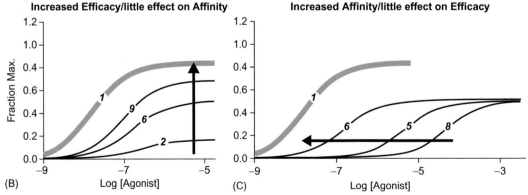

FIGURE 14.1 Agonist concentration-response curves. (A) Concentration-response curves of the agonists described by data in Table 14.1. Gray curve (compound 1) is the standard agonist, "activone." (B) Compounds 9, 6, and 2 basically have the same pEC_{50} values but differ in maximal response. Therefore, the differences in structure between these analogues constitute structures that change only efficacy. (C) Compounds 6, 5, and 8 have the same maximal response (equal efficacy); therefore, the differences in structure between these compounds relate only to changes in affinity.

TABLE 14.2 Agonist Date for Predicting Agonism *In vivo*

	Identifier	R_1	R_2	Maximum	pEC_{50}
1	activone			1	7.1
2	ACS238465	t-butyl	methyl	0.17	6
3	ACS238469	propyl	methyl	0.3	3.5

Answer: The main determinant of agonism in any tissue is efficacy. Affinity affects only the potency of an agonist and not whether it will produce agonist response (unless the concentration of the agonist is below the affinity, in which case there is not enough agonist in the receptor compartment to induce effect). Therefore, the molecule with the highest efficacy (irrespective of affinity and potency) will be the one to produce the most robust and widespread agonism in all tissues. Thus, agonist 3, although not very potent, has the higher efficacy (greater maximal response) and, assuming the concentration that ensures adequate binding of the agonist to the receptor can be attained, will produce the greater agonism in all tissues.

14.2.3 "Super Agonists"

Question: There is no rule to indicate that a natural ligand should have the highest efficacy for a given target. It is well known that, ounce for ounce, Splenda and saccharin are "sweeter" than natural sugar. What would be the optimal system to detect a "super agonist," that is, one that has a higher efficacy for the target than the natural agonist? What systems would not show super-agonism?

Answer: An agonist is a full agonist in any system where one of the biochemical reactions in the cascade of reactions, beginning with drug stimulation and ending with total cellular response, is saturated. The maximal response to any one target (receptor) in the tissue may or may not be the system maximum. If it is the system maximum, then a super agonist will not look different from any other strong agonist, since both will produce the same maximal response (i.e., the target and system maximum) (Figure 14.2A). However, if the target maximum is below the system maximum, then the possibility exists that a super agonist (red curve) could produce a greater maximal response than the previously known standard full agonist (black curve); Figure 14.2B. For example, if a low expression level of β-adrenoceptor were present in a cell line, then a full agonist such as isoproterenol may

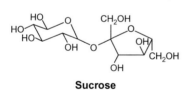

Sucrose

Sucralose 'Splenda'

Saccharin

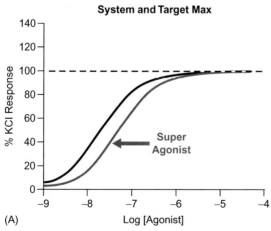

(A)

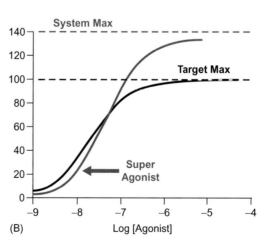

(B)

FIGURE 14.2 "Super agonists." The synthetic sugar analogues sucralose and saccharin are known to be "sweeter" than natural sugar ounce for ounce. (A) The system maximal response (highest response capable of the assay system to any agonist for any target) is equal to the maximal response mediated by the target of interest. In this system, an agonist of higher efficacy than the natural agonist ("super agonist") would produce the system maximal response and would not be distinguishable from the natural agonist. (B) The target maximal response is lower than what the assay system is capable of. Under these circumstances, it might be possible to stimulate the target and detect a greater maximal response, but no element of the response cascade for the target of interest can be saturated in the stimulus-response cascade for this to occur.

produce a lower cyclic AMP maximal response than a full cyclic AMP activator such as forskolin (which acts directly at the adenylate cyclase enzyme to produce maximal stimulation). Under these circumstances, there is a possibility that a super-β-adrenoceptor agonist would produce a maximal response greater than isoproterenol (one that approaches forskolin). However, if the β-adrenoceptor-specific elements of the cyclic AMP machinery become saturated at stimulus levels produced by isoproterenol, then no increased maximum will be produced by the super agonist.

14.2.4 Atypical Agonists

Question: A classical method of determining the specificity of agonism is to block the agonist effect with low concentrations of a specific antagonist for that receptor. In recombinant systems, an additional test is to determine that agonism is observed only in cells that contain the target of interest. The following profile was observed for alcuronium in a recombinant system containing muscarinic m2 receptors mediating inhibition of cyclic AMP. The system demonstrated classical muscarinic m2 agonism as determined by the responses to the muscarinic standard agonist carbachol, and the inhibition thereof by the muscarinic antagonist QNB. These responses were not observed in cells not transfected with cDNA for muscarinic m2 receptors (i.e., that did not express the m2 receptor). Alcuronium produced responses only in cells expressing m2 receptors as well. However, QNB was completely ineffective in blocking this response. What could be happening?

Answer: Alcuronium produces agonism by activation of the m2 receptor through an allosteric site. Binding of alcuronium at this site stabilizes a receptor conformation that activates G_i-protein to inhibit cyclic AMP (as does carbachol). However, whereas carbachol and QNB compete for the same binding site (their interaction is orthosteric), the sites for QNB and alcuronium are not interactive, and binding of QNB has no effect on the binding and subsequent activation of the receptor by alcuronium (see Figure 14.3). Thus, the muscarinic specificity of alcuronium was confirmed by need of the target to gain effect but was not confirmed by the standard method of blockade by an antagonist.

14.2.5 Ordering of Affinity and Efficacy in Agonist Series

Question: A set of agonists, labeled 1 to 5, produce some agonism in two systems (see data in Table 14.3). System A is very well coupled (high receptor density), and system B is poorly coupled. What are the rank orders of efficacy and affinity for these agonists? Hint: This question

cannot be answered completely from the data given. What other experiments should be done to furnish the complete answer?

Answer: Since potencies of full agonists (as seen in system A, Figure 14.4) are complex functions of both affinity and efficacy, the pEC_{50} value cannot be used as a direct measure of either. The key is the activity shown in system B (Figure 14.4). The curves in system B can be used to estimate the relative efficacy of the compounds through their relative maximal response values $(5 > 2 > 4 > 1 > 3)$. In terms of affinity, the rank order among the compounds that produce a curve is $2 > 4 > 5$. The fact that compound 3 produces no response allows it to be used as an antagonist in system B in separate experiments. As shown in the curves on the left, chosen concentrations of the compounds that produce little response produce antagonism of responses to the agonist compound 5. This antagonism is then used to estimate affinity with Schild analysis. The estimates of pA_2s from the curves are 5.7 (cmpd 3), 6.0 (cmpd 1), and 4.5 (cmpd 4). The pEC_{50} value for cmpd 4 correlates well with the pA_2; see Figure 14.4. The order of affinity is $1 > 3 > 2 > 4 > 5$.

14.2.6 Kinetics of Agonism

Question: The Fluorometric Imaging Plate Reader (FLIPR) system for measuring agonist responses in cells measures the transient intracellular release of calcium. While it is a universal platform for measuring physiological response, it is limited by the fact that it captures only the first few seconds of physiological signal. An allosteric agonist is known to bind to the receptor with a $pK_i = 6.3$. However, when tested for agonism in a calcium agonist assay (FLIPR), the pEC_{50} is 4.1 (Figure 14.5A). Thus, it appears that the agonist does not activate the receptors until it occupies nearly >90% of the receptors! Interestingly, when the same agonist is tested in a reporter assay, the pEC_{50} is 6.1, coinciding well with the binding curve (Figure 14.5B). What could be the reason that the agonist curve was shifted so far to the right of the binding curve in FLIPR?

Answer: A clue to what might be happening is the fact that the agonist is allosteric (and therefore might have a very long requirement for onset) and that FLIPR records only the first few seconds of response (calcium responses are transient; see Figure 14.6A). In contrast, reporter assays allow the compound to produce activation over a 24-hour period; therefore, in this assay format, equilibration time for complete activation of the receptor population is not an issue (Figure 14.6B). Therefore, if the agonist has a slow rate of onset and the assay captures only the first seconds of receptor

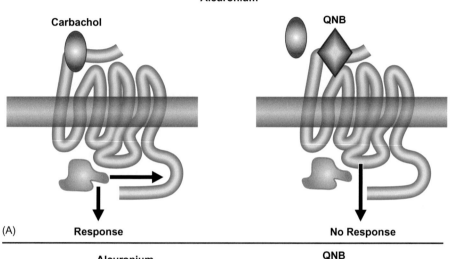

Alcuronium

FIGURE 14.3 Atypical agonists.
Panel A shows the activation of the muscarinic receptor by the orthosteric agonist carbachol and blockade by the orthosteric antagonist QNB. Panel B shows activation of the same receptor through the allosteric agonist alcuronium and lack of blockade of this effect by QNB.

Carbachol

QNB

(A)   Response   No Response

Alcuronium

QNB

(B)   Response   Response

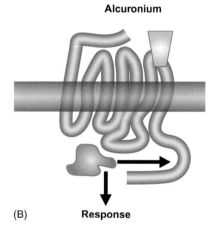

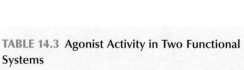

TABLE 14.3 Agonist Activity in Two Functional Systems

		R =	System A		System B	
			Max%	pEC$_{50}$	Max%	pEC$_{50}$
ACS38715	1	t-Butyl	100	8	9	N/A
ACS38866	2	Benzyl	100	7.5	50	4.8
ACS39500	3	Ethyl	100	7.3	0	N/A
ACS36414	4	Propyl	100	7	25	4.5
ACS35780	5	Methyl	100	6.7	82	3.7

activation, a considerable shortfall in agonism can be obtained in the temporally insensitive assay. The fact that the curve "appears" at high concentrations agrees with this scenario since the rate of onset is first order and increases with concentration. Therefore, the temporal shortfall becomes less of an issue at higher concentrations (see Figure 14.6C, D).

14.2.7 Affinity-Dominant versus Efficacy-Dominant Agonists

Question: Chemists refer to this as the "case of the disappearing agonism." In a well-coupled recombinant system

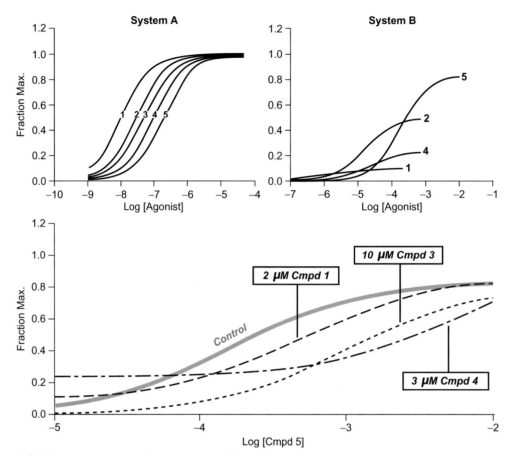

FIGURE 14.4   (A) Concentration-response curves for agonism of compounds listed in Table 14.3 in the more sensitive system A. (B) Concentration-response curves to the same agonists in the less responsive system B. Graph below these shows the effects of the three lowest efficacy agonists (agonists 1, 3, and 4) on the concentration-response curve to the most efficacious agonist 5. The dextral displacement produced by the low-efficacy agonists can be used to calculate a dose ratio that, in turn, can be used to calculate a pA_2 (surrogate pK_B) value to define affinity.

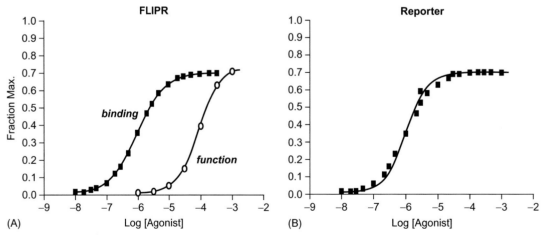

FIGURE 14.5   Effect of the kinetics of agonist production on location of agonist concentration-response curves.   (A) Concentration-response and binding curves for an allosteric agonist in a Fluorometric Image Plate Reader (FLIPR) format where only the first few seconds of response are measured. The functional agonist curve is shifted to the right by a factor of 100 from the receptor occupancy curve calculated by the known affinity and the adsorption isotherm. (B) This same agonist is tested in a format where the kinetics of response collection does not limit observation of agonism (reporter). In this case, the functional and binding curves coincide.

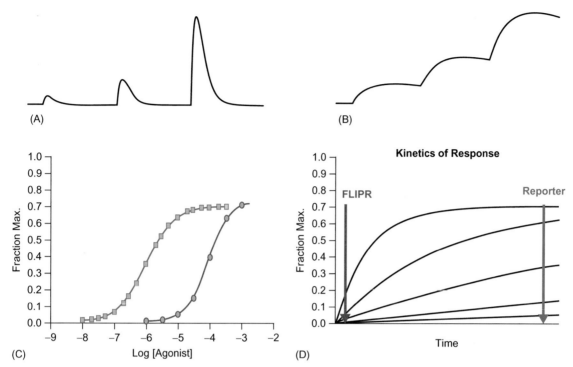

FIGURE 14.6 Reponses to the agonist in the FLIPR (panel A) versus the responses in the nonkinetically limited assay (panel B). Panel C shows the equilibrium response in blue and the early response captured by FLIPR in red. Panel D shows the complete kinetics of response production and the temporal difference between the early transient response (panel A) and equilibrium response (panel B).

with a high level of target expression, ACS332881 produces a potent full agonism (pEC$_{50}$ 9.3; max = 100%). In fact, in this system, ACS332881 is even more potent than the standard, Normolysin (pEC$_{50}$ = 8.7; max = 100%; see Figure 14.7 top panel). Confident in the activity, the team progressed ACS332881 into the natural cell system. To their dismay, there was *no* agonism to AC332881 (in fact, it was an antagonist with pIC$_{50}$ = 7.92; see Figure 14.7 bottom panel). The system seemed to be responding well since Normolysin produced 100% maximal response with a pEC$_{50}$ of 6.0. What could be happening?

Answer: In keeping with the tenet that efficacy drives agonism while affinity and efficacy both drive potency, the divergent profiles of ACS332881 and Normolysin stem from the fact that the former is a high-affinity, low-efficacy agonist while the latter is a low-affinity, high-efficacy agonist (as are most natural neurotransmitters). Thus, in a highly coupled system where even a low-efficacy ligand can produce agonism, AC332881 is potent due to its high affinity. In the more poorly coupled system, ACS332881 does not have the efficacy to produce any agonism yet binds to the receptor according to its high affinity. This latter fact makes it a good antagonist in this assay. These effects are shown in Figure 14.7. These data are consistent with AC332881 having 1/30 times the intrinsic efficacy of Normolysin but 100 times the affinity (ACS332881 pK$_A$ = 8.0; Normolysin pK$_A$ = 6.0). The divergence in agonism occurs because

there is a 2000-fold reduction in the sensitivity when going from the recombinant system to the natural system. These data also do not augur well for ACS332881 producing useful therapeutic agonism if the natural system is a reflection of the efficiency of receptor coupling *in vivo*. In fact, the worst could happen, namely that ACS332881, by virtue of its high affinity, could produce potent antagonism of any normal physiological tone.

14.2.8 Agonist Affinities and Potencies Do Not Correlate

Question: A series of agonists were tested in a binding assay and their affinities estimated through displacement of an antagonist radioligand in a whole-cell assay. The most active are listed in order of increasing affinity (1 to 5) in Table 14.4. However, the resulting relative potency of the agonists did not match the relative order of affinity. Thus, while all the compounds produced full agonism, the − log of the molar concentrations that produced 50% maximal response (pEC$_{50}$ values) presented a different relative order of potency. What could be happening? Which data are most relevant to the therapeutic system?

Answer: The binding assay yielded estimates of the affinity of the agonists but not the efficacy, which has a separate structure-activity relationship. The compounds have the following values of relative efficacy:

FIGURE 14.7 Loss of agonism to a high-affinity, low-efficacy agonist (ACS332881). Top panel shows the effects of the agonists ACS332881 and Normolysin in a highly sensitive system. Bottom panel shows effects in a much less sensitive system (not dextral displacement of the Normolysin curve). In this system, ACS332881 produces no agonism.

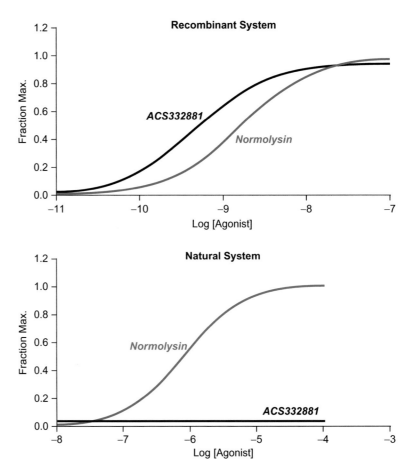

TABLE 14.4 Correlating Agonist Potency and Affinity

		pK_A	pEC_{50}
1	ACS888241	4.00	6.70
2	ACS889313	4.52	6.00
3	ACS887333	5.30	7.82
4	ACS888714	5.70	7.30
5	ACS889992	7.00	7.52

Compound	Relative Efficacy
ACS888241	500
ACS889313	50
ACS887333	190
ACS889992	25
ACS888714	30

It can be seen that the agonist with the lowest affinity also had the highest efficacy (much like natural neurotransmitters that have low affinity but very high efficacy). The potency of full agonists is a complex amalgam of affinity and efficacy as given by the operational model of agonism shown as follows:

$$\text{Response} = \frac{([\text{Agonist}]/K_A\tau)E_{max}}{([\text{Agonist}]/K_A)(1+\tau)+1}, \qquad (14.1)$$

where τ is a measure of efficacy and the efficiency of the system in translating occupancy to response, and K_A is the equilibrium dissociation constant of the agonist-receptor complex (1/affinity). From this equation it can be seen that potency (as a pEC_{50} value) is given by:

$$pEC_{50} = -\text{Log}\frac{K_A}{(1+\tau)}. \qquad (14.2)$$

The functional potency data are the relevant data since the functional activity will behave according to the operational model. It can be seen that high-efficacy values lead to high pEC_{50} values irrespective of the affinity. Therefore, the order of affinities shown to follow produces the different order of functional potencies shown (Figure 14.8).

14.2.9 Lack of Agonist Effect

Question: A recombinant β-adrenoceptor cell line was required for a cardiovascular drug discovery program. Accordingly, several clones were prepared and stable cell lines derived from them. Since the receptors were tagged

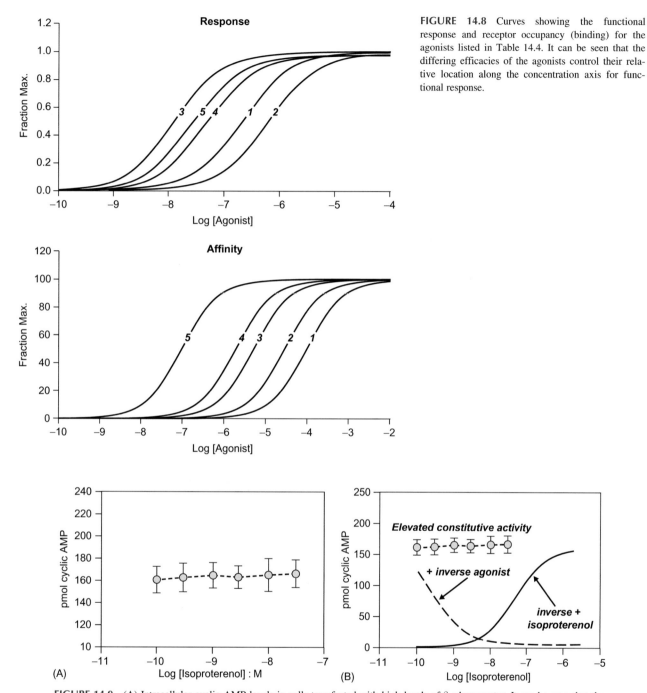

FIGURE 14.8 Curves showing the functional response and receptor occupancy (binding) for the agonists listed in Table 14.4. It can be seen that the differing efficacies of the agonists control their relative location along the concentration axis for functional response.

FIGURE 14.9 (A) Intracellular cyclic AMP levels in cells transfected with high levels of β-adrenoceptor. It can be seen that the powerful β-adrenoceptor agonist isoproterenol produces no visible effect. (B) Same cells treated with an inverse agonist; this produces a decrease in the elevated baseline, which can then be elevated again with isoproterenol.

with labels that allowed surface expression to be quantified, the team members were able to choose the clone with the highest level of receptor expression. It was felt that this would be the most sensitive. The concentration-response curve to the powerful β-adrenoceptor agonist isoproterenol was disappointing to say the least (see Figure 14.9A). What could have gone wrong, and how could this be elucidated further?

Answer: The fact that the system does not respond to isoproterenol, a powerful agonist, suggests either that the expressed receptor is damaged and insensitive to stimulation or that the system is unable to respond to stimulation. In cases where the receptor is not damaged, it could be that the system is already fully stimulated. Under these circumstances, further effects of isoproterenol agonism would not be observed. The key here is the high receptor

TABLE 14.5 Assay-Specific Agonism

Compound	Response in FLIPR		Response in Reporter	
	pEC$_{50}$	%MAX	pEC$_{50}$	%MAX
PTH	7.1	100	8.4	100
ACS333887	6.3	75	6.1	5
ACS442776	5.7	23	6.2	45
ACS998446	6.7	85	6.9	3
ACS222997	5.7	15	6.2	45

expression level for the β_2-adrenoceptors. Receptors are known to spontaneously produce active states (albeit at a low level). Under conditions of receptor overexpression, there can be an adequate level of ambient active state receptor present at the cell surface to produce significant spontaneous elevation of basal response (see Section 3.10 on constitutive activity). In extreme cases, these elevations in basal response can attain maximal levels for cellular stimulation. Thus, the high expression of β-adrenoceptors could have produced an already maximal level of elevated cyclic AMP, leaving the cell insensitive to further agonism.

This potential scenario can be uncovered by treating the cell with a β-adrenoceptor inverse agonist such as propranolol or ICI118,551 (see Figure 14.9B). If a maximal constitutive activity is present, an inverse agonist will decrease the basal response in a concentration-dependent manner. Furthermore, after selective depression of the basal response with an inverse agonist, the receptor will regain sensitivity to an agonist such as isoproterenol (although with diminished potency, since the inverse agonist will also be an antagonist of the agonism). Thus, elevations in cyclic AMP will be produced by high concentrations of isoproterenol in the presence of the inverse agonist. As for utility in testing, such a constitutively active system would not be useful for agonist studies.

14.2.10 Assay-Specific Agonism

Question: Synthetic agonists of the parathyroid hormone receptor (PTH) for an osteoporosis program were tested in two recombinant PTH receptor agonist assays: calcium transient response (FLIPR) and a reporter assay. The most sensitive cell line was used for both assays. The characteristics for the natural agonist, PTH, indicated that both assays were robust and sensitive. However, the profile for agonism, shown in Table 14.5, was obtained leaving the team puzzled as to why some powerful agonists in the FLIPR assay (reputedly a lower sensitivity assay than the reporter assay; see data for PTH, Table 14.5) showed low activity in the more sensitive reporter assay. For example, ACS998446 lost a great deal of activity in the reporter assay. Also, some relative weak agonists in the FLIPR assay showed comparable activity (certainly not diminished) in the reporter assay (i.e., see ACS222997, Table 14.5, which showed greater agonist activity in the reporter assay); see Figure 14.10. What could be the reason for this discrepancy?

Answer: The difference in agonism could be due to the real time versus stop time format. Specifically, the FLIPR system measures the calcium transient response in real time, thereby allowing the peak to be measured. In contrast, the reporter format measures the historical effects of the agonist over a period of time. This corresponds to the integral of the real time curve over time (Figure 14.11A). If the system has basal activity, then an agonist response is measured as an increase in the historical response over basal for a given period of time. If the response is sustained, the integral is substantial and a change is recorded. However, if the response is transient, then the historical signal may be insignificant (Figure 14.11B). A series of transient responses may not demonstrate a concentration-response behavior, in contrast to a series of sustained responses. Sustained and transient response patterns may be rooted in physiology. For example, a G-protein receptor response can be powerful but rapid (transient), whereas a β-arrestin-based signal may be of a lower level but sustained. Therefore, a real time assay may more faithfully represent the former response and a stop-time system (i.e.,

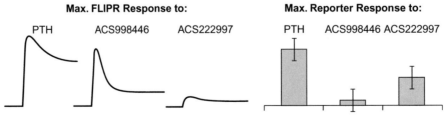

FIGURE 14.10 Two types of response measured for PTH receptor activation. The FLIPR format captures peak effect and shows that ACS998446 produces a greater peak effect than does ACS222997. The reporter format captures the historical response over time and is more sensitive to prolonged effects than transient peak responses. Under these circumstances, the sustained response to ACS222997 produces a greater overall response than the transient ACS998446.

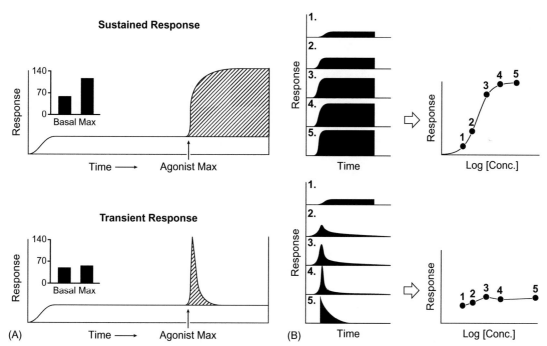

Sustained Response

Transient Response

(A) Time ——→ Agonist Max   (B) Time   Log [Conc.]

FIGURE 14.11 (A) Responses to two agonists; one produces a sustained response while the other produces a transient fading response. If the response is taken from the integral of the temporal curves (i.e., reporter history of cyclic AMP production), then the sustained agonist response will be faithfully reflected by the area under the curve (historical response). In contrast, the transient peak responses (that do not generate sustained areas under the curve) will not be reflected in the reporter response, and the transient agonist will appear to be inactive in this assay format.

reporter) the latter. Therefore, the pattern of response is consistent with ACS998446 producing a G-protein-based response and ACS222997 producing a sustained β-arrestin-based response. Thus, the reporter will record a more robust response for ACS222997, and the real time FLIPR assay will record a more robust peak effect due to ACS998446.

14.3 ANTAGONISM

14.3.1 Antagonist Potency and Kinetics: Part A

Question: A methyl analogue (R = Me) of a muscarinic competitive antagonist shows a pA_2 value of 9.55 in the FLIPR assay with a 20 min pre-incubation of cells with antagonist. All SAR in this series indicate that increasing the size of the R group should increase potency. However, when R = tBut, the pA_2 is 9.6. The chemists are puzzled and demand a retest. Things become more complicated when the retest is done in a reporter functional assay and it is found that the R = Me compound has a pA_2 of 9.7 and the R = tBut compound now has a pA_2 of 10.25. What could be happening?

Background: The program is a stage where structure activity relationships for increasing potency are being tracked with estimates of antagonist potency. Due to resource constraints, biologists are determining the minimal concentration required to shift an agonist concentration-response curve by a factor of 2 (i.e., pA_2) in accordance with the belief that this concentration is a good estimate of the minimal concentration required to be present at the target to cause blockade (i.e., an estimate of K_B, the concentration binding to 50% of the receptors — see Figure 11.27).

Answer: The short (20 min) pre-incubation time of the cells with the antagonist is the key. The true K_B of the antagonist with R = Me is 0.17 nM ($pK_B = 9.7$). This is a ratio of the rate of offset (5×10^{-4} s^{-1}) and onset (3×10^6 s^{-1} mol^{-1}). The effects of a range of concentrations of this antagonist at 20 min are shown in Figure 14.12A along with the resulting Schild regression (Figure 14.12B). The observed pA_2 indicates potency a little lower than the true K_B because 20 min is insufficient equilibration time; the error is quite small and equals $1.8 \times K_B = 0.3$ nM for a pA_2 of 9.5. In contrast, the equilibration time is not an issue in the reporter assay since acquisition of the agonist response requires 24 hours. Under these circumstances, the antagonist is present in the media for a great deal longer than is required for receptor onset, and insufficient onset is not a problem. However, the other side of the coin is that reporter assays may subject the tissue to toxic effects of new compounds, thereby causing an overestimation of antagonist potency (i.e., receptor blockade + toxic effect). In the case of the

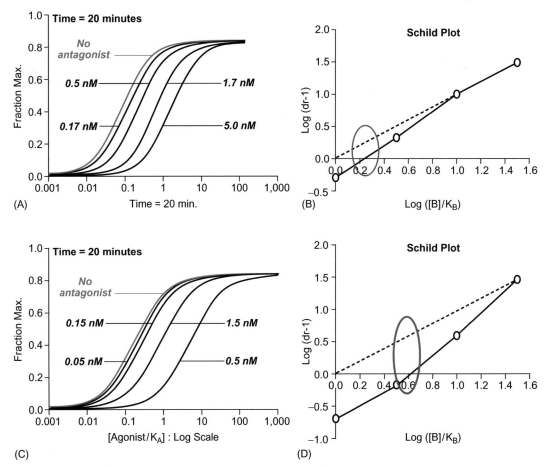

FIGURE 14.12 Effect of equilibration time on observed potency of antagonists. (A) R = Me analogue muscarinic antagonist in FLIPR assay; effects of various concentrations on agonist concentration-response curves when antagonist equilibrated with the assay for 20 min. (B) Schild regression for the antagonist shown in panel A. It can be seen that, at 20 min, the effects of lower concentrations of antagonist are underestimated to a greater extent than those of higher concentrations causing the Schild regression to have a steep slope (slope >1). The red circle indicates the effects of concentrations near the pA_2; these are affected most by the short equilibration times. (C) Effects of the tBut antagonist on muscarinic agonist concentration-response curves. (D) Schild regression for the tBut analogue. It can be seen that the temporal effects seen in panel B are exacerbated for the slower tBut antagonist.

R = Me compound, toxicity is not an issue, and the true K_B (0.17 nM) is reflected in the observed pA_2 in the reporter assay of 9.7 (a close estimate of the true pK_B of 9.8). The same is not true of the R = tBut compound. The change in structure, predicted by the chemists to increase potency, in fact does just that, in accordance with the general finding that increased potency results from a decrease in the rate of offset of the molecule from the receptor (as opposed to an increase in the rate of onset, since this usually reaches a diffusion limit). In this case, the change from R = Me to R = tBut decreases the rate of offset by a factor of 6 (to $1.67 \times 10^{-4} \, s^{-1}$) and decreases the rate of onset by a factor of 3. While this increases the potency threefold (to K_B = (rate of offset)/(rate of onset) = $(0.5 \times 10^{-4} \, s^{-1})/(1 \times 10^6 \, s^{-1} \, mol^{-1} = 0.05$ nM), it also increases the error due to the shortfall in equilibration time in the FLIPR assay,

since it takes longer for this antagonist to come to equilibrium with the receptors. The effects of a range of concentrations of this antagonist at 20 min are shown in Figure 14.12C along with the resulting Schild regression (Figure 14.12D). The observed pA_2 is now 4.5 times the true K_B, yielding a value of 4.5×0.05 nM = 0.25 nM for a pA_2 of 9.6. Kinetics are not an issue in the reporter assay, and an observed potency near the true K_B of 0.05 nM (pA_2 = 10.3) is observed in that assay. The kinetic effect is differentially more important for the slower offset, more potent R = tBut compound.

General Lessons Learned: Low concentrations of antagonists (i.e., near the K_B) are most sensitive to kinetics of onset. Insufficient time of equilibration can lead to underestimation of competitive antagonist potency and can be detected by retesting at a longer time or determination of a Schild regression (slope > 1 may indicate inadequate equilibration time).

14.3.2 Antagonist Potency in pIC_{50} Format (Kinetics Part B)

Question: It is worth reconsidering the previous exercise in terms of using an IC_{50} format for tracking antagonism. Under these circumstances, a constant concentration of agonist is present in the assay and then a range of concentrations of antagonist is added until complete blockade of the response is achieved. The concentration of antagonist that produces 50% blockade of the response is designated the IC_{50} (more correctly, $-\log IC_{50}$ values are used in the form of pIC_{50}s). This is some constant multiple of the true K_B. As long as the same concentration of agonist is used for the series of antagonists, the ratios of the IC_{50} values can be used as accurate surrogates for the ratios of the K_B values, and changes in antagonist potency can be tracked rapidly.

The same two antagonists (R = Me and R = tBut) presented in the previous question are tested in pIC_{50} mode. The methyl analogue muscarinic competitive antagonist shows a pIC_{50} value of 9.0 in the FLIPR assay with a 20 min pre-incubation of cells with antagonist. As noted previously, all SAR in this series indicated that increasing the size of the R group should increase the potency. However, when R = tBut, the pIC_{50} is also 9.0. A retest is done in a reporter functional assay and it is found that the R = Me compound has a pIC_{50} of 9.1 and the R = tBut compound now has a pIC_{50} of 9.6. What could be happening?

Answer: The short (20 min) pre-incubation time of the cells with the antagonist is the key in this format as well. The true K_B of the antagonist with R = Me is 0.17 nM, and this translates to a pIC_{50} value of 9.0. The pIC_{50} curves for 20, 30, 60, and 200 min are shown in Figure 14.13A. It can be seen that the curve at 20 min is steeper (Hill coefficient

> 1) and shifted to the right of the curves at longer times, but the effects are minor because this is a relatively fast-acting antagonist. The 20 min pre-equilibration underestimates the potency of the antagonist. There is a slight increase in potency for this antagonist at greater equilibration times, which finally reflect the true potency of the antagonist (at 200 min pIC_{50} = 9.1). The effect of equilibration time on a slower acting antagonist such as the R = tBut compound is more profound. The change in structure did increase potency in accordance with the general finding that increased potency results from a decrease in the rate of offset of the molecule from the receptor. In this case, the change from R = Me to R = tBut decreases the rate of offset by a factor of 6 (to 1.67×10^{-4} s^{-1}) with a concomitant decrease in the rate of onset of 3. While this increases the potency threefold (to K_B = (rate of offset)/(rate of onset) = $(0.5 \times 10^{-4}$ s$^{-1})/(1 \times 10^6$ s^{-1} mol^{-1} = 0.05 nM)), it also increases the error due to the shortfall in equilibration time in the FLIPR assay, since it takes longer for this antagonist to come to equilibrium with the receptors. This is reflected in the pIC_{50} curves for this antagonist as shown in Figure 14.13B. Here it can be seen that the curve at 20 min is even steeper and shifted farther to the right than for the antagonist of faster offset (Figure 14.13A). The observed pIC_{50} at 20 min is 9.0 due to the suboptimal equilibration time. At 200 min, the true potency of the antagonist is reflected in the more potent pIC_{50} value of 9.6.

Greater Lessons Learned: In the absence of any other information, the chemists were presented with the following scenario: the change from Me to tBut did not change potency, a finding contrary to previous data and confusing to the known SAR for this series. However, the Hill coefficient of the pIC_{50} curve of > 1 suggests that temporal inequilibrium may have been a factor. Increasing the equilibration time of the antagonist with the assay yielded a completely different scenario; namely, one where the change from Me to tBut increased the

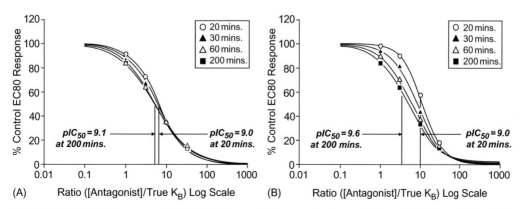

(A) Ratio ([Antagonist]/True K_B) Log Scale

(B) Ratio ([Antagonist]/True K_B) Log Scale

FIGURE 14.13 Inhibition curves for the R = Me muscarinic antagonist shown in Figure 14.12A (panel A) and the R = tBut antagonist shown in Figure 14.12C (panel B). It can be seen that the pIC_{50} at 20 min underestimates the potency of both antagonists but that the error is larger for the tBut analogue.

potency by a factor of 3 (pIC$_{50}$ changes from 9.1 to 9.6; factor = $10^{0.5}$ = 3).

14.3.3 Mechanism of Antagonist Action (Kinetics Part C)

Question: This question is based on data from the previous question. A perspicacious chemist recalled that the R = Me compound produced noncompetitive antagonism in the FLIPR assay. The pattern of the curves (control and curve in the presence of 5 nM antagonist after 2 hours equilibration) is shown in Figure 14.14A. This produced consternation among the chemist ranks until the biologist assured them it was expected. The chemists then asked what the pattern was for the R = tBut compound. If the biologist was correct, which panel would you predict would be the pattern for a slightly lower concentration (2 nM) of the R = tBut compound: panel B, C, or D? Why? Which antagonist would give the better target coverage? Why?

Answer: The R = tBut antagonist most likely will give a pattern shown in panel D. In most cases, the FLIPR assay causes slow offset antagonists to produce a truncated agonist curve, thus yielding a depressed maximum noncompetitive effect. This is because the FLIPR captures an early-phase transient response for calcium release. Therefore, if the agonist and antagonist cannot equilibrate according to their true equilibrium dissociation constants within the time allowed for measurement of response (which with FLIPR is very short), then responses requiring a greater agonist-receptor occupancy (i.e., near the maximum) will be disproportionately more inhibited, thereby producing a depressed maximal response. This effect is more pronounced with slower antagonists. Since the rate of offset of the R = tBut antagonist is slower than that of the R = Me antagonist, it would be expected that the R = tBut antagonist will produce even greater depression of the maximal response in this assay. *Target coverage* refers to binding of the molecule to the target in an open system. The slower the offset, the more persistent the binding. Thus, since the rate of offset of the R = tBut antagonist is slower, it should be more persistent and thus give better target coverage than the R = Me compound.

14.3.4 Mechanism of Antagonist Action: Curve Patterns

Question: A close examination of the concentration-response curves for the antagonist in a reporter system revealed the pattern shown in Figure 14.15. Both the chemists and the biologists agreed that the antagonist appeared to produce simple competitive antagonism in this system. What features of the pattern indicate this?

Answer: The model for simple competitive antagonism has the following prerequisites: The antagonist must

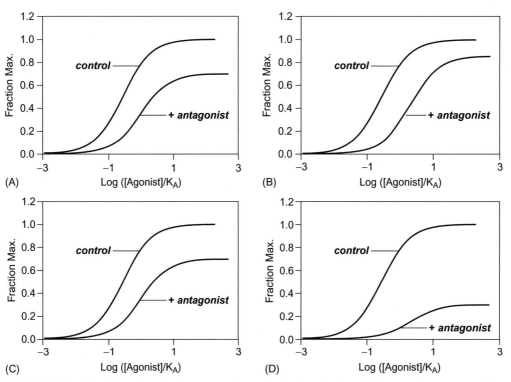

FIGURE 14.14 The effects of various insurmountable antagonists in a hemi-equilibrium-sensitive assay (FLIPR) where slow offset from the receptor leads to a depression of the maximal response. In general, the slower the offset, the more depression is seen for a given degree of receptor occupancy.

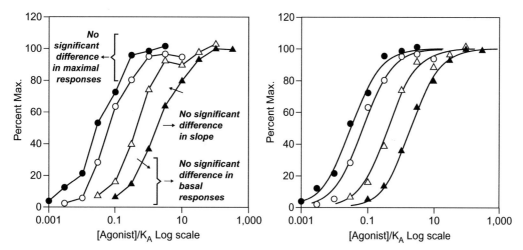

FIGURE 14.15 Patterns of antagonism. A series of curves with an apparent common maximal response; basal starting point and slope can be refit to a model of curves with common maxima, basal, and slope. This is indicative of simple competitive antagonism.

produce parallel shifts to the right of the agonist concentration-response curves with no change in the basal or maximal levels of response (see Figure 14.15). Hypothesis testing (F-test) can be used to determine if the data can be fit to parallel curves with common maxima and basal effects to fulfill the requirement for being *consistent with*, not necessarily *proof of*, simple competitive antagonism. It should be noted that there are many instances of allosteric and physiological antagonism mediated through separate receptors known to provide identical patterns.

14.3.5 Mechanism of Action: Incomplete Antagonism

Question: Two ligands in a related series block the functional effects of histamine in a cyclic AMP assay (see Table 14.6). However, while ACS444876 completely blocks the effects of 100 nM histamine, ACS444751, a more potent antagonist, blocks only half of the maximal histamine response. What are two target-related and mechanism-based actions of these antagonists that could be causing this divergence? It should be assumed that nonspecific off-target effects have been excluded; that is,

both ACS444876 and ACS444751 produce no cellular effects in the absence of histamine receptors.

Answer: One possibility for the pattern of incomplete antagonism produced by ACS444751 is that the antagonist is a partial agonist producing a low-level (approximately 33% max) agonist response. Therefore, the compound produces blockade of a full agonist (and thus a depression of response to yield a pIC_{50}), but this blockade stops when the effect of the partial agonist takes over at high antagonist concentration. At this point, maximal levels of antagonist yield the partial agonist effects of the antagonist, and the pIC_{50} curve tops out at 33% response (Figure 14.16). In contrast, ACS444876 has no partial agonist activity and thus produces no response of its own. Under these circumstances, the pIC_{50} curve continues to 0%.

A second possibility for this pattern of incomplete antagonism is that ACS444751 is an allosteric modulator that produces a maximal fivefold shift to the right of the agonist concentration-response curve ($\alpha = 0.2$) while ACS444876 is either a neutral orthosteric antagonist or an allosteric modulator that produces a greater degree of maximal modulation ($\alpha = 0.01$; maximal 100-fold shift to the right of the agonist curve). At the concentration of agonist used to construct the pIC_{50} curves, the maximal fivefold shift to the right produced by ACS444751 results in a pIC_{50} curve that has a maximal inhibition of 50−60%; see Figure 14.17. The much larger shift to the right produced by ACS444876 allows this antagonist to reduce the response in the pIC_{50} curve to 0% as would be seen with a normal orthosteric neutral antagonist (see Figure 14.17). If different concentrations of agonist were to be used to construct the pIC_{50} curves, then the plateau maxima of the inhibition curves could be different. For example, if a concentration of 1 μM were to be used for the pIC_{50} curves (instead of 100 nM), then the maximal

TABLE 14.6 Incomplete Antagonism

	R	pIC_{50}	Max Inhib
ACS444876	tBut	5.5	98%
ACS444751	Benzyl	6.5	53%

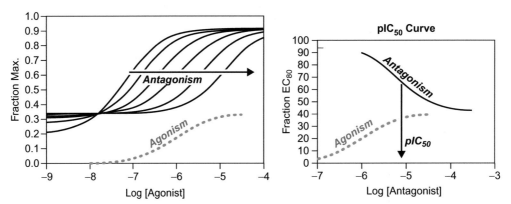

FIGURE 14.16   Effects of a partial agonist on responses to a full agonist. The partial agonist produces shifts to the right of the curve to the full agonist as well as an elevated basal (due to the intrinsic agonism produced by the partial agonist). The blue line indicates the direct effects of the partial agonist on the system. The panel to the right shows an inhibition curve to the partial agonist producing inhibition of a concentration of full agonist that produces 80% maximal effect. It can be seen that the concentration-dependent inhibition defines a curve the midpoint of which is the pIC_{50} of the partial agonist. However, the inhibition curve does not reduce the EC_{80} response to basal levels; instead, the curve is reduced only to the maximal level of response caused by the partial agonist.

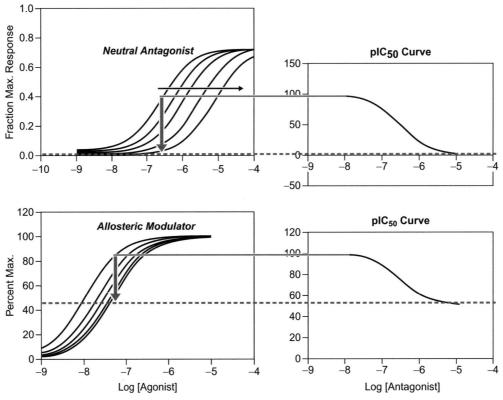

FIGURE 14.17   Inhibition curves produced by an orthosteric competitive antagonist (top panels) and an allosteric modulator that produces a fivefold shift to the right of the agonist concentration-response curves (bottom panels). The top panel shows the effect of the antagonist inhibiting a concentration of the full agonist that normally produces 50% maximal response. The antagonist reduces the response to basal levels. In contrast the allosteric modulator blocks the effects of the full agonist (a concentration that normally produces an 80% maximal response) to a level that is elevated above basal. This is because the maximal effect of the modulator does not displace the agonist, but, rather, it simply reduces the affinity of the receptor for the agonist by a factor of 5. Under these circumstances, the inhibition curves demonstrate an elevated basal response.

TABLE 14.7 Antagonism below Baseline

	R	pIC_{50}	Max Inhib
ACS449433	Et	7.5	101%
ACS448111	Propyl	6.2	154%(− 54%)*

Response fell 54% below basal value.

inhibition for ACS444751 would be 42% and for ACS444876 would be 90% (see Figure 4.8 for examples).

Approaches to Differentiate Partial Agonism from Allosterism: An obvious next experiment to determine which of these mechanisms could be operative is to test the antagonists for direct agonist activity. If no direct agonism is observed, then the allosteric mechanism can be best determined by observing the effects of a range of concentrations of antagonist on full agonist concentration-response curves. This would show the saturation of effect made obvious by the cessation of the shifts to the right of the agonist concentration-response curves at high antagonist concentrations.

14.3.6 pIC_{50} Mode: Antagonism Below Basal

Question: Two ligands in a related series block the functional effects of acetylcholine (inhibition of Forskolin-induced cyclic AMP production; see Table 14.7). The pIC_{50} values for both ACS449443 and ACS448111 indicate potent antagonism. However, while ACS449433 completely blocks the effects of a concentration of acetylcholine producing 80% maximal response, the pIC_{50} inhibition curve for ACS448111 shows a dramatic negative effect with the inhibition curve producing a maximal effect 54% *below* the basal effect. What could be happening, and what experiments could be done to elucidate whether such a mechanism is operative?

Answer: If an antagonist drops the baseline below the starting point in a pIC_{50} format, it suggests either that the antagonist has a toxic effect that reduces a physiologically elevated baseline, or that the system is constitutively active due to spontaneous receptor activity and that the antagonist is an inverse agonist (see Figure 14.18). The inverse agonist property reduces the receptor-mediated constitutive activity. Nonspecific depressant effects can be observed through testing the antagonist on the tissue

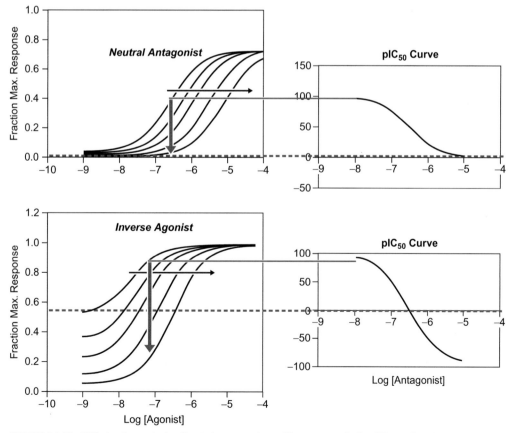

FIGURE 14.18 Effects of a neutral orthosteric antagonist and inverse agonist in pIC_{50} mode. A neutral antagonist reduces an EC_{80} concentration of agonist to basal levels. An inverse agonist reduces the EC_{80} concentration below basal as shown in the bottom panels.

where the basal response is elevated through another mechanism. If no depression is observed, then a receptor-specific effect (i.e., specific inverse agonism) is indicated.

14.3.7 Secondary Effects of Antagonists

Question: In a functional system, an antagonist shifts the agonist curves to the right in a concentration-dependent manner. However, as the curves shift, the maximal response is depressed and this too is antagonist concentration dependent. This is a frequent occurrence in functional experiments on whole-cell systems. The pattern of antagonism to this antagonist is shown in Figure 14.19A. What could be happening, and what experiments could be designed to elucidate further?

Answer: Biphasic agonist concentration-response curves are often encountered in experimental pharmacology. There are two general mechanisms for such behavior: It can be agonist specific or related to the strength of receptor activation. The first mechanism is where a specific agonist has a secondary property that inhibits the ability of the tissue to respond to the agonist (agonist A in Figure 14.19B). In contrast, agonist B does not have

this specific property causing depression of response. Alternatively, a tissue or specific receptor could be refractory to intense stimulation, and thus response will wane for any agonist. In cases where a receptor desensitizes rapidly, then bell-shaped concentration-response curves can be observed. Thus, there will be a region of agonist stimulation (see Figure 14.19C) where any response will be diminished as an antagonist shifts the concentration-response curves into regions where the response is diminished (bell-shaped curves caused by signal-strength-related depression of maximal response). This would be observed for agonism-specific depression. In the latter case, all antagonists that produce dextral displacement of concentration-response curves would cause depression of maximal response.

14.3.8 Antagonist Potency Variably Dependent on Agonist Concentration

Question: Two scaffolds with histamine receptor antagonist activity were in the process of being optimized with a histamine functional assay; see Figure 14.20. It was known that the assay was somewhat variable (i.e.,

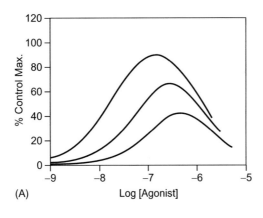

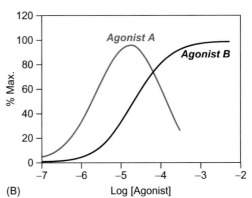

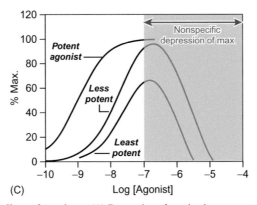

FIGURE 14.19 Secondary effects of agonists. (A) Depression of maximal response to agonist in the presence of increasing concentrations of antagonist. (B) Depression of maxima (bell-shaped curves) may be agonist specific. (C) Bell-shaped curves can be stimulation-strength dependent whereby maximal stimulation of the target by any agonist causes reversal of response. This could be through a nonspecific effect or specific target-related effect.

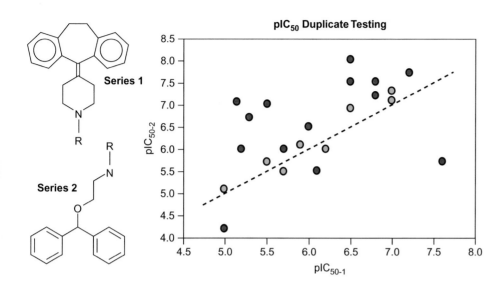

pIC$_{50}$ Duplicate Testing

Series 1

Series 2

FIGURE 14.20 Retests of antagonists in pIC$_{50}$ mode with single concentration analysis. The potency of series 2 (red) varies considerably between tests, whereas there is better agreement within series 1 (blue circles).

histamine varies in potency from day to day), but it was considered suitable for antagonist SAR through the determination of pIC$_{50}$ values for the experimental antagonists. Interestingly, it was found that the pIC$_{50}$ values for blockade of a concentration of histamine that produced 80% maximal response varied a great deal more for one scaffold (series 2; red circles on graph) than another series (series 1; blue circles). Figure 14.20 shows the effect of duplicate-testing the antagonists on separate days. What could be the reason for this?

Answer: These data are consistent with one of the scaffolds (series 2) being more sensitive to variance in agonism of the system than the other. This can occur if the members of series 2 are competitive antagonists (and thus are sensitive to the strength of signal used in the assay). The "correction" for this (Cheng–Prusoff correction [1]) is a linear function between the K_B (true antagonist potency) and the IC$_{50}$ (see Figure 14.21 for competitive antagonists). The other compounds (series 1) are noncompetitive antagonists. This latter class of antagonist depresses the concentration-response curves to the agonist and is quite insensitive to the strength of signal put into the assay (see Figure 14.21 for noncompetitive antagonists). Therefore, the change in stimulation level would affect the observed potency estimate of the competitive antagonist but not the noncompetitive antagonist. This variance in sensitivity to input signal can be seen in the expressions for IC$_{50}$ for competitive versus noncompetitive antagonists. For competitive antagonists:

$$IC_{50} = K_B([A]/K_A)(1 + \tau) + 1. \qquad (14.3)$$

For noncompetitive antagonists the corresponding expression is:

$$IC_{50} = K_B(([A]/K_A)(1 + \tau) + 1)/(([A]/K_A) + 1), \quad (14.4)$$

where K_B is the equilibrium dissociation constant of the antagonist-receptor complex, [A] the concentration of

agonist, and τ the sensitivity of the system. Both K_B and [A] are constant so it is most likely variability will be found in τ, the sensitivity of the system (i.e., variance on receptor density, efficiency of stimulus-response coupling, etc.). Figure 14.22A shows the variability factor for a given concentration of agonist ([A]/K_A = 5) as a function of τ; the shaded area is an example where τ values vary five-fold from day to day. It can be seen that this causes much more variance for the competitive antagonist than it does for the noncompetitive antagonist (see Figure 14.22B).

14.4 *IN VITRO–IN VIVO* TRANSITIONS AND GENERAL DISCOVERY

14.4.1 "Silent Antagonism"

Question: A program was initiated to produce "silent antagonism" of leukotriene effect in asthma (no agonist effect, only inhibition of natural agonist in the system). Accordingly, a human leukotriene receptor was expressed in Chinese hamster ovary (CHO) cells; this system responded to the natural agonist but it was noted that the natural agonist was not as potent in this recombinant system as it was in samples of human airway tissue. Chemists produced a series of antagonists with the potencies shown in Table 14.8. After consideration of ADME properties and acute potency, ACS663992 (pK_B = 7.0) was chosen for further study in an animal model of hyper-reactive airways. Upon injection of ACS663992, the animal experienced severe bronchospasm and had to be quickly removed from the test chamber. Thus, a compound that should have provided protection against leukotriene-induced bronchospasm itself produced bronchospasm. What could be happening, and what experiments could be designed to confirm the mechanism?

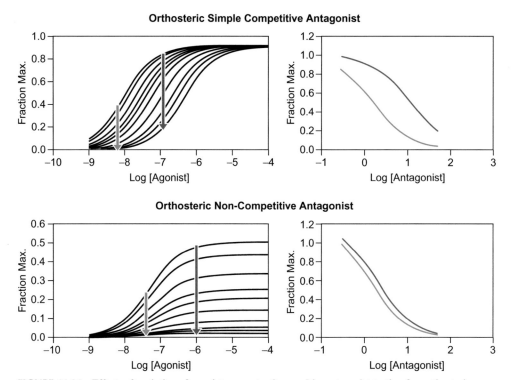

FIGURE 14.21   Effects of variation of agonist concentration used in antagonist testing for orthosteric competitive antagonist (top panels) and orthosteric noncompetitive antagonist (bottom panels). Testing in pIC_{50} mode for the competitive antagonist (at level EC_{40}, blue; and EC_{80}, red) results in a considerable difference in the inhibition curves (coded red and blue, top right panel. In contrast, for noncompetitive antagonists, blocking an EC_{40} versus EC_{80} makes little difference to the location of the inhibition curve (bottom right panel).

Answer: The main clue to the divergent activity of these assays is the fact that the natural ligand is less potent in the recombinant system. Whether this is due to a less efficient receptor expression in the CHO cell line or a less efficient coupling of the expressed receptors, this lower sensitivity may preclude detection of weak positive efficacy that could otherwise produce agonism in more sensitive systems. This appears to be the case for ACS663992. The model for asthma may involve hyper-reactive airways, which could be much more sensitive to low-efficacy leukotriene agonism. In this instance, ACS663992 is a low-efficacy partial agonist with a 100 nM affinity ($pK_B = 7.0$). Figure 14.23 shows the effects of 150 nM ACS663992 on concentration-response curves to leukotriene in the recombinant system (no agonism observed; 4.5-fold shift to the right of the concentration-response curve) and the hyper-reactive airway system (40% agonism; twofold shift to the right of the concentration-response curve). ACS663992 has 0.03 times the intrinsic efficacy of leukotriene. The natural system has 1000 times greater sensitivity to leukotriene than does the recombinant system; therefore, the compound is able to demonstrate overt agonism in the more sensitive system.

14.4.2 Loss of Activity

Question: A test molecule emerged as a potent β-blocker in β-adrenoceptor binding studies with a $pK_B = 9.2$ (i.e., 50% receptor bound at a concentration of 0.6 nM). The program team felt extremely confident about the binding assay yielding accurate measures of β-adrenoceptor blocking activity; therefore, the critical path progressed straight from the binding assay to an *in vivo* assay for β-blockade in a model of cardiac function. The team was dismayed to find that the molecule with $pK_B = 9.2$ was a very weak β-blocker *in vivo* in spite of the fact that it was administered intravenously and drug concentration at the site of action was not an issue. The biologists then tested the compound in an *in vitro* cardiac model (papillary muscle) and found that it was very weak as well. What could be the reason for the dissociation of activity of the compound in binding and functional assays? What additional experiments could be done to elucidate the reason for the dissimulation?

Answer: It is clear that the molecule has another property that cancels β-blockade *in vivo* or in functional systems; a likely scenario is a potentiation of β-adrenoceptor

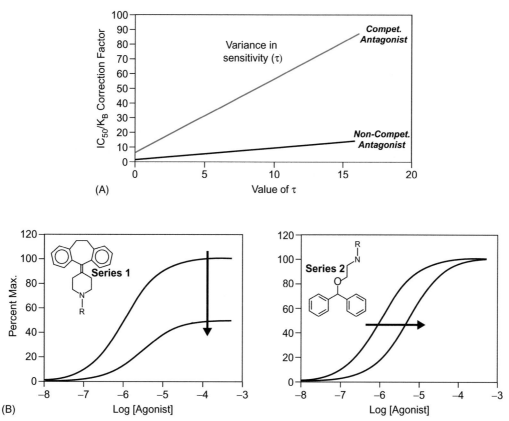

FIGURE 14.22 Effect of the efficacy, receptor number, and efficiency of receptor coupling on the agonist to estimates of potency of competitive and noncompetitive antagonists (Equations 14.3 and 14.4); panel A. Area of agonist concentration generally used for screening is ($[A]/K_A = 5$); it can be seen that the observed competitive antagonist potency varies more with changing τ (variable receptor number and/or coupling efficiency) for competitive versus noncompetitive antagonists. Panel B (left) shows the effect of a noncompetitive antagonist (series 1) on the agonist concentration-response curve. Panel B (right) shows the effect of a competitive antagonist (series 2) on the agonist concentration-response curves.

TABLE 14.8 "Silent Antagonism"

Compound	pK$_B$	Agonist Max
ACS686372	6.8	12%
ACS776339	5.4	0%
ACS663992	7.0	0%
ACS556887	7.8	33%
ACS332774	6.1	15%

agonism. Since β-adrenoceptor agonism in cardiac muscle results in elevation of cellular cyclic AMP, and since a common control mechanism for cardiac cells is degradation of cyclic AMP by cardiac phosphodiesterases, one possibility is the concomitant blockade of phosphodiesterase by the β-blocker. This would have the effect of potentiating β-agonism, while the receptor effect of the antagonist would have the effect of reducing agonism; a

net cancellation of effect would result (see Figure 14.24). In the binding assay, phosphodiesterase is not an issue and only the receptor effect is observed. One approach to differentiating and elucidating concomitant effects is to take advantage of kinetics. If the rates of onset of two effects are different, then observation of the onset of the ligand could show each effect as it approaches equilibrium (*vide infra*).

14.4.3 Marking Relevant Agonism

Question: A discovery program seeks antagonists for the chemokine receptor CCR5 for treatment of rheumatoid arthritis. The functional system used to determine functional antagonism is a highly sensitive melanophore assay. The chemokine CCL3L1 is used as the agonist, and the reference antagonists are Met-RANTES and AOP-RANTES, two peptide analogues of natural chemokines known to be silent antagonists in other *in vivo* systems. The team noticed that a substantial agonism (70% and 59% maximal effect) was produced in the assay in

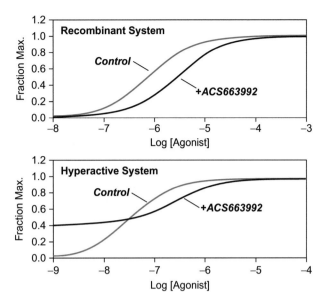

FIGURE 14.23 The effect of variable system sensitivity on very-low-efficacy antagonists. Top panel: ACS663992 produces "silent" competitive antagonism of agonist responses in a system of low sensitivity (EC$_{50}$ of agonist = 1 μM). Bottom panel: This same antagonist, when tested in a system of higher sensitivity (EC$_{50}$ of agonist = 30 nM) now reveals partial agonism.

contrast to the known silent antagonist activity of this peptide in *in vivo* models of rheumatoid arthritis; see Table 14.9. A survey of the best synthetic antagonists in the program yielded a disturbing agonism, leading to fears of inducing damaging inflammation and chemotaxis *in vivo*. From the list of antagonists, which compounds would be most prone to possibly producing inflammatory effects, and which might be taken into *in vivo* models with minimal fear of inducing such effects? Why?

Answer: Since maximal response is the only parameter solely dependent on agonist efficacy, then a calibration between the *in vitro* and *in vivo* systems is a useful approach to predicting *in vivo* response. Therefore, since

TABLE 14.9 Marking Significant Agonism for Prediction *In vivo*

	pEC$_{50}$	Max
AOP-RANTES	8.9	70%
Met-RANTES	8.1	59%
ACS333299	7.4	68%
ACS229493	8.1	45%
ACS999661	7.4	85%
ACS226554	8	33%

it has been established that AOP-RANTES and Met-RANTES do not produce agonism *in vivo*, then it may be assumed that ligands producing maximal responses equal to or less than those agonists in the *in vitro* systems will not produce agonism *in vivo* as well. Thus, no agonism can be expected to be observed *in vivo* with ACS333299, ACS229493, and ACS226554 (max <59%). It is possible that some agonism may be seen with ACS999661 since the maximal response to this agonist was greater than that observed with AOP-RANTES and Met-RANTES.

14.4.4 *In vitro–In vivo* Correspondence of Activity

Question: ACS999881 is part of a series of potent phosphodiesterase (PDE) III inhibitors; it has a pK$_I$ = 8.9. The discovery team felt extremely comfortable with the causal relationship shown in other studies between *in vivo* cardiac contractility and PDE III blockade, and the critical path for this program led straight from *in vitro* enzyme blockade to an *in vivo* model of cardiac failure. The team

FIGURE 14.24 Self-cancellation of effect. The antagonist blocks receptors to cause a shift to the right of the agonist concentration-response curve (blue) but also potentiates agonism to shift curves to the left (red). The result is a curve that closely resembles the control, giving the impression that the antagonist is not active.

was rewarded with ACS999881; the compound was a potent positive inotropic compound *in vivo*. The team progressed this molecule to candidate status and an investigational new drug (IND) report was initiated. For completeness, data from an *in vitro* cardiac contractility preparation were to be included. The team was surprised and chagrined to find that ACS999881 did not show positive inotropic activity in an *in vitro* cardiac preparation. This posed a difficult question for the IND that the Food and Drug Administration (FDA) would surely like an answer to before the compound was approved. What could be the cause of the dissimulation, and what experiment could be done to obviate the problem?

Answer: In the case of enzyme antagonists, a basal stimulation of the system may be required to observe any effect of enzyme inhibition. In this case, the enzyme is phosphodiesterase (PDE), which hydrolyzes elevated levels of cytosolic cyclic AMP. *In vivo*, the heart is under a tonic sympathetic β-adrenoceptor stimulation, but the cardiotonic effect of this stimulation is kept to a subthreshold level by the hydrolysis of the resulting cyclic AMP by PDE. Inhibition of this braking effect through inhibition of PDE allows the cyclic AMP levels in the cell to be elevated with a resulting positive inotropic effect. Without this stimulation of the system, no effect of PDE blockade will be observed. In terms of system stimulation, a PDE inhibitor will potentiate the effects of a β-adrenoceptor agonist. If the *in vitro* assay is placed under a subthreshold level of β-adrenoceptor stimulation, then blockade of PDE will potentiate the subthreshold effect to a visible effect, that is, a curve will appear with PDE blockade (see Figure 14.25). Therefore, the *in vitro* cardiac preparation should be carried out with a subthreshold level of β-adrenoceptor stimulation to better simulate *in vivo* conditions.

14.4.5 Divergent Agonist-Dependent Antagonism

Question: ACS555213 (Figure 14.26) is a potent muscarinic receptor antagonist as demonstrated by a competitive blockade of the agonist carbachol in a variety of functional assays ($pK_B = 9.1$). However, when ACS555213 was tested *in vivo*, the experiment had to be aborted as severe bradycardia (slow heart rate), respiratory distress, and muscle tremor were observed. The antagonist was then tested under more physiological conditions in an *in vitro* system. In these experiments, the natural neurotransmitter acetylcholine was used as the agonist. To the team's surprise, it was observed that ACS555213 was a very weak antagonist of acetylcholine response ($pK_B = 6.8$). The Schild plot for ACS555213 with acetylcholine as the agonist was inordinately steep with a slope of 1.6. Moreover, the temporal kinetics of response showed a complex pattern of blockade of acetylcholine response (initial increase in response beyond control followed by a diminution of response) that was not evident for carbachol (see patterns in Figure 14.26). What could be the mechanism of action of ACS555213?

Answer: There are numerous reasons why antagonists may show differing activity *in vitro* versus *in vivo* (pharmacokinetics often plays a role). However, in this case, a key element is the difference in agonists involved. Specifically, the agonist used *in vitro* is a stable molecule (carbachol), while the agonist involved *in vivo* is the neurotransmitter acetylcholine. Upon noting that the antagonist was ineffective *in vivo*, the appropriate experiment was to return to the *in vitro* setting and test the relevant agonist; namely, acetylcholine. The fact that ACS555213 was equally ineffective *in vitro* when acetylcholine was the agonist strongly suggested that the agonist was the

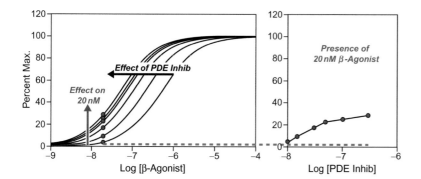

FIGURE 14.25 A phosphodiesterase (PDE) inhibitor produces shifts to the left of the concentration-response curve to a β-adrenoceptor agonist. Red circles represent the observed effect of a low concentration of β-adrenoceptor agonist present in the assay as PDE inhibitor is added. It can be seen that, in the absence of the PDE inhibitor, no effect is seen. However, as the PDE inhibitor produces increasing levels of phosphodiesterase blockade, the effects of the previously subthreshold concentration of agonist become manifest themselves as response. The response observed to the PDE inhibitor, in the presence of a low level of β-adrenoceptor agonist, is shown in the panel on the right. An experimental version of this is shown in Figure 10.14.

FIGURE 14.26 **Muscarinic antagonism with secondary properties.** ACS555213 produces a two-phase effect on acetylcholine response; an initial potentiation is followed by a sustained blockade (panels A and B). In panels C and D, the corresponding effects on carbachol are shown; these data indicate that the complex effect is seen only with acetylcholine and not the surrogate agonist carbachol.

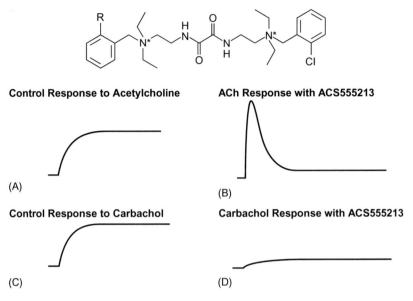

Control Response to Acetylcholine

(A)

ACh Response with ACS555213

(B)

Control Response to Carbachol

(C)

Carbachol Response with ACS555213

(D)

relevant factor. One difference between carbachol and acetylcholine is that the latter molecule is a substrate for the enzyme acetylcholinesterase (ACherase). This enzyme is present in the synaptic cleft and controls the concentration of acetylcholine at the synapse. Specifically, it hydrolyzes acetylcholine to terminate its action in neurons.

The data in total suggest that ACS555213, in addition to being a muscarinic receptor blocker (as shown by its ability to block carbachol responses), is also an inhibitor of ACherase. This latter property would potentiate the action of acetylcholine as it would prevent the natural degradation of the agonist at nerve endings. The concomitant enzyme inhibition (acetylcholine potentiation) and muscarinic receptor blockade would tend to cancel and make ACS555213 a weak antagonist of acetylcholine both *in vivo* and *in vitro* (see similar effect in Figure 14.24). The ACherase activity would be irrelevant for carbachol. There are other observations consistent with this hypothesis. The first is the temporal complex response *in vitro* with acetylcholine. There is no reason to suppose that the rate of onset of ACS555213 for ACherase and the receptor should be equal, and in cases of dual activities, the onset kinetics often can separate the two effects. In this case, the acetylcholine response was actually potentiated beyond the level of control before it was reduced (see Figure 14.26). This suggests that the rate of onset for the enzyme is faster than that for the receptor. As the enzyme is blocked, the concentration of acetylcholine reaching the receptor increases; as the receptor becomes blocked, the response declines. Also, the effects of ACherase tend to be more pronounced on lower concentrations of acetylcholine. The fact that the Schild regression with acetylcholine as the agonist has a slope greater than unity suggests that, as the receptor blockade caused the concentration-response curve to be shifted to higher

concentrations where ACherase ceases to become a factor, the receptor blockade becomes more important (causing an increased slope of the Schild regression). Finally, the symptoms observed *in vivo* (bradycardia, muscle tremor, respiratory distress) are classic signs of ACherase poisoning. This example is based on actual data with the dual muscarinic antagonist/ACherase inhibitor ambenonium (structure of ACS555213 with R = Cl). The dual effects of ACherase inhibition and receptor blockade can be differentiated with kinetics for ambenonium [2]. In a tissue where ACherase reduces receptor compartment concentrations of acetylcholine, ACherase blockade by drugs such as neostigmine produces potentiation of responses to acetylcholine (Figure 14.27A). Under these conditions, ambenonium can be shown to produce potentiation of effect followed by receptor blockade (inhibition of response) with low levels of receptor stimulation (1 μM and 10 μM acetylcholine); the differential kinetics allow separation of these two effects (Figure 14.27B and C).

14.5 SAR EXERCISES

14.5.1 Surrogate Screens

Question: A therapeutically advantageous approach to potentiating failing responses, such as those of neurons in Alzheimer's disease, is to allosterically potentiate the neural response. This has the advantage of preserving the complex patterns of stimulation found in the brain. In a high-throughput screen for cholinergic receptor potentiating agents, a surrogate cholinergic receptor agonist; namely, arecoline, was used. It is a stable analogue of the natural neurotransmitter, acetylcholine, and much better suited to the requirements of a screening process. The

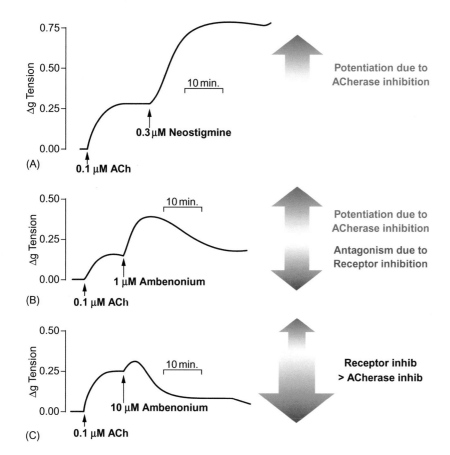

FIGURE 14.27 **Complex effects of ambenonium revealed through differential kinetics of onset.** (A) The response to 1 μM acetylcholine is potentiated by blockade of acetylcholinesterase with neostigmine. (B) The effect to the same concentration of acetylcholine is initially potentiated but then blocked by ambenonium at 1 μM. (C) The potentiation is less and blockade more pronounced at higher concentrations of ambenonium (10 μM). Ambenonium is a known dual inhibitor of muscarinic receptors and acetylcholinesterase. Data redrawn from [2].

compound ACS555667 was found to potentiate arecoline by a factor of 15 and thus was considered to be a viable lead for the program. Secondary testing with a variety of arecoline response systems and binding assays confirmed the initial activity, and it was clear that ACS555667 was a powerful potentiator of arecoline response and binding. However, testing in electrophysiological studies with intact neuron systems was disappointing to say the least. In fact, ACS555667 appeared to block acetylcholine neuronal function in natural systems. What could the problem have been, and what could early experiments have done to determine this?

Answer: This is a classic example of allosteric probe dependence and is, in fact, based on actual data. Specifically, ACS555667 is a close analogue of the allosteric muscarinic receptor modulator eburnamonine (But = Et for eburnamonine). This modulator is known to potentiate arecoline by a factor of 15 but to actually block the effects of acetylcholine by a factor of 3 [3]. In general, if the scaffolds of interest are allosteric, then the primary activity must be confirmed with the physiologically relevant agonist. A functional assay with acetylcholine as the agonist should have been inserted into the critical path before the animal model was tested (Figure 14.28).

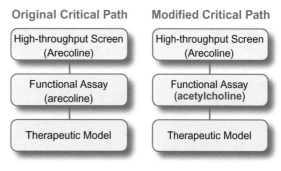

FIGURE 14.28 **Surrogate testing for potentiation of cholinergic receptor function.** The original critical path uses arecoline as the agonist and would confirm the original screening activity. The modified critical path uses acetylcholine to confirm the potentiating activity to confirm that the potentiation will extend to the physiologically relevant agonist, acetylcholine. The fact that allosteric effect (potentiation) can be probe dependent opens the possibility that a molecule that potentiates arecoline will not produce concomitant potentiation of acetylcholine and thus will be therapeutically inactive.

14.6 PHARMACOKINETICS

14.6.1 Clearance

Question: *In vitro* studies in hepatocytes can be used to predict *in vivo* clearance. In this case, prazosin was incubated with human hepatocytes for varying periods of time

FIGURE 14.29 **Disappearance of prazosin upon incubation in a hepatocyte preparation.** A time-dependent degradation of prazosin is observed (66% degraded over 6 hours), which resembles a first-order degradation.

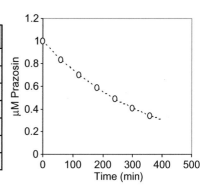

Human Hepatocytes : Prazosin Clearance

For low concentration of prazosin (<<Km of hepatocyte system)

t (min)	μM	Ln(μM)
0	1.000	0
60	0.835	−0.18
120	0.698	−0.36
180	0.583	−0.54
240	0.487	−0.72
300	0.407	−0.9
360	0.340	−1.08

(see Figure 14.29) and samples withdrawn to measure remaining drug in solution. From these data and the following information, estimate the *in vivo* clearance in humans for prazosin (assuming clearance for this drug is mainly hepatic).

Additional information:

- Hepatocellularity $= 120 \times 10^6$ cell/g.
- Liver weight $= 21$ g/kg body weight.
- $Q_H =$ liver blood flow $= 20$ mL/min/kg body weight.
- Assume no protein binding ($f_u = 1$).

Answer: The first step is to determine the half life of prazosin. The first-order curve shown in Figure 14.29 is replotted with natural logarithmic ordinates to produce a straight line; see Figure 14.30. Then the intrinsic clearance for this hepatocyte preparation is calculated from:

$$\text{Intrinsic clearance} = CL_{int} = \frac{\ln2 \times (100\mu L/mL)}{t_{1/2} \times (\text{cell} \times 10^6/mL)}.$$
$$= 3.0 ml/min/10^6 cells$$
(14.5)

This calculation is then carried out for the whole liver:

$$CL_{int(\text{whole liver})} = CL_{int} \times \text{hepatocellularity} \times \text{liver weight},$$
(14.6)

where hepatocellularity $= 120 \times 10^6$ cell/g and liver weight is 21 g/kg body weight. $CL_{int(\text{whole liver})} = 3$ mL/min/10^6 cells $\times 10^6$ cell/g $\times 21$ g/kg $= 7.56$ mL/kg/min.

At this point, the standard equation for hepatic clearance (see Equations 9.9 and 9.12) is used to convert CL_{int} to *in vivo* human clearance ($CL_{H(calc)}$):

$$CL_{H(calc)} = \frac{Q_H \times f_u \times CL_{int(\text{whole liver})}}{Q_H \times f_u \times CL_{int(\text{whole liver})}},$$
(14.7)

where Q_H is liver blood flow (20 mL/min/kg body weight) and f_u is the fraction of drug not bound by protein (assumed in this case to be 1). This leads to the calculation for *in vivo* hepatic clearance of:

$$CL_{H(calc)} = \frac{(20 \text{ mL/kg/min}) \times (7.56 \text{ mL/min/kg})}{(20 \text{ mL/kg/min}) + (7.56 \text{ mL/min/kg})}.$$
$$= 5.49 \text{ ml/min/kg}$$
(14.8)

FIGURE 14.30 Data in Figure 14.29 plotted as a semi-logarithmic plot produces a linear relationship between ln (remaining concentrations of prazosin) and time. The linear relationship yields a $t_{1/2}$ of 231 min.

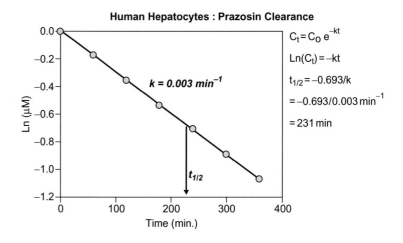

Human Hepatocytes : Prazosin Clearance

$k = 0.003$ min^{-1}

$t_{1/2}$

$C_t = C_0 e^{-kt}$

$Ln(C_t) = -kt$

$t_{1/2} = -0.693/k$

$= -0.693/0.003$ min^{-1}

$= 231$ min

14.6.2 Drug-Drug Interactions

Question: Diazepam has low but significant hepatic clearance; the concentration-time relationships for i.v. and oral dosing are shown in Figure 14.31A. How would these curves change after the patient receives cimetidine, a known CYP450 inhibitor?

Answer: The half time for elimination would increase due to decreased hepatic elimination; this effect would be seen both for i.v. and oral dosing. The latter condition might also show an increased maximal concentration (C_{max}) due to reduced first pass effect (reduced metabolism upon oral absorption and passage through the liver); see Figure 14.31B.

14.6.3 Distribution I

Question: 80 mg of drug D is administered to an 80 kg man and the immediate concentration is found to be 5 mg/L. From the apparent volume of distribution, would you conclude that drug D is:

- Highly bound to plasma proteins?
- Distributed in total body water?
- Confined to the extracellular fluid?
- Confined to the plasma?

Answer: The volume of distribution is V = 80 mg/ 5 mg/L = 16 L, which, referring to Table 14.10, is 20% of an 80 kg man. Therefore, the drug is confined to the extracellular space.

14.6.4 Distribution II

Question: Drug E is given to a 70 kg man and confined to plasma; the concentration at time zero is 50 mg/kg. What was the initial dose of drug?

Answer: Referring to Table 14.10, the plasma volume is 3 L. Therefore, the initial dose of drug was 50 mg/ L × 3 L = 150 mg.

14.6.5 Half Life I

Question: Drug A achieves a concentration of 3 mg/L plasma concentration with a single dose of 30 mg (see Figure 14.32). What dose of drug A, and how often during a 24-hour period, should drug A be given to achieve a steady state level of 6 mg/L (C_{ss})?

Answer: From Figure 14.32 it can be seen that the $t_{1/2}$ for drug A is approximately 8 hours. If drug A is given at a dose of 20 mg every $t_{1/2}$ (8 hours), a steady state

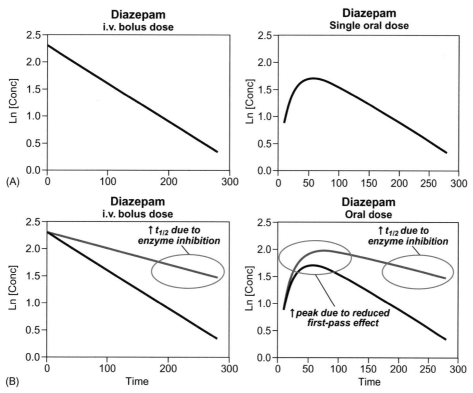

FIGURE 14.31 Effects of a CYP450 inhibitor (cimetidine) on plasma levels of diazepam given by the intravenous route (left panels) and oral route (right panels). Blockade of metabolism prolongs elimination (increased $t_{1/2}$) and, in the case of oral administration, blocks first pass metabolism to allow more diazepam to be absorbed and enter the circulation (increased peak concentration and $t_{1/2}$).

TABLE 14.10 Volumes of Specific Compartments in the Body

Compartment	Volume L/kg	Liter in 70 kg Male	% Total Body Weight
Plasma Water	0.045	3	4.5
Extracellular Water	0.2	14	20
Intracellular Water	0.42	28	41
Total Body Water	0.6	42	60

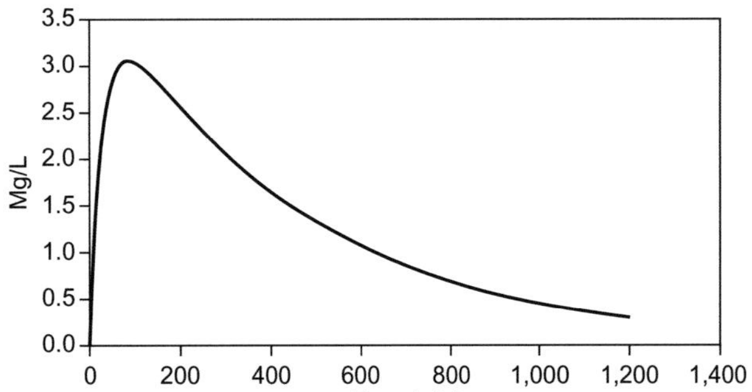

FIGURE 14.32 Drug A is given by the oral route to give a peak concentration of 3 mg/L^{-1} and demonstrates the kinetics shown in the figure.

concentration of 2×3 mg/L = 6 mg/L will be achieved by the end of 4 to 5 half times. Therefore, 20 mg given three times a day will achieve a C_{ss} of 6 mg/L.

14.6.6 Half Life II

Question: A dose of 300 mg of drug C is given i.v., and after 1 hour, 150 mg remains. How long after the initial injection will there be only 37 mg remaining in the body?

Answer: The half life of drug C is 1 hour (300 mg to 150 mg in 1 hour). After another half life, there will be 75 mg, and after another half life there will be 37.5 mg. Therefore, 3 half times = 3 hours after the injection, there will be 37 mg remaining.

14.6.7 Half Life III

Question: Drug B is injected intravenously and achieves an instantaneous concentration of 100 mg/L. Previously it had been noted that the rate of clearance was the same for a range of concentrations. After 5 min, the concentration is 10 mg/L. At what time will the drug be 99% eliminated from the body?

Answer: The fact that the rate of elimination is independent of concentration indicates that the drug is eliminated by a first-order process characterized by the relation $C_t = C_0 \ e^{-kt}$, where C_t and C_0 refer to

concentrations at time t and zero, respectively, and k is the rate constant for first-order elimination. The logarithmic metameter of this equation is:

$$\text{Log } C_t = \text{Log } C_0 - kt/2.303. \qquad (14.9)$$

Substituting 100 mg/L for C_0 (Log $C_0 = 2$) and 10 mg/L at 5 min for C_t (Log $C_t = 1$) yields a rate constant for elimination of $(2-1) \times 2.303/5$ min = 0.46 min^{-1}. Therefore, substituting $C_t = 1$ (1% of 100 mg/L; Log $C_t = 0$) into Equation 14.9 yields a time of 10 min. Therefore, after 10 min, there will be 1% of the drug remaining (99% elimination).

14.6.8 Renal Clearance I

Question: Trevor, a graduate student earning money in a clinical trial, checked into the clinic every afternoon to give urine samples for clearance measurements of drug G, known to be cleared primarily by the kidney. One day he changed this routine to an early morning visit. The data are shown in Table 14.11. What could be the cause of the aberrant reading?

Answer: Trevor liked to start his mornings with a stop at the local coffee bar to have a double shot of espresso coffee. The amount of caffeine present in the coffee was sufficient to increase Trevor's urine volume, thereby increasing his renal clearance through the relation $CL_r = (C_u \times U)/C_p$, where C_u and C_p are concentration of drug in the urine and plasma, respectively, and U is the volume of urine. By the afternoon (normal time for sampling), the effects of the caffeine waned and urine volume was back to normal.

14.6.9 Renal Clearance II

Question: Drug H has a clearance rate of 400 mL/min in people with normal renal function. What can be determined about the renal excretion mechanism (note that GFR is 125 mL/min)?

Answer: Since this clearance is considerably higher than glomerular filtration, it is clear that drug H is actively secreted by the renal tubules.

TABLE 14.11 Indirect Measures of Urine Flow in a Clinical Trial

Time of Day	mL/min
PM	20
PM	21
PM	18.5
AM	38
PM	19.5
PM	20.6

14.6.10 Renal Clearance III

Question: Drug I, which is 50% protein bound, has a clearance rate of 65 mL/min in people with normal renal function. What can be determined about the renal excretion mechanism (note that GFR is 125 mL/min)?

Answer: Protein binding prevents filtration, thus the rate of clearance is 1/2 GFR. Were the drug not protein bound, the clearance would be nearly exactly GFR; therefore, the drug is filtered and not significantly secreted or reabsorbed or the drug is secreted and reabsorbed to an equal extent.

14.6.11 Absorption

Question: For rapid absorption following oral administration, a drug should be given:

(a) Just after a meal, because concurrent absorption of nutrients maximizes drug absorption.
(b) Between meals, as the stomach empties more rapidly when filled with food.
(c) Between meals, because there will be no delayed emptying due to food.
(d) With meals, because gastric emptying will be delayed by food.

Answer: (a) This will have little effect. (b) This is incorrect, since the stomach empties more slowly when filled with food. (d) Incorrect, since the drug is mainly absorbed in the intestine, not the stomach; therefore, the faster it reaches the site of absorption, the sooner it will be absorbed. The correct answer is (c).

14.6.12 Predictive Pharmacokinetics I

Question: Drug A has a volume of distribution of 500 L; 10% is excreted unchanged with a total clearance of 80 L/hour. Liver blood flow is normal (90 L/hour). What is the relative renal and hepatic clearance of drug A, the hepatic extraction ratio, and the predicted maximum oral bioavailability?

Answer: The fraction of drug A excreted by the kidney (f_e) = renal clearance/total clearance. Since 10% of the drug is excreted unchanged $(f_e = 0.1)$, it can be assumed that renal clearance = 0.1×80 L/hour = 8 L/hour. Assuming that $Cl_{total} = Cl_{renal} + Cl_{hepatic}$, the hepatic clearance is 80 L/hour − 8 L/hour = 72 L/hour. The hepatic extraction ratio is given by the hepatic clearance divided by the hepatic blood flow, which, in this case, is E_H = 72 L/hour/90 L/hour = 0.8. The maximal predicted oral bioavailability (F) is given by the product of the fractional hepatic clearance (f_H), which is 1 minus the hepatic extraction ratio E_H $(1 − 0.8 = 0.2)$ and the fractional oral absorption (f_o), assumed in this case to be unity (maximal case). Therefore, $F = 0.2 \times 1 = 0.2$.

14.6.13 Predictive Pharmacokinetics II

Question: Drug B has a total clearance of 3 L/hour and a volume of distribution of 25 L; 10% is excreted unchanged. Assuming liver blood flow is normal (90 L/hour), what is this drug's half life, what is its likely dosing schedule per day, and how long will it take to get this drug's level to a steady state?

Answer: The half life can be obtained from the equation $t_{1/2} = 0.693 \times V/Cl$ (see Equation 9.19), which, in this case, is $t_{1/2} = 0.693 \times 25$ L/hour/3 L/hour = 5.78 hours (approximately 6 hours). This drug needs to be given approximately every half time, which, in this case, would be 24 hours/6 hours = 4 times a day. A steady state will be achieved after approximately 5 half times, which, in this case, is 5×6 hours = 30 hours.

14.6.14 Predictive Pharmacokinetics III

Question: Drug C has a total clearance of 7 L/hour, a volume of distribution of 420 L, and a rate of excretion unchanged of 80%. Will drug levels of this drug be affected by induction and/or inhibition of liver metabolism, compromised liver blood flow due to cardiovascular disease, or the presence of liver disease? Would renal disease affect levels of drug C?

Answer: Since 80% of this drug is excreted unchanged, its major route of excretion is the kidney. Therefore, changes in liver function (enzyme function through induction or inhibition), liver blood flow through cardiovascular output would not be expected to change the excretion of drug C substantially. However, renal disease would have serious effects on the clearance of drug C.

14.6.15 Log D and Pharmacokinetics

Question: The primary activity SAR for a series of molecules is leading to progressively increasing lipophilicity. What may be the pharmacokinetic consequences of this trend? (Evaluate all answers.)

(a)　Increased absorption.
(b)　Increased volume of distribution.
(c)　Decreased $t_{1/2}$.
(d)　Increased renal excretion.

Answer:

(a)　Yes: Usually, increased lipophilicity will increase the ability of a molecule to traverse lipid membranes.

(b)　Yes: There could be increased tissue binding and sequestration into compartments, thereby reducing the central compartment concentration and increasing volume of distribution.

(c)　No: The drug most likely will be more readily reabsorbed in the distal tubule, and thus renal excretion may be reduced.

(d)　No: The increased volume of distribution will lead to a decreased clearance. The drug will not be as available to clearance mechanisms, and the $t_{1/2}$ will be longer.

14.7 CONCLUSIONS

This chapter is designed to give readers some experience in applying the methods and theories of pharmacodynamics and pharmacokinetics within the context of practical problems encountered in the evaluation of multiple compounds in discovery and development programs. A recurrent theme in the pharmacodynamic problems is the influence of different assay systems on the data and how, if an assay-independent measure of activity could be found, this can alleviate this problem. The pharmacokinetic questions illustrate how simple formulae relating clearance, volume of distribution, and $t_{1/2}$ enable most if not all conclusions to be made about the pharmacokinetics of the drugs involved.

REFERENCES

[1] Cheng YC, Prusoff WH. Relationship between the inhibition constant (K_i) and the concentration of inhibitor which causes 50 percent inhibition (I_{50}) of an enzymatic reaction. Biochem Pharmacol 1973;22:3099−108.

[2] Kenakin TP, Beek D. Self-cancellation of drug properties as a mode of organ selectivity: the antimuscarinic effects of ambenonium. J Pharmacol Exp Ther 1985;232:732−40.

[3] Jakubic J, Bacakova L, Lisa V, El-Fakahany EE, Tucek S. Positive cooperativity of acetylcholine and other agonists with allosteric ligands on muscarinic acetylcholine receptors. Mol Pharmacol 1997;52:172−9.

Appendices

A.1 STATISTICAL TABLES OF USE FOR ASSESSING SIGNIFICANT DIFFERENCE

1. t-distribution
2. F-distribution ($p < 0.05$)
3. F-distribution ($p < 0.025$)
4. F-distribution ($p < 0.01$)

A.1.1 t-Distribution

To determine the 0.05 critical value from t-distribution with 5 degrees of freedom, look in the 0.05 column at the fifth row: $t_{(.05,5)} = 2.015048$.

TABLE A.1.1 t-Table with Right-Tail Probabilities

df/p	0.40	0.25	0.10	0.05	0.025	0.01	0.005	0.0005
1	0.324920	1.000000	3.077684	6.313752	12.70620	31.82052	63.65674	636.6192
2	0.288675	0.816497	1.885618	2.919986	4.30265	6.96456	9.92484	31.5991
3	0.276671	0.764892	1.637744	2.353363	3.18245	4.54070	5.84091	12.9240
4	0.270722	0.740697	1.533206	2.131847	2.77645	3.74695	4.60409	8.6103
5	0.267181	0.726687	1.475884	2.015048	2.57058	3.36493	4.03214	6.8688
6	0.264835	0.717558	1.439756	1.943180	2.44691	3.14267	3.70743	5.9588
7	0.263167	0.711142	1.41924	1.894579	2.36462	2.99795	3.49948	5.4079
8	0.261921	0.706387	1.396815	1.859548	2.30600	2.89646	3.35539	5.0413
9	0.260955	0.702722	1.383029	1.833113	2.26216	2.82144	3.24984	4.7809
10	0.260185	0.699812	1.372184	1.812461	2.22814	2.76377	3.16927	4.5869
11	0.259556	0.697445	1.363430	1.795885	2.20099	2.71808	3.10581	4.4370
12	0.259033	0.695483	1.356217	1.782288	2.17881	2.68100	3.05454	4.3178
13	0.258591	0.693829	1.350171	1.770933	2.16037	2.65031	3.01228	4.2208
14	0.258213	0.692417	1.345030	1.761310	2.14479	2.62449	2.97684	4.1405
15	0.257885	0.691197	1.340606	1.753050	2.13145	2.60248	2.94671	4.0728
16	0.257599	0.690132	1.336757	1.745884	2.11991	2.58349	2.92078	4.0150
17	0.257347	0.689195	1.333379	1.739607	2.10982	2.56693	2.89823	3.9651
18	0.257123	0.688364	1.330391	1.734064	2.10092	2.55238	2.87844	3.9216
19	0.256923	0.687621	1.327728	1.729133	2.09302	2.53948	2.86093	3.8834
20	0.256743	0.686954	1.325341	1.724718	2.08596	2.52798	2.84534	3.8495
21	0.256580	0.686352	1.323188	1.720743	2.07961	2.51765	2.83136	3.8193
22	0.256432	0.685805	1.321237	1.717144	2.07387	2.50832	2.81876	3.7921
23	0.256297	0.685306	1.319460	1.713872	2.06866	2.49987	2.80734	3.7676

(Continued)

TABLE A.1.1 (Continued)

df/p	0.40	0.25	0.10	0.05	0.025	0.01	0.005	0.0005
24	0.256173	0.684850	1.371836	1.710882	2.06390	2.49216	2.79694	3.7454
25	0.256060	0.684430	1.316345	1.708141	2.05954	2.48511	2.78744	3.7251
26	0.255955	0.684043	1.314972	1.705618	2.05553	2.47863	2.77871	3.7066
27	0.255858	0.683685	1.313703	1.703288	2.05183	2.47266	2.77068	3.6896
28	0.255768	0.683353	1.312527	1.701131	2.04841	2.46714	2.76326	3.6739
29	0.255684	0.683044	1.311434	1.699127	2.04523	2.46202	2.75639	3.6594
30	0.255605	0.682756	1.310415	1.697261	2.04227	2.45726	2.75000	3.6460
inf	0.253347	0.674490	1.281552	1.644854	1.95996	2.32635	2.57583	3.2905

A.1.2 F-Distribution

By convention, the numerator degrees of freedom are always given first (switching the order of degrees of freedom changes the distribution, that is, $F_{(10,12)}$ does not equal $F_{(12,10)}$). For the following F-tables, *rows represent denominator degrees of freedom and columns represent numerator degrees of freedom.*

TABLE A.1.2 F-Table for $\alpha = 0.05$

df2/df1	1	2	3	4	5	6	7	8	9	10	12	15	20	24	30	40	60	120	INF
1	161.4476	199.5000	215.7073	224.5832	230.1619	233.9860	236.7684	238.8827	240.5433	241.8817	243.9060	245.9499	248.0131	249.0518	250.0951	251.1432	252.1957	253.2529	254.3144
2	18.5128	19.0000	19.1643	19.2468	19.2964	19.3295	19.3532	19.3710	19.3848	19.3959	19.4125	19.4291	19.4458	19.4541	19.4624	19.4707	19.4791	19.4874	19.4957
3	10.1280	9.5521	9.2766	9.1172	9.0135	8.9406	8.8867	8.8452	8.8123	8.7855	8.7446	8.7029	8.6602	8.6385	8.6166	8.5944	8.5720	8.5494	8.5264
4	7.7086	6.9443	6.5914	6.3882	6.2561	6.1631	6.0942	6.0410	5.9988	5.9644	5.9117	5.8578	5.8025	5.7744	5.7459	5.7170	5.6877	5.6581	5.6281
5	6.6079	5.7861	5.4095	5.1922	5.0503	4.9503	4.8759	4.8183	4.7725	4.7351	4.6777	4.6188	4.5581	4.5272	4.4957	4.4638	4.4314	4.3985	4.3650
6	5.9874	5.1433	4.7571	4.5337	4.3874	4.2839	4.2067	4.1468	4.0990	4.0600	3.9999	3.9381	3.8742	3.8415	3.8082	3.7743	3.7398	3.7047	3.6689
7	5.5914	4.7374	4.3468	4.1203	3.9715	3.8660	3.7870	3.7257	3.6767	3.6365	3.5747	3.5107	3.4445	3.4105	3.3758	3.3404	3.3043	3.2674	3.2298
8	5.3177	4.4590	4.0662	3.8379	3.6875	3.5806	3.5005	3.4381	3.3881	3.3472	3.2839	3.2184	3.1503	3.1152	3.0794	3.0428	3.0053	2.9669	2.9276
9	5.1174	4.2565	3.8625	3.6331	3.4817	3.3738	3.2927	3.2296	3.1789	3.1373	3.0729	3.0061	2.9365	2.9005	2.8637	2.8259	2.7872	2.7475	2.7067
10	4.9646	4.1028	3.7083	3.4780	3.3258	3.2172	3.1355	3.0717	3.0204	2.9782	2.9130	2.8450	2.7740	2.7372	2.6996	2.6609	2.6211	2.5801	2.5379
11	4.8443	3.9823	3.5874	3.3567	3.2039	3.0946	3.0123	2.9480	2.8962	2.8536	2.7876	2.7186	2.6464	2.6090	2.5705	2.5309	2.4901	2.4480	2.4045
12	4.7472	3.8853	3.4903	3.2592	3.1059	2.9961	2.9134	2.8486	2.7964	2.7534	2.6866	2.6169	2.5436	2.5055	2.4663	2.4259	2.3842	2.3410	2.2962
13	4.6672	3.8056	3.4105	3.1791	3.0254	2.9153	2.8321	2.7669	2.7144	2.6710	2.6037	2.5331	2.4589	2.4202	2.3803	2.3392	2.2966	2.2524	2.2064
14	4.6001	3.7389	3.3439	3.1122	2.9582	2.8477	2.7642	2.6987	2.6458	2.6022	2.5342	2.4630	2.3879	2.3487	2.3082	2.2664	2.2229	2.1778	2.1307
15	4.5431	3.6823	3.2874	3.0556	2.9013	2.7905	2.7066	2.6408	2.5876	2.5437	2.4753	2.4034	2.3275	2.2878	2.2468	2.2043	2.1601	2.1141	2.0658
16	4.4940	3.6337	3.2389	3.0069	2.8524	2.7413	2.6572	2.5911	2.5377	2.4935	2.4247	2.3522	2.2756	2.2354	2.1938	2.1507	2.1058	2.0589	2.0096
17	4.4513	3.5915	3.1968	2.9647	2.8100	2.6987	2.6143	2.5480	2.4943	2.4499	2.3807	2.3077	2.2304	2.1898	2.1477	2.1040	2.0584	2.0107	1.9604
18	4.4139	3.5546	3.1599	2.9277	2.7729	2.6613	2.5767	2.5102	2.4563	2.4117	2.3421	2.2686	2.1906	2.1497	2.1071	2.0629	2.0166	1.9681	1.9168
19	4.3807	3.5219	3.1274	2.8951	2.7401	2.6283	2.5435	2.4768	2.4227	2.3779	2.3080	2.2341	2.1555	2.1141	2.0712	2.0264	1.9795	1.9302	1.8780
20	4.3512	3.4928	3.0984	2.8661	2.7109	2.5990	2.5140	2.4471	2.3928	2.3479	2.2776	2.2033	2.1242	2.0825	2.0391	1.9938	1.9464	1.8963	1.8432
21	4.3248	3.4668	3.0725	2.8401	2.6848	2.5727	2.4876	2.4205	2.3660	2.3210	2.2504	2.1757	2.0960	2.0540	2.0102	1.9645	1.9165	1.8657	1.8117
22	4.3009	3.4434	3.0491	2.8167	2.6613	2.5491	2.4638	2.3965	2.3419	2.2967	2.2258	2.1508	2.0707	2.0283	1.9842	1.9380	1.8894	1.8380	1.7831
23	4.2793	3.4221	3.0280	2.7955	2.6400	2.5277	2.4422	2.3748	2.3201	2.2747	2.2036	2.1282	2.0476	2.0050	1.9605	1.9139	1.8648	1.8128	1.7570
24	4.2597	3.4028	3.0088	2.7763	2.6207	2.5082	2.4226	2.3551	2.3002	2.2547	2.1834	2.1077	2.0267	1.9838	1.9390	1.8920	1.8424	1.7896	1.7330
25	4.2417	3.3852	2.9912	2.7587	2.6030	2.4904	2.4047	2.3371	2.2821	2.2365	2.1649	2.0889	2.0075	1.9643	1.9192	1.8718	1.8217	1.7684	1.7110

(Continued)

TABLE A.1.2 (Continued)

df2/df1	1	2	3	4	5	6	7	8	9	10	12	15	20	24	30	40	60	120	INF
26	4.2252	3.3690	2.9752	2.7426	2.5868	2.4741	2.3883	2.3205	2.2655	2.2197	2.1479	2.0716	1.9898	1.9464	1.9010	1.8533	1.8027	1.7488	1.6906
27	4.2100	3.3541	2.9604	2.7278	2.5719	2.4591	2.3732	2.3053	2.2501	2.2043	2.1323	2.0558	1.9736	1.9299	1.8842	1.8361	1.7851	1.7306	1.6717
28	4.1960	3.3404	2.9467	2.7141	2.5581	2.4453	2.3593	2.2913	2.2360	2.1900	2.1179	2.0411	1.9586	1.9147	1.8687	1.8203	1.7689	1.7138	1.6541
29	4.1830	3.3277	2.9340	2.7014	2.5454	2.4324	2.3463	2.2783	2.2229	2.1768	2.1045	2.0275	1.9446	1.9005	1.8543	1.8055	1.7537	1.6981	1.6376
30	4.1709	3.3158	2.9223	2.6896	2.5336	2.4205	2.3343	2.2662	2.2107	2.1646	2.0921	2.0148	1.9317	1.8874	1.8409	1.7918	1.7396	1.6835	1.6223
40	4.0847	3.2317	2.8387	2.6060	2.4495	2.3359	2.2490	2.1802	2.1240	2.0772	2.0035	1.9245	1.8389	1.7929	1.7444	1.6928	1.6373	1.5766	1.5089
60	4.0012	3.1504	2.7581	2.5252	2.3683	2.2541	2.1665	2.0970	2.0401	1.9926	1.9174	1.8364	1.7480	1.7001	1.6491	1.5943	1.5343	1.4673	1.3893
120	3.9201	3.0718	2.6802	2.4472	2.2899	2.1750	2.0868	2.0164	1.9588	1.9105	1.8337	1.7505	1.6587	1.6084	1.5543	1.4952	1.4290	1.3519	1.2539
inf	3.8415	2.9957	2.6049	2.3719	2.2141	2.0986	2.0096	1.9384	1.8799	1.8307	1.7522								

TABLE A.1.3 Table for $\alpha = 0.025$

df2/df1	1	2	3	4	5	6	7	8	9	10	12	15	20	24	30	40	60	120	INF
1	647.7890	799.5000	864.1630	899.5833	921.8479	937.1111	948.2169	956.6562	963.2846	968.6274	976.7079	984.8668	993.1028	997.2492	1001.414	1005.598	1009.800	1014.020	1018.258
2	38.5063	39.0000	39.1655	39.2484	39.2982	39.3315	39.3552	39.3730	39.3869	39.3980	39.4146	39.4313	39.4479	39.4562	39.465	39.473	39.481	39.490	39.498
3	17.4434	16.0441	15.4392	15.1010	14.8848	14.7347	14.6244	14.5399	14.4731	14.4189	14.3366	14.2527	14.1674	14.1241	14.081	14.037	13.992	13.947	13.902
4	12.2179	10.6491	9.9792	9.6045	9.3645	9.1973	9.0741	8.9796	8.9047	8.8439	8.7512	8.6565	8.5599	8.5109	8.461	8.411	8.360	8.309	8.257
5	10.0070	8.4336	7.7636	7.3879	7.1464	6.9777	6.8531	6.7572	6.6811	6.6192	6.5245	6.4277	6.3286	6.2780	6.227	6.175	6.123	6.069	6.015
6	8.8131	7.2599	6.5988	6.2272	5.9876	5.8198	5.6955	5.5996	5.5234	5.4613	5.3662	5.2687	5.1684	5.1172	5.065	5.012	4.959	4.904	4.849
7	8.0727	6.5415	5.8898	5.5226	5.2852	5.1186	4.9949	4.8993	4.8232	4.7611	4.6658	4.5678	4.4667	4.4150	4.362	4.309	4.254	4.199	4.142
8	7.5709	6.0595	5.4160	5.0526	4.8173	4.6517	4.5286	4.4333	4.3572	4.2951	4.1997	4.1012	3.9995	3.9472	3.894	3.840	3.784	3.728	3.670
9	7.2093	5.7147	5.0781	4.7181	4.4844	4.3197	4.1970	4.1020	4.0260	3.9639	3.8682	3.7694	3.6669	3.6142	3.560	3.505	3.449	3.392	3.333
10	6.9367	5.4564	4.8256	4.4683	4.2361	4.0721	3.9498	3.8549	3.7790	3.7168	3.6209	3.5217	3.4185	3.3654	3.311	3.255	3.198	3.140	3.080
11	6.7241	5.2559	4.6300	4.2751	4.0440	3.8807	3.7586	3.6638	3.5879	3.5257	3.4296	3.3299	3.2261	3.1725	3.118	3.061	3.004	2.944	2.883
12	6.5538	5.0959	4.4742	4.1212	3.8911	3.7283	3.6065	3.5118	3.4358	3.3736	3.2773	3.1772	3.0728	3.0187	2.963	2.906	2.848	2.787	2.725
13	6.4143	4.9653	4.3472	3.9959	3.7667	3.6043	3.4827	3.3880	3.3120	3.2497	3.1532	3.0527	2.9477	2.8932	2.837	2.780	2.720	2.659	2.595
14	6.2979	4.8567	4.2417	3.8919	3.6634	3.5014	3.3799	3.2853	3.2093	3.1469	3.0502	2.9493	2.8437	2.7888	2.732	2.674	2.614	2.552	2.487
15	6.1995	4.7650	4.1528	3.8043	3.5764	3.4147	3.2934	3.1987	3.1227	3.0602	2.9633	2.8621	2.7559	2.7006	2.644	2.585	2.524	2.461	2.395
16	6.1151	4.6867	4.0768	3.7294	3.5021	3.3406	3.2194	3.1248	3.0488	2.9862	2.8890	2.7875	2.6808	2.6252	2.568	2.509	2.447	2.383	2.316
17	6.0420	4.6189	4.0112	3.6648	3.4379	3.2767	3.1556	3.0610	2.9849	2.9222	2.8249	2.7230	2.6158	2.5598	2.502	2.442	2.380	2.315	2.247
18	5.9781	4.5597	3.9539	3.6083	3.3820	3.2209	3.0999	3.0053	2.9291	2.8664	2.7689	2.6667	2.5590	2.5027	2.445	2.384	2.321	2.256	2.187
19	5.9216	4.5075	3.9034	3.5587	3.3327	3.1718	3.0509	2.9563	2.8801	2.8172	2.7196	2.6171	2.5089	2.4523	2.394	2.333	2.270	2.203	2.133
20	5.8715	4.4613	3.8587	3.5147	3.2891	3.1283	3.0074	2.9128	2.8365	2.7737	2.6758	2.5731	2.4645	2.4076	2.349	2.287	2.223	2.156	2.085
21	5.8266	4.4199	3.8188	3.4754	3.2501	3.0895	2.9686	2.8740	2.7977	2.7348	2.6368	2.5338	2.4247	2.3675	2.308	2.246	2.182	2.114	2.042
22	5.7863	4.3828	3.7829	3.4401	3.2151	3.0546	2.9338	2.8392	2.7628	2.6998	2.6017	2.4984	2.3890	2.3315	2.272	2.210	2.145	2.076	2.003

(Continued)

TABLE A.1.3 (Continued)

df2 / df1	1	2	3	4	5	6	7	8	9	10	12	15	20	24	30	40	60	120	INF
23	5.7498	4.3492	3.7505	3.4083	3.1835	3.0232	2.9023	2.8077	2.7313	2.6682	2.5699	2.4665	2.3567	2.2989	2.239	2.176	2.111	2.041	1.968
24	5.7166	4.3187	3.7211	3.3794	3.1548	2.9946	2.8738	2.7791	2.7027	2.6396	2.5411	2.4374	2.3273	2.2693	2.209	2.146	2.080	2.010	1.935
25	5.6864	4.2909	3.6943	3.3530	3.1287	2.9685	2.8478	2.7531	2.6766	2.6135	2.5149	2.4110	2.3005	2.2422	2.182	2.118	2.052	1.981	1.906
26	5.6586	4.2655	3.6697	3.3289	3.1048	2.9447	2.8240	2.7293	2.6528	2.5896	2.4908	2.3867	2.2759	2.2174	2.157	2.093	2.026	1.954	1.878
27	5.6331	4.2421	3.6472	3.3067	3.0828	2.9228	2.8021	2.7074	2.6309	2.5676	2.4688	2.3644	2.2533	2.1946	2.133	2.069	2.002	1.930	1.853
28	5.6096	4.2205	3.6264	3.2863	3.0626	2.9027	2.7820	2.6872	2.6106	2.5473	2.4484	2.3438	2.2324	2.1735	2.112	2.048	1.980	1.907	1.829
29	5.5878	4.2006	3.6072	3.2674	3.0438	2.8840	2.7633	2.6686	2.5919	2.5286	2.4295	2.3248	2.2131	2.1540	2.092	2.028	1.959	1.886	1.807
30	5.5675	4.1821	3.5894	3.2499	3.0265	2.8667	2.7460	2.6513	2.5746	2.5112	2.4120	2.3072	2.1952	2.1359	2.074	2.009	1.940	1.866	1.787
40	5.4239	4.0510	3.4633	3.1261	2.9037	2.7444	2.6238	2.5289	2.4519	2.3882	2.2882	2.1819	2.0677	2.0069	1.943	1.875	1.803	1.724	1.637
60	5.2856	3.9253	3.3425	3.0077	2.7863	2.6274	2.5068	2.4117	2.3344	2.2702	2.1692	2.0613	1.9445	1.8817	1.815	1.744	1.667	1.581	1.482
120	5.1523	3.8046	3.2269	2.8943	2.6740	2.5154	2.3948	2.2994	2.2217	2.1570	2.0548	1.9450	1.8249	1.7597	1.690	1.614	1.530	1.433	1.310
inf	5.0239	3.6889	3.1161	2.7858	2.5665	2.4082	2.2875	2.1918	2.1136	2.0483	1.9447								

TABLE A.1.4 **F-Table for** $\alpha = 0.05$

df2/ df1	1	2	3	4	5	6	7	8	9	10	12	15	20	24	30	40	60	120	INF
1	4052.181	4999.500	5403.352	5624.583	5763.650	5858.986	5928.356	5981.070	6022.473	6055.847	6106.321	6157.285	6208.730	6234.631	6260.649	6286.782	6313.030	6339.391	6365.864
2	98.503	99.000	99.166	99.249	99.299	99.333	99.356	99.374	99.388	99.399	99.416	99.433	99.449	99.458	99.466	99.474	99.482	99.491	99.499
3	34.116	30.817	29.457	28.710	28.237	27.911	27.672	27.489	27.345	27.229	27.052	26.872	26.690	26.598	26.505	26.411	26.316	26.221	26.125
4	21.198	18.000	16.694	15.977	15.522	15.207	14.976	14.799	14.659	14.546	14.374	14.198	14.020	13.929	13.838	13.745	13.652	13.558	13.463
5	16.258	13.274	12.060	11.392	10.967	10.672	10.456	10.289	10.158	10.051	9.888	9.722	9.553	9.466	9.379	9.291	9.202	9.112	9.020
6	13.745	10.925	9.780	9.148	8.746	8.466	8.260	8.102	7.976	7.874	7.718	7.559	7.396	7.313	7.229	7.143	7.057	6.969	6.880
7	12.246	9.547	8.451	7.847	7.460	7.191	6.993	6.840	6.719	6.620	6.469	6.314	6.155	6.074	5.992	5.908	5.824	5.737	5.650
8	11.259	8.649	7.591	7.006	6.632	6.371	6.178	6.029	5.911	5.814	5.667	5.515	5.359	5.279	5.198	5.116	5.032	4.946	4.859
9	10.561	8.022	6.992	6.422	6.057	5.802	5.613	5.467	5.351	5.257	5.111	4.962	4.808	4.729	4.649	4.567	4.483	4.398	4.311
10	10.044	7.559	6.552	5.994	5.636	5.386	5.200	5.057	4.942	4.849	4.706	4.558	4.405	4.327	4.247	4.165	4.082	3.996	3.909
11	9.646	7.206	6.217	5.668	5.316	5.069	4.886	4.744	4.632	4.539	4.397	4.251	4.099	4.021	3.941	3.860	3.776	3.690	3.602
12	9.330	6.927	5.953	5.412	5.064	4.821	4.640	4.499	4.388	4.296	4.155	4.010	3.858	3.780	3.701	3.619	3.535	3.449	3.361
13	9.074	6.701	5.739	5.205	4.862	4.620	4.441	4.302	4.191	4.100	3.960	3.815	3.665	3.587	3.507	3.425	3.341	3.255	3.165
14	8.862	6.515	5.564	5.035	4.695	4.456	4.278	4.140	4.030	3.939	3.800	3.656	3.505	3.427	3.348	3.266	3.181	3.094	3.004
15	8.683	6.359	5.417	4.893	4.556	4.318	4.142	4.004	3.895	3.805	3.666	3.522	3.372	3.294	3.214	3.132	3.047	2.959	2.868
16	8.531	6.226	5.292	4.773	4.437	4.202	4.026	3.890	3.780	3.691	3.553	3.409	3.259	3.181	3.101	3.018	2.933	2.845	2.753
17	8.400	6.112	5.185	4.669	4.336	4.102	3.927	3.791	3.682	3.593	3.455	3.312	3.162	3.084	3.003	2.920	2.835	2.746	2.653
18	8.285	6.013	5.092	4.579	4.248	4.015	3.841	3.705	3.597	3.508	3.371	3.227	3.077	2.999	2.919	2.835	2.749	2.660	2.566
19	8.185	5.926	5.010	4.500	4.171	3.939	3.765	3.631	3.523	3.434	3.297	3.153	3.003	2.925	2.844	2.761	2.674	2.584	2.489
20	8.096	5.849	4.938	4.431	4.103	3.871	3.699	3.564	3.457	3.368	3.231	3.088	2.938	2.859	2.778	2.695	2.608	2.517	2.421
21	8.017	5.780	4.874	4.369	4.042	3.812	3.640	3.506	3.398	3.310	3.173	3.030	2.880	2.801	2.720	2.636	2.548	2.457	2.360
22	7.945	5.719	4.817	4.313	3.988	3.758	3.587	3.453	3.346	3.258	3.121	2.978	2.827	2.749	2.667	2.583	2.495	2.403	2.305
23	7.881	5.664	4.765	4.264	3.939	3.710	3.539	3.406	3.299	3.211	3.074	2.931	2.781	2.702	2.620	2.535	2.447	2.354	2.256
24	7.823	5.614	4.718	4.218	3.895	3.667	3.496	3.363	3.256	3.168	3.032	2.889	2.738	2.659	2.577	2.492	2.403	2.310	2.211
25	7.770	5.568	4.675	4.177	3.855	3.627	3.457	3.324	3.217	3.129	2.993	2.850	2.699	2.620	2.538	2.453	2.364	2.270	2.169
26	7.721	5.526	4.637	4.140	3.818	3.591	3.421	3.288	3.182	3.094	2.958	2.815	2.664	2.585	2.503	2.417	2.327	2.233	2.131

(Continued)

TABLE A.1.4 (Continued)

df2/ df1	1	2	3	4	5	6	7	8	9	10	12	15	20	24	30	40	60	120	INF
27	7.677	5.488	4.601	4.106	3.785	3.558	3.388	3.256	3.149	3.062	2.926	2.783	2.632	2.552	2.470	2.384	2.294	2.198	2.097
28	7.636	5.453	4.568	4.074	3.754	3.528	3.358	3.226	3.120	3.032	2.896	2.753	2.602	2.522	2.440	2.354	2.263	2.167	2.064
29	7.598	5.420	4.538	4.045	3.725	3.499	3.330	3.198	3.092	3.005	2.868	2.726	2.574	2.495	2.412	2.325	2.234	2.138	2.034
30	7.562	5.390	4.510	4.018	3.699	3.473	3.304	3.173	3.067	2.979	2.843	2.700	2.549	2.469	2.386	2.299	2.208	2.111	2.006
40	7.314	5.179	4.313	3.828	3.514	3.291	3.124	2.993	2.888	2.801	2.665	2.522	2.369	2.288	2.203	2.114	2.019	1.917	1.805
60	7.077	4.977	4.126	3.649	3.339	3.119	2.953	2.823	2.718	2.632	2.496	2.352	2.198	2.115	2.028	1.936	1.836	1.726	1.601
120	6.851	4.787	3.949	3.480	3.174	2.956	2.792	2.663	2.559	2.472	2.336	2.192	2.035	1.950	1.860	1.763	1.656	1.533	1.381
inf	6.635	4.605	3.782	3.319	3.017	2.802	2.639	2.511	2.407	2.321	2.185	2.039	1.878	1.791	1.696	1.592	1.473	1.325	1.000

A.2 MATHEMATICAL FITTING FUNCTIONS

$$y = \text{Basal} + \frac{E_{max} - \text{Basal}}{1 + 10^{(\text{LogEC}_{50} + \text{Log}[A])^n}}$$

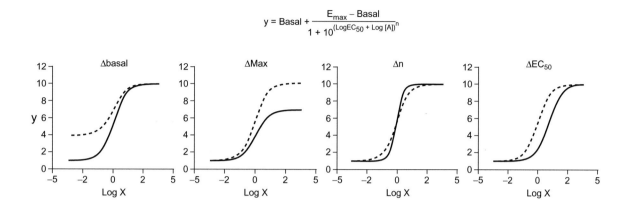

$$y = A + Bx + Cx^2$$

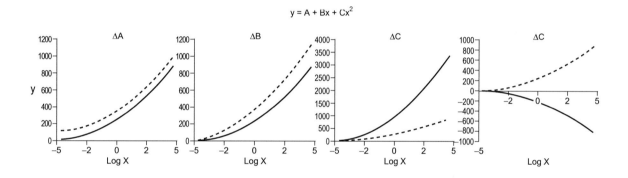

$$y = Ae^{-\left[\frac{(x-B)}{C}\right]}$$

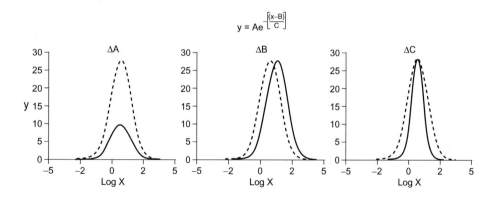

$$y = Ae^{-Bx} + C$$

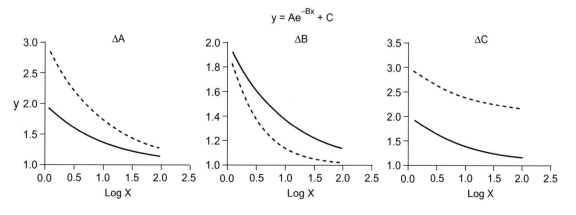

$$y = B\,(1 - e^{-Ax}) + C$$

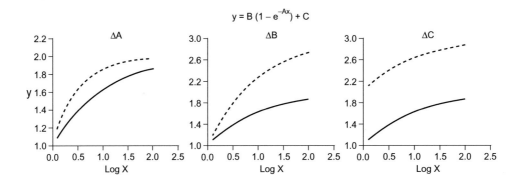

$$y = C + B\left[1 - \left[\frac{x}{x + A}\right]\right]$$

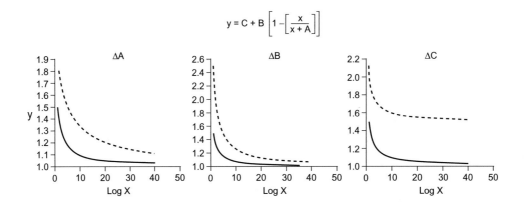

$$y = A + \frac{B}{x}$$

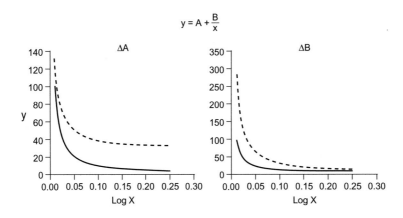

$$y = e^{A + B\cdot Log\,(x) + C\cdot(Log(X))^2}$$

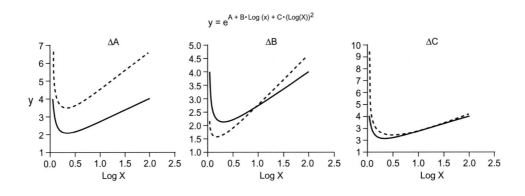

$$y = A + B \cdot x^C$$

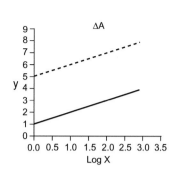

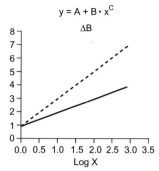

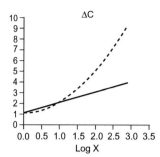

$$Y = C + B \cdot 10^{Ax}$$

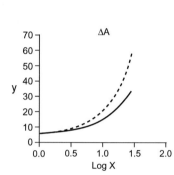

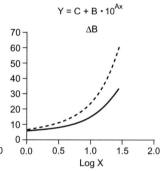

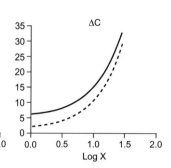

$$Y = B + A \cdot 10^{Log(x)}$$

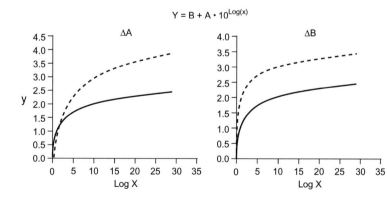

$$y = \frac{(C-D)}{1+\left(\frac{10^X}{10^A}\right)^B} + D$$

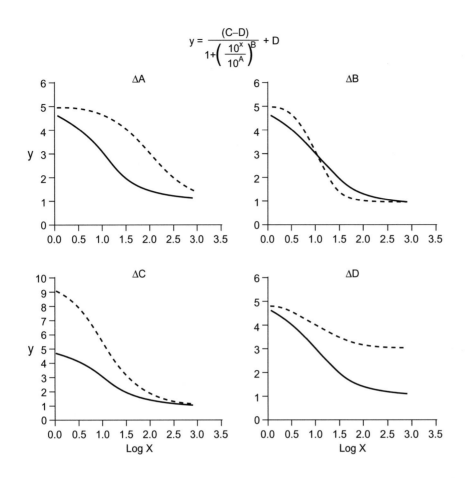

$$y = basal + \frac{Max - basal}{1 + 10^{(pEC_{50} + Log[A])^n}}$$

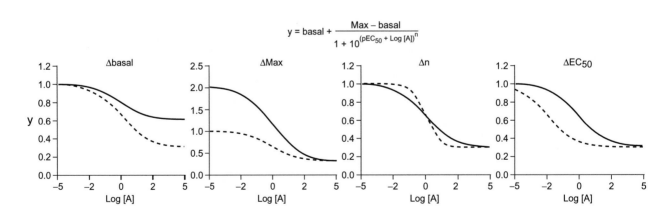

GLOSSARY OF PHARMACOLOGICAL TERMS

Affinity/affinity constant ligands reside at a point of minimal energy within a binding locus of a protein according to a ratio of the rate that the ligand leaves the surface of the protein (k_{off}) and the rate it approaches the protein surface (k_{on}). This ratio is the equilibrium dissociation constant of the ligand–protein complex (denoted $K_{eq} = k_{off}/k_{on}$) and defines the molar concentration of the ligand in the compartment containing the protein where 50% of the protein has ligand bound to it at any one instant. The "affinity" or attraction of the ligand for the protein is the reciprocal of K_{eq}.

Agonist a molecule that produces physiological response through activation of a receptor.

Alkylating agent a reactive chemical that forms a covalent bond with chemical moieties on the biological target (usually a protein). For instance, β-haloalkylamines generate an aziridinium ion in aqueous base that inserts into $-SH$, $-CHOH$, or other chemical structures in peptides. Once inserted, the effects of the alkylating agent are irreversible.

Allele different forms of a gene at a given locus.

Allosteric modulators unlike competitive antagonists that bind to the same domain on the receptor as the agonist, allosteric modulators bind to their own site on the receptor and produce an effect on agonism through a protein conformational change. Allosteric modulators can affect the affinity or the responsiveness of the receptor to the agonist. A hallmark of allosteric interaction is that the effect reaches a maximal asymptote corresponding to saturation of the allosteric sites on the receptor. For example, an allosteric modulator may produce a maximal tenfold decrease in the affinity of the receptor for a ligand upon saturation of the allosteric sites.

Allosterism (allosteric) the imposition of an effect on a protein through interaction of a molecule with a site on the protein distinct from the natural binding locus for the endogenous ligand for that protein. Interactions between the allosteric molecule and the endogenous ligand occur through the protein and not through direct steric interaction.

Analysis of variance (ANOVA) a statistical procedure that quantifies differences between means of samples and the extent of variances within and between those means to determine the probability of there being a difference in the samples.

Antagonist a molecule that interferes with the interaction of an agonist and a receptor protein or a molecule that blocks the constitutive elevated basal response of a physiological system.

Association constant the ratio of the rate of onset of a molecule to a receptor binding site and the rate of dissociation of the molecule away from that site (reciprocal of K_{eq}; see *Affinity*).

B_{max} a term denoting the maximal binding capacity of an experimental binding system, usually a preparation containing receptors (membranes, cells). The magnitude is most often expressed in number of receptors per cell or molar concentration of receptors per milligram protein.

cDNA complementary DNA copied from a messenger RNA coding for a protein; it is inserted into surrogate host cells to cause them to express the protein.

Cheng–Prusoff correction published by Cheng and Prusoff (Biochem Pharmacol 22, 3099–3108, 1973), this method is used to derive the equilibrium dissociation constant of a ligand-receptor (or enzyme) pair from the experimentally observed IC_{50} (concentration that produces 50% reduction in effect) for that molecule; see Equation 4.11.

Clone identical cells (with respect to genetic constitution) derived from a single cell by asexual reproduction. Receptors can be cloned into cells by inserting a gene into the cell line; a colony of cells results that are identical and all have the expressed receptor.

Competitive antagonist by definition, competitive antagonists compete with the agonist for the same binding domain on the receptor. Therefore, the relative affinities and quantities of the agonist and antagonist dictate which ligand dominates. Under these circumstances, the concentration of agonist can be raised to the point where the concomitant receptor occupancy by the antagonist is insignificant. When this occurs, the maximal response to the agonist is observed, that is, surmountable antagonism results.

Concentration ratio the ratio of molar concentrations of agonist that produce equal levels of response in a given pharmacological preparation (usually the ratio of EC_{50} concentrations). This term is used most often when discussing antagonism (equiactive concentration of agonist in the absence and presence of an antagonist).

Concentration-response curve a more specific (and technically correct) term for a dose-response curve done *in vitro*. This curve defines the relationship between the concentrations of a given molecule and the observed pharmacological effect.

Constitutive receptor activity receptors spontaneously produce conformations that activate G-proteins in the absence of agonists. This activity, referred to as *constitutive activity*, can be observed in systems in which the receptor expression levels are high and the resulting levels of spontaneously activating receptor species produce a visible physiological response. An inverse agonist reverses this constitutive activity and thus reduces, in a dose-dependent manner, the spontaneously elevated basal response of a constitutively active receptor system.

Cooperativity the interaction of molecules on a protein resulting from the mutual binding of those molecules. The cooperativity may be positive (whereby the binding of one of the substances facilitates the interaction of the protein with the other molecule) or negative (binding of one molecule decreases the interaction of the protein with the other molecule).

415

Cooperativity factor   an allosteric ligand has an effect on a receptor protein mediated through the binding of that ligand to the allosteric binding domain. The intensity of that effect, usually a change in the affinity of the receptor for other ligands or the efficacy of a ligand for the receptor, is quantified by the cooperativity factor. Denoted α, a positive value for α defines a potentiation. Conversely, a fractional value denotes an inhibition. Thus if $\alpha = 0.1$, a tenfold decrease in the affinity of a tracer ligand for the receptor is produced by the allosteric modulator. Magnitudes of the α factor for a given allosteric molecule are unique for the tracer for receptor function/binding used to measure the interaction; see Chapter 7, Section 7.4.

Coupling   processes that cause the interaction of molecules with membrane receptors to produce an observable cellular response; see Chapter 2, Section 2.2.

Cubic ternary complex model   a molecular model (J Ther Biol 178, 151−167, 1996a; 178, 169−182, 1996b; 181, 381−397, 1996c) describing the coexistence of two receptor states that can interact with both G-proteins and ligands. The receptor/G-protein complexes may or may not produce a physiological response; see Chapter 3, Section 3.11.

Degrees of freedom   statistical term for the number of choices that can be made when fixing values of expected frequency leading to the number of independent comparisons that can be made in a sample of observations.

Desensitization   the reduction in response to an agonist or other physiological stimulation upon repeated instance of stimulation or continued presence of an agonist. Also referred to as *tachyphylaxis*.

Dissociation constant   the ratio of the rate of offset of ligand away from a receptor divided by the rate of onset of the ligand approaching the receptor. It has the units of concentration and specifically is the concentration of ligand that occupies 50% of the total number of sites available for ligand binding at equilibrium (see *Affinity*).

Domain   sequence of amino acids in a protein that can be identified as controlling a specific function, that is, recognition of ligands.

Dose ratio   the concentration of agonist producing the same response in the presence of a given concentration of antagonist divided by the concentration of agonist producing the same response in the absence of the antagonist. For instance, if the control EC_{50} for an agonist dose-response curve is 10 nM and the EC_{50} in the presence of a given concentration of antagonist is 30 nM, then the dose ratio in this case is 3 (see *Concentration ratio*).

Downregulation   the reduction in the number of biological targets (e.g., cell surface receptors, enzymes) usually occurring with repeated stimulation of the system. For example, repeated stimulation of receptors by an agonist can lead to uncoupling of the receptors from stimulus-response mechanisms (due to phosphorylation of the receptors) followed by internalization of the receptor protein into the cell. This latter process is referred to as *downregulation of receptors*; see Chapter 2, Section 2.6, and Chapter 5, Figure 5.7.

EC_{50}/ED_{50}   the "effective concentration" of an agonist producing (in this case) 50% maximal response to that particular drug (not necessarily 50% of the maximal response of the system). Other values can be quantified for other levels of response in which case the subscript denotes the response level (i.e., EC_{25}

refers to the concentration of agonist producing 25% maximal response to that agonist). ED_{50} is the *in vivo* counterpart of EC_{50} referring to the dose of an agonist that produces 50% maximal effect.

Efficacy   historically, this term was given to agonists to define the property of the molecule that causes the production of a physiological response. However, with the discovery of negative efficacy (inverse agonists) and efficacy related to other properties of receptors that do not involve a physiological response, a more general definition of efficacy is that property of a molecule that causes the receptor to change its behavior toward the host.

E_{max}   conventional term for the maximal response capable of being produced in a given system.

Equiactive dose ratios   ratios of molar concentrations of drug (usually agonists) that produce the same response in a given system; also referred to as EMR and EPMR; see Chapter 10, Section 10.2.3.

Equiactive (equieffective) molar concentration (potency) ratios (EMR, EPMR)   variants of the term *dose ratio* or *equiactive dose ratios*. Usually pertaining to agonists, these are the molar concentrations that produce the same response in a given system. These ratios are dependent on the affinity and efficacy of the agonists and thus are system independent, that is, characterize agonists and receptors in all systems. Care must be taken that the maximal responses of the agonists concerned are equal.

Equilibrium (dissociation) constant   reciprocal of the association constant and affinity; characterizes the binding of a molecule to a receptor. Specifically, it is the ratio of the rate of offset of the molecule away from the receptor divided by the rate of onset toward the receptor. It also is a molar concentration that binds to 50% of the receptor population.

Extended ternary complex model   a modification of the original ternary complex model for GPCRs (J Biol Chem 268, 4625−4636, 1993) in which the receptor is allowed to spontaneously form an active state that can then couple to G-proteins and produce a physiological response due to constitutive activity.

Fade   the time-dependent decrease in response upon prolonged exposure of a biological system to an agonist. Originally, this was defined as the characteristic peak contraction followed by relaxation produced by guinea pig vas deferentia, but the term has also been generalized to include all forms of real-time observed loss of responsiveness (often termed *tachyphylaxis*). It can be due to desensitization of the receptor or other factors. Fade is generally thought of as a case of decline of response in the continued presence of agonist as opposed to frequent stimulation.

Full agonist   name given to an agonist that produces the full system maximal response (E_{max}). It is a system-dependent phenomenon and should not necessarily be associated with a particular agonist, as an agonist can be a full agonist in some systems and a partial agonist in others.

Functional antagonism   reduction in the responsiveness to a given agonist by activation of cellular mechanisms that produce a counterstimulus to the cell.

Furchgott analysis   a technique (in Advances in Drug Research, Vol. 3, pp. 21−55, N. J. Harper and A. B. Simmonds, Eds., Academic Press, London, 1996) used to measure the affinity of a full agonist in a functional assay (see Chapter 5, Section 5.6.2, and Chapter 12, Section 12.2.3).

Gaddum analysis, Gaddum (method of) this method (Q J Exp Physiol 40, 49–74, 1955) compares equiactive concentrations of an agonist in the absence and presence of a concentration of noncompetitive antagonist that depresses the maximal agonist response. These are compared in a double reciprocal plot (or variant thereof) to yield the equilibrium dissociation constant of the noncompetitive antagonist-receptor complex (see Chapter 6, Section 6.4, and Chapter 12, Section 12.2.8).

Gaddum equation (competitive antagonism) the pivotal simple equation (see Chapter 6, Sections 6.2 and 6.8.1) describing the competition between two ligands for a single receptor site. It forms the basis for Schild analysis.

Gaddum equation (noncompetitive antagonism) this technique measures the affinity of a noncompetitive antagonist based on a double reciprocal plot of equiactive agonist concentrations in the absence and presence of the noncompetitive antagonist. The antagonist must depress the maximal response to the agonist for the method to be effective; see Chapter 6, Section 6.4.

Gene the sequence of DNA that codes for a complete protein.

Genetic polymorphism polymorphism due to two or more alleles in a gene leading to more than one phenotype with respect to biological target reactivity to drugs.

Genome the set of genes for an organism that determines all inherited characteristics. In general, the sequence and location of every gene responsible for coding every protein.

Genotype the pattern of genes inherited by an individual. The makeup of a biological target due to coding of the gene for that target.

G-proteins trimeric membrane-bound proteins that have intrinsic GTPase activity and act as intermediaries between 7TM receptors and a host of cellular effectors; see Chapter 2, Section 2.2.

Hemi-equilibria a pseudoequilibrium that can occur when a fast-acting agonist equilibrates with a receptor system where a slow-acting antagonist is present. The agonist will occupy the nonantagonist-bound receptors quickly and then must equilibrate with antagonist-bound receptors; this latter process can be extremely slow so as to be essentially irreversible within the time frame of some experiments. Under these conditions, a slow-acting competitive antagonist may appear to be an irreversibly acting antagonist.

Heptahelical receptors another name for 7TM receptors or G-protein-coupled receptors. It refers to the motif of the helices of the protein crossing the cell membrane seven times to form intracellular and extracellular domains.

Hyperbola (hyperbolic) a set of functions defining nonlinear relationships between abscissae and ordinates. This term is used loosely to describe nonlinear relationships between the initial interaction of molecules and receptors and the observed response (i.e., stimulus-response cascades of cells).

IC$_{50}$ the concentration (usually molar) of an inhibitor (receptor, enzyme antagonist) that blocks a given predefined stimulus by 50%. It is an empirical value in that its magnitude varies with the strength of the initial stimulus to be blocked.

Insurmountable antagonism a receptor blockade that results in depression of the maximal response. Under these circumstances, unlike competitive antagonism, no increase in the concentration of agonist will regain the control maximal response in the presence of the antagonist.

Intrinsic activity a scale of agonist activity devised by Ariens (Arch Int Pharmacodyn Ther 99, 32–49, 1954) referring to the fractional maximal response to an agonist relative to a standard "full agonist" in the same system (where a full agonist produces the full system maximal response). Thus, a partial agonist that produces a maximal response 50% that of a full agonist has an intrinsic activity (denoted α) of 0.5. Full agonists have $\alpha = 1$ and antagonists $\alpha = 0$.

Intrinsic efficacy the term *efficacy*, as defined originally by Stephenson (Br Pharmacol 11, 379–393, 1956), involved agonist and system components. Intrinsic efficacy (as given by Furchgott: Advances in Drug Research, Vol. 3, pp. 21–55, N. J. Harper and A. B. Simmonds, Eds., Academic Press, London, 1966) was defined to be a solely agonist-specific quantification of the ability of the agonist to induce a physiological or pharmacological response. Thus, efficacy is the product of intrinsic efficacy multiplied by the receptor density (see Chapter 3, Section 3.5).

Inverse agonist these ligands reverse constitutive receptor activity. Currently it is thought that this occurs because inverse agonists have a selectively higher affinity for the inactive versus the active conformation of the receptor. It is important to note that while inverse agonist activity requires constitutive activity to be observed, the property of the molecule responsible for this activity does not disappear when there is no constitutive activity. In these cases, inverse agonists function as simple competitive antagonists.

In vitro Latin *in vitro veritas* (in glass lies the truth) referring to experiments conducted in an artificial environment (i.e., organ bath, cell culture) leading to conditions of fewer and more controllable variables.

In vivo with reference to *in vitro,* referring to experiments conducted in whole living organisms.

Irreversible antagonists irreversible ligands have negligible rates of offset (i.e., once the ligand binds to the receptor it essentially stays there). Under these circumstances, receptor occupancy does not achieve a steady state but, rather, increases with increasing exposure time to the ligand. Thus, once a receptor is occupied by the irreversible antagonist, it remains inactivated throughout the course of the experiment.

IUPHAR an acronym for International Union of Pharmacology, a nongovernment organization of national societies functioning under the International Council of Scientific Unions.

k_1 referring to the rate of onset of a molecule to a receptor with units of $s^{-1} \, mol^{-1}$.

$k_2(k_{-1})$ referring to the rate of offset of molecule from a receptor in units of s^{-1}.

K_A standard pharmacologic convention for the equilibrium dissociation constant of an agonist-receptor complex with units of M. It is the concentration that occupies half the receptor population at equilibrium. It also can be thought of as the reciprocal of affinity.

K_B convention for the equilibrium dissociation constant of an antagonist-receptor complex usually determined in a functional assay denoting antagonism of a physiological response, although it can be associated with an antagonist when it is used in other types of experiments. It has units of M and is the concentration that occupies half the receptor population at equilibrium. It also can be thought of as the reciprocal of affinity.

K_d convention for the equilibrium dissociation constant of a radioligand-receptor complex.

K_I basically the K_B for an antagonist but specifically measured in a biochemical binding study (or enzyme assay).

Ligand   a molecule that binds to a biological receptor.

Ligand binding   a biochemical technique that measures the physical association of a ligand with a biological target (usually a protein); see Chapter 4, Section 4.2.

Logistic function   generally yields a sigmoidally shaped line similar to that defined by drug dose-response relationships in biological systems. It is defined by $y = (1 + e^{-(a+bx)})^{-1}$. Substituting a as $\log(EC_{50})$ and x as $\log [A]$ leads to the Langmuir adsorption isotherm form of dose-response curves $y = [A]^b/([A]^b + (EC_{50})^b)$.

Log normal distribution   the distribution of a sample that is normal only when plotted on a logarithmic scale. The most prevalent cases in pharmacology refer to drug potencies (agonist and/or antagonist) that are estimated from semilogarithmic dose-response curves. All parametric statistical tests on these must be performed on their logarithmic counterparts, specifically their expression as a value on the p-scale ($-$log values); see Chapter 1, Section 1.11.2.

Mass action   this law states that the rate of a chemical reaction is proportional to the concentration (mass) of the reactants.

Michaelis-Menten kinetics   in 1913 L. Michaelis and M. Menten realized that the rate of an enzymatic reaction differed from conventional chemical reactions. They postulated a scheme whereby the reaction of a substrate plus enzyme yields enzyme plus substrate and placed it into the form of the equation: reaction velocity = (maximal velocity of the reaction $\times$ substrate concentration)/(concentration of substrate $+$ a fitting constant K_m). The K_m (referred to as the Michaelis$-$Menten constant) is the concentration of the substrate at which the reaction rate is half the maximal value; it also characterizes the tightness of the binding between substrate and enzyme.

Negative efficacy   by definition, *efficacy* is that property of a molecule that causes the receptor to change its behavior toward the biological host. *Negative efficacy* refers to the property of selective affinity of the molecule for the inactive state of the receptor; this results in inverse agonism. Negative efficacy causes the active antagonism of constitutive receptor activity but is observed only in systems that have a measurably elevated basal response due to constitutive activity. It is a property of the molecule and not the system.

Noncompetitive antagonism   if an antagonist binds to the receptor and precludes agonist activation of that receptor by its occupancy, then no amount of agonist present in the receptor compartment can overcome this antagonism and it is termed *noncompetitive*. This can occur either by binding to the same binding domain as the agonist or another (allosteric) domain. Therefore, this definition is operational in that it does not necessarily imply a molecular mechanism, only a cause and effect relationship. The characteristic of noncompetitive antagonism is eventual depression of the maximal response; however, parallel displacement of agonist dose-response curves, with no diminution of maximal response, can occur in systems with receptor reserve for the agonist; see Chapter 6, Section 6.4.

Nonlinear regression   a technique that fits a specified function of x and y by the method of least squares (i.e., the sum of the squares of the differences between real data points and calculated data points is minimized).

Nonspecific binding (nsb)   binding of a traceable (i.e., radioactive) ligand (in a binding assay designed to measure the specific binding of the ligand) that binds to other components of the experimental system (i.e., other nonrelated proteins, wall of the vessel). It is defined operationally as the amount of ligand not displaced by an excess (approximately $100 \times K_B$) of a selective antagonist for the biological target; see Chapter 4, Section 4.2.

Null method   physiological or pharmacological effects are translations of biochemical events by the cell. The null method assumes that equal responses emanate from equal initial stimulation of the receptor; therefore, when comparing equal responses, the complex translation is cancelled and statements about the receptor activity of agonists can be made. Relative potencies of agonists producing equal responses thus are interpreted to be measures of the relative receptor stimuli produced by the agonists at the receptor; see Chapter 5, Section 5.6.2.

Occupancy   the probability that a molecule will be bound to a receptor at a given concentration. For example, an occupancy of 50% states that, at any one instant, half of the receptors will have a molecule bound and half will not. This is a stochastic process, and the actual receptors that are bound change constantly with time. However, at any one instant, the total fraction bound will be the fractional occupancy.

Operational model   devised and published by James Black and Paul Leff (Proc R Soc Lond Biol 220, 141$-$162, 1983), this model uses experimental observation to describe the production of a physiological response by an agonist in general terms. It defines affinity and the ability of a drug to induce a response as a value of τ, which is a term describing the system (receptor density and efficiency of the cell to convert an activated receptor stimulus into a response) and the agonist (efficacy). It has provided a major advance in the description of functional effects of drugs; see Chapter 3, Section 3.6 for further discussion.

Orphan receptor   a gene product that is predicted to be a receptor through structure and spontaneous interaction with G-proteins but for which there is no known endogenous ligand or physiological function.

Outliers   observations that are very inconsistent with the main sample of data, that is, apparently significantly different from the rest of the data. While there are statistical methods to test whether these values may be aberrant and thus should be removed, caution should be exercised in this practice as these data may also be the most interesting and indicative of a rare but important occurrence.

Partial agonist   whereas a full agonist produces the system maximal response, a partial agonist produces a maximal response that is below that of the system maximum (and that of a full agonist). As well as producing a submaximal response, partial agonists produce antagonism of more efficacious full agonists.

pA$_2$/pA$_x$ this negative logarithm of the molar concentration of an antagonist produces a twofold (for a pA$_2$) shift to the right of an agonist dose-response curve. If the shift is different from 2, then it may be defined as pA$_x$, where the degree of the shift of the dose-response curve is x (i.e., pA$_5$ is the $-$log concentration that produces a fivefold shift to the right of the agonist dose-response curve). The pA$_2$ is by far the most prevalent value determined, as this also may have meaning on a molecular level (i.e., under certain conditions the pA$_2$ is also the pK$_B$ for an antagonist).

pD$_2$ historical term for the negative logarithm of the EC$_{50}$ for an agonist in a functional assay, not often used in present-day pharmacology.

Phenotype characteristics that result from the expression of a genotype.

pK$_B$ negative logarithm of the K$_B$. This is the common currency of antagonist pharmacology, as pK$_B$ values are log normally distributed and thus are used to characterize receptors and antagonist potency.

pK$_I$ negative logarithm of the K$_I$, the equilibrium dissociation constant of an antagonist-receptor complex measured in a biochemical binding or enzyme study (also log normally distributed).

Polymorphisms in pharmacology, these are associated with genetic polymorphisms of biological targets (see *Genetic polymorphisms*).

Potency the concentration (usually molar) of a drug that produces a defined effect. Often, potencies of agonists are defined in terms of EC$_{50}$ or pEC$_{50}$ values. The potency usually does not involve measures of maximal effect but rather only in locations along the concentration axis of dose-response curves.

Potentiation the increase in effect produced by a molecule or procedure in a pharmacological preparation. This can be expressed as an apparent increase in efficacy (i.e., maximal response), potency, or both.

Pseudoirreversible antagonism true irreversible antagonism involves a covalent chemical bond between the antagonist and the receptor (such that the rate of offset of the antagonist from the receptor is zero). However, on the timescale of pharmacological experiments, the rate of offset of an antagonist can be so slow as to be essentially irreversible. Therefore, although no covalent bond is involved, the antagonist is for all intents and purposes bound irreversibly to the receptor.

Receptor reserve in highly efficiently coupled receptor systems, high-efficacy agonists may produce excess stimulus that saturates cellular stimulus-response mechanisms. Under these conditions, these agonists produce the system maximal response through activation of only a fraction of the existing receptor population. The remaining fraction is thus "spare" or a "reserve" in that irreversible removal of this fraction will cause a shift to the right of the agonist dose-response curve but no diminution of maximum. For example, in a system where the maximal response to an agonist can be attained by activation of 5% of the receptor population, there will be a 95% receptor reserve.

Receptors in theoretical terms, a receptor is a biological recognition unit that interacts with molecules of other stimuli (i.e., light) to translate information to cells. Receptors technically can be any biological entity such as enzymes, reuptake recognition sites, and genetic material such as DNA; however, the term usually is associated with proteins on the cell surface that transmit information from chemicals to cells. The most therapeutically relevant receptor class is G-protein-coupled receptors, presently comprising 45% of all existing drug therapies.

Recombinant DNA this is DNA containing new genetic material in an order different from the original. Genetic engineering can be used to do this deliberately to produce new proteins in cells.

Relative intrinsic activity this actually is redundant, as intrinsic activity itself is defined only in relative terms, that is, the maximal response of an agonist as a fraction of the maximal response to another agonist.

Relative potency absolute agonist potency is the product of receptor stimulus (brought about by agonist affinity and

efficacy) and the processing of the stimulus by the cell into an observable response. Because this latter process is system (cell type) dependent, absolute potencies are system-dependent measures of agonist activity. However, when comparing two agonists in the system, null procedures cancel these effects; therefore, the relative potency of agonists (provided both are full agonists) are system-independent estimates of agonist activity that can be compared across systems; see Chapter 10, Section 10.2.3.

Resultant analysis this procedure, developed by James Black and colleagues (Br J Pharmacol 84, 561−571, 1985), allows measurement of the receptor affinity of a competitive antagonist, which has secondary properties that obscure the receptor antagonism; see Chapter 6, Section 6.6 for further discussion.

Saturation binding a biochemical procedure that quantifies the amount of traceable ligand (i.e., radioligand) to a receptor protein. It yields the affinity of the ligand and the maximal number of binding sites (B$_{max}$); see Chapter 4, Section 4.2.1.

Scatchard analysis a common linear transformation of saturation binding data used prevalently before the widespread availability of nonlinear fitting software. The Scatchard transformation (see Chapter 4, Section 4.2.1), while easy to perform, can be misleading and lead to errors.

Schild analysis this powerful method of quantifying the potency of a competitive antagonist was developed by Heinz Schild (Br J Pharmacol 14, 48−58, 1959; see Chapter 6, Section 6.3). It is based on the principle that the antagonist-induced dextral displacement of a dose-response curve is due to its potency (K$_B$ value) and its concentration in the receptor compartment. Because the antagonism can be observed and the concentration of antagonist is known, the K$_B$ can be calculated.

Schild plot the relationship between antagonism and concentration is loglinear according to the Schild equation. The tool to determine if this is true experimentally is the Schild plot, namely a regression of log (DR−1 values (where DR is the dose ratio for the agonist in the presence and absence of antagonist)) upon the logarithm of the molar concentration of the antagonist. If this regression is linear with unit slope, then the antagonism adheres to the simple competitive model and the intercept of regression is the pK$_B$. For further discussion, see Chapter 6, Section 6.3.

Second messenger these are molecules produced by cellular effectors that go on to activate other biochemical processes in the cell. Some examples of second messengers are cyclic AMP, inositol triphosphate, arachidonic acid, and calcium ion (see Chapter 2, Section 2.2).

Selectivity the difference in activity a given biologically active molecule has for two or more processes. Thus, if a molecule has a tenfold (for example) greater affinity for process A over process B, then it can be said to have selectivity for process A. However, the implication is that the different activity is not absolute, that is, given enough molecule, the activation of the other process(es) will occur.

Sigmoid the characteristic "S-shaped" curves defined by functions such as the Langmuir isotherm and logistic function (when plotted on a logarithmic abscissal scale).

Spare receptors another term for receptor reserve (see *Receptor reserve*).

Specificity this can be thought of as an extreme form of selectivity (see *Selectivity*) where, in this case, no increase in the concentration of the molecule will be sufficient to activate the other process(es). This term is often used erroneously in that the extremes of concentration have not been tested (or cannot be tested due to chemical, toxic, or solubility constraints in a particular system) to define what probably is only selectivity.

Stimulus   this is quanta of initial stimulation given to the receptor by the agonist. There are no units to stimulus, and it is always utilized as a ratio quantity comparing two or more agonists. Stimulus is not an observable response but is processed by the cell to yield a measurable response.

Stimulus-response coupling   another term for receptor coupling. It describes the series of biochemical reactions that link the initial activation of the receptor to the observed cellular (or organ) response.

Subtype   often refers to a receptor and denotes a variation in the gene product such that the endogenous ligand is the same (i.e., neurotransmitter, hormone) but the function, distribution, and sensitivity of the receptor subtypes differ. Antagonists often can distinguish receptor subtypes.

Surmountable antagonism   an antagonist-induced shift to the right of an agonist dose-response curve with no diminution of the maximal response to the agonist (observed with simple competitive antagonists and some types of allosteric modulators).

Tachyphylaxis   the progressive reduction in response due to repeated agonist stimulation (see *Desensitization* and *Fade*).

The maximal response to the agonist is reduced in tachyphylaxis (whereas the sensitivity is reduced with tolerance).

Ternary complex (model)   this model describes the formation of a complex among a ligand (usually an agonist), a receptor, and a G-protein. Originally described by De Lean and colleagues (J Biol Chem 255, 7108−7117, 1980), it has been modified to include other receptor behaviors (see Chapter 3, Sections 3.8 to 3.11), such as constitutive receptor activity.

Transfection   the transfer of DNA from one cell into another cell. This DNA then replicates in the acceptor cell.

Two-state model   a model of proteins that coexists in two states controlled by an equilibrium constant. Molecules with selective affinity for one of the states will produce a bias in that state upon binding to the system. Two-state theory was conceived to describe the function of ion channels but also has relevance to receptors (see Chapter 3, Section 3.7).

Uncompetitive antagonism   form of inhibition (originally defined for enzyme kinetics) in which both the maximal asymptotic value of the response and the equilibrium dissociation constant of the activator (i.e., agonist) are reduced by the antagonist. This differs from noncompetitive antagonism where the affinity of the receptor for the activating drug is not altered. Uncompetitive effects can occur due to allosteric modulation of receptor activity by an allosteric modulator (see Chapter 6, Section 6.4).

Index

Note: Page numbers followed by "*f*" and "*t*" refer to figures and tables, respectively.

A

Absorption, of drug, 213–214, 218–243, 227*f*, 229*f*, 401
Acebutolol, 184*f*
ACE-NEP inhibitors, 282*f*, 298–300
Acetohexamide, 239–240, 240*f*
Acetaminophen, 261–262
Acetylcholine, 71*t*, 159, 160*t*, 161–162, 364–368, 389–390, 395–396
Acid-base properties, of druglike molecules, 213–214, 224*t*
Activity. *See* Drug activity
Acyclovir, 221*t*, 226–227
Administration route, of drug, 225–227, 233–234
β-Adrenoceptor agonists, 23, 23*f*, 31, 75, 75*f*, 88–89, 88*f*, 100–101, 100*f*, 225, 285, 286*f*, 294, 295*f*, 296*f*, 300, 395
α-Adrenoceptor antagonists, 347
β-Adrenoceptor antagonists, 344–345, 344*f*
β-Adrenoceptor bronchodilators, 6
Adrenocortical steroids, 9
Adsorption, of drug molecules, 38–40
Adverse drug effects. *See* Side effects, of drugs
Affinity, 6–7, 9–18, 18*f*
    of agonists, 72–75, 98–101, 110–114, 131–133, 151–152, 359–361, 379–380
    allosteric modulator effect on, 162–175
    of allosteric modulators, 195–196, 364
    of antagonists, 122–138, 357–358, 361–369
    constitutive receptor activity and, 53–55
    EC50 relationship to, 114–115
    efficacy correlation with, 313–314, 314*f*, 373
    in extended ternary complex model, 52–53
    functional assays for measurement of, 95–96, 115, 355–357, 359–361
    G-protein coupling effect on, 82
    measurement of, 72–75, 351–353
    modeling of, 47–48, 47*f*
    in multistate receptor models and probabilistic theory, 15–16
    ordering of, in agonist series, 376
Affinity-dependent potency, 98–101
Affinity-dominant agonists, 377–379
Aflatoxin, 270–271
Agonism. *See also* Allosteric agonism; Inverse agonism
    classical model of, 49–50
    exercises in, 373

marking relevancy of, 393–394
quantifying, 96–102
    affinity-dependent v. efficacy-dependent potency, 98–101
    secondary and tertiary testing of agonists, 101–102
Agonist-antagonist hemi-equilibria, 122, 126, 127*f*, 138–139, 193
Agonist-dependent antagonism, divergent, 395–396
Agonists. *See also* Full agonists; Partial agonists
    affinity and EC50 relationship of, 114–115
    affinity of, 72–75, 98–101, 110–114, 131–133, 151–152, 359–361, 379–380
    antagonist potency dependency on concentration of, 390–391
    binding of, 9–11, 11*f*
    efficacy of, 27–28, 28*f*, 29*f*, 72–75, 97, 107–115, 375
    functional assays of, 85–96, 107–110, 114–115
    indirectly acting, 114–116
    ordering of efficacy and affinity in series of, 376
    potency of, 110–114, 128–133
    secondary and tertiary testing of, 101–102
    system effects on response of, 27–30
    toxic effects of high concentrations of, 127–128
β-Agonists, 8
Albuterol, 88*f*
Alcuronium, 71, 71*f*, 71*t*, 160*t*, 169, 176, 176*f*, 307–308, 376
Allometric scaling, 247–249
Allosteric agonism, 101–102, 166, 198–199, 376
Allosteric antagonism, 119–120, 120*f*, 126, 128, 128*f*, 155
    affinity of, 167–168, 196, 364–368
    derivations, 178–179
    detection of, 368–369
    functional study of, 162–175
    introduction to, 155
    methods for detecting, 175–177
    nature of, 155–158
    negative allosteric modulators (NAMs), 166, 168–172
    optimal assays for, 174–175
    orthosteric antagonism v, 163*t*, 175–177
    positive allosteric modulators (PAMs), 166, 172–174

phenotypic profiles, 166
properties of allosteric modulators, 160*t*, 162
Schild analysis for, 176*f*, 179
summary of, 177
unique effects of, 158–162
Allosteric competitive antagonism, 387–389
Allosteric insurmountable antagonism, 193–194, 210, 362–363
Allosteric interactions, 37–38
    in displacement binding, 68–71, 69*f*, 71*f*, 71*t*, 72*f*, 80
    kinetic binding studies of, 71
    maximal inhibition of binding in, 81
    partial agonism v., 389
Allosteric ligands, efficacy response to, 178–179
Allosteric model, of receptor activity, 178
Allosteric modulators, 160*t*, 396–397
    functional study of, 162–175
    in high-throughput screening, 313
    properties of, 163*t*
    unique effects of, 158–162
Alprenolol, 184*f*, 234*t*
Ames test, 272–273, 272*f*
Ambenonium, 395–396
Amiloride, 221*t*
Aminoglycosides, 246–247, 303
Amiodarone, 298
Amitriptyline, 230–231, 298, 299*f*
Amoxicillin, 222–223, 244, 246
Ampicillin, 303, 305*f*
Amplification
    of stimulus, 27–30, 86
    by successive rectangular hyperbolic , equations, 41
Amylin, 73, 74*f*, 290–291, 290*f*
Analysis of covariance, 342–345
Andrews binding energy, 313
Angiotensin converting enzyme (ACE) inhibitors, 222–223, 263*t*, 296, 298–300
Animal models, 296
Animal studies, for target validation, 284–285
Antagonism. *See also* Allosteric antagonism; Competitive antagonism; Insurmountable antagonism; Noncompetitive antagonism; Surmountable antagonism
    divergent agonist-dependent, 395–396
    exercises in, 383–391
    incomplete, 387–389
    saturable, 119, 127–128
    silent, 391–392
    unsaturable, 119

Antagonist
  affinity of, 122–138, 357–358, 361–369
  binding of, 9–11, 11f, 155–158
  determining mode of action of, 192–193
  high-throughput screening for, 311–313
  pA$_2$ and, 131
  potency of, 121f, 122–134, 136–137, 136f,
    140, 191–192, 196, 357–358,
    363–371, 383–385, 390–391
  receptor coverage
    kinetics of dissociation, 110–114
    with hemi-equilibria, 114
  secondary testing of, 195–196
  toxic effects of high concentrations of,
    127–128
Antagonist offset, kinetics of, 386
Antedrugs, 227
Anti-allergic drug, 261–262
Anticholinergics, 8–9, 243t
Anticonvulsants, 246–247, 269–270
Antidepressants, 243t, 298, 299f
Antihistamines, 224–225, 298–300, 301f
Antipyrene, 221t
Antiviral drugs, 263t
Aplaviroc, 157–158, 157f, 159f, 160f, 177,
    177f, 196, 196f
Arabinoside, 303
Arecoline, 71t, 155, 160t, 161–162, 161f,
    307–308, 396–397
β-Arrestin, 33–35, 90, 90f, 102, 102f
Artemisinin, 302–303
Aspirin, 9, 234t, 261–262
Assays. See also Binding assays; Functional
    assays
  in cellular context, 294–296
  comparison of assays with range of ligands,
    346t
  for drug detection, 311–314
  for estimating drug toxicity, 276–278
  for measuring drug activity, 37
  pharmacokinetic, in drug discovery and
    development, 249–252
  for screening for molecules with biological
    activity, 285–286
Assay-specific agonism, 382–383
Astemizole, 230–231, 261–262
Asymmetrical dose-response curves, 341–342
Atenolol, 36f, 184f, 344–345, 344f, 345t
Atipamezole, 5
Atorvastatin, 294
Atorvastin, 230–231
Atropine, 3–4, 71, 71f, 71t, 140, 140f, 160t,
    170–171, 363–364
Atypical agonists, 376
Autonomic receptor profiling, 273–274

B
Barbiturates, 8–9, 227–228, 235, 269–270
Barlow, Scott, and Stephenson method, for
    measuring affinity of partial agonists,
    107–110, 115, 355–356
Baseline, antagonism below, 389–390
Benzodiazepines, 8–9, 218f
Betaxolol, 184f
Bethanechol, 71, 71t, 160t

Bias, 103–104
Biased signaling, 102–107
  receptor selectivity, 107
Binding, 9–11, 11f. See also Displacement
    binding; Saturation binding
  of antagonists, 9–11, 11f, 155–158
  in classical model of receptor function, 46,
    49–50
  cooperativity in, 342–343, 344f
  of drug to protein, 227–228, 401
  in extended ternary complex model, 52–53,
    60–61
  high-affinity, 72–75
  of HIV, 48–49, 49f, 58–59, 156–158, 157f,
    159f, 160f, 162, 177, 177f, 283–285,
    285f, 308, 310f
  in operational model of receptor function,
    50–51, 59–60
  to receptors, 9–19, 11f, 17f, 57–58
  specific, 64–67
  in ternary complex model, 52
  two-stage, 81–82
  in two-state theory, 51–52, 60
Binding assays, 63, 351–353
  binding theory and experiment, 63–71
  complex binding phenomena: agonists
    affinity from binding curves, 72–75
  derivations, 79–82
  displacement binding, 64, 67–71, 79–80,
    351–353
  dissociation of activity between functional
    assays and, 392
  of drug activity, 37
  experimental prerequisites for correct
    application of, 75–78
  functional studies v., 85–86
  for high-throughput screening, 312
  kinetic binding studies, 64, 71
  lack of correlation between agonist affinity
    and potency in, 379–380
  saturation binding, 64–67, 351
Binding curves, 72–77, 82
Bioavailability, of drug, 228–229, 242–243,
    247, 248f, 252f, 401
Biochemical nature, of stimulus-response
    cascade, 23–25
Biological targets, 286–291
Biomarkers, 296–297
Biopharmaceutics, 213–214
Biopharmaceutics Classification System (BCS),
    217
Bisoprolol, 36f, 184f
Bisphosphonate, 242–243
Black-Leff operational model of agonism,
    96–102
  affinity-dependent versus efficacy-dependent,
    98–101
  secondary and tertiary testing of agonists,
    101–102
α-Blockers, 8–9
β-Blockers, 8–9, 33–35, 184, 184f, 218f, 303,
    304f, 314, 392
B$_{max}$. See Maximal binding
Brefeldin A, 313
Bronchodilators, 8–9

Brucine, 160t
Bucindolol, 36f
Budesonide, 293–294
Bulaquine, 256f
Bupropion, 299f
Burimamide, 251–252, 252f, 284

C
Caffeine, 227–228, 400
Calcitonin, 27–30, 32–33, 33f, 65, 66f, 67,
    67f, 87–89, 88f, 92, 93f, 290–291,
    323–325, 327, 328t
Calcium, 31, 87
Calcium antagonists, 8–9
Calcium channel blockers, 306–307, 308f
Camptothecin, 313
Capacity-limited metabolism, 244
Captopril, 296, 298–300, 303
Carbachol, 71t, 97, 100f, 125, 126f, 140f, 176,
    176f, 357–358, 376, 395–396
Carbamazepine, 228, 244, 269–270
Carbon tetrachloride, 270–271
Carbutamide, 304, 305f
Carvedilol, 36f, 184, 184f
Catecholamines, 303
CCR5, 196, 196f, 285–286, 287f, 393–394
  in HIV binding, 48–49, 49f, 58–59,
    157–158, 159f, 160f, 170, 171f, 177,
    283–285, 308, 310f
CD4, in HIV binding, 48–49, 49f, 58–59
Ceftriaxone, 221t
Cellular context, assays in, 294–296
Cellular functional studies, of drug activity.
    See Functional assays
Cellular response, to receptor stimulus, 30–35
Cellular screening systems, for drug discovery,
    291–296
Cellular veil, drug response through, 27–30
Cephalexin, 222–223
Cephalosporins, 303
Cephalosporium cryptosporium, 303
Cerivastatin, 294
Channels, two-state theory of, 46, 51–52, 60
Chemical antagonism, 115
  agonist concentration, abstraction of,
    153–154
  antagonist concentration, abstraction of, 154
Chemical libraries. See High-throughput
    screening (HTS)
Chemical sources, for potential drugs,
    302–307
Chemical tools, 283–285
Chemistry, of druglike molecules, 214–218
Cheng-Prusoff relationship, 68, 68f, 189–190,
    353, 354f, 369–371
Chiral center, 218
Chloramphenicol, 213, 221t
Chloropractolol, 132–133, 133f, 359–361
Chloroquine, 235t, 238, 239f, 302–303
Cholestyramine, 243
Cimetide, 284
Cimetidine, 11, 12f, 252f, 399
Cisapride, 230–231
Citalopram, 299f
Clark plot, 133

Index

423

Classical model of receptor function, 46, 49–50
Clearance, 228–229, 232–234, 247–249, 248f, 252f, 397–398, 401. See also Hepatic clearance; Renal clearance
Clinical development, 283–284, 317t
Clinical feedback, in drug discovery, 296–297
Clinical testing, 274–278, 316–318
Clinical use of drugs, adverse side effects associated with, 258t
Clomipramine, 299f
Clonidine, 296
Clozapine, 261–262, 272, 298
Cocaine, 270–271, 303, 304f, 305f
Codeine, 230–231, 234t, 302–303
Coefficient of variation, 323
Combinatorial techniques. See High-throughput screening (HTS)
Compartments, volume of distribution of, 234–240, 400t
Competitive antagonism, 120–122, 390–391. See also Allosteric competitive antagonism; Insurmountable competitive antagonism; Orthosteric competitive antagonism; Orthosteric surmountable competitive antagonism; Surmountable competitive antagonism
affinity of, 357–358, 363–364
curve patterns of, 386
Gaddum method for measurement of, 149
IC50 correction factors for, 209
measurement of pKB from pIC50, 369–371
pA2 and pKB relationship for, 209–210
pIC50 curves of, 189–190, 191f
Competitive displacement, 68–71, 68f, 71f, 79–81
Complex binding phenomena, 72–75
Concentration
of agonist, antagonist potency dependency on, 390–391
determination of equiactive concentrations on dose-response curves, 353–355
of drug, 38–40, 218–247, 401
of protein, binding curve response to, 75–77, 82
Concentration-dependent antagonism, 119
Concentration-response curves. See Dose-response curves
Confidence limits, 324–325
for pIC50 measurements of potential drugs, 199–200, 202f, 204f
Confirmation, of drug leads, 315, 316f
Conformation
of proteins, 15–16, 313–314
of receptors, 155, 162–175
Conformational selection, 15–16, 20
Constitutive receptor activity, 53–55, 61, 128–131, 191, 192f, 389–390
Cooperative behavior, in binding, 57–58, 342–343, 344f
Cooperativity constant, of allosteric antagonists, 364–368
Correlation, 327–329
Correlation coefficient, 328–329
Coumarin, 227–228

Coupling efficiency, 27–31
Crystallization, of drug, 38–39
Cubic ternary complex model, 55–56, 61
Curve fitting, 330–345
of asymmetrical curves, 341–342
detecting different curves in, 340
good practice, 332–333
of incomplete curves, 336
outliers and weighting data points, 334–336
Curves. See Dose-response curves
Cyanopindolol, 38
Cyclic AMP, 23–25, 25f, 26f, 31, 87, 294, 376
Cyclosporine, 230–231, 246–247, 304
Cyclosporins, 303
CypHer-5, 90
Cyproheptadine, 298–300, 301f
Cytochrome P450, 261–262
Cytotoxicity, 255–257, 271–272

D

Data sets, pairing of, 325–326
Data variability band, 309–311
Density, of receptors, 32–33, 61
Description data, 2
Descriptive statistics. See Statistics
Desensitization, 35–37, 93–96, 96f, 138
Desipramine, 221t, 234t, 299f
Desmethylclozapine, 298
Detection, of allosteric drug antagonism, 175–177
Development, of drugs, 314–316
pharmacokinetic assays in, 249–252
tri-level testing in, 101–102, 101t, 291–293, 292f
Dexamethasone, 293–294
Diacetylmorphine, 226–227, 226f
Diazepam, 228, 230–231, 233–234, 234t, 236–237, 237f, 245, 246f, 399
Diclofenax, 270–271
Dicloxacillin, 244
Digitoxin, 227–228, 234t, 243
Digoxin, 221t, 235, 235f, 237f, 238, 239f, 242–243, 246–247, 263t
Dihydropyridine, 306–307, 308f
Diltiazem, 217, 233
Dimerization, of receptors, 287–289, 288f, 289t, 298–300, 300f
Dioxin, 272–273
Dimethylsulfoxide, 217
Dipivalylepinephrine, 226–227, 227f
Discovery. See Drug discovery
Disopyramide, 244
Displacement binding, 64, 67–71, 77–80, 82, 351–353
Displacement curves, 73, 75–77, 82
Dissimulation
in drug concentration, 38–39
of functional assays over time, 93–95
Distribution, of drug, 219, 228, 228f, 252f, 399. See also Volume of distribution, of drug
Dofetilide, 263t
Dobutamine, 184f, 300
Dopamine, 226–227, 298, 299f
Dopamine agonists, 8–9, 85–86

Dosage. See also Concentration
drug clearance effect on, 232–234
volume of distribution for determination of, 236–237
Dose ratios (DRs), 122–134, 362–363
Dose-response curves, 14–19, 14f, 259f. See also Curve fitting
adsorption process effect on, 40
of affinity-dependent v. efficacy dependent agonists, 98–101
allosteric agonist effect on, 101–102
antagonism effects on, 119, 192–193
asymmetrical, 341–342
biphasic, 390
choice of model for fitting, 330–345
in classical model of receptor function, 49–50
desensitization effect on, 35–37, 95–96, 96f
detection of differences in, 340
determination of equiactive concentrations on, 353–355
for determining kinetics of agonism, 376
for determining kinetics of antagonist offset, 386
drug insolubility effect on, 38–39
for estimating insurmountable antagonist affinity, 362–363, 368–369
examples of hypothesis testing with, 337–339
for full agonists, 110–111, 111f, 113, 356–357
of incomplete antagonism, 387–389
of inverse agonism, 128, 130f, 131
for measurement of affinity and maximal allosteric constant of surmountable allosteric modulation, 364–368
for measuring competitive antagonist affinity, 357–358, 363–364
for measuring noncompetitive antagonist affinity, 361–362
for measuring pKB from pIC50 for competitive antagonists, 369–371
mechanism of antagonist action and patterns of, 386
of new drug, establishment of, 101f, 291–293, 292f
in operational model of receptor function, 50–51, 59–60, 98–101
for ordering efficacy and affinity in agonist series, 376
for partial agonists, 98f, 107–111, 111f, 131–133, 355–356, 359–361
receptor occupancy effect on, 27–30
in Schild analysis, 122–134
simple competitive antagonist effect on, 190f
timing of measurement of, 93, 94f
in two-state theory, 51–52
Dosing
exercises in, 399, 401
multiple, 244–247, 246f
Double reciprocal plot, 65–67
Doxepin, 234t, 299f
DRs. See Dose ratios
Drug activity
discrimination of, in system-based drug discovery, 291, 292f

Drug activity (*Continued*)
  loss of, 392−393
  measurement of, 37
  in vitro-in vivo correspondence of, 394−395
Drug concentration. *See* Concentration
Drug development, 314−316
  early discovery phase, 317*t*
  lead optimization phase, 317*t*
  clinical development phase, 317*t*
Drug discovery
  chemical sources for potential drugs,
      302−307
  clinical testing, 274−278
  drug discovery and development, 314−316
  in vivo systems, biomarkers, and clinical
      feedback, 296−297
  pharmacodynamics and high-throughput
      screening, 307−314
  pharmacokinetic assays in, 249−252
  pharmacology in, 300−302
  process of, 281
      biological targets, defining, 286−291
      recombinant systems, 285−286
      system-based approach v., 291−296
      target validation and chemical tools,
          283−285
  safety pharmacology, 255−261
  system-based, 291−296
  target-based, 282−291
  tri-level testing in, 101−102, 101*t*, 291−293,
      292*f*
  types of therapeutically active ligands,
      297−300
Drug parameters, system-independent
  affinity, 6−7, 9−18, 18*f*
  efficacy, 6−7, 9−11, 15−18, 18*f*, 20
Drug efficacy, 182−188
Drug protein binding, 228, 400
Drug receptors. *See* Receptors
Drug response. *See* Response
Drug-drug interactions, 231, 261−270, 263*t*,
      399
Drug-induced mutagenicity, 272−273, 272*f*
Druglike molecules, 214−218, 283, 302, 306
Drug-receptor activity, through cellular veil,
      27−30
Drug-receptor interaction, kinetics of, 120−122
Drug-receptor theory, 45
  classical model of receptor function, 46,
      49−50
  constitutive receptor activity, 53−55, 57
  cubic ternary complex model, 55−57
  derivations, 57−61
  extended ternary complex model, 52−53,
      60−61
  introduction to, 46
  mathematical model use in, 47
  multistate receptor models and probabilistic
      theory, 56−57
  operational model of receptor function,
      46−49, 59−60, 98−101
  ternary complex model, 46, 52
  two-state theory, 46, 51−52, 60
Drugs, positive property of, 255
Drugs, toxicity in, 255−257

E

Eadie plot. *See* Scatchard plot
Eadie-Hofsted plot. *See* Scatchard plot
Eburnamonine, 160*t*, 161−162, 161*f*, 397
EC_{50}, 17−19, 18*f*
  affinity relationship to, 114−115
  allosteric effects on, 170, 170*f*
  of full agonists, 110−114
  functional studies of, 91, 92*f*
  of partial agonists, 97, 107−110, 131−133
  in two-state theory, 51−52
Efavirenz, 157, 157*f*
Efficacy, 6−7, 9−11, 15−18, 18*f*, 20
  affinity correlation with, 314, 314*f*, 373−374
  agonist lack of, 380−382
  of agonists, 27−28, 28*f*, 29*f*, 72−75, 97,
      107−114, 116, 375
  allosteric ligand effect on, 178−179
  allosteric modulator effect on, 162−175
  in classical model of receptor function,
      49−50
  constitutive receptor activity and, 53−55
  -dependent potency, 98−101
  -dominant agonists, 377−379
  in extended ternary complex model, 52−53
  in multistate receptor models and
      probabilistic theory, 15−16
  negative, 28*f*, 53−54
  in operational model of receptor function,
      50−51
  ordering of, in agonist series, 376
  receptor reserve relationship to, 22−23, 23*f*
Efficiency
  coupling, 27−31
  of ligands, 313
Egualen sodium, 256*f*
Elimination, 228, 228*f*, 229*f*, 234−237, 247,
      248*f*, 399. *See also* Clearance
  by kidney, 240−242, 400−401
  by liver, 232−234, 401
  saturation of, 243
Elimination rate constant, 234−235, 238, 247,
      248*f*
EMRs. *See* Equimolar potency ratios
Enalapril, 217, 226−227
Enzyme reactions, kinetics of, 25−26
Epinephrine, 4, 4*f*, 226−227, 227*f*
EPMRs. *See* Equipotent molar potency ratios
Equiactive concentrations, on dose-response
      curves, 353−355
Equilibration phase, of antagonism, 120−121
Equilibrium
  antagonist potency dependency on, 383−385
  in functional assays, 93, 95, 95*f*
  between two ligands, importance of
      equilibrium time for, 77−78
Equilibrium dissociation constant (K_A)
  in classical model of receptor function, 49
  of competitive antagonists, 122−125
  of full agonists, 97, 113−114
  in operational model of receptor function,
      50−51, 59−60
  of partial agonists, 97
  in two-state theory, 51−52

Equilibrium dissociation constant of antagonist-
      receptor complex (K_B), 209
Equilibrium dissociation constant of
      nonradioactive ligand-receptor complex
      (K_B), 351−353, 361−362
Equilibrium dissociation constant of
      radioligand-receptor complex (K_d), 351
Equimolar potency ratios (EMRs), 110−111
Equipotent molar potency ratios (EPMRs),
      110−111, 114
Estradiol, 230−231, 235−236
Ethosuximide, 239*f*
Etodolac, 309*f*
Eudismic index, 218
Exemestane, 256*f*
Experimental data, model consistency with,
      330−345
  analysis of covariance for determining
      number of regression lines, 343−345
  asymmetrical dose-response curves,
      341−342
  choice of model for data comparison,
      330−332
  comparison of assays with range of ligands,
      347
  comparison of means by two methods or in
      two systems, 346−347
  curve fitting good practices, 332−333
  data comparison to linear models, 342
  detection of differences in curves, 340
  hypothesis testing with dose-response curve
      examples, 337−339
  outliers and weighting data points, 334−336
  overextrapolation of data, 336
  regression linearity, 342−343
Experimental design, 321
  comparison of samples with standard values,
      346−347
  experimental data and model consistency,
      329−330
  comparison of assays with range of ligands,
      347
  comparison of means by two methods or in
      two systems, 346−347
  introduction to, 321
  quality control and, 347−350
  statistics for comparing sample data,
      321−330
  summary of, 350
Experimental pharmacology, 197−199
Experimental prerequisites, for correct
      application of binding techniques,
      75−78
Extended ternary complex model, 52−53, 55,
      60−61
External receptor kinase signal, 33−35
Extraction ratio, 232−234
Extrapolation, of data, 336

F

F value, 326−327, 332, 337−339
Famotidine, 217
Felodipine, 230−231, 269−270
Fenoximone, 294−295, 295*f*
Fexofenadine, 263*t*

First pass effect, 242–243
Flucytosine, 239f
Fluoxetine, 299f
Fluphenazine, 226–227
Fluvastatin, 221t
Fluvoxamine, 299f
Formulation, of drug, 213–214
Forskolin, 294–295, 295f, 375–376
Free concentration, of drug, 40, 42
Frovatriptan, 256f
Full agonists, 27–30
    affinity of, 110–115, 356–357
    analysis of, 110–114
    fitting data to operational model, 97
    partial agonists v., 111, 111f
    potency ratios for, 110–112, 111f
    system independence of, 115
Functional assays, 353–371
    of allosteric drug antagonism, 162–175
    Barlow, Scott, and Stephenson method for
        measuring affinity of partial agonists,
        107–110, 115, 355–356
    binding assays vs., 85–86
    choice of, 86–90
    derivations, 114–116
    determination of equiactive concentrations
        on dose-response curves, 353–355
    dissimulation in, 93–95
    dissociation of activity between binding
        assays and, 392
    of drug activity, 37–38
    estimates of relative efficacy of agonists in,
        110, 115
    for estimating insurmountable antagonist
        affinity, 362–363, 368–369
    functional pharmacological experiments,
        85–86
    Furchgott method for measuring affinity of
        full agonists, 110–115, 356–357
    Gaddum method for measurement of
        noncompetitive antagonist affinity, 152,
        361–362
    for high-throughput screening, 298f, 310t,
        312
    for kinetics of antagonist offset, 141–142
    measurement of affinity and maximal
        allosteric constant of surmountable
        allosteric modulation in, 364–368
    measurement of agonist affinity in,
        107–110, 115–116, 356–357,
        359–361
    for measurement of pK_B from pIC50 for
        competitive antagonists, 369–371
    real time v. stop time experiments in, 95–96
    recombinant cell systems for, 90–92
    resultant analysis for measuring affinity of
        competitive antagonists with multiple
        properties, 363–364
    Schild analysis for measurement of
        competitive antagonist affinity,
        357–358
    Stephenson method for partial agonist
        affinity measurement, 152, 359–361
    summary of, 114
Furchgott method, 113–116, 113f, 114f,
    356–357

Furmethide, 71t
Furosemide, 217, 304, 305f

G

Gaddum method, 122, 149, 152, 361–362
Gallamine, 155–156, 164–166, 166f, 366
Gaussian distribution, 322
General pharmacokinetics, 227–229
General pharmacology, 274
Gentamicin, 242, 244
Gleevec, 286–287
Glomerular filtration, of drug, 240–241, 400
Glucocorticoids, 8–9, 269–270, 293–295
Glycerol trinitrate, 242–243
Glyceryl trinitrate, 233–234
Gompertz function, 341f, 342
gp120, in HIV binding, 48–49, 49f, 58–59,
    158, 159f
GPCRs. See G-protein-coupled receptors
G-protein-coupled receptors (GPCRs), 4–5, 46
    activation of, 102, 102f
    agonist affinity in, 82
    binding curves for agonists in systems of,
        72–75
    constitutive receptor activity and, 53–55, 61
    cubic ternary complex model of, 55–56, 61
    dimerization of, 287–289
    ERK activation v., 33–35
    extended ternary complex model of, 52–53,
        60–61
    in functional assays, 87, 90, 90f
    in recombinant functional systems, 91–92,
        92f, 286, 287f
    in stimulus-response cascade, 24–25, 24f
    ternary complex model of, 46, 52
Griseofulvin, 244
Guanabenz, 221t

H

H_2 antagonists, 251–252, 252f, 284
Half life, of drug, 228–229, 234–240,
    244–245, 248f, 249–250, 399–401
β-Haloalkylamine, 144–146
Haloperidol, 249f, 274
Hanes plot, 65
Hemi-equilibrium
    agonist-antagonist, 122, 126, 127f, 138–139,
        193–194
Hepatic clearance, 232–234, 401
Hepatic metabolism, 229–232
Hepatocytes, 231–232, 232t, 397–398
Hepatotoxicity, 261–271
    drug-drug interactions, 261–270
    direct, 270–271
Herceptin, 297
hERG activity, 273
Heterodimerization, of receptors, 287–289,
    288f, 289t
Heterogeneity, of receptors, 343–344, 344f
High-affinity binding, 72–75
High-throughput screening (HTS), 297–298,
    298f, 306–314
    for antagonists, 312
    binding assays for, 307
    pharmacodynamics and, 307–314

Hildebrand-Benesi plot. See Hanes plot
Hill equation, for asymmetrical curves, 341f, 342
Histamine, 22–23, 23f, 355, 387
Histamine antagonists, 8–9, 11, 12f
Histamine receptor antagonists, 9
Hit optimization. See Lead optimization
HIV binding, 48–49, 49f, 156–158, 157f,
    159f, 160f, 162, 283–285, 285f
    effect of variation in model of, 58–59
    high-throughput screening for, 308, 310f
Homodimerization, of receptors, 287, 288f,
    289–290, 289t
5-HT agonists, 11, 11f, 38, 298–300, 304f
HTS. See High-throughput screening
Hydantoins, 8–9
Hydrochlorthiazide, 217
Hydrophilic character, of druglike molecules,
    215–216
Hydroxyhexamide, 239–240, 241f
Hydroxyzine hydrochloride, 215
Hydroxyzine pamoate, 215
Hyperbolic functions
    series, single hyperbolic function modeling
        of, 41
    successive rectangular, amplification by, 41
Hypothesis testing, 331, 337–339

I

IC_{50}. See also pIC_{50}
    of allosteric antagonists, 69, 81
    of competitive antagonists, 68f, 69, 80–81,
        209
    of competitive v. noncompetitive
        antagonism, 391
    correction factors, 209
    of insurmountable antagonists, 368–369
    of inverse agonists, 130
Ifenprodil, 170–171, 196, 197f
Imatinib, 284
Imigran, 309f
Imipramine, 228, 233, 235t, 243, 299f
In vitro–in vivo transitions
    divergent agonist-dependent antagonism,
        395–396
    exercises in, 391–396
    in vitro-in vivo correspondence of activity,
        394–395
    loss of activity in, 392–393
    marking relevant agonism, 393–394
In vivo systems, for drug discovery, 296–297
Incomplete antagonism, 387–389
Independent variable, drug concentration as,
    38–40
Indomethacin, 234t, 309f
Inhibition, of agonist response. See Antagonist
Inositol triphosphate, 89–90
Insolubility, of drug, 38–39
Insurmountable antagonism, 119–122, 136,
    136f, 193f. See also Allosteric
        insurmountable antagonism; Orthosteric
        insurmountable antagonism
    estimating affinity of, 362–363, 368–369
    orthosteric v. allosteric, 194
    pA_2 and pKB relationship in, 153
    patterns of, 193f

Insurmountable competitive antagonism, 191*f*
Insurmountable allosteric antagonism, 210
Insurmountable orthosteric antagonism, 209–210
Interfacial inhibition, 313
Intravenous dosing, 232–233, 236, 245*f*
Inverse agonism, 28*f*, 53–55, 128–131, 193, 389–390
  antagonism from, 192*f*
  in constitutively active receptor systems, 128–131
  functional effects of, 150–151
  IC_{50} of, 130
  pA_2 measurement for, 151
  Schild analysis for, 130*f*, 131
Inverse agonist, 54–55
Irreversible antagonism, 114–115
Irreversible enzyme inhibition, 269*f*
Isoproterenol, 23, 23*f*, 31, 37*f*, 91, 92*f*, 100–101, 101*f*, 125, 126*f*, 133*f*, 234*t*, 300, 302*f*, 344–345, 344*f*, 360, 375–376, 380–382
Itraconazole, 264
Iterative least squares weighting, 334–336
Ivermectin, 303

J
Jaborandi, 3–4

K
K_A. *See* Equilibrium dissociation constant
Kaumann and Marano method, for measuring partial agonist affinity, 360–361
K_B. *See* Equilibrium dissociation constant of antagonist-receptor complex; Equilibrium dissociation constant of nonradioactive ligand-receptor complex
K_d. *See* Equilibrium dissociation constant of radioligand-receptor complex
Ketamine, 218
Ketoprofen, 217–218
Kidney, drug elimination by, 240–242, 400–401
Kinetic binding studies, 64, 71
Kinetics
  of agonism, 376–377
  of antagonism, 383–385
  of drug binding, 13–15
  of drug elimination and redistribution, 240*f*
  of drug-receptor interaction, 120–122
  of enzyme reactions, 25–26

L
Labetalol, 36*f*, 184*f*, 217
β-Lactam antibiotics, 222–223
Langmuir adsorption isotherm, 13–15, 17, 49, 50*f*, 60–61, 331, 341–342
Lansoprazole, 221*t*
Lead criteria, 317*t*
Lead confirmation, 315–316
Lead identification, 313
Lead optimization, 201*t*, 203*t*, 255, 283, 317*t*
Lemoine and Kaumann method, for measuring partial agonist affinity, 360–361

Leukotriene, 391
Leukotriene antagonists, 9
Levodopa, 226–227
Levofloxacin, 263*t*
Lew and Angus method, for surmountable competitive antagonism, 133–134
Lidocaine, 233, 234*t*, 235*t*, 246–247
Ligand bias, 103–104
Ligands
  comparison of assays with range of, 347
  importance of time for reaching equilibrium between, 77–78
  types of therapeutically active, 360–361
Ligand-target validation, 176*f*, 315, 316*f*
Limited solubility, of drug, 38–39
Linear models, data comparison to, 342
Linear pharmacokinetics, 243–244
Linearity, of regression, 342–343
Lineweaver Burk plot, 65, 263*f*
Lipophylic character, of druglike molecules, 215–216
Liver, 278
  drug clearance by, 232–234, 401
  drug metabolism by, 229–232
Loading dosage, 236, 244–245, 245*f*
Log D, pharmacokinetics and, 401–402
Loperamide, 263*t*
Loratadine, 224–225
Losartan, 104–105, 306–307, 310*f*
Lovastatin, 156, 156*f*, 294, 303
Luvox, 261–262

M
Macroaffinity, 56–57
MAD (maximal absorbable dose), 217
MAOI. *See* Monoamine oxidase inhibitor
Maprotiline, 299*f*
Margin of safety, 255–257, 259*f*
Mathematical approximation, of stimulusresponse mechanism, 25–27
Mathematical models, of drug-receptor theory, 45
  classical model of receptor function, 46, 49–50
  constitutive receptor activity, 53–55, 61
  cubic ternary complex model, 55–56, 61
  derivations, 57–61
  extended ternary complex model, 52–53, 60–61
  introduction to, 45–46
  multistate receptor models and probabilistic theory, 56–57
  operational model of receptor function, 46, 50–51, 59–60, 97, 115
  ternary complex model, 46, 52
  two-state theory, 46, 51–52, 60
  use of, 47–49
Maximal allosteric constant, 364–368
Maximal binding (B_{max}), 64–67, 75–76
Maximal constitutive activity, in cubic ternary complex model, 55–56
Maximal final response, of two agonists saturating stimulus-response cascade, 41–42
Maximal inhibition, 81

Maximal response, 17–18, 47
  of agonist-antagonist hemi-equilibria, 138–139
  of agonists in operational model, 96–97
  estimating relative efficacy of agonists with, 110
  functional studies of, 91, 92*f*
  on incomplete curves, 336
  in noncompetitive antagonism, 134–138
  of partial agonists, 107, 115
Means, comparison of, 322–324, 326–327, 346–347
Mechanism of action
  of antagonists, 192–195, 386–389
Mefloquine, 302–303
Meperidine, 234*t*
Metabolism, of drug, 219, 229–232, 251*t*
Methadone, 230–231
Methotrexate, 228
Methoxamine, 294–295, 295*f*
Methylfurmethide, 71, 71*t*
Methyl-N-scopolamine, 71*t*
Methyl-QNB, 71, 71*f*
Metiamide, 251–252, 252*f*, 284
Metoclopramide, 243*t*
Metoprolol, 223*f*
Mevastatin, 303
Michaelis–Menten equation, 263*f*
Michaelis–Menten kinetics, of enzyme reactions, 25–26
Microsomes, 231–232, 232*t*
Minima, in curve fitting, 331–332
Models, experimental data consistency with, 330–345
  analysis of covariance for determining number of regression lines, 343–345
  asymmetrical dose-response curves, 341–342
  choice of model for data comparison, 330–332
  comparison of assays with range of ligands, 347
  comparison of means by two methods or in two systems, 346–347
  curve fitting good practices, 332–333
  data comparison to linear models, 342
  detection of differences in curves, 340
  hypothesis testing with dose-response curve examples, 337–339
  outliers and weighting data points, 334–336
  overextrapolation of data, 336
  regression linearity, 342–343
Molecular weight, of druglike molecules, 214, 217–218, 218*f*
Monoamine oxidase inhibitor (MAOI), 225–226
Monocrotaline, 270–271
Morphine, 226–227, 226*f*, 230–231, 233, 234*t*, 238, 239*f*, 242, 302–303
Moxifloxacin, 249, 249*f*
Multicompartment system, drug elimination from, 235–236, 236*f*, 238–239, 240*f*
Multiple dosing, 244–247, 248*f*
Multiple populations, single populations v., 329–330

Multistate receptor models, probabilistic theory and, 56–57
Multivariate SAR, 201–202, 204f
Mutagenicity, drug-induced, 262f, 272–273

N

Nadolol, 217, 256f
Nalidixic acid, 228
Naloxone, 225–226
Naltrindole, 298–300, 301f
Naproxen, 215–217, 221t
Narcotics, 243t
Natural products, for potential drugs, 302–303
Negative allosteric modulators (NAMs), 166, 168–172
Negative efficacy, 28f, 53–54
Nelfinavir, 303
Nevirapine, 156–157, 157f
Nifedipine, 308f
Nisoldipine, 230–231
Nitrates, 8–9, 225–226, 242–243
Nitrendipine, 230–231
Nitroglycerin, 234t
Noncompetitive antagonism, 120–122, 126, 127f, 134–138, 391
    Gaddum method for measurement of, 149, 152, 361–362
    pA2 and pKB relationship for, 209–210
    pIC50 curves of, 189, 191f
Noncompetitive displacement, 68, 69f, 79–80
Non-linear pharmacokinetics, 243–244, 247, 248f
Nonlinear regressional analysis, for surmountable competitive antagonism, 133–134
Nonspecific binding (nsb), 64–67, 351, 353
Nonsteroidal anti-inflammatory drugs (NSAIDs), 9, 270–271, 285
Norepinephrine, 298, 299f, 303, 305f, 342–345, 344f
Norgestrel, 303, 305f
Normal distribution. See Gaussian distribution
Normolysin, 377–379
Nortriptylene, 217, 230–231, 234t, 235t, 299f
NSAIDs. See Nonsteroidal anti-inflammatory drugs
nsb. See Nonspecific binding
Nucleation, of drug, 38–39
Null analyses of agonism, 107–114
    partial agonists, 107–110
    full agonists, 110–114

O

Observation bias, 103–104
Offset
    rate of, 196–197, 197f, 198f
Olanzapine, 298
One-compartment system, drug elimination from, 238–239, 240f
One-way analysis of variance, 326–327
Operational model of receptor function, 46, 50–51, 59–60
    fitting data to, 97
    inverse agonism in, 151
    partial agonism in, 151
Opioid agonists, 8–9

Opium, 302–303
Oral absorption, of drug, 213–214, 401
Oral bioavailability, 242–243
Organs, drug clearance by, 232–234
Orphan receptors, 287
Orthosteric agonism, 101–102, 166
Orthosteric antagonism, 119, 195–196
    antagonist receptor coverage, kinetics of dissociation, 141–143
    agonist-antagonist hemi-equilibria, 122, 126, 127f, 138–139, 193f
    allosteric antagonism v., 163t, 175–177
    chemical antagonism, 146–147
    derivations, 149–154
    irreversible antagonism, 144–146
    indirectly acting agonists, blockade of, 144
    introduction to, 119–120
    kinetics of drug-receptor interaction, 120–122
    resultant analysis, 139–140
    summary of, 148–149
Orthosteric competitive antagonism, 193, 387–389
Orthosteric insurmountable antagonism, 194, 209–210, 362–363
Orthosteric molecules, 158
Orthosteric noncompetitive antagonism, 120–122, 126, 127f, 134–138
Orthosteric surmountable competitive antagonism, 122–134
Ouabain, 227–228
Outliers, 334–336, 347–348
Overexpression, of receptors, 53–55, 381–382
Overextrapolation, of data, 336
Oxotremorine, 72–73, 73f, 97, 99f, 113, 113f, 356–357
Oxprenolol, 256f
Oxymetazoline, 114, 114f, 185
Oxytocin, 9

P

pA2 measurement
    for antagonism, 370f
    for insurmountable antagonism, 152–153, 209–210, 362–363
    for inverse agonism, 151
    for partial agonism, 151–152
Paired data sets, 325–326
Papaverine, 302–303
Paroxetine, 299f
Partial agonists, 27–30, 194f
    analysis of, 107
    antagonist as, 190–191, 192f, 193, 387–389
    fitting data to operational model, 97
    full agonists v., 110–111, 111f
    functional assays for measurement of affinity of, 107–110, 115
    functional effects of, 151
    maximal response and efficacy of, 107–110, 115
    pA2 measurement for, 151
    Stephenson method for measuring affinity of, 152, 359–361
    in surmountable competitive antagonism, 131–133
Paxil, 261–262

PDE inhibitors, 294–295, 295f, 394–395
Penicillin, 227–228, 242, 246, 263t, 303, 305f, 307
Penicillin G, 244
Penicillium chrysogenum, 303
Pentazocine, 234t
Permeability
    in vitro assays for estimation of, 250t
    of membrane to drug, 221–222, 221t, 222f, 223f
Perospirone, 256f
Pharmacodynamics, 1–2, 214f
    exercises in, 373
        agonism, 373–383
        antagonism, 383–391
        conclusions, 402
        introduction to, 373
        pharmacokinetics, 397–402
        structure-activity relationship, 397f
    in vitro-in vivo transitions and general discovery, 391–396
    high-throughput screening and, 307–314
Pharmacokinetics, 1–2, 213
    allometric scaling, 247–249
    assays in drug discovery and development, 249–252
    bioavailability of drug, 228–229, 242–243, 247, 248f, 252f, 401
    biopharmaceutics, 213–214
    chemistry of druglike character, 214–218
    clearance of drug, 228–229, 232–234, 247, 248f, 249–250, 252f, 397–398, 401
    drug absorption, 213–214, 219–227, 228f, 229f, 401
    drug administration route, 225–227, 233–234
    exercises in, 373
        absorption, 401
        agonism, 373–383
        antagonism, 383–391
        clearance, 397–398
        conclusions, 402
        distribution, 399
        drug-drug interactions, 399
        half life, 399–400
        introduction to, 373
        Log D and pharmacokinetics, 401–402
        predictive, 385–386
        renal clearance, 400–401
        structure-activity relationship, 396–397
    in vitro–in vivo transitions and general discovery, 391–396
    general, 227–229
    half-life of drug, 228–229, 234–240, 244–247, 248f, 399–401
    introduction to, 213
    metabolism of drug, 219, 229–232, 251t
    multiple dosing, 244–247, 248f
    non-linear, 243–244, 247, 248f
    practical pharmacokinetics, 247–249
    renal clearance, 240–242, 401
    summary of, 252–253
    volume of distribution, 228–229, 234–240, 247, 248f, 399
Pharmacological assay formats. See Binding assays; Functional assays

Pharmacological experiments, 181
optimal design of, 181–197
drug efficacy, 182–188
affinity, 188–195
orthosteric vs. allosteric mechanisms, 195–196
target coverage, 196–197
null experiments, 197–199
fitting data to models, 197–199
experimental data, interpretation of, 199–202
therapeutic activity, predicting, 202–208
predicting agonism, 203–204
predicting binding, 204–206
target coverage, kinetics of, 206
drug combinations, 206–208
Pharmacological intervention, therapeutic landscape and, 8–9, 10t
Pharmacological methods. See Binding assays; Functional assays
Pharmacological test systems, 5–7, 6f
Pharmacology, 1
data driven drug-based, 198
definition of, 1–3
dose-response curves, 14–19, 14f
in drug discovery, 300–302
introduction to study of, 1
Langmuir adsorption isotherm, 13–15, 17, 45
mathematical models of drug-receptor theory, 45
classical model of receptor function, 46, 49–50
constitutive receptor activity, 53–55, 61
cubic ternary complex model, 55–56, 61
derivations, 57–61
extended ternary complex model, 52–53, 60–61
introduction to, 45–46
multistate receptor models and probabilistic theory, 56–57
operational model of receptor function, 46, 50–51, 59–60, 97, 115
ternary complex model, 46, 52
two-state theory, 46, 51–52, 60
use of, 47–49
pharmacological test systems of, 5–7, 6f
receptors in, 3–5, 4f, 7–9, 7f, 10t
safety in, 255–261
summary of, 19–20
system-independent drug parameters
affinity, 6–7, 9–15, 17–18, 18f
efficacy, 6–7, 9–11, 15–18, 18f, 20
Pheniramine, 257f
Phenobarbital, 230–231, 234t
Phenoxybenzamine (POB), 22–23, 23f, 114, 144–146, 356–357
Phentolamine, 302f, 342, 342f
Phenylbutazone, 227–228, 244
Phenylpropanolamine, 214–215, 215f
Phenytoin, 217, 228, 244, 244f, 259f, 269–270
Phospholipidosis, 270
Physostigmine salicylate, 215
Physostigmine sulfate, 215

pIC_{50}
antagonism below basal, 389–390
antagonist potency in format of, 385
of competitive antagonists, measurement of pKB from, 369–371
of drug leads, 199, 201f, 204f
of incomplete antagonism, 387–389
pIC_{50} curves, 189–191, 387–389
Pilocarpine, 3–4, 161, 161f, 284
Pimozide, 230–231
Pindolol, 184f, 295–296, 296f
Pirbuterol, 295–296, 296f
Pirenzepine, 125, 125f
pK_a, of druglike molecules, 214–215, 215f, 224t
pK_B
of antagonists, 191–192
of competitive antagonists, from pIC50, 369–371
for insurmountable allosteric antagonism, 210
for insurmountable orthosteric antagonism, 153, 209–210
Polycyclic hydrocarbons, 269–270
Polypharmacology, of therapeutically active ligands, 360–361
Population analysis, 329–330
Populations, 322–324, 329–330
Positive allosteric modulators (PAMs), 166, 172–174
Potency, 17–18, 47
affinity-dependent v. efficacy-dependent, 98–101
agonist affinity not correlating with, 379–380
of agonists, 110–114, 128–133
of antagonists, 119–120, 121f, 122–125, 128–131, 136, 136f, 139–140, 196–197, 357–358, 363–371, 383–385, 391
estimation of, 48–49, 49f
functional studies of, 85, 86f, 90–92, 92f
incomplete curves for measurement of, 336
p-scales and representation of, 18–19
in surmountable allosteric modulation, 164–166
Potency ratios, for full agonists, 110–112, 111f, 115
Power analysis, 348–350
Practical pharmacokinetics, 247–249
Practolol, 302f
Pravastatin, 293–294
Prazosin, 5, 397–398, 398f
Precipitation. See Nucleation, of drug
Predictive data, 2
Predictive pharmacokinetics, 401
Prednisolone, 293–294
Prenalterol, 27–28, 28f, 31, 37f, 99f, 100–101, 101f, 294–296, 295f, 296f
Primidone, 230–231
Privileged structure, 306–307, 306f
Probabilistic theory
in high-throughput screening, 314–315, 316f
multistate receptor models and, 56–57

Probe specificity, of allosteric modulators, 158, 175–177, 196, 397
Probenecid, 227–228
Procainamide, 234t, 239–240, 263t
Procaine, 303, 305f
Prodrugs, 226–227, 226f, 227f
Progamide, 226–227, 226f
Propoxyphene, 234t
Propranolol, 33–35, 184f, 217, 228, 234t, 242, 303, 304f, 314, 380–382
Protein binding, to drug, 227–228, 401
Protein-protein receptor interactions, 290–291, 290f
Proteins
concentration of, binding curve response to, 75–77, 82
conformations of, 15–16, 313–314
receptors as, 7–8, 7f
Protriptyline, 299f
Prozac, 261–262
p-Scales, representation of potency with, 18–19

Q

Q-test, 348, 348t
Quality control, experimental design and, 347–350
Quinacrine, 227–228, 235
Quinidine, 221t, 234t, 235t
Quinine, 227–228, 302–303

R

Racemic mixture, 218
Radioligands, 57–58, 63, 86
Ranitidine, 217, 221t
RANTES, 170, 171f, 177f, 196, 196f, 285–286, 286f, 393–394
Rapamycin, 293–294, 303
Rate of receptor offset, 196, 197f, 198f
Reabsorption, of drug by kidney, 240–241, 401
Real time experiments, stop time experiments v., 95–96, 382–383
Reboxetine, 299f
Receptor allosterism, nature of, 155–158
Receptor antagonism, 147
Receptor offset, 196, 197f, 198f
Receptor reserve, 22–23, 35–37, 122, 134–138
Receptors
allosteric model of activity of, 178
classical model of, 46, 49–50
concept of, 3–5, 4f
conformation of, allosteric antagonist effects on, 155, 158–175
definition of, 1–2
density of, 32–33, 61, 90–91, 92f
desensitization of, 35–37
dimerization of, 57, 287–290, 288f, 298–300, 300f
dose-response curves of, 14–19, 14f
drug affinity for, 6–7, 9–18, 18f
drug efficacy for, 6–7, 9–11, 15–18, 18f, 20

heterogeneity in, 343−344
in human body, 8−9, 10t
nature of, 7−8, 7f
occupancy of, 21−23, 134−136, 141−142, 162−175
operational model of, 46, 50−51, 59, 97
orphan, 287
overexpression of, 54, 381−382
pharmacological test systems for, 5−7, 6f
polymorphisms of, 285, 285f
tachyphylaxis of, 35−37
Recombinant cell systems, 5, 6f, 32−33, 90−92, 285−286, 380−382, 391−392
Reductionist approach. *See* Target-based drug discovery
Re-equilibration phase, of antagonism, 120−122
Regression, 327−329
analysis of covariance for determining number of regression lines, 343−345
linearity of, 342−343
Relative efficacy, of agonists, 110, 115, 376
Relenza, 303
Relevancy, of agonism, 393−394
Renal clearance, 240−242, 400−401
Renin inhibitors, 218f
Renin-angiotensin inhibitors, 8−9
Reporter assays, 89−90, 95, 95f, 376−377, 382−385
Reserve. *See* Receptor reserve
Response, 10, 11f, 47, 182. *See also* Maximal response
of agonists, system effects on, 27−30
allosteric ligand effect on, 178−179
in classical model of receptor function, 49−50
differential cellular, 30−35
of inverse agonists, 128−131
in noncompetitive antagonism, 134−138
in operational model of receptor function, 50−51, 59
in presence of antagonist, 120−122
rate of, 93
tissue processing of, 21
assay format advantages and disadvantages, 37−38
biochemical nature of stimulusresponse cascade, 23−25
derivations, 41−42
differential cellular response to receptor stimulus, 30−35
drug concentration as independent variable, 38−40
drug response as seen through cellular veil, 21−23
mathematical approximation of stimulus-response mechanism, 25−27
measurement of drug activity, 37
receptor desensitization and tachyphylaxis, 35−37
system effects on agonist response: full and partial agonists, 27−30
Response pathway, choice of, 31
Resultant analysis, 139−140, 153, 363−364
Reversible kinetics, 146
Riboflavin, 244

Richards function, 341−342
Rifampin, 269−270
Rituximab, 297
Rolipram, 293−294
Rosuvasatin, 294
Route, of drug administration, 225−227, 233−234

S

Safety pharmacology, 255−261
hepatotoxicity, 261−271
drug-drug interactions, 261−270
direct, 270−271
cytotoxicity, 271−272
mutagenicity, 272−273
hERG activity, 273
Torsades de Pointes, 273
autonomic receptor profiling, 273−274
general pharmacology, 274
Salbutamol, 225−226, 303, 344−345, 344f
Salicylamide, 244
Salicylates, 9, 215, 225, 227−228
Salicylic acid, 228, 234t, 244
Salmonella tryphimurium, 272−273
Salvarsan, 307
Sample data
comparison of, 321
confidence intervals, 324−325
detection of single v. multiple populations, 329−330
Gaussian distribution, 322
one-way analysis of variance, 326−327
paired data sets, 325−326
populations and samples, 322−324
regression and correlation, 327−329
two-way analysis of variance, 327
detection of differences in, 347−348
standard values comparisons with, 346−347
Samples, 322−324, 348−349
Saquinavir, 230−231
SAR. *See* Structure-activity relationship
Saturable antagonism, 119, 127f
Saturation
of allosteric modulators, 161−162, 175, 195−196
of elimination, 243
of stimulus-response cascade by two agonists, 41−42
Saturation binding, 64−67, 351
Saturation curve, protein concentration effect on, 75−76, 82
Scaling, allometric, 247−249
Scatchard plot, 65, 66f, 67f
Schild analysis, 139−140
for allosteric antagonism, 176f, 178−179
best practice for use of, 127−128
derivation of, 149
dose-response curves precluding use of, 126−127
for inverse agonists in constitutively active receptor systems, 130f, 131
for measuring competitive antagonist affinity, 357−358, 363−364
for partial agonists, 131−132, 132f

in resultant analysis, 153
for surmountable antagonism, 193
competitive, 122−134
Schild regression
analysis of covariance of, 343−345
as indicator of insufficient equilibration time, 383−385
linearity of, 342−343
Scopolamine, 140, 357−358, 364
Scott plot. *See* Hanes plot
Screening, surrogate, 396−397
Screening systems, for drug discovery, 291−297, 298f
Second messengers
in functional assays, 86, 89, 95, 95f
in stimulus-response cascade, 23−25, 26f, 31
Secondary effects, of antagonists, 390
Secondary testing, of agonists, 101−102
Secretion, of drug by kidney, 240−241, 400
Selegiline, 225−226
Sensitivity
to classical antagonists, 175−177
of high-throughput screening, 312
Separation band, 309−311
Series hyperbolae, single hyperbolic function modeling of, 41
Serotonin. *See* 5-HT
Sertraline, 299f
Side effects, of drugs, 255−261, 304, 305f
Sildanefil, 230−231
Silent antagonism, 391−396
Simvastatin, 294
Single populations, multiple populations v., 111−112
Slope. *See* Variable slope
Solubility
of drug, 38−39
of druglike molecules, 214, 216f, 217
Sotalol, 184f
Specific binding, 64−67
Specificity, of allosteric modulators, 158−162, 175−177, 195−196, 260, 397
Spironolactone, 243
Spiropiperidines, 306−307, 310f
Spongothymidine, 303
Spongouridine, 303
Standard values, sample comparisons with, 346−347
Statins, 294, 297
Statistics, 321
for comparing sample data, 321−330
confidence intervals, 324−325
detection of single v. multiple populations, 329−330
Gaussian distribution, 322
one-way analysis of variance, 326−327
paired data sets, 325−326
populations and samples, 322−324
regression and correlation, 327−329
two-way analysis of variance, 327
comparison of samples with standard values, 346−347
experimental data and model consistency, 330−345

Statistics (*Continued*)
    analysis of covariance for determining
        number of regression lines, 343–345
    asymmetrical dose-response curves,
        341–342
    choice of model for data comparison,
        330–332
    comparison of assays with range of
        ligands, 347
    comparison of means by two methods or
        in two systems, 346–347
    curve fitting good practices, 332–333
    data comparison to linear models, 342
    detection of differences in curves, 340
    hypothesis testing with dose-response
        curve examples, 337–339
    outliers and weighting data points,
        334–336
    overextrapolation of data, 336
    regression linearity, 342–343
  experimental design and quality control,
    347–350
  introduction to, 321
  summary of, 350
Staurosporine, 284
Stephenson method, for partial agonist affinity
    measurement, 152, 359–361
Stimulus, 10, 11*f*
  amplification of, 27–30, 86–87
  in classical model of receptor function,
    49–50
  differential cellular response to, 30–35
  target-mediated trafficking of, 33–35
Stimulus pathway, augmentation or modulation
    of, 31
Stimulus-response cascade
  biochemical nature of, 23–25
  maximal final response of two agonists
    saturating, 41–42
  receptor density differences, 32–33
  response pathway selection, 31
  stimulus pathway augmentation or
    modulation, 31
  target-mediated trafficking of stimulus,
    33–35
Stimulus-response mechanism, 10, 11*f*, 26
Stop time experiments, real time experiments
    v., 95–96, 382–383
Streptomycin, 227–228
Structure-activity relationship (SAR), 199,
    201–202, 201*t*, 202*f*, 203*t*, 204*f*, 255
  agonism and, 373–374
  EMRs and EPMRs in determination of,
    110–112, 111*f*
  exercises in, 396–397
Strychnine, 71, 160*t*
Successive rectangular hyperbolic equations,
    amplification by, 41
Sulfanilamide, 304, 305*f*
Sulfasalazine, 221*t*
Sulfonamides, 227–228
Sulfonylureas, 9
Sulindac, 270–271
Sum of least squares, for assessing curve fit,
    331, 334, 337–339

Sumitryptan, 298–300
Super agonists, 375–376
Surmountable allosteric modulation, 193,
    364–368
Surmountable antagonism, 119–120, 122–134,
    193
Surmountable competitive antagonism,
    122–134
Surrogate screening, 308–309, 310*f*, 396–397
Drug discovery process, 281
  assays in cellular context, 294–296
  challenges for, 281–282
  summary of, 318
  target-based approach v., 291
System bias, 103–104
System-independent drug parameters
  affinity, 6–7, 9–18, 18*f*
  efficacy, 6–7, 9–11, 15–16, 18*f*, 20

T

t value, 346–347, 350
Tachyphylaxis, of receptors, 35–37, 100–101
Talindolol, 263*t*
Target coverage, 196, 197*f*, 198*f*, 386
Target validation, 283–285
Target-based drug discovery, 282–291
  target validation and chemical tools,
    283–285
  recombinant systems, 285–286
  biological targets, defining, 286–291
Target-mediated trafficking, of stimulus,
    33–35
Targets, biological, definition of, 286–291
T-distribution, 324
Terbutaline, 88*f*
Terfenadine, 230–231, 261–262
Ternary complex model, 46, 52
Tertiary testing, of agonists, 101–102
Tetracyclines, 227–228, 243, 243*t*, 303
Theophylline, 8–9, 227–228, 234*t*, 235*t*, 242,
    244, 246–247, 255–257, 259*f*
Therapeutic landscape, pharmacological
    intervention and, 8–9, 10*t*
Thiopental, 235
Timing, in functional assays, 93–96
Timolol, 36*f*, 184*f*
Tissue processing, of drug response, 21
  assay format advantages and disadvantages,
    37–38
  biochemical nature of stimulus-response
    cascade, 23–25
  through cellular veil, 21–23
  derivations, 41–42
  differential cellular response to receptor
    stimulus, 30–35
  drug concentration as independent variable,
    38–40
  mathematical approximation of stimulus-
    response mechanism, 25–27
  measurement of drug activity, 37
  receptor desensitization and tachyphylaxis,
    35–37
  system effects on agonist response: full and
    partial agonists, 27–30

Tolbutamide, 234*t*, 235*t*, 242, 304, 305*f*
Torsades de pointes, as drug side effect,
    230–231, 260–261, 273*f*
Total binding, 64–67, 351–352
Toxicity, 255–257
  of drug leads, 255–261
  of high concentrations of agonist or
    antagonist, 127–128
  effects classifications, 259*t*
Trafficking, target-mediated, 33–35
Transitions, between in vitro and in vivo,
    391–396
Tricyclic antidepressants, 8–9, 243*t*
Triglycerides, 270
Tri-level testing, in drug discovery and
    development, 101*t*
Trimipramine, 299*f*
Troglitazone, 249, 249*f*, 255–257, 270
t-test, 323*t*, 325*t*, 326
Two-compartment system, drug elimination
    from, 235–236, 236*f*, 240*f*
Two-stage binding reactions, 81–82
Two-state theory, 46, 51–52, 60
Two-way analysis of variance, 327
Tyramine, 144

U

Unsaturable antagonism, 119

V

Valaciclovir, 226–227
Valproic acid, 224–225, 228, 234*t*, 243, 270
Variability, in sample data, 322–324
Variable slope, in pharmacological models,
    59–60
Variation, in HIV-1 binding model, 58–59
Vasodilators, 8–9, 295*f*, 303
Venlafaxine, 299*f*
Verapamil, 221–222, 221*t*, 223*f*, 223*t*, 228,
    242–243, 263*t*
Vinca alkaloids, 302–303
Vincamine, 160*t*
Vioxx, 255–257
Volume of distribution, of drug, 228, 234–240,
    247, 248*f*, 399

W

Warfarin, 228, 234*t*, 235*t*, 246–247
Water solubility, of druglike molecules, 214,
    216–217, 216*f*
Weighting, of data points, in fitting
    experimental data to models, 334–336
Wortmannin, 293

Y

Yohimbine, 4–5, 71, 72*f*, 298, 299*f*

Z

β-Zearalenol, 293–294
Zearalenone, 293–294
Zofenopril, 256*f*, 306, 307*f*
Zofran, 309*f*

Printed in the United States
By Bookmasters